Ovarian Toxicology

SECOND EDITION

Ovarian Toxicology

SECOND EDITION

Edited by

Patricia B. Hoyer

The University of Arizona, College of Medicine, Tucson, USA

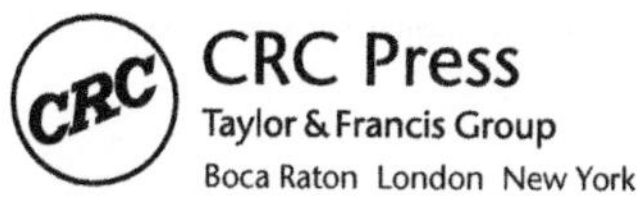

CRC Press is an imprint of the
Taylor & Francis Group, an **informa** business

CRC Press
Taylor & Francis Group
6000 Broken Sound Parkway NW, Suite 300
Boca Raton, FL 33487-2742

First issued in paperback 2017

ISBN-13: 978-1-4665-0406-6 (hbk)
ISBN-13: 978-1-138-19985-9 (pbk)

Library of Congress Cataloging-in-Publication Data

Ovarian toxicology / editor, Patricia B. Hoyer. -- Second edition./
p. ; cm.
Includes bibliographical references and index.
Summary: "Today, we are exposed to an ever-growing number of chemicals in the environment and there is an increasing awareness of the effects of these chemicals on the ovaries. As such, the potential for xenobiotic-induced infertility needs to be better understood. Additionally, menopause-associated disorders are of growing health concern in view of the fact that by the year 2025, 19.5% of the population of the U.S. will be menopause-aged women. Exploring research into chemicals that have the potential to cause early menopause by destroying pre-antral ovarian follicles, this book is an essential resource for researchers in academia, regulatory agencies, and industry"--Provided by publisher.
ISBN 978-1-4665-0406-6 (hardcover : alk. paper)
I. Hoyer, Patricia B., 1942- editor of compilation.
[DNLM: 1. Ovary--drug effects. 2. Environmental Pollutants--toxicity. 3. Ovarian Neoplasms--chemically induced. 4. Xenobiotics.

RG441 WP 320]
618.1'1071--dc23 2013028520

Visit the Taylor & Francis Web site at
http://www.taylorandfrancis.com

and the CRC Press Web site at
http://www.crcpress.com

Contents

Preface

Since the latter part of the twentieth century in this country, there has been an increase in the number of working women and a tendency for women to postpone the start of a family. These trends have heightened an awareness of the impact of environmental chemicals in the workplace on reproductive function. A variety of considerations can affect fertility in women who are older when beginning a family, and women with fertility problems may not discover them until their reproductive life span is waning. In addition to a generally reduced quality of oocytes with age, more years of exposure to environmental influences can also have a potential harmful effect. A better understanding of the effect of these influences on ovarian function is of particular importance since a healthy ovary is critical to normal reproduction.

Reproductive function in women can be compromised by exposure to toxic chemicals. Reproductive toxicants can act via direct alterations in steroid hormone production (in the ovary) or by interference with steroid hormone action (in the hypothalamus, pituitary, and/or reproductive tract). Alternatively, the effects of ovarian toxicants can result in ovarian failure caused by extensive oocyte destruction. As a result of extensive follicular damage, neuroendocrine feedback is disrupted and circulating levels of gonadotropins, follicle-stimulating hormone (FSH), and luteinizing hormone (LH) rise. Therefore, follicle destruction can ultimately disrupt endocrine balance by causing a reduction in ovarian production of estrogen and progesterone and an elevation in FSH and LH.

Since the first edition of this book was published, there has been a substantial increase in information related to the impact of a variety of xenobiotic chemicals on ovarian function. This has contributed to an expansion of the original chapters and mechanistic information that can be reviewed. The book is divided into four parts: Ovarian Function, Ovotoxic Chemical Classes, Ovarian Cancer, and Risk Assessment. This book represents a compilation of chapters prepared by researchers who have substantially contributed to our understanding of the impact of xenobiotics and environmental factors on ovarian function. Additionally, issues associated with epidemiology and risk assessment testing as regards the ovary have also been addressed. This book will prove equally interesting and useful to scientists in academic, industrial, and regulatory settings.

Patricia B. Hoyer, PhD

Editor

Patricia B. Hoyer, PhD, is a professor in the Department of Physiology at the University of Arizona, Tucson, Arizona. Her research specializes in the effects of environmental chemicals on ovarian function. Her professional activities have included membership in professional societies such as the Society of Toxicology and the Society for Study of Reproduction. She has also served as a panel member as well as chair for the NIH and the American Cancer Society study sections. She currently serves on the editorial boards of *Toxicology and Applied Pharmacology*, *Biology of Reproduction*, and *Experimental Biology and Medicine*. In 2010, she organized the XVII International Ovarian Workshop. She has authored or coauthored 115 peer-reviewed scientific publications, 30 invited book chapters, and reviews in such texts as *Comprehensive Toxicology* and *Casarett & Doull's Toxicology*. During her career, she has delivered numerous presentations at national/international meetings and symposia. Dr. Hoyer has trained over 25 PhD and master's students and postdoctoral fellows. These efforts have earned her the 2011 Trainee Mentoring Award for the Society for Study of Reproduction and the 2013 Mentoring Award for Women in Toxicology at the annual meeting of the Society of Toxicology.

Contributors

S.K. Agarwal
Department of Reproductive Medicine
University of California, San Diego
San Diego, California

Ahmed Y. Ali
Department of Cellular and Molecular Medicine
University of Ottawa
and
Chronic Disease Program
Ottawa Hospital Research Institute
Ottawa, Ontario, Canada

Janice M. Bahr
University of Illinois at Urbana-Champaign
Urbana, Illinois

Sakhila K. Banu
Department of Veterinary Integrative Biosciences
Texas A&M University
College Station, Texas

Sanguine Byun
Department of Agricultural Biotechnology
College of Agriculture and Life Sciences
Seoul National University
Seoul, Republic of Korea

and

Harvard Medical School
Harvard University
Boston, Massachusetts

and

Cutaneous Biology Research Centre
Massachusetts General Hospital
Charlestown, Massachusetts

Kathryn Coe
Richard M. Fairbanks School of Public Health
Indiana University-Purdue University
Indianapolis, Indiana

and

The University of Arizona
Tucson, Arizona

Ralph L. Cooper
Endocrine Toxicology Branch
Toxicity Assessment Division
National Health and Environmental Effects Research Laboratory
United States Environmental Protection Agency
Research Triangle Park, North Carolina

Zelieann R. Craig
Department of Comparative Biosciences
College of Veterinary Medicine
University of Illinois at Urbana-Champaign
Urbana, Illinois

Timothy P. DelValle
Department of Comparative Biosciences
College of Veterinary Medicine
University of Illinois at Urbana-Champaign
Urbana, Illinois

Lee Farrand
Department of Agricultural Biotechnology
College of Agriculture and Life Sciences
Seoul National University
Seoul, Republic of Korea

Jodi A. Flaws
Department of Comparative Biosciences
University of Illinois at Urbana-Champaign
Urbana, Illinois

Warren G. Foster
Department of Obstetrics and Gynecology
McMaster University
Hamilton, Ontario, Canada

S. Ganesan
Department of Animal Science
Iowa State University
Ames, Iowa

Anne M. Gannon
Department of Obstetrics and Gynecology
McMaster University
Hamilton, Ontario, Canada

Jerome M. Goldman
Endocrine Toxicity Branch
Toxicity Assessment Division
National Health and Environmental Effects Research Laboratory
United States Environmental Protection Agency
Research Triangle Park, North Carolina

Katlyn S. Hafner
Department of Comparative Biosciences
College of Veterinary Medicine
University of Illinois at Urbana-Champaign
Urbana, Illinois

Patrick Hannon
Department of Comparative Biosciences
University of Illinois at Urbana-Champaign
Urbana, Illinois

Wafa Harrouk
Center for Drug Evaluation and Research
U.S. Food and Drug Administration
Silver Spring, Maryland

Lisa M. Hess
Richard M. Fairbanks School of Public Health
Indiana University-Purdue University
Indianapolis, Indiana

Kendra Hodgkinson
Department of Cellular and Molecular Medicine
University of Ottawa
and
Centre for Cancer Therapeutics
Ottawa Hospital Research Institute
Ottawa, Ontario, Canada

Patricia B. Hoyer
Department of Physiology
The University of Arizona
Tucson, Arizona

Claude L. Hughes
Cardiovascular and Metabolic Unit
Quintiles, Inc.
and
Department of Mathematics
North Carolina State University
and
Department of Obstetrics and Gynecology
Duke University Medical Center
Durham, North Carolina

Akechai Im-Aram
Department of Agricultural Biotechnology
College of Agriculture and Life Sciences
Seoul National University
Seoul, Republic of Korea

Aileen F. Keating
Department of Animal Science
Iowa State University
Ames, Iowa

Ji Young Kim
Chronic Disease Program
Ottawa Hospital Research Institute
Ottawa, Ontario, Canada

and

Department of Agricultural Biotechnology
College of Agriculture and Life Sciences
Seoul National University
Seoul, Republic of Korea

Hyong Joo Lee
Department of Agricultural Biotechnology
College of Agriculture and Life Sciences
Seoul National University
Seoul, Republic of Korea

Elaine Lai-Han Leung
Macau Institute for Applied Research in Medicine and Health
and
State Key Laboratory of Quality Research in Chinese Medicine
and
Faculty of Chinese Medicine
Macau University of Science and Technology
Taipa, Macau, People's Republic of China

Ulrike Luderer
Division of Occupational and Environmental Medicine
Department of Medicine
and
Department of Developmental and Cell Biology
University of California, Irvine
Irvine, California

Ronit Machtinger
Department of Obstetrics, Gynecology and Reproductive Biology
Sheba Medical Center
Sackler School of Medicine
Ramat Gan, Israel

J.A. Madden
Department of Animal Science
Iowa State University
Ames, Iowa

Susan L. Makris
National Center for Environmental Assessment
U.S. Environmental Protection Agency
Washington, District of Columbia

Connie J. Mark-Kappeler
WIL Research
Ashland, Ohio

Krista M. Milich
Institute of Mind and Biology
University of Chicago
Chicago, Illinois

Catherine Racowsky
Department of Obstetrics, Gynecology and Reproductive Biology
Brigham and Women's Hospital
Harvard Medical School
Boston, Massachusetts

Katherine F. Roby
Department of Anatomy and Cell Biology
Institute for Reproductive Health and Regenerative Medicine
University of Kansas Medical Center
Kansas City, Kansas

J.C. Sadeu
Department of Obstetrics and Gynecology
McMaster University
Hamilton, Ontario, Canada

G. Marie Swanson
Richard M. Fairbanks School of Public Health
Indiana University-Purdue University
Indianapolis, Indiana

Benjamin K. Tsang
Department of Cellular and Molecular Medicine
and
Department of Obstetrics and Gynecology
University of Ottawa
and
Chronic Disease Program
Ottawa Hospital Research Institute
Ottawa, Ontario, Canada

and

Department of Agricultural Biotechnology
College of Agriculture and Life Sciences
Seoul National University
Seoul, Republic of Korea

Barbara C. Vanderhyden
Department of Cellular and Molecular Medicine
and
Department of Obstetrics and Gynecology
University of Ottawa
and
Centre for Cancer Therapeutics
Ottawa Hospital Research Institute
Ottawa, Ontario, Canada

Wei Wang
Department of Comparative Biosciences
University of Illinois at Urbana-Champaign
Urbana, Illinois

Part I

Ovarian Function

1 Ovarian Physiology

Janice M. Bahr and Krista M. Milich

CONTENTS

1.1 INTRODUCTION

In this chapter, we present the basic function and physiology of the ovary. This information is needed to study ovarian toxicology, especially because one must first know what is normal before one can understand the impact of toxicants. This chapter presents a broad overview of ovarian physiology and concludes with suggestions for how toxicants may impact the function of the ovary.

1.2 SEXUAL DEVELOPMENT OF THE GONADS

Despite their obvious differences, the ovary and the testis are sibling structures that originate from the same primordial tissue or genital ridges, which are a pair of thickened rows of coelomic epithelial cells along the inner surface of the mesonephric. A number of genes controlling embryonic development of the gonads have been identified. Most progress has been made in understanding the genetic control of testis formation. In 1990, a single gene on the Y chromosome, *SRY*, was identified to be necessary and sufficient to induce testis formation. For many years, ovary formation was considered to be the default process, which occurred in the absence of SRY expression. However, we now know that ovary development in the fetus is actively controlled by a number of genes, which antagonize the testis formation pathway and promote ovarian formation (Figure 1.1). The ovary-specific

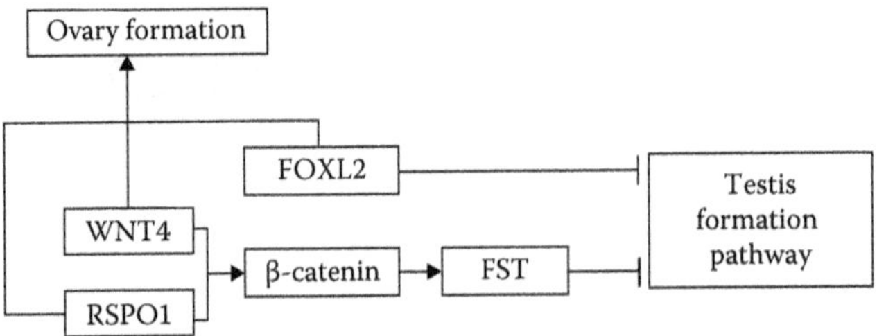

FIGURE 1.1 Putative pathways for ovary formation in the mouse embryo. Two somatic cell derived factors, RSPO1 and WNT4, activate β-catenin pathway in XX somatic cells in an autocrine or paracrine manner. β-catenin induces expression of follistatin (FST), which blocks the pathways resulting in testis formation. Forkhead transcription factor (FOXL2) also blocks the testis formation pathway. (Compliments of HH Yao.)

factors responsible for the development of the ovary, R-spondin1 (RSPO1), WNT4, beta-catenin, FOXL2, and follistatin (FST), have been identified in the mouse, see Liu et al. (2010); Ungewitter and Yao (2010).

1.3 OOGENESIS

The ovary performs two primary functions—the production of gametes (oocytes) and the production of hormones. The process of producing oocytes is called oogenesis. This process begins during the development of the fetus at which time the female produces all of the oocytes that she will use during her entire life. In this way, oogenesis is very different from spermatogenesis in which males continually produce sperm.

Oogenesis occurs through the process of mitosis and meiosis. Initially, oogonia undergo mitosis to produce oocytes. The oocyte then undergoes the initial stages of meiosis, but that process is arrested at the diplotene stage of prophase 1. The cell stays at this stage until menarche. The luteinizing hormone (LH) surge prior to ovulation causes resumption of meiosis 1. Thus, during ovulation, the primary oocyte develops into the secondary oocyte.

Immediately following the completion of the first meiotic division, the second meiotic cycle begins. However, the second meiotic division is also arrested. Meiosis II stops in the second meiotic metaphase until fertilization occurs (provided the oocyte is fertilized). When the spermatozoon enters the oocyte, meiosis II is resumed.

Oogenesis is most notable in that all of the oocytes that a female produces in her lifetime are produced as a fetus and continually decline throughout the female's life. At 20 weeks of gestation in humans, a female has 14 million oocytes. This number drops significantly by the time of birth to only 1.5 million oocytes. At puberty, there are a mere 300,000 of these oocytes remaining. By the time a woman is 52 and nearing the age of menopause, she has approximately 100 oocytes. Meanwhile, a woman only ovulates on average 400–500 oocytes in her lifetime. Thus, the majority of oocyte loss is not associated with ovulation.

1.4 FOLLICULOGENESIS

The ovary is a compartmentalized tissue consisting of germ cells and somatic cells, the latter are the source of steroid and protein hormones (Figure 1.2). In the mouse, primordial germ cells migrate from the yolk sac into the genital ridge 10.5–11.5 days postconception (dpc) where they reside as clusters or nests of interconnected oogonia. Within a day after this migration (12.5 dpc), pregranulosa cells form from somatic cell precursors, a process controlled by a number of extrinsic and internal signals. One of the earliest markers present in pregranulosa cells is FOXL2, which suppresses expression of the genes, e.g., StAR and Cyp19a1, involved in terminal differentiation of granulosa cells. As nests of oocytes are broken down, primordial follicles are formed, which consist of an oocyte and a single layer of flattened granulosa cells surrounded by the basal lamina. At this time in development, the oocyte in the primordial follicle progresses from mitosis to meiosis, being arrested at meiosis 1 in prophase 1 until the oocyte is exposed to the preovulatory surge of LH, which may be months or years later, depending on the species. The formation of follicles is absolutely dependent upon the presence of germ cells, which suggests that some signal is produced by germ cells which causes granulosa cells to form. The nests of oocytes and subsequent formation of follicles occur in the cortex of the ovary. The medulla is generally devoid of oocytes, instead consisting of blood vessels, nerves, and connective tissue. For further information regarding follicular assembly, see Pepling (2012).

The next step in follicular development is the formation of primary follicles, which occurs several days after birth in the mouse. Primary follicles are surrounded by cuboidal granulosa cells and a basal lamina. A noncellular layer called the zona pellucida is produced between the oocyte and the granulosa cells. The granulosa

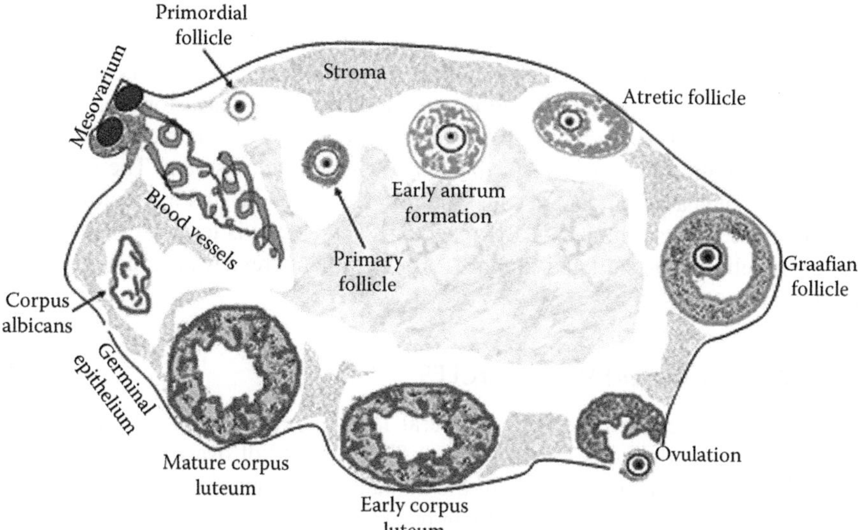

FIGURE 1.2 The human ovary showing the stages of folliculogenesis, ovulation, and luteal formation and demise.

cells make contact with the oocyte by sending microvilli through the zona pellucida, forming gap junctions with the oocyte.

Secondary follicles are present around day 14 after birth in the mouse and consist of distinct granulosa and theca layers. These follicles are also called pre-antral because the granulosa cells form a solid mass of cells around the oocyte. The granulosa cells proliferate forming multilayers within the basal lamina. It is at this time in folliculogenesis that the theca layer forms. The cellular origin of theca cells has not been identified, but it is proposed that theca cells are recruited from the ovarian stroma by factors secreted by the activated follicle. It has been clearly shown that growth differentiation factor 9, a member of the transforming growth factor-β super family, produced by the oocyte is one factor responsible for the formation of theca cells. The theca layer provides support for the follicle, contains blood vessels and nerves, and is the primary site of androgen production in the mammalian follicle. The outer layer of the theca layer, called the theca externa, consists mainly of blood vessels, nerves, and connective tissue. The inner layer, called the theca interna, contains steroid-producing cells, which at one time were called interstitial cells. The final stage of growth from the secondary follicle to the antral follicle requires follicle-stimulating hormone (FSH).

The largest follicle, called the antral or Graafian follicle, is a highly differentiated endocrine structure, is dependent upon FSH and LH, and is the primary site of steroid and protein hormone synthesis. The granulosa cells proliferate further and can be differentiated into three types. The corona radiata is a single layer of granulosa cells immediately next to the zona pellucida and maintains gap junctions with the oocyte. It is through the corona radiata that signals, nutrients, and chemical messengers are transferred between the oocyte and the surrounding follicle. The cumulus oophorus, a multilayer of granulosa cells, surrounds the corona radiata. The cumulus oophorus and corona radiata stay attached to the oocyte at the time of ovulation and can be clearly seen in the oviduct immediately after ovulation. As the connections break down between the granulosa cells forming the corona radiata and the more distal or mural granulosa cells, serum-like fluid is secreted into the space forming a cavity called an antrum. The fluid, called follicular fluid, is very rich in steroids and also contains a significant percentage of the constituents of blood serum. The granulosa cells next to the basal lamina are called mural granulosa cells and in the mature follicle have the highest number of LH receptors. The oocyte is tethered to the mural granulosa cells via the cumulus oophorus. For an in-depth review of folliculogenesis, see Rajkovic et al. (2006).

1.5 FATE OF OVARIAN FOLLICLES

An ovarian follicle can have one of several fates, namely become atretic, form a cyst, or ovulate and form a corpus luteum. The majority of ovarian follicles never ovulate but rather undergo atresia. In the human, only 1 out of every 1000 oocytes present at birth will ovulate. Atresia can occur at any stage of folliculogenesis, but usually occurs in pre-antral follicles. Atretic follicles are easily visible in histologic preparations of ovaries. The atretic follicles instead of the usual round appearance are irregular in shape. The oocyte's membrane becomes wrinkled and the granulosa cells have a pyknotic appearance, with a shrunken, degenerating nucleus with dense, formless chromatin. The granulosa cells undergo apoptosis, whereas the theca cells are thought to dedifferentiate into stromal cells and may redifferentiate as new follicles are formed. The cause of atresia may be due to a lack of adequate gonadotropin support, which could be caused by inadequate blood supply to these follicles.

Besides atretic follicles, a number of follicles may stop growing as either secondary or tertiary follicles and form a cyst filled with fluid. Cysts do not usually ovulate, because generally there is not the usual rapid increase in estradiol to trigger an LH surge. The relative tonic concentrations of ovarian steroids in the blood act in a negative feedback manner to prevent the secretion of gonadotropin releasing hormone (GnRH) and LH by the hypothalamus and pituitary, respectively. Cysts are associated with certain ovarian diseases such as polycystic ovary.

1.6 OVULATION

A number of follicles will ovulate each cycle depending upon the species, usually one in humans or more in litter bearing animals. As the follicle grows and becomes a Graafian follicle, the granulosa cells secrete copious amounts of estradiol. This rapid increase in estradiol, through a positive feedback mechanism, triggers the release of GnRH from the cyclic center in the hypothalamus, which in turn causes the release of a large preovulatory LH surge. The massive LH release causes a decrease in estradiol secretion, an increase in secretion of progesterone by the granulosa cells, and an increase in the synthesis of the progesterone receptor. LH activates cyclooxygenase-2 (COX-2), which increases the production of vasoactive substances, e.g., prostaglandin E2 (PgE2). Progesterone also activates the production of A disintegrin and metalloproteinase with thrombospondin motifs-1 (ADAMTS-1) enzymes involved in inflammation. These vasoactive substances move to the theca layers, causing the dilatation of capillaries, increasing the vascular compartment, i.e., a hyperemic response, similar to inflammation. As capillaries become more porous, serum proteins exude into the interstitial space of the follicle. Serum proteins activate quiescent fibroblasts in the theca and tunica albuginea to proliferate. Activated fibroblasts secrete metalloproteinases (MMP-1), which degrade the extracellular matrix of the collagenous connective tissue. Also in preparation for ovulation, gap junctions breakdown between the granulosa cells and the oocyte removing the meiotic inhibition, allowing the oocyte to progress from prophase of meiosis 1 to diplotene of meiosis 2. The first polar body is formed resulting in a haploid oocyte. After these biochemical changes, the stigma forms and rupture occurs. The oocyte rapidly exits the follicle with the cumulus oophorus and corona radiata still attached to the oocyte. If the female was mated, fertilization of the oocyte occurs in the oviduct. For an in-depth review of ovulation, see Espey and Richards (2006).

1.7 CORPUS LUTEUM (CL)

Following ovulation, the remaining granulosa and theca cells are transformed morphologically and biochemically into the CL. This temporary endocrine structure on the ovary primarily synthesizes large amounts of progesterone necessary for preparation of the uterus if pregnancy is to occur. Immediately following ovulation, the follicle fills with blood and is called the corpus hemorrhagicum. As the follicle transitions to the CL, blood vessels and nerves penetrate the basal lamina and surround the granulosa cells. Based on findings in the ruminants, granulosa cells become large luteal cells whereas the theca cells form small luteal cells. The large luteal cells with few LH receptors produce basal progesterone concentrations. The small luteal cells have large numbers of LH receptors and are very responsive to LH and secrete large amounts of progesterone in response to LH stimulation via the adenylyl cyclase second-messenger system. Luteal cells have many low-density lipid (LDL) and high-density lipid (HDL) receptors to enable the cells to take up large amounts of cholesterol from the blood. Luteal cells have PgE2 receptors; and in species that are dependent upon prolactin for a functional CL, such as the rodent, there are many membrane prolactin receptors. Progesterone receptors within the CL are absolutely essential for a functional CL as shown by preventing progesterone receptors to bind progesterone, i.e., use of RU 486, a progesterone receptor antagonist which results in luteolysis.

There are different CL formed based on their functions. For example, in humans and animals with long cycles, e.g., cows; pigs; sheep, the CL that forms following ovulation is fully functional during the luteal phase of the cycle. The lifespan of the CL will only be extended if there is signal from the fetus (maternal recognition of pregnancy) to extend the lifespan of the CL. In contrast in rodents, if ovulation occurs without mating, the CL formed is not functional and produces very low amounts of progesterone. However, if the female was mated by a sterile male, the female will become pseudopregnant and the CL will be functional for about one-half the length of pregnancy. In the case of a fertile mating, the CL will be functional throughout the entire pregnancy.

After a certain period of time, the CL undergoes luteolysis and the remaining tissue is called the corpus albicans (white body). The length of the CL lifespan, as well as the cause of luteolysis, varies greatly with species. In the rodent, luteolysis occurs because progesterone is metabolized to an inactive progestin, 20α-hydroxyprogesterone. In ruminants, oxytocin produced by the large luteal cells and released in response to uterine prostaglandin F2α (PgF2α) decreases blood flow to the CL and prevents LH from signaling steroidogenesis. In humans, the cause of luteolysis is not clearly defined, but may be caused by local production of PgF2α in the CL.

1.8 HORMONES PRODUCED BY THE OVARY

The second function of the ovary is to produce hormones. This section will first discuss the synthesis of steroids followed by that of proteins. The ovary is one of the primary sites of steroidogenesis. Steroids act within the ovary as well as numerous target sites, e.g., brain; pituitary; uterus; cervix; vagina; mammary gland; adipose tissue; skin; liver; and kidney. The steroids are responsible for the menstrual/estrous cycles.

The major products of steroidogenesis in the ovary are progesterone and estrogens (estradiol 17β and estrone) and to a lesser extent androstenedione and testosterone. These steroids interact with specific receptors in target tissues. The synthesis of steroids, regulated by specific enzymes called cytochrome P450 enzymes, starts with cholesterol. Cholesterol is taken up from the peripheral circulation in the form of HDL and LDL and can also be stored in steroidogenic cells as cholesterol esters. This 27-carbon molecule enters mitochondria with the assistance of the steroidogenic acute regulatory protein (StAR) where cholesterol is converted into pregnenolone, a 21-carbon molecule. The enzyme, P450 side-change cleavage enzyme (CYP 11A), is rate-limiting and is a key site of regulation. Pregnenolone diffuses from the mitochondria into the cytoplasm where, in the presence of the smooth endoplasmic reticulum, pregnenolone is converted by 3β-hydroxsteroid dehydrogenase (3βHSD)/Δ5-Δ4 isomerase into progesterone. Pregnenolone, via the Δ5 pathway, can also be converted into 17α-OH-pregnenolone by CYP17, which is then converted into a weak androgen, dehydroepiandrosterone (DHEA). This androgen is converted into androstenedione by 3βHSD. Progesterone, a C21 steroid molecule, is converted to a C19 androgen, androstenedione by CYP17. Testosterone is produced from androstenedione by 17βHSD. Androstenedione and testosterone are irreversibly converted to estrone and estradiol-17β by aromatase, CYP19, respectively. For a detailed discussion of steroidogenesis, see Strauss (2009).

The primary steroid product of the preovulatory follicle is estradiol-17β, secreted by the granulosa cells, first in response to the stimulation of FSH and later by LH. However, steroidogenesis in the follicle is dependent upon the interaction of both the theca and the granulosa cells, hence called the two-cell-two gonadotropin theory (Figure 1.3). The theca layer expresses LH receptors and steroidogenic enzymes, CYP11A, 3βHSD, and CYP17, enabling the theca layer to convert cholesterol into androgens, which then diffuse across the basal lamina into the granulosa cells. In these cells, under the stimulation of CYP19 (aromatase) by FSH, estradiol and estrone are produced. As the follicles approach ovulation, the granulosa cells increase the synthesis of progesterone, needed for ovulation and the initiation of luteinization.

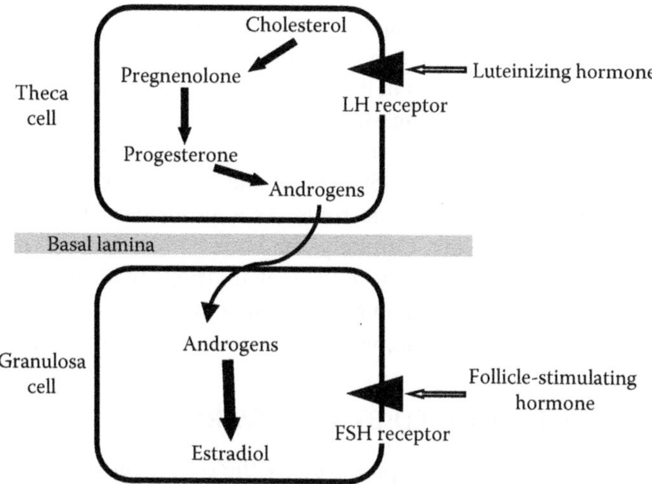

FIGURE 1.3 The two-cell, two gonadotropin theory of ovarian steroidogenesis.

1.9 METABOLISM OF STEROIDS

One aspect of steroidogenesis is understanding how steroids are synthesized and bring about a response in target cells, but equally important is an understanding of how steroids are metabolized and what internal and external factors can modify their metabolism. Steroid concentrations in the blood and the amount of steroids available to target tissues are equally dependent upon the rates of synthesis and metabolism. Toxins and other substances in our environment can directly affect the synthesis and metabolism of steroids, which in turn affect the function of the body.

Steroids in the blood exist either as free steroids or as conjugated steroids. The choice of the word "free" implies the structure of the steroid allows the steroid to enter the cell, bind to its appropriate receptor, and bring about a cellular change. In the blood, ~96% of the free steroids are bound to serum-binding proteins, e.g., albumin and sex binding globulins. In contrast, a large proportion of the steroids in the blood are conjugated steroids in which either a glucuronide or sulfate group is reversibly attached at carbon 3. Conjugated steroids do not enter cells and can easily be unconjugated by glucuronidase or sulfatase to form a free steroid. Conjugated steroids are excreted into the urine whereas active steroids are found in the feces.

To understand the metabolism of steroids, knowledge of the enterohepatic circulation of steroids is paramount (Figure 1.4). Enterohepatic circulation of steroids implies the circulation of conjugated steroids from the gut to the liver and back to the gut. Conjugated steroids entering the gut, either from the bile or ingested, are unconjugated by bacteria in the gut, allowing the free steroid to be taken up by the epithelium of the gut. In the gut epithelial cells, the free steroids are reconjugated and enter the hepatic portal vein. Free steroids coming from the ovary and adrenal gland will also be in the hepatic portal vein, which transports these steroids to the liver. In the liver, the majority of the free steroids will be conjugated, many of which will enter the bile. The remaining free and conjugated steroids will exit the liver and enter the general circulation. The enterohepatic circulation is essential to extend the half-life of free steroids in the blood. However, the enterohepatic circulation can easily be altered by the ingestion or injection of antibiotics, diet, xenobiotics, toxicants, alcohol, and other factors. In an effort to detoxify these substances, the liver increases the synthesis of the P450 cytochrome enzymes, which detoxify toxins and increase the metabolism of free steroids. As a result, steroid concentrations in the blood decrease significantly. Certainly, the book "*Silent Spring*," published by Rachel Carson (1962), clearly demonstrated how toxicants in the environment were interfering with steroid metabolism in birds, causing them to lay eggs either without or with very thin shells, so no young were hatched—hence the silent spring.

1.10 PROTEINS PRODUCED BY THE OVARY

There is a broad array of proteins produced by the ovary, but this chapter focuses on inhibin, activin, follistatin, Müllerian-inhibiting factor (MIS), and insulin-like growth factor (IGF) I and II. Inhibin and activin are members of the TGF-β

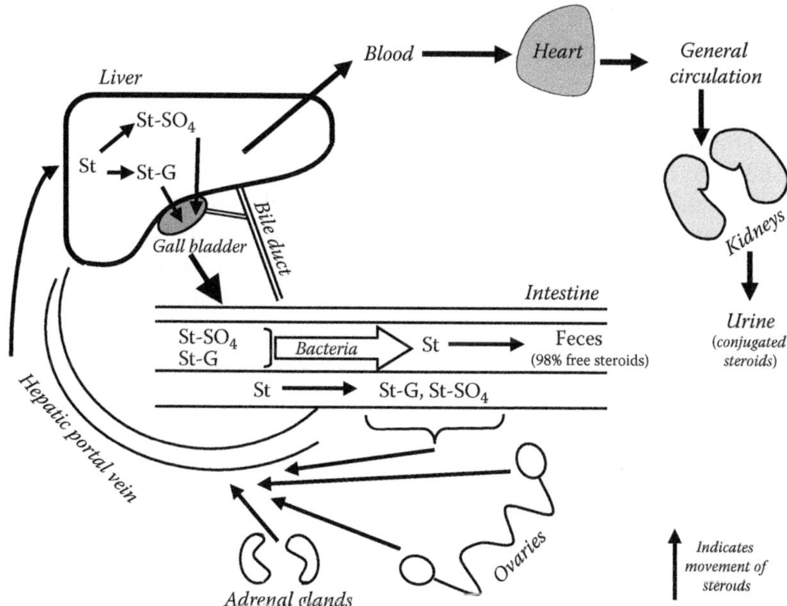

FIGURE 1.4 Enterohepatic circulation of steroids. Free androgens and estrogens produced by the ovary and adrenal glands are conjugated in the liver via the P450 cytochrome enzymes. The majority of the conjugated steroids enter the gall bladder where they are secreted in the bile into the small intestine along with conjugated steroids. In the small intestine, conjugated steroids are deconjugated by gut bacteria, enter the gut epithelium where steroids are reconjugated, enter the hepatic portal vein and are transported to the liver. A change in the P450 cytochrome enzymes induced by toxicants can either decrease or increase the concentrations of free steroids in the blood and feces.

superfamily. Inhibin has endocrine, paracrine, and autocrine functions. Inhibin is a heterodimeric 32-kDa glycoprotein consisting of two subunits linked by disulfide bonds. Inhibin consists of α inhibin, and either βA or βB, and is secreted by the granulosa cells. An endocrine hormone, inhibin, inhibits FSH secretion from the pituitary gland. In the ovary, inhibin increases LH- and IGF-stimulated androgen production by thecal cells.

Activin is a dimer of two β subunits, either βAβB, βBβB, or βAβB. Whereas activin can increase FSH secretion from cultured pituitary cells *in vivo,* activin is irreversibly bound to follistatin hence inactivating activin. The primary action of activin is intraovarian, where its action on follicular maturation and granulosa cell function is stage-dependent. Follistatin is produced by small antral and preovulatory follicles.

IFG-I and II are low molecular weight, single-chain polypeptide growth factors. IFG-I enters the follicular fluid from the systematic circulation, whereas IGF-2 is produced by granulosa and theca cells of small follicles. IGF-I's role in ovarian function has been extensively studied. In mice lacking IGF-I, follicular maturation is arrested, granulosa cell proliferation is reduced, and the response of the follicle to estradiol is impaired. Actions of IGF-I and II are primarily regulated by local production of IGF-binding proteins, which are produced by the granulosa cells of the dominant follicles.

Müllerian-inhibiting substance (MIS) (or anti-Müllerian hormone-AMH), another ovarian protein hormone, is a dimeric glycoprotein produced by granulosa cells of small follicles. Mice lacking MIS have accelerated depletion of follicles because MIS inhibits the recruitment of primary follicles into the growing pool of follicles. Also MIS causes a reduction in the response of the growing follicle to FSH.

Interleukins and tumor necrosis factor-α are also present in the ovary. Interleukin-1 (IL-I) is produced by macrophages. In the rodent, there is a compartmentalized, hormonally dependent intraovarian IL-I system with ligands, receptors, and antagonists. In mice and pigs, IL-I decreases functional and morphological luteinization of granulosa cells. Tumor necrosis factor-α may also have a role in luteolysis, with macrophages secreting this factor.

1.11 OVARIAN CYCLE: ESTROUS AND MENSTRUAL CYCLES

The ovary, via all of the changes in hormones mentioned earlier, creates the reproductive cycle unique to each female species. In some cases, the cycle is called the estrous cycle; and in the case of humans and other primates, the cycle is called the menstrual cycle. The term used to designate the cycle refers to the means by which the first day of the cycle is identified. In the case of domestic animals with long cycles, e.g., pigs; cows; sheep, the first of the cycle is the first day the female displays heat and will allow the male to mate. In humans and other primates, where mating is not restricted to one time of the cycle, the first day of menstruation is identified as the first day of the cycle. In the rodent, which has a 4–5 day cycle, no day is designated as day one of the cycle; rather the day of the cycle is indicated by the morphology of the cells found in a vaginal lavage. In contrast, induced ovulators, such as the rabbit, ferret, do not have distinct cycles, but rather periods of follicular growth with increasing concentrations of estradiol in the blood inducing the female to accept the male for mating.

Spontaneous ovulators (not requiring mating to ovulate), regardless of the length of the cycle, have a follicular and a luteal phase punctuated by ovulation. In the rodent, follicular growth occurs quickly and the rodent's ovary produces antral follicles, competent to ovulate every 4–5 days. In pigs, cows, and sheep, etc., the follicular phase is very short, is usually only 4–5 days followed by ovulation and a long luteal phase of 12–15 days. In the human, the follicular phase can be variable followed by ovulation and a luteal phase of usually 14 days. In humans, the length of the menstrual cycle can be quite variable, but the luteal phase is relatively constant.

During the estrous and menstrual cycles, the ovary undergoes remarkable changes first as rapid follicular growth, followed by ovulation and then the conversion of the empty follicle (after the exit of the oocyte) into a functional CL. These morphological and biochemical changes are driven by signals, i.e., photoperiod, feedback of hormones, etc., impinging on the hypothalamus, which in turn communicates via the secretion of GnRH to the anterior pituitary causing the secretion of FSH and LH.

Other factors, such as body weight, stress, xenobiotics, toxicants, etc., can also influence the response of the hypothalamus and the anterior pituitary to the feedback of steroids and protein hormones from the ovary.

In conclusion, the ovary is truly a remarkable and complex organ. Probably, no other organ in the body undergoes such dramatic cellular and hormonal changes in such a rapid, precise manner day after day. Because of this complex and rapidly changing nature, the ovary is impacted by environmental factors, which is the focus of this book. This basic knowledge of the ovary is necessary to understand how toxicants can affect the formation and function of the ovary, see Strauss and Williams (2009).

REFERENCES

Carson, R. (1962) *Silent Spring*. Houghton Mifflin, Boston, MA.

Espey, L.L. and Richards, J.S. (2006) Ovulation, In: *Knobil and Neill's Physiology of Reproduction*, 3rd edn., J.D. Neill, ed., Elsevier, Amsterdam, the Netherlands, pp. 425–474.

Liu, C.F., Liu, C., and Yao, H.H.-C. (2010) Building pathways for ovary organogenesis in mouse embryos. In: *Current Topics in Developmental Biology*, vol. 90, Academic Press, London, U.K., pp. 263–283.

Pepling, M.E. (2012) Follicular assembly: mechanisms of action. *Reproduction* 143:139–149.

Rajkovic, A., Pangas, S.A., and Matzuk, M.M. (2006) Follicular development: Mouse, sheep, and human models, In: *Knobil and Neill's Physiology of Reproduction*, 3rd edn., J.D. Neill, ed., Elsevier, Amsterdam, the Netherlands, pp. 383–423.

Strauss, J.F. (2009) The synthesis and metabolism of steroid hormones, In: *Yen and Jaffe's Reproductive Endocrinology*, 6th edn., J.F. Strauss and R.L. Barbieri, eds., Saunders, Philadelphia, PA, pp. 79–104.

Strauss, J.F. and Williams, C.J. (2009) The ovarian life cycle, In: *Yen and Jaffe's Reproductive Endocrinology*, 6th edn., J.F. Strauss and R.L. Barbieri, eds., Saunders, Philadelphia, PA, pp. 155–190.

Ungewitter, E.K. and Yao, H.H.-C. (2012) How to make a gonad: Cellular mechanisms governing formation of the testes and ovaries. *Sexual Development*, DOI:10.1159/000338612.

2 Ovarian Metabolism of Xenobiotics

S. Ganesan, J.A. Madden*, and Aileen F. Keating*

CONTENTS

2.1 INTRODUCTION

The mammalian ovary is the major female gonad with two primary functions: production of a viable germ cell and generation of the sex steroid hormones. Both of these functions are performed by follicular structures, in which the oocyte (germ cell) is surrounded by granulosa cells and eventually also by theca cells. Interaction between the granulosa cell layer and oocyte maintains oocyte viability, while interaction between the granulosa and theca cells results in steroid hormone production; thus, anything that disrupts follicular health will impair fertility. Follicles are present within the ovary at a variety of different developmental stages, the most immature of which is the primordial follicle. Females are born with a finite number of primordial follicles, composed of a meiotically arrested oocyte surrounded by flattened granulosa cells, which serve as the ovarian follicular reserve (Hirshfield, 1991). Once depleted, primordial follicles cannot be replaced, and the ovary eventually undergoes ovarian failure, commonly known as menopause (Hoyer and Sipes, 1996; Hoyer, 2001, 2005). Postmenopausal women are at an increased risk for developing cardiovascular disease, osteoporosis, Alzheimer's disease, and colorectal and ovarian cancer (Hoyer and Sipes, 1996; Hoyer, 2001, 2005); thus,

* These authors contributed equally and should be considered co-first authors.

a longer time frame spent in the postmenopausal state is detrimental for not only reproductive but also overall female health.

A number of chemical classes can destroy ovarian follicles and/or alter steroidogenesis including, but not limited to, environmental, industrial, chemotherapeutic, and xenoestrogenic chemicals (Bhattacharya and Keating, 2011). Follicles at any stage of development can be impacted by xenobiotic exposures leading to deleterious effects on follicle development, oocyte competence and ovulation, and hormone production (Hoyer and Sipes, 1996; Hoyer, 2001, 2005; Hoyer et al., 2001; Bhattacharya and Keating, 2011, 2012a). The reproductive impact of a chemical exposure depends on what follicular development stage is targeted: If the large or antral follicles are depleted, temporary interruptions to reproductive function are observed since these follicles can ultimately be replaced by recruitment from the ovarian reserve. However, chemicals that destroy primordial follicles are more insidious and lead to permanent infertility and premature ovarian failure (POF) since the ovarian reserve is irreplaceable.

The level and duration of exposure to an environmental toxicant can also influence the reproductive impact. Chronic, low-dose exposures, likely to be environmental in nature, are difficult to identify because their ovarian impact may go unrecognized for years. Ongoing selective damage of small preantral follicles may not initially raise concern until the onset of POF that may occur years later. Further, the age at which exposure occurs can impact the outcome. Higher numbers of primordial follicles that are present during childhood and prepubertally mean that a chemical exposure during this life stage may not result in the same extent of follicle loss as that which would be observed postpubertally. However, damage to oocytes by chemical exposures *in utero* and/or during childhood does present a significant concern, since these effects would not be detected until the reproductive years.

Thus, ovotoxic xenobiotic exposures represent a significant health risk for females. In addition to toxicity caused by the parent chemical, metabolites formed in hepatic and extrahepatic tissues (including the ovary itself) can have detrimental ovarian effects. The ovary therefore requires the capacity to metabolize both the primary form and secondary metabolites to inactive compounds in order both to preserve the ovarian follicular pool and to ensure that ovarian function is not compromised.

Ovarian metabolism of xenobiotics greatly impacts the ovotoxic outcome of a chemical exposure. Chemicals for which knowledge of the impact of ovarian metabolism is available will be described in this chapter—trichloroethylene (TCE), 7,12-dimethylbenz(a)anthracene (DMBA), 4-vinylcyclohexene (VCH), and cyclophosphamide (CPA). In addition, the role of regulatory factors on ovarian metabolism will be discussed, and the involvement of phosphatidylinositol-3 kinase (PI3K) signaling on regulation of xenobiotic metabolism gene expression will be described.

2.1.1 Biotransformation Enzymes

A number of enzymes capable of chemical biotransformation have emerged as having critical roles in ovarian metabolism and are discussed throughout this chapter.

A brief summary of their function relative to different chemical classes is provided here as an introduction for those studies in which they are found to impact the extent of ovotoxicity that occurs.

The cytochrome P450 (CYP) enzymes comprise a large family that play critical roles in phase I metabolism of a wide variety of xenobiotics. CYP enzymes are found in all tissues, and they can be involved in chemical activation or detoxification, depending on the chemical substrate (Parkinson and Ogilve, 2008). Another group of phase I biotransformation enzymes are the epoxide hydrolases (EH), which catalyze the addition of water to alkene epoxides and arene oxides. There are five forms of EH, including the isoform under discussion in this chapter, microsomal epoxide hydrolase (mEH). mEH has a wide alkene epoxide and arene oxide substrate range but has a preference for monosubstituted epoxide structures (Parkinson and Ogilve, 2008).

Glutathione (GSH) is a ubiquitous antioxidant compound, present in all cells, and is composed of glycine, cysteine, and glutamic acid. The formation of GSH occurs in two steps catalyzed by γ-glutamylcysteine (γ-Gcl) and glutathione synthetase (Gss). The conjugation of GSH to a chemical represents a phase II modification. GSH is the most abundant intracellular thiol present in cells and detoxifies reactive oxygen species (ROS) by either spontaneous or enzyme-catalyzed reduction (Dalton et al., 2004). Interestingly, the ovary has high concentrations of GSH (Mattison et al., 1983; Lopez and Luderer, 2004), and ovulated oocytes have the highest GSH concentration of any cell type (Calvin et al., 1986). Additionally, ovarian GSH synthesis is regulated by gonadotropins (Luderer et al., 2001), and oocytes from aged mice (42–45 week old) have decreased concentrations of GSH compared to young mice (Hamatani et al., 2004; Brink et al., 2009). GSH xenobiotic conjugation is catalyzed by the glutathione *S*-transferase (GST) family of enzymes, which include the isoforms alpha, pi, mu, omega, and theta and comprise about 10% of total cellular protein (Parkinson and Ogilve, 2008).

Two key transcription factors that are documented to activate numerous xenobiotic metabolism enzymes are the aryl hydrocarbon receptor (AHR) and nuclear factor erythroid 2-related factor 2 (NRF2). AHR is a member of the basic helix–loop–helix (bHLH) DNA binding protein family (Okey et al., 1994). AHR is important for transcription of genes involved in not only xenobiotic metabolism but also regulation of cell cycle, apoptosis, and oxidative stress genes (Denison and Heath-Pagliuso, 1998; Nebert et al., 2000). Under normal conditions, AHR is located in the cytoplasm in a complex with heat shock protein (HSP) 90. Upon activation, this protein complex dissociates, and AHR translocates to the nucleus, where it dimerizes with the AHR nuclear translocator (ARNT) and binds to the xenobiotic response element (XRE) in target gene promoters (Hankinson, 1995). NRF2 is a member of the CNC-bZip (cap "n" collar basic leucine zipper) subfamily of leucine zipper transcription factors (Nguyen et al., 2004). NRF2 is bound to KEAP1 protein in the cytoplasm of cells until the cell is exposed to a stress that requires NRF2 action (Itoh et al., 1999). NRF2 is particularly important in regulation of the phase II xenobiotic metabolism enzymes, including the GSTs (Itoh et al., 1997).

2.2 TRICHLOROETHYLENE

The lipophilic nature and low boiling point of TCE make it an ideal chemical for a number of processes including metal degreasing and dry cleaning (Weiss, 1996). Products such as wood stains, adhesives, lubricants, and paint removers contain TCE (Wu and Berger, 2007). Due to this widespread use, TCE is a common water contaminant (Davidson and Beliles, 1991), and human exposures occur through drinking, inhalation, or transdermal absorption (EPA, 1985). TCE is approximately three times more detectable in rural compared to urban regions in the United States (Wu and Schaum, 2000).

TCE causes reproductive toxicity by affecting fertilization—female rats exposed to TCE via inhalation (1700 ppm, 2 h/day, 5 day/week) displayed altered oocyte plasma membrane composition resulting in decreased oocyte fertilizability (Berger and Horner, 2003). Oocytes from female rats exposed orally to TCE (0.45% TCE in 3% Tween) for 4, 5, or 14 days also displayed less capacity for binding and fertilization by unexposed rat sperm, compared to control oocytes (Wu and Berger, 2007).

TCE induces ovotoxicity through bioactivation by the CYP-dependent and GSH-conjugating pathways; however, whether these biotransformation events occur in ovarian tissue remains unclear but plausible based on the following literature. CYP enzyme-mediated oxidation of TCE through the action of CY1 A1/2, CYP 2B1/2, CYP 2C11/6, and CYP 2E1 (Nakajima et al., 1988, 1990, 1992a,b; Guengerich et al., 1991a; Guengerich and Turvy, 1991b) results in formation of trichloroethanol (TCOH), which can further be metabolized via glucuronidation to TCOH glucuronide (Cummings and Lash, 2000). TCE can also be metabolized to dichloroacetic acid (DCA) and monochloroacetic acid (MCA) (Cummings and Lash, 2000). In addition to the effects of the parent compound, mouse oocytes exposed *in vitro* to TCAA, DCA, and TCOH display reduced fertilization rates (Cosby and Dukelow, 1992), and these TCE metabolites have been detected in the rat ovary following TCE exposure through drinking water (0.45% for 2 weeks) (Wu and Berger, 2007). CYP 2E1 has the highest affinity for TCE (Nakajima et al., 1988, 1990, 1992a,b, 1993; Guengerich et al., 1991a; Guengerich and Turvy, 1991b; Cummings and Lash, 2000), and increased ovarian CYP 2E1 activity has been demonstrated in rats exposed to TCE, suggesting ovarian TCE metabolism may occur through the CYP-dependent oxidative pathway (Reinke and Moyer, 1985).

In extraovarian tissues, the second route of TCE metabolism is through GSH conjugation that results in formation of S-(1,2-dichlorovinyl)glutathione (DCVG) (Lash et al., 1995, 1998). Dipeptidase (DPT) and γ-glutamyltransferase (GTT) then convert DCVG to *S*-(1,2-dichlorovinyl)-L-cysteine (DCVC), which can be further metabolized to form *N*-acetyl-DCVC (NAcDCVC) (Lash et al., 1995, 1998) by the cysteine *S*-conjugate *N*-acetyl-*S*-transferase (Adjei and Weinshilboum, 2002). Generally, GSH conjugation represents a detoxification modification to a chemical, since GSH conjugates become more water soluble, resulting in more rapid excretion of the chemical from the body. In the case of TCE, however, *in vitro* exposure of rat oocytes to the metabolite that results from GSH conjugation, DCVC (5 mM; 4 h), reduced zona pellucida-free oocyte fertilizability (Wu and Berger, 2008), indicating that GSH addition is a bioactivating modification.

2.3 7,12-DIMETHYLBENZ(A)ANTHRACENE

Polycyclic aromatic hydrocarbons (PAHs) are atmospheric pollutants that consist of fused aromatic rings, and human exposure arises from by-products of organic matter burning. PAHs have carcinogenic, mutagenic, and teratogenic effects (Shimada, 2006).

It has long been recognized that cigarette smoking accelerates entry of females into the postmenopausal physiological state (Jick and Porter, 1977). Cigarette smoke contains high level of the PAHs, DMBA, benzo(a)pyrene (BaP), and 3-methylcholanthrene (3-MC) (Mattison et al., 1983; Vahakangas et al., 1985). *In vivo* exposure of mice and rats has demonstrated that DMBA, 3-MC, and BaP deplete primordial follicles (Mattison and Schulman, 1980b; Mattison et al., 1983; Borman et al., 2000) and induce ovarian tumor formation (Krarup, 1967, 1969). Mice treated with BaP, 3-MC, or DMBA (80 mg/kg) also showed signs of necrosis in primordial follicles (Mattison and Schulman, 1980a), with the level of toxicities being DMBA > 3-MC > BaP (Mattison and Thorgeirsson, 1978). This section will describe studies on ovarian DMBA metabolism as a model PAH.

DMBA destroys all ovarian follicle types in mice and rats (Matikainen et al., 2001; Rajapaksa et al., 2007b; Igawa et al., 2009) in a dose-dependent manner (Rajapaksa et al., 2007b; Igawa et al., 2009). DMBA-induced follicle destruction is initiated by oocyte loss followed by somatic cell apoptosis (Morita and Tilly, 1999). Due to the loss of all follicle types, a reduction in ovarian volume typically occurs (Mattison and Schulman, 1980b; Weitzman et al., 1992).

PAHs require metabolism to produce reactive ovotoxic metabolites (Mattison et al., 1983) that bind to cellular macromolecules including DNA, RNA, and protein (Sims and Grover, 1974). In hepatic tissue, DMBA undergoes extensive metabolism to form bioactive metabolites (Bengtsson et al., 1983a). The metabolism pathway begins with DMBA oxidation to DMBA-3,4-diol by CYP 1B1 and hydrolysis by mEH. The 3,4-diol metabolite undergoes further epoxidation by CYP1A1 and CYP1B1 to form the carcinogen, DMBA-3,4-diol-1,2-epoxide (Kleiner et al., 2004; Shimada and Fujii-Kuriyama, 2004).

Early studies determined that bioactivation was also necessary for induction of ovotoxicity by DMBA. DMBA-induced oocyte destruction *in vivo* was inhibited by treatment with alpha-naphthoflavone (ANF; 10 μg/ovary) (Shiromizu and Mattison, 1985). ANF is an AHR antagonist and thereby prevents activation of a number of metabolism enzymes. Intraovarian injection of mice with DMBA (10 μg/ovary) resulted in oocyte destruction (95%) (Shiromizu and Mattison, 1985). AHR-deficient mice are resistant to DMBA-induced primordial follicle destruction (Matikainen et al., 2001), and co-treatment with DMBA and ANF (80 mg/kg intraperitoneal (IP)) prevented ovarian follicle destruction in mice (Shiromizu and Mattison, 1985). Induction of xenobiotic metabolism enzymes in response to DMBA involves the action of AHR. *AhR* mRNA and protein are increased in response to ovarian DMBA exposure prior to the onset of follicle loss (Bhattacharya and Keating, 2012b), further supporting a role for AHR in DMBA-induced activation of *Cyp 1b1, meh*, and *Gstp* (Bhattacharya and Keating, 2012b). Thus, the action of ovarian enzymes is required for DMBA-induced ovotoxicity.

A role for CYP 1B1 involvement in DMBA-induced ovotoxicity has been determined. While a modest DMBA-induced increase (0.4-fold) in *Cyp 1b1* mRNA was detected in mouse ovaries (Shimada et al., 2003), inhibition of CYP 1B1 activity in isolated ovarian microsomes using an anti-CYP 1B1 antibody decreased DMBA metabolism (Otto et al., 1992), while no effect of an anti-CYP 1A1 antibody on DMBA metabolism was demonstrated (Otto et al., 1992).

Utilizing a whole ovary culture model to study metabolism of DMBA has further supported the capacity of the ovary for bioactivation of DMBA (Igawa et al., 2009). Cultured rat ovaries were exposed to DMBA or DMBA-3,4-diol at concentrations ranging from 12.5 to 1000 nM for 15 days. Primordial follicle loss occurred at a concentration of 75 nM DMBA and 12.5 nM DMBA-3,4-diol. Small primary follicle loss followed a similar pattern, with follicle destruction occurring at 375 nM DMBA and 75 nM DMBA 3,4-diol (Igawa et al., 2009). Therefore, the lower concentrations required to cause follicle loss indicate that 3,4-diol metabolite is more ovotoxic than the DMBA parent compound.

The involvement of mEH in DMBA bioactivation has been investigated in mice and rats using this system. DMBA (1 μM) induced primordial and small primary follicle loss after 6 h in cultured mouse ovaries (Rajapaksa et al., 2007b) but not until 4 days in cultured rat ovaries (Igawa et al., 2009). mEH protein is localized in ovarian granulosa cells (Rajapaksa et al., 2007b; Igawa et al., 2009), and mEH catalytic activity has been demonstrated in granulosa cells and microsomal fractions from corpora lutea (Hattori et al., 2000). mEH is induced by DMBA both at the transcriptional and translational levels in both species prior to the onset of follicle loss (Rajapaksa et al., 2007b; Igawa et al., 2009). In mice, although there is DMBA-induced primordial follicle loss after 6 h, upregulation of mEH mRNA levels after 2 days was followed by a full-fold increase in follicle loss thereafter on day 4 (Rajapaksa et al., 2007b). Additionally, inhibition of mEH activity using the competitive inhibitor, cyclohexene oxide (CHO), demonstrated that when mEH was blunted in mouse ovaries, there was a reduction in DMBA-induced loss of primordial and small primary follicles (Rajapaksa et al., 2007b). mEH's role in DMBA bioactivation has also been confirmed in rats (Igawa et al., 2009). Inhibition of mEH with CHO was unable to prevent ovotoxicity caused by the 3,4-diol intermediate, which bypasses mEH bioactivation of DMBA (Figure 2.1; Igawa et al., 2009). Thus, mEH ovarian expression and activity are essential for DMBA bioactivation to the ovotoxic metabolite.

Thus, the data from ovarian studies support DMBA conversion via CYP 1B1 to DMBA-3,4-epoxide, which is then hydrolyzed to DMBA-3,4-diol by the action of mEH. DMBA-3,4-diol then undergoes epoxidation by CYP 1A1 or CYP 1B1 to form DMBA-3,4-diol-1,2-epoxide, which is the ultimate ovotoxic metabolite.

Although DMBA detoxification has not been characterized as well as that of bioactivation, a role for GSH-mediated detoxification of DMBA is supported (Tsai-Turton et al., 2007; Bhattacharya and Keating, 2012b). Supplementation of cultured preovulatory follicles with GSH during DMBA exposure protects against apoptosis (Tsai-Turton et al., 2007). Also, GSTP-null mice have increased DMBA-induced skin tumor formation compared to their wild-type littermates (Henderson et al., 1998) indicating that GSTP may mediate catalysis of GSH conjugation to DMBA.

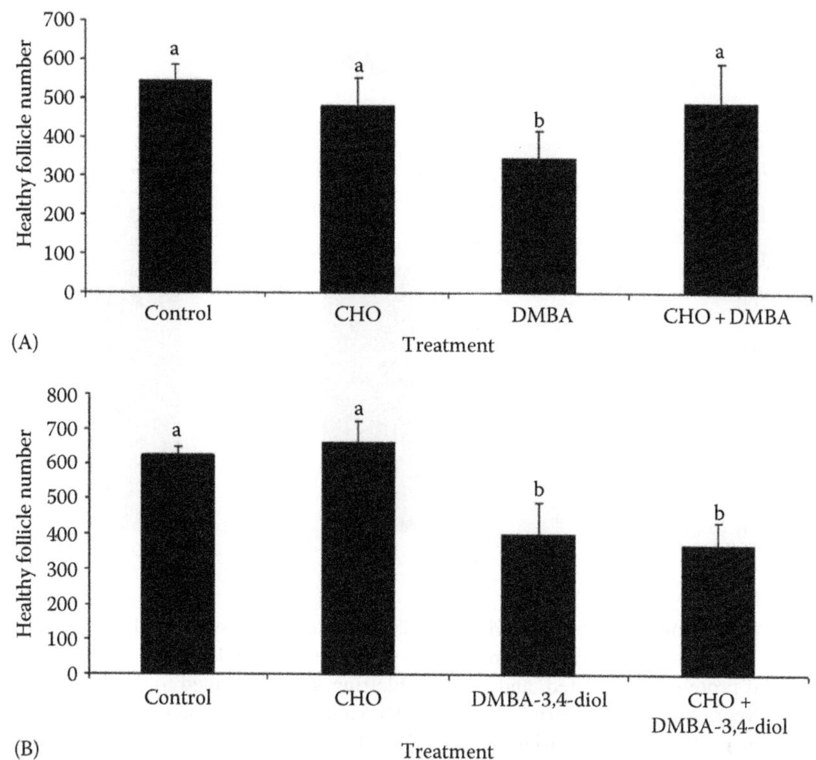

FIGURE 2.1 Effect of mEH inhibition on DMBA- or DMBA-3,4-diol-induced follicle loss. Ovaries from PND4 Fischer 344 rats were cultured with (A) vehicle control or media containing DMBA (1 μM) ± CHO (mEH inhibitor; 2 mM) for 4 days or (B) vehicle control or media containing DMBA-3,4-diol (75 nM) ± CHO (2 mM) for 4 days. Following incubation, ovaries were collected and processed for histological evaluation, and healthy follicles were counted. Values are mean ± SE total follicles counted/ovary, n = 5. (Reproduced from Igawa, Y. et al., *Toxicol. Appl. Pharmacol.*, 234, 361, 2009. With permission.)

Gstp mRNA and protein expression are increased in PND4 cultured rat ovaries exposed to DMBA at a time point prior to DMBA-induced follicle loss (Figure 2.2; Bhattacharya and Keating, 2012b); thus, GSTP is likely to be involved in the ovarian response to DMBA exposure.

NRF2-deficient mice are more sensitive to and have increased incidence of DMBA-induced skin tumors (Xu et al., 2006; Becks et al., 2010). NRF2 can bind to an enhancer element in the *Gstp* gene promoter to activate its transcription (Ikeda et al., 2004). Also, NRF2-deficient mice have only 3%–20% of hepatic GST expression relative to their wild-type littermates (Chanas et al., 2002). Thus, these studies support a role for NRF2 in DMBA detoxification, potentially through the action of GSTP.

There are three major mitogen-activated protein kinase (MAPK) members: extracellular signal-regulated kinase (ERK), c-Jun N-terminal kinase (JNK), and p38 MAPK. The three are regulated independently and control many processes involved

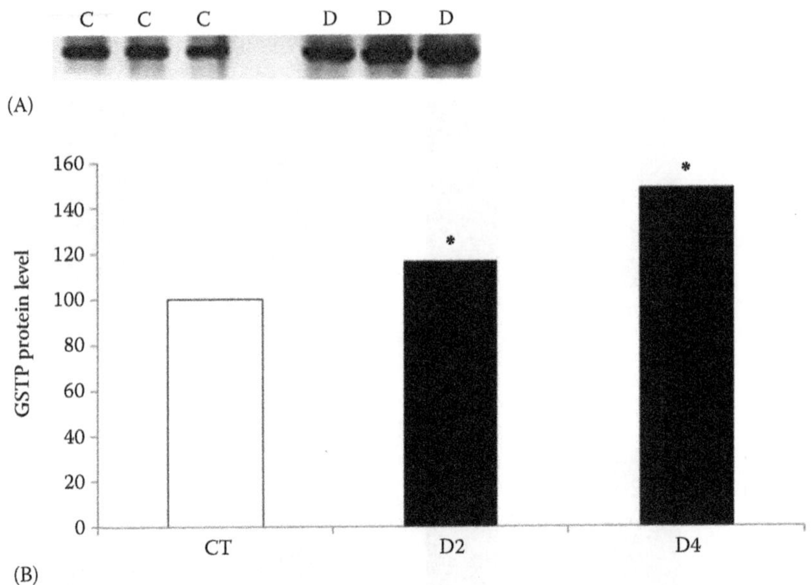

FIGURE 2.2 Temporal effect of DMBA on GSTP protein expression. PND4 F344 rat ovaries were cultured in media containing vehicle control (C) or DMBA (D; 1 μM) for 2 or 4 days. Total protein was isolated, and Western blotting was performed to detect GSTP protein. (A) Representative Western blot day 4. (B) Values are expressed as a percentage of control mean ± SE, n = 3 (10 ovaries per pool). $^*P < 0.05$, different from control. (Reproduced from Bhattacharya, P. and Keating, A.F., *Toxicol. Appl. Pharmacol.*, 260, 201, 2012. With permission.)

in cell survival, growth, and death (Marshall, 1995; Whitmarsh and Davis, 1996; Dunn and Klaassen, 1998). The ERK pathway is generally involved in cell growth and proliferation (Hill and Treisman, 1995), while JNK and p38 mediate the stress response and apoptosis (Xia et al., 1995; Johnson et al., 1996; Zanke et al., 1996; Rincon et al., 1998). A role for GST enzymes in negatively regulating the action of JNK has recently been supported in extraovarian tissues (Adler et al., 1999). This is also the case in the ovary. GSTP forms an ovarian protein complex with JNK (Keating et al., 2010) and increased GSTP in response to DMBA exposure results in increased binding of JNK by GSTP and prevention of JNK phosphorylation of its downstream substrate c-Jun (Figure 2.3; Bhattacharya and Keating, 2012b). Thus, it appears that GSTP provides a further protective role against DMBA-induced apoptosis, using this mechanism of antiapoptotic protein regulation.

2.4 4-VINYLCYCLOHEXENE

VCH is a by-product of the pesticide, rubber, plastic, and flame retardant industries (Rappaport and Fraser, 1977), and human exposures are largely occupational in nature through either dermal or oral intake (Program, 1989; Bevan et al., 1996). VCH selectively destroys primordial and small primary follicles leading to POF

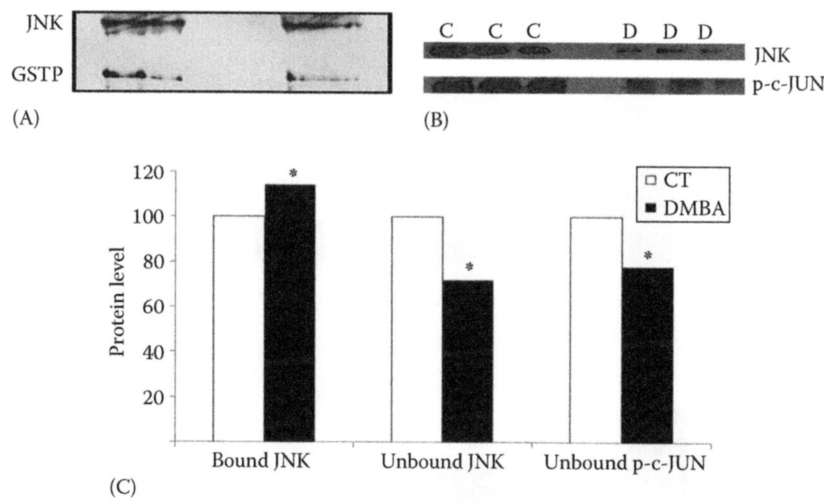

FIGURE 2.3 Impact of DMBA exposure on ovarian GSTP:JNK protein complex association. PND4 F344 rat ovaries were cultured in media containing vehicle control (C) or DMBA (D; 1 μM) for 4 days, followed by total protein isolation. (A) Immunoprecipitation using an anti-GSTP antibody, followed by Western blotting to detect JNK protein. (B) Western blotting was performed on the unbound protein fraction to detect JNK and p-c-JUN proteins. (C) Quantification of the amount of JNK protein bound to GSTP and unbound JNK and p-c-JUN protein level. Values are expressed as a percentage of control mean ± SE, n = 3 (20 ovaries per pool). *$P<0.05$, different from control. (Reproduced from Bhattacharya, P. and Keating, A.F., *Toxicol. Appl. Pharmacol.*, 260, 201, 2012. With permission.)

in mice and rats (Flaws et al., 1994; Doerr et al., 1995; Springer et al., 1996a,b; Hoyer et al., 2001).

VCH can be bioactivated to the ultimate diepoxide ovotoxic metabolite, 4-vinylcyclohexene diepoxide (VCD), through the action of ovarian expressed CYP 2E1 (Rajapaksa et al., 2007a). Mice dosed with vehicle, VCH (7.4 mmol/kg/day), or VCD (0.57 mmol/kg/day) for 15 days (IP) had increased ovarian CYP 2E1 mRNA, protein, and activity (Cannady et al., 2003). Further investigations have shown that CYP 2E1-null mice suffer less follicle loss relative to their wild-type littermates (Rajapaksa et al., 2007a); thus, CYP2E1 appears to be involved in VCH bioactivation to VCD. Ovarian CYP 2A is also increased in mouse ovaries following VCH (7.4 mmol/kg/day) and VCD (0.57 mmol/kg/day) exposures (15 days; IP), while the CYP 2B isoform responds only to VCD exposure (Cannady et al., 2003). These data indicate an involvement of CYP 2A and 2B in VCH and VCD biotransformation.

Ovarian expressed mEH is involved in detoxification of VCD. VCD induces mEH mRNA and protein expression both *in vivo* (Flaws et al., 1994; Cannady et al., 2002) and *in vitro* (Keating et al., 2008; Bhattacharya et al., 2012c) prior to follicle loss in mice and rats. Inhibition of mEH using CHO during VCD exposure resulted in greater follicle loss relative to VCD-treated ovaries, further supporting a detoxification role for mEH during VCD-induced ovotoxicity (Figure 2.4; Bhattacharya et al., 2012).

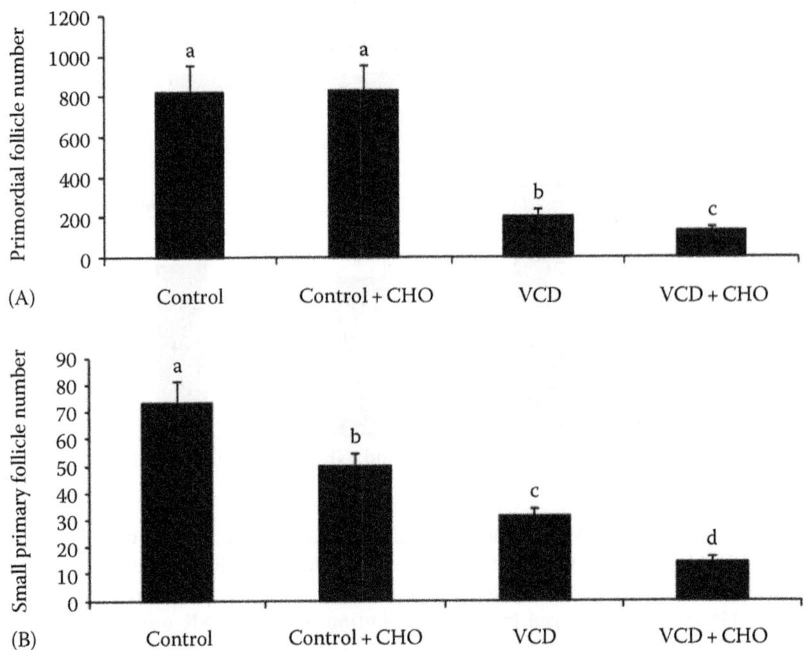

FIGURE 2.4 Effect of mEH inhibition on VCD-induced follicle loss. PND4 F344 rat ovaries were cultured in media containing vehicle control or VCD (30 μM) ±CHO (2 mM) for 8 days. Ovaries were processed for histological evaluation, and healthy follicles were classified and counted. Values are expressed as mean ± SE total follicles counted/ovary, n = 5. Different letters indicate significant difference; $P<0.05$. (Reproduced from Bhattacharya, P. et al., *Toxicol. Appl. Pharmacol.*, 258, 118, 2012. With permission.)

mEH protein is abundantly distributed in the mouse ovary (Cannady et al., 2002). Therefore, it has the potential to be actively involved in mediating ovarian responses to xenobiotic chemicals. Whereas mEH is involved in bioactivation of DMBA, it can catalyze detoxification of VCD. The concentration of DMBA required to induce loss of approximately 50% of primordial follicles is 1 μM, and loss occurs after 4 days of exposure in the ovarian culture system (Igawa et al., 2009). In contrast, VCD induces the same amount of primordial follicle loss at a concentration of 30 μM and after a longer time of exposure, 6 days (Keating et al., 2009). Thus, this difference in mEH function during DMBA and VCD exposures is likely to provide at least partial explanation for the increased ovotoxicity of DMBA compared to VCD.

In addition to DMBA, a protective role for ovarian GSTP is hypothesized to occur during VCD exposure (Keating et al., 2010). *Gstp* mRNA and protein are increased in response to VCD. In a similar manner to that during DMBA-induced ovotoxicity, GSTP forms a protein complex with JNK and inhibits JNK action, as evidenced by reduced phosphorylation of the JNK target, c-Jun (Keating et al., 2010). Additionally, the mu isoform of the GST family (GSTM) forms an ovarian protein complex with apoptosis stress-related kinase 1 (ASK1) (Bhattacharya et al.,

Under Review). ASK1 is pro-apoptotic and is an upstream regulator of JNK activity (Ichijo et al., 1997). *Ask1* mRNA is increased at the time of VCD-induced follicle loss, and in a similar manner to that of GSTP, during VCD exposure, the amount of ASK1 protein bound to GSTM is increased, thus indicating an antiapoptotic protective role for ovarian GSTM (Bhattacharya et al., Under Review). In this way, the combined action of GSTP and GSTM is increased in a protective response in the ovary during VCD exposure. It should be noted, however, that deciphering the specific contribution of GSTP and GSTM in conjugating GSH to VCD remains to be determined.

NRF2 is thought to also play a role in regulation of the xenobiotic metabolism response to VCD. Mice lacking NRF2 were more sensitive to VCD-induced ovotoxicity than their wild-type counterparts (Hu et al., 2006). Whether this action of NRF2 was at the level of the liver or ovary, however, has not been determined.

2.5 CHEMOTHERAPEUTICS

It is estimated that over 1.6 million people in the United States will be diagnosed with cancer in 2012 (Siegel et al., 2012). Compared to 1977 when the 5-year survival rate was 49%, 67% of cancer patients will now survive at least 5 years postdiagnosis (Siegel et al., 2012). Early detection and advanced medical treatments are likely attributable to factors responsible for these enhanced survival rates. However, as cancer survival rates increase, a growing number of survivors are facing the consequences of their treatment, which unfortunately for many women includes POF and infertility.

A number of antineoplastic agents can cause female infertility, including busulfan, cisplatin, and CPA. In 1956, the first observed ovotoxic chemotherapy effects were induced by busulfan, which caused all patients ($n = 4$) to be premenopausal three months into therapy (Louis et al., 1956). Busulfan is an alkylating agent, which acts by cross-linking DNA to interfere with cell replication (Jackson et al., 1959).

Cisplatin (cis-diamminedichloroplatinum (II): CDDP), a nonalkylating agent, is also an ovotoxic antineoplastic chemical. CDDP is a platinum-based chemotherapy that, similar to alkylating agents, reacts with DNA, inhibiting DNA synthesis and causing apoptosis. CDDP is used to treat a variety of cancers including breast, ovarian, lung, and head and neck cancers with side effects that include nephrotoxicity and ovotoxicity (Dobyan et al., 1980; Nakai et al., 1982; Wallace et al., 1989). Studies in rats have demonstrated that a single dose of CDDP decreased primordial follicles by 25%–35% and increased follicular cysts and apoptosis (Borovskaya et al., 2004). Repeated CDDP exposure in rats depleted the total number of follicles, increased postimplantation loss rates, and decreased litter number (Matsuo et al., 2007; Nozaki et al., 2009). There is evidence that CDDP causes DNA laddering, chromatin condensation, and arrest of the cell cycle at the G2 phase (Barry et al., 1990; Boersma et al., 1996; Schmitt et al., 2004). Additionally, *in vivo* and *in vitro* studies reported that CDDP induced the production of ROS (Kopke et al., 1997; Satoh et al., 2003), which may also contribute to CDDP-induced ovarian damage.

The metabolism of CDDP is slowly being deciphered, and while it remains unclear if CDDP is enzymatically biotransformed, it is hypothesized that CDDP-containing chloride ligands are displaced by water yielding a positive charged platinum compound that reacts with DNA, thus cross-linking the strands and inhibiting DNA synthesis (Oswald et al., 1990a,b), which ultimately leads to cell apoptosis involving the Bcl-2 and Bax pathways (Barry et al., 1990; Boersma et al., 1996; Schmitt et al., 2004).

CPA is an antineoplastic prodrug that acts as an alkylating agent to treat, alone or in combination, a variety of cancers and autoimmune disorders. CPA was FDA approved in 1959 and is also known by its brand names: Cytoxan, Clafen, and Neosar. CPA is administered orally or intravenously to patients of all ages and has a wide range of side effects including alopecia, nausea, immunosuppression, and infertility (Fraiser et al., 1991). Infertility is particularly concerning for females because CPA destroys primordial follicles (Plowchalk and Mattison, 1991).

In a similar manner as that of DMBA, CPA is inactive until it is metabolized, primarily by hepatic CYP enzymes, inducing production of a number of active and inactive metabolites. The bioactivation step that contributes greatly to CPA-induced ovotoxicity is the C-4 oxidation of CPA to form 4-hydroxycyclophosphamide (4-HC), followed by interconversion to the open-ring form, aldophosphamide, which fragments to phosphoramide mustard (PM) and acrolein (Ludeman, 1999; Pinto et al., 2009). Previous research has found 4-HC to be an ovotoxic metabolite of CPA, because 4-HC can easily pass through the cell membrane and produce PM intracellularly (Ludeman, 1999; Desmeules and Devine, 2006). PM is known to be the antineoplastic metabolite of CPA (Shulman-Roskes et al., 1998), and its formation is required for ovotoxicity *in vitro* (Plowchalk and Mattison, 1991) and *in vivo* (Desmeules and Devine, 2006). However, PM can undergo another spontaneous reaction to form the volatile, cytotoxic metabolite chloroethylaziridine (CEZ) (Rauen and Norpoth, 1968; Shulman-Roskes et al., 1998), which, due to its higher cell permeability (Hata and Watanabe, 1994) and longer half-life compared to PM (Lu and Chan, 2006), may also contribute to CPA-induced ovotoxicity (Desmeules and Devine, 2006).

Previous studies have demonstrated that *in vitro* CPA and/or PM exposures target primordial follicles in mice (Plowchalk and Mattison, 1991) and antral follicles in rats (Desmeules and Devine, 2006) at concentrations relevant to human exposures (Struck et al., 1987; Desmeules and Devine, 2006). The specific ovarian cell-type targeted depend on the follicle type, such that in smaller follicles, oocytes are being targeted, while in larger follicles, it is the granulosa cells (Desmeules and Devine, 2006). Granulosa cells of primary follicles are stained positively for caspase-3 and terminal deoxynucleotidyl transferase dUTP nick end labeling (TUNEL) (evidence of apoptosis) following PM exposure; thus, it was concluded that apoptosis is responsible for those cells' death (Desmeules and Devine, 2006). However, it is acknowledged that due to the close interaction and communication between the granulosa cells and the oocyte, it is difficult to determine exactly which cell type is the initial ovotoxic target (Desmeules and Devine, 2006).

Evidence suggests that the detoxification of CPA and its metabolites occurs by NADPH oxidation via aldehyde dehydrogenases and GSH conjugation via the GSTs, with the precise mechanisms remaining to be determined (Pinto et al., 2009). Further, these mechanisms may vary between follicle types (Desmeules and Devine, 2006). Studies also suggest that a spontaneous GSH conjugation to PM can occur, thus lessening both the toxic and therapeutic effects of CPA (Colvin et al., 1993; Colvin, 1994; Dirven et al., 1994; Shulman-Roskes et al., 1998). The stability of CEZ has also been demonstrated to decrease with excess GSH (Shulman-Roskes et al., 1998), supporting detoxification roles for GSH conjugation to CPA, PM, and CEZ.

2.6 PHOSPHATIDYINOSITOL-3 KINASE

The PI3K signaling pathway is critical for maintaining the viability of primordial follicles that comprise the ovarian reserve (Reddy et al., 2005; Liu et al., 2006; Jagarlamudi et al., 2009). Kit ligand (KitL) expressed in the granulosa cells of primordial follicles (Ismail et al., 1996) binds to an oocyte-expressed receptor, c-Kit (Manova et al., 1990; Orr-Urtreger et al., 1990; Horie et al., 1991), leading to c-Kit autophosphorylation. Once phosphorylated, the action of c-Kit eventually results in PI3K activation (Roskoski, 2005). PI3K are lipid kinases that phosphorylate the 3′-OH group on the inositol ring of inositol phospholipids. Activation of PI3K results in conversion of the plasma membrane lipid phosphatidylinositol-4,5-bisphosphate (PIP_2) to phosphatidylinositol-3,4,5-triphosphate (PIP_3), and PIP_3 recruits proteins that have lipid-binding domains from the cytoplasm to the plasma membrane where they become phosphorylated (Pawson and Nash, 2000). Two examples of such proteins are the serine/threonine kinases 3′-phosphoinositide-dependent kinase-1 (PDK1) and AKT (Cantley, 2002). Mice with oocyte-specific depletion of PDK1 had accelerated oocyte loss and were depleted of oocytes within 8 weeks after birth (Reddy et al., 2009). Follicle destruction was determined to occur at the primordial follicle stage, indicating a role for PDK1 in primordial follicle viability (Reddy et al., 2009). Downstream of PDK1, phosphorylated AKT (pAKT) can translocate to the nucleus, where it regulates a number of cellular responses such as growth, survival, and cell cycle entry and, thus, is largely a pro-survival gene (Datta et al., 1999). Mice lacking oocyte-specific expression of AKT were infertile with loss of primordial follicles by PND90 (Brown et al., 2010).

This pathway also plays a "gatekeeper" role in determining activation of primordial follicles from their dormant state and entry into the growing follicular pool (Liu et al., 2006; Jagarlamudi et al., 2009; Reddy et al., 2010). The forkhead transcription factor family member, FOXO3, is negatively regulated by pAKT. Mice lacking FOXO3 expression experience POF due to global activation of the primordial follicle pool (Castrillon et al., 2003). In contrast, oocyte-specific overexpression of FOXO3 results in infertility in mice due to complete lack of primordial follicle activation (John et al., 2008). Thus, FOXO3 has been implicated as a critical regulator of primordial follicle activation.

It is noteworthy to stress the importance of this phenomenon since overactivation of primordial follicles into the growing follicular pool does not culminate in additional ovulated oocytes; instead, these follicles are destroyed by apoptosis, and entrance into POF is accelerated. This is especially relevant when considering chemical exposures that deplete the primordial follicle pool.

2.6.1 PI3K Regulation of Xenobiotic Metabolism Gene Expression

The PI3K pathway's importance both as a target for ovotoxicants (Keating et al., 2009, 2011; Mark-Kappeler et al., 2011; Sobinoff et al., 2011) and as a regulator of xenobiotic metabolism has recently emerged (Bhattacharya and Keating, 2012b; Bhattacharya et al., 2012). VCD reduces PI3K signaling in primordial and small primary oocytes as a mechanism of inducing ovotoxicity (Keating et al., 2011). Decreased phosphorylation of c-KIT (Mark-Kappeler et al., 2011) and oocyte-expressed pAKT (Keating et al., 2011) occurs rapidly after VCD exposure in PND4 cultured rat ovaries. Both of these events can collectively compromise oocyte viability. There is also a decrease in oocyte FOXO3 in the follicles targeted by VCD (Keating et al., 2011). This likely accelerates entry of primordial follicles into the growing follicular pool, thus committing these follicles to a fate of destruction. *Kitl* mRNA is upregulated in response to VCD, which may be a protective response induced by the ovary in response to VCD exposure, and, in fact, exogenous addition of KITL during VCD exposure significantly attenuates VCD-induced follicle loss (Fernandez et al., 2008). Therefore, PI3K activity is reduced by VCD to cause primordial and small primary follicular destruction.

PND4 mouse ovaries exposed to DMBA also display altered PI3K signaling. Increased pAKT with a concomitant decrease in pFOXO3 was observed in DMBA-treated primordial follicle oocytes, both of which would compromise oocyte viability and accelerate POF (Sobinoff et al., 2011). Additionally, phosphorylation of the PI3K downstream signaling component, mammalian target of rapamycin (mTOR) consistent with mTOR activation was observed (Sobinoff et al., 2011).

The ovotoxic outcomes of DMBA and VCD exposures are altered when PI3K is inhibited—follicle loss by VCD is lessened, while that of DMBA is accelerated (Keating et al., 2009). As detailed in the sections on DMBA and VCH metabolism, mEH bioactivates DMBA but detoxifies VCD. PI3K signaling is involved in insulin-induced hepatic regulation of mEH (Kim and Novak, 2007), and it has also been demonstrated that C/EBPα and C/EBPβ, transcription factors involved in mEH induction, are activated through PI3K signaling (Ki and Kim, 2008). For these reasons, it is logical to consider that altered mEH expression may occur during PI3K inhibition and may contribute to the altered ovotoxic impact of PI3K inhibition during VCD and DMBA exposures.

Ovarian expressed mEH mRNA and protein are increased during PI3K inhibition (Figure 2.5; Bhattacharya et al., 2012); thus, when PI3K action is blunted, the increased amount of ovarian expressed mEH would detoxify VCD and bioactivate DMBA to greater extents, which is supported by the enhanced follicular loss from DMBA as compared to VCD (Keating et al., 2011). Furthermore, inhibition of PI3K

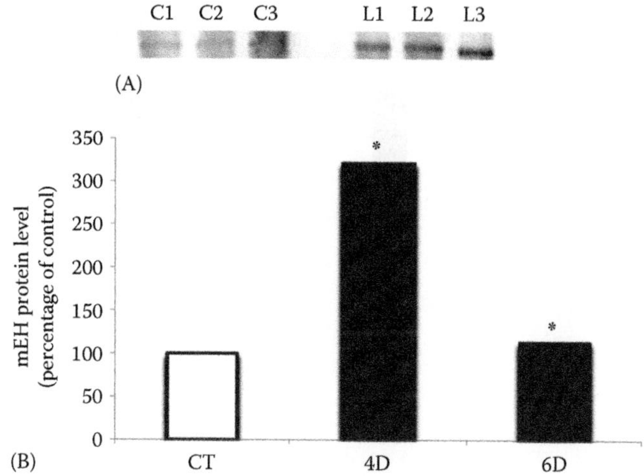

FIGURE 2.5 Temporal effect of PI3K inhibition on mEH protein. PND4 F344 rat ovaries were cultured in media containing vehicle control (CT) ±20 μM LY294002 for 4 or 6 days. Total protein was isolated, and Western blotting was performed to detect mEH protein. (A) Representative Western blot is shown on day 4; control = C; LY294002 = L. (B) Values are expressed as a percentage of control mean ± SE, n = 3 (10 ovaries per pool). $^{*}P < 0.05$, different from control. (Reproduced from Bhattacharya, P. et al., *Toxicol. Appl. Pharmacol.*, 258, 118, 2012. With permission.)

signaling has been demonstrated to increase expression of *AhR*, *Nrf2*, *Gstp*, and *Gstm* at the mRNA and protein levels (Figure 2.6; Bhattacharya and Keating, 2012b; Bhattacharya et al., Under Review).

Taken together, these data demonstrate the involvement of PI3K signaling in regulation of transcription factors or enzymes that are directly involved in ovarian xenobiotic metabolism. Thus, new roles for this signaling pathway are emerging, and since this pathway is amenable to manipulation through chemical means, therapeutic interventions may become possible in the future.

2.7 CONCLUSION

The action of ovarian expressed enzymes is critical in determination of whether a chemical exposure is ovotoxic or not. It is both interesting and concerning that enzymes can mediate either bioactivation or detoxification of xenobiotics depending on the chemical to which the tissue is exposed. Clearly, further research on ovarian detoxification schemes for chemicals is needed. Until such a time that we better understand ovarian biotransformation processes, potential POF, infertility, and other negative reproductive outcomes caused by environmental exposures remain a concern, and development of therapeutic strategies to prevent such negative consequences will be limited.

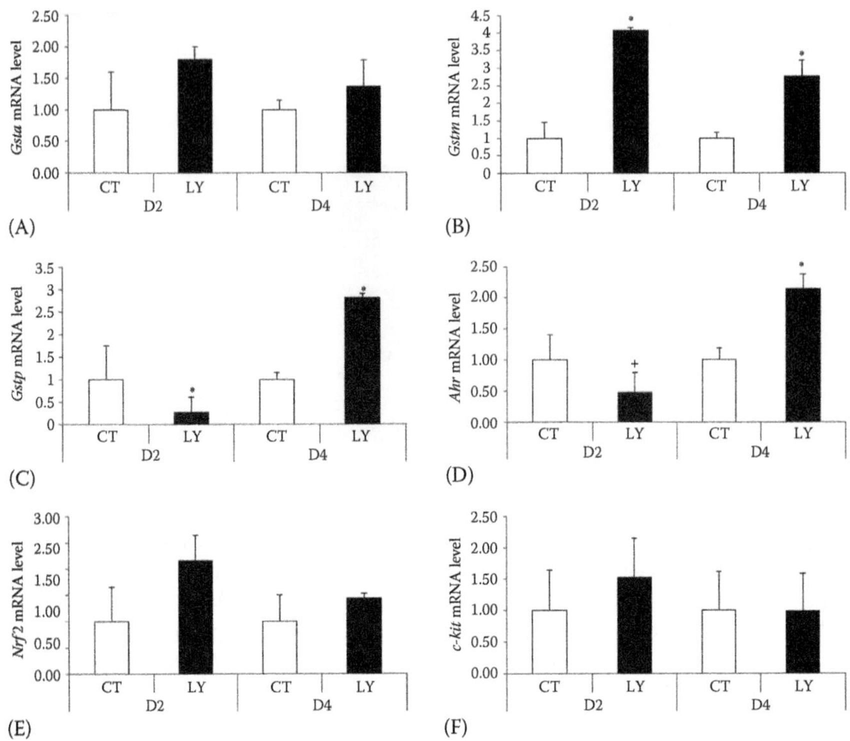

FIGURE 2.6 Regulation of *Gsta*, *Gstm*, *Gstp*, *Ahr*, *Nrf2*, and *c-kit* mRNA by PI3K signaling. PND4 F344 rat ovaries were cultured in media containing vehicle control (CT) ±LY294002 (LY; 20 μM) for 2 or 4 days. Following incubation, total RNA was isolated and RT-PCR used to quantify mRNA levels of (A) *Gsta*, (B) *Gstm*, (C) *Gstp*, (D) *Ahr*, (E) *Nrf2*, and (F) *c-kit*. Values are expressed as mean fold change ± SE, n = 3 (10 ovaries per pool). *$P < 0.05$, different from control. (Reproduced from Bhattacharya, P. and Keating, A.F., *Toxicol. Appl. Pharmacol.,* 260, 201, 2012. With permission.)

ACKNOWLEDGMENTS

The project described was supported by the National Institutes of Environmental Health Sciences R00ES016818 to A.F.K. The content is solely the responsibility of the authors and does not necessarily represent the official views of the National Institute of Environmental Health Sciences or the National Institutes of Health.

REFERENCES

Adjei AA, Weinshilboum RM. 2002. Catecholestrogen sulfation: Possible role in carcinogenesis. *Biochem Biophys Res Commun* 292:402–408.

Adler V, Yin Z, Fuchs SY et al. 1999. Regulation of JNK signaling by GSTp. *Embo J* 18:1321–1334.

Barry MA, Behnke CA, Eastman A. 1990. Activation of programmed cell death (apoptosis) by cisplatin, other anticancer drugs, toxins and hyperthermia. *Biochem Pharmacol* 40:2353–2362.

Becks L, Prince M, Burson H et al. 2010. Aggressive mammary carcinoma progression in Nrf2 knockout mice treated with 7,12-dimethylbenz[a]anthracene. *BMC Cancer* 10:540.

Bengtsson M, Montelius J, Mankovitz L et al. 1983a. Metabolism of polycyclic aromatic hydrocarbons in the rat ovary. *Biochem Pharmacol* 32:129–136.

Berger T, Horner CM. 2003. In vivo exposure of female rats to toxicants may affect oocyte quality. *Reprod Toxicol* 17:273–281.

Bevan C, Stadler JC, Elliott GS et al. 1996. Subchronic toxicity of 4-vinylcyclohexene in rats and mice by inhalation exposure. *Fund Appl Toxicol* 32:1–10.

Bhattacharya P, Keating AF. 2011. Ovarian metabolism of xenobiotics. *Exp Biol Med* 236:765–771.

Bhattacharya P, Keating AF. 2012a. Impact of environmental exposures on ovarian function and role of xenobiotic metabolism during ovotoxicity. *Toxicol Appl Pharmacol* 261:227–235.

Bhattacharya P, Keating AF. 2012b. Protective role for ovarian glutathione S-transferase isoform pi during 7,12-dimethylbenz[a]anthracene-induced ovotoxicity. *Toxicol Appl Pharmacol* 260:201–208.

Bhattacharya P, Sen N, Hoyer PB et al. 2012c. Ovarian expressed microsomal epoxide hydrolase: Role in detoxification of 4-vinylcyclohexene diepoxide and regulation by phosphatidylinositol-3 kinase signaling. *Toxicol Appl Pharmacol* 258:118–123.

Bhattacharya P, Madden JA, Sen N et al. 2013. Glutathione S-transferase class mu regulation of apoptosis signal-related kinase 1 protein during VCD-induced ovotoxicity in neonatal rat ovaries. *Toxicol Appl Pharmacol* 267:49–56.

Boersma AW, Nooter K, Oostrum RG et al. 1996. Quantification of apoptotic cells with fluorescein isothiocyanate-labeled annexin V in chinese hamster ovary cell cultures treated with cisplatin. *Cytometry* 24:123–130.

Borman SM, Christian PJ, Sipes IG et al. 2000. Ovotoxicity in female Fischer rats and B6 mice induced by low-dose exposure to three polycyclic aromatic hydrocarbons: Comparison through calculation of an ovotoxic index. *Toxicol Appl Pharmacol* 167:191–198.

Borovskaya TG, Goldberg VE, Fomina TI et al. 2004. Morphological and functional state of rat ovaries in early and late periods after administration of platinum cytostatics. *Bull Exp Biol Med* 137:331–335.

Brink TC, Demetrius L, Lehrach H et al. 2009. Age-related transcriptional changes in gene expression in different organs of mice support the metabolic stability theory of aging. *Biogerontology* 10:549–564.

Brown C, LaRocca J, Pietruska J et al. 2010. Subfertility caused by altered follicular development and oocyte growth in female mice lacking PKB alpha/Akt1. *Biol Reprod* 82:246–256.

Calvin HI, Grosshans K, Blake EJ. 1986. Estimation and manipulation of glutathione levels in prepubertal mouse ovaries and ova: Relevance to sperm nucleus transformation in the fertilized egg. *Gamete Res* 14:265–275.

Cannady EA, Dyer CA, Christian PJ et al. 2002. Expression and activity of microsomal epoxide hydrolase in follicles isolated from mouse ovaries. *Toxicol Sci* 68:24–31.

Cannady EA, Dyer CA, Christian PJ et al. 2003. Expression and activity of cytochromes P450 2E1, 2A, and 2B in the mouse ovary: The effect of 4-vinylcyclohexene and its diepoxide metabolite. *Toxicol Sci* 73:423–430.

Cantley LC. 2002. The phosphoinositide 3-kinase pathway. *Science* 296:1655–1657.

Castrillon DH, Miao L, Kollipara R et al. 2003. Suppression of ovarian follicle activation in mice by the transcription factor Foxo3a. *Science* 301:215–218.

Chanas SA, Jiang Q, McMahon M et al. 2002. Loss of the Nrf2 transcription factor causes a marked reduction in constitutive and inducible expression of the glutathione S-transferase Gsta1, Gsta2, Gstm1, Gstm2, Gstm3 and Gstm4 genes in the livers of male and female mice. *Biochem J* 365:405–416.

Colvin OM. 1994. Mechanisms of resistance to alkylating agents. *Cancer Treat Res* 73:249–262.

Colvin OM, Friedman HS, Gamcsik MP et al. 1993. Role of glutathione in cellular resistance to alkylating agents. *Adv Enz Regul* 33:19–26.

Cosby NC, Dukelow WR. 1992. Toxicology of maternally ingested trichloroethylene (TCE) on embryonal and fetal development in mice and of TCE metabolites on in vitro fertilization. *Fundam Appl Toxicol* 19:268–274.

Cummings BS, Lash LH. 2000. Metabolism and toxicity of trichloroethylene and S-(1,2-dichlorovinyl)-L-cysteine in freshly isolated human proximal tubular cells. *Toxicol Sci* 53:458–466.

Dalton TP, Chen Y, Schneider SN et al. 2004. Genetically altered mice to evaluate glutathione homeostasis in health and disease. *Free Radic Biol Med* 37:1511–1526.

Datta SR, Brunet A, Greenberg ME. 1999. Cellular survival: A play in three Akts. *Genes Dev* 13:2905–2927.

Davidson IW, Beliles RP. 1991. Consideration of the target organ toxicity of trichloroethylene in terms of metabolite toxicity and pharmacokinetics. *Drug Metab Rev* 23:493–599.

Denison MS, Heath-Pagliuso S. 1998. The Ah receptor: A regulator of the biochemical and toxicological actions of structurally diverse chemicals. *Bull Env Contam Toxicol* 61:557–568.

Desmeules P, Devine PJ. 2006. Characterizing the ovotoxicity of cyclophosphamide metabolites on cultured mouse ovaries. *Toxicol Sci* 90:500–509.

Dirven HA, Venekamp JC, van Ommen B et al. 1994. The interaction of glutathione with 4-hydroxycyclophosphamide and phosphoramide mustard, studied by 31P nuclear magnetic resonance spectroscopy. *Chem Biol Interact* 93:185–196.

Dobyan DC, Levi J, Jacobs C et al. 1980. Mechanism of cis-platinum nephrotoxicity: II. Morphologic observations. *J Pharmacol Exp Ther* 213:551–556.

Doerr JK, Hooser SB, Smith BJ et al. 1995. Ovarian toxicity of 4-vinylcyclohexene and related olefins in B6C3F1 mice: role of diepoxides. *Chem Res Toxicol* 8:963–969.

Dunn RT 2nd, Klaassen CD. 1998. Tissue-specific expression of rat sulfotransferase messenger RNAs. *Drug Metab Dispos* 26:598–604.

Environmental Protection Agency. 1985. *Health Assessment Document for Tricholoroethylene.* Final Report. EPA/600/8-82/006F. Washington, DC: Environmental Protection Agency, Office of Health and Environmental Assessment.

Fernandez SM, Keating AF, Christian PJ et al. 2008. Involvement of the KIT/KITL signaling pathway in 4-vinylcyclohexene diepoxide-induced ovarian follicle loss in rats. *Biol Reprod* 79:318–327.

Flaws JA, Doerr JK, Sipes IG et al. 1994. Destruction of preantral follicles in adult rats by 4-vinyl-1-cyclohexene diepoxide. *Reprod Toxicol* 8:509–514.

Fraiser LH, Kanekal S, Kehrer JP. 1991. Cyclophosphamide toxicity. Characterising and avoiding the problem. *Drugs* 42:781–795.

Guengerich FP, Kim DH, Iwasaki M. 1991a. Role of human cytochrome P-450 IIE1 in the oxidation of many low molecular weight cancer suspects. *Chem Res Toxicol* 4:168–179.

Guengerich FP, Turvy CG. 1991b. Comparison of levels of several human microsomal cytochrome P-450 enzymes and epoxide hydrolase in normal and disease states using immunochemical analysis of surgical liver samples. *J Pharmacol Exp Therap* 256:1189–1194.

Hamatani T, Falco G, Carter MG et al. 2004. Age-associated alteration of gene expression patterns in mouse oocytes. *Hum Mol Genet* 13:2263–2278.

Hankinson O. 1995. The aryl hydrocarbon receptor complex. *Ann Rev Pharmacol Toxicol* 35:307–340.

Hata Y, Watanabe M. 1994. Metabolism of aziridines and the mechanism of their cytotoxicity. *Drug Metab Rev* 26:575–604.

Hattori N, Fujiwara H, Maeda M et al. 2000. Epoxide hydrolase affects estrogen production in the human ovary. *Endocrinology* 141:3353–3365.

Henderson CJ, Smith AG, Ure J et al. 1998. Increased skin tumorigenesis in mice lacking pi class glutathione S-transferases. *Proc Natl Acad Sci U S A* 95:5275–5280.

Hill CS, Treisman R. 1995. Transcriptional regulation by extracellular signals: Mechanisms and specificity. *Cell* 80:199–211.

Hirshfield AN. 1991. Development of follicles in the mammalian ovary. *Int Rev Cytol* 124:43–101.

Horie K, Takakura K, Taii S et al. 1991. The expression of c-kit protein during oogenesis and early embryonic development. *Biol Reprod* 45:547–552.

Hoyer PB. 2001. Reproductive toxicology: Current and future directions. *Biochem Pharmacol* 62:1557–1564.

Hoyer PB. 2005. Damage to ovarian development and function. *Cell Tiss Res* 322:99–106.

Hoyer PB, Devine PJ, Hu X et al. 2001. Ovarian toxicity of 4-vinylcyclohexene diepoxide: A mechanistic model. *Toxicol Pathol* 29:91–99.

Hoyer PB, Sipes IG. 1996. Assessment of follicle destruction in chemical-induced ovarian toxicity. *Annu Rev Pharmacol Toxicol* 36:307–331.

Hu X, Roberts JR, Apopa PL et al. 2006. Accelerated ovarian failure induced by 4-vinyl cyclohexene diepoxide in Nrf2 null mice. *Mol Cell Biol* 26:940–954.

Ichijo H, Nishida E, Irie K et al. 1997. Induction of apoptosis by ASK1, a mammalian MAPKKK that activates SAPK/JNK and p38 signaling pathways. *Science* 275:90–94.

Igawa Y, Keating AF, Rajapaksa KS et al. 2009. Evaluation of ovotoxicity induced by 7,12-dimethylbenz[a]anthracene and its 3,4-diol metabolite utilizing a rat in vitro ovarian culture system. *Toxicol Appl Pharmacol* 234:361–369.

Ikeda H, Nishi S, Sakai M. 2004. Transcription factor Nrf2/MafK regulates rat placental glutathione S-transferase gene during hepatocarcinogenesis. *Biochem J* 380:515–521.

Ismail RS, Okawara Y, Fryer JN et al. 1996. Hormonal regulation of the ligand for c-kit in the rat ovary and its effects on spontaneous oocyte meiotic maturation. *Mol Reprod Dev* 43:458–469.

Itoh K, Chiba T, Takahashi S et al. 1997. An Nrf2/small Maf heterodimer mediates the induction of phase II detoxifying enzyme genes through antioxidant response elements. *Biochem Biophys Res Comm* 236:313–322.

Itoh K, Wakabayashi N, Katoh Y et al. 1999. Keap1 represses nuclear activation of antioxidant responsive elements by Nrf2 through binding to the amino-terminal Neh2 domain. *Genes Dev* 13:76–86.

Jackson H, Fox BW, Craig AW. 1959. The effect of alkylating agents on male rat fertility. *Br J Pharmacol Chemother* 14:149–157.

Jagarlamudi K, Liu L, Adhikari D et al. 2009. Oocyte-specific deletion of Pten in mice reveals a stage-specific function of PTEN/PI3K signaling in oocytes in controlling follicular activation. *PLoS One* 4:e6186.

Jick H, Porter J. 1977. Relation between smoking and age of natural menopause. Report from the Boston Collaborative Drug Surveillance Program, Boston University Medical Center. *Lancet* 1:1354–1355.

John GB, Gallardo TD, Shirley LJ et al. 2008. Foxo3 is a PI3K-dependent molecular switch controlling the initiation of oocyte growth. *Dev Biol* 321:197–204.

Johnson NL, Gardner AM, Diener KM et al. 1996. Signal transduction pathways regulated by mitogen-activated/extracellular response kinase kinase kinase induce cell death. *J Biol Chem* 271:3229–3237.

Keating AF, Fernandez SM, Mark-Kappeler CJ et al. 2011. Inhibition of PIK3 signaling pathway members by the ovotoxicant 4-vinylcyclohexene diepoxide in rats. *Biol Reprod* 84:743–751.

Keating AF, Mark-Kappeler CJ, Sen N et al. 2009. Effect of phosphatidylinositol-3 kinase inhibition on ovotoxicity caused by 4-vinylcyclohexene diepoxide and 7,12-dimethylbenz[a] anthracene in neonatal rat ovaries. *Toxicol Appl Pharmacol* 241:127–134.

Keating AF, Sen N, Sipes IG et al. 2010. Dual protective role for glutathione S-transferase class pi against VCD-induced ovotoxicity in the rat ovary. *Toxicol Appl Pharmacol* 247:71–75.

Keating AF, Sipes IG, Hoyer PB. 2008. Expression of ovarian microsomal epoxide hydrolase and glutathione S-transferase during onset of VCD-induced ovotoxicity in B6C3F(1) mice. *Toxicol Appl Pharmacol* 230:109–116.

Ki SH, Kim SG. 2008. Phase II enzyme induction by alpha-lipoic acid through phosphatidylinositol 3-kinase-dependent C/EBPs activation. *Xenobiotica* 38:587–604.

Kim SK, Novak RF. 2007. The role of intracellular signaling in insulin-mediated regulation of drug metabolizing enzyme gene and protein expression. *Pharmacol Therapeut* 113:88–120.

Kleiner HE, Vulimiri SV, Hatten WB et al. 2004. Role of cytochrome p4501 family members in the metabolic activation of polycyclic aromatic hydrocarbons in mouse epidermis. *Chem Res Toxicol* 17:1667–1674.

Kopke RD, Liu W, Gabaizadeh R et al. 1997. Use of organotypic cultures of Corti's organ to study the protective effects of antioxidant molecules on cisplatin-induced damage of auditory hair cells. *Am J Otol* 18:559–571.

Krarup T. 1967. 9:10-Dimethyl-1:2-benzantracene induced ovarian tumours in mice. *Acta Pathol Mirco Scand* 70:241–248.

Krarup T. 1969. Oocyte destruction and ovarian tumorigenesis after direct application of a chemical carcinogen (9:0-dimethyl-1:2-benzanthrene) to the mouse ovary. *Int J Cancer* 4:61–75.

Lash LH, Qian W, Putt DA et al. 1998. Glutathione conjugation of trichloroethylene in rats and mice: sex-, species-, and tissue-dependent differences. *Drug Metab Disp* 26:12–19.

Lash LH, Xu Y, Elfarra AA et al. 1995. Glutathione-dependent metabolism of trichloroethylene in isolated liver and kidney cells of rats and its role in mitochondrial and cellular toxicity. *Drug Metab Disp* 23:846–853.

Liu K, Rajareddy S, Liu L et al. 2006. Control of mammalian oocyte growth and early follicular development by the oocyte PI3 kinase pathway: new roles for an old timer. *Dev Biol* 299:1–11.

Lopez SG, Luderer U. 2004. Effects of cyclophosphamide and buthionine sulfoximine on ovarian glutathione and apoptosis. *Free Rad Biol Med* 36:1366–1377.

Louis J, Limarzi LR, Best WR. 1956. Treatment of chronic granulocytic leukemia with myleran. *AMA Arch Intern Med* 97:299–308.

Lu H, Chan KK. 2006. Pharmacokinetics of N-2-chloroethylaziridine, a volatile cytotoxic metabolite of cyclophosphamide, in the rat. *Canc Chemo Pharmacol* 58:532–539.

Ludeman SM. 1999. The chemistry of the metabolites of cyclophosphamide. *Curr Pharma Des* 5:627–643.

Luderer U, Kavanagh TJ, White CC et al. 2001. Gonadotropin regulation of glutathione synthesis in the rat ovary. *Reprod Toxicol* 15:495–504.

Manova K, Nocka K, Besmer P et al. 1990. Gonadal expression of c-kit encoded at the W locus of the mouse. *Development* 110:1057–1069.

Mark-Kappeler CJ, Sen N, Lukefahr A et al. 2011. Inhibition of ovarian KIT phosphorylation by the ovotoxicant 4-vinylcyclohexene diepoxide in rats. *Biol Reprod* 85:755–762.

Marshall CJ. 1995. Specificity of receptor tyrosine kinase signaling: transient versus sustained extracellular signal-regulated kinase activation. *Cell* 80:179–185.

Matikainen T, Perez GI, Jurisicova A et al. 2001. Aromatic hydrocarbon receptor-driven Bax gene expression is required for premature ovarian failure caused by biohazardous environmental chemicals. *Nat Genet* 28:355–360.

Matsuo G, Ushijima K, Shinagawa A et al. 2007. GnRH agonist acts as ovarian protection in chemotherapy induced gonadotoxicity: An experiment using a rat model. *Kurume Med J* 54:25–29.

Mattison DR, Nightingale MS, Shiromizu K. 1983. Effects of toxic substances on female reproduction. *Environ Health Perspect* 48:43–52.

Mattison DR, Schulman, JD. 1980a. How xenobiotic chemicals can destroy oocytes. *Am J Ind Med* 4(15):157–169.

Mattison DR, Schulman JD. 1980b. How xenobiotic chemicals can destroy oocytes. *Contemp Obstet Gynecol* 15:157.

Mattison DR, Shiromizu K, Pendergrass JA et al. 1983. Ontogeny of ovarian glutathione and sensitivity to primordial oocyte destruction by cyclophosphamide. *Pediatr Pharmacol* 3:49–55.

Mattison DR, Thorgeirsson SS. 1978. Smoking and industrial pollution, and their effects on menopause and ovarian cancer. *Lancet* 1:187–188.

Morita Y, Tilly JL. 1999. Oocyte apoptosis: Like sand through an hourglass. *Dev Biol* 213:1–17.

Nakai Y, Konishi K, Chang KC et al. 1982. Ototoxicity of the anticancer drug cisplatin. An experimental study. *Acta Oto-laryngologica* 93:227–232.

Nakajima T, Okino T, Okuyama S et al. 1988. Ethanol-induced enhancement of trichloroethylene metabolism and hepatotoxicity: difference from the effect of phenobarbital. *Toxicol Appl Pharmacol* 94:227–237.

Nakajima T, Wang RS, Elovaara E et al. 1992a. A comparative study on the contribution of cytochrome P450 isozymes to metabolism of benzene, toluene and trichloroethylene in rat liver. *Biochem Pharmacol* 43:251–257.

Nakajima T, Wang RS, Elovaara E et al. 1993. Cytochrome P450-related differences between rats and mice in the metabolism of benzene, toluene and trichloroethylene in liver microsomes. *Biochem Pharmacol* 45:1079–1085.

Nakajima T, Wang RS, Katakura Y et al. 1992b. Sex-, age- and pregnancy-induced changes in the metabolism of toluene and trichloroethylene in rat liver in relation to the regulation of cytochrome P450IIE1 and P450IIC11 content. *J Pharmacol Exp Therap* 261:869–874.

Nakajima T, Wang RS, Murayama N et al. 1990. Three forms of trichloroethylene-metabolizing enzymes in rat liver induced by ethanol, phenobarbital, and 3-methylcholanthrene. *Toxicol Appl Pharmacol* 102:546–552.

Nebert DW, Roe AL, Dieter MZ et al. 2000. Role of the aromatic hydrocarbon receptor and [Ah] gene battery in the oxidative stress response, cell cycle control, and apoptosis. *Biochem Pharmacol* 59:65–85.

Nguyen T, Yang CS, Pickett CB. 2004. The pathways and molecular mechanisms regulating Nrf2 activation in response to chemical stress. *Free Rad Biol Med* 37:433–441.

Nozaki Y, Furubo E, Matsuno T et al. 2009. Collaborative work on evaluation of ovarian toxicity. 6) Two- or four-week repeated-dose studies and fertility study of cisplatin in female rats. *J Toxicol Sci* 34 Suppl 1:SP73–SP81.

Okey AB, Riddick DS, Harper PA. 1994. The Ah receptor: mediator of the toxicity of 2,3,7,8-tetrachlorodibenzo-p-dioxin (TCDD) and related compounds. *Toxicol Letts* 70:1–22.

Orr-Urtreger A, Avivi A, Zimmer Y et al. 1990. Developmental expression of c-kit, a proto-oncogene encoded by the W locus. *Development* 109:911–923.

Oswald CB, Chaney SG, Hall IH. 1990a. Inhibition of DNA synthesis in P388 lymphocytic leukemia cells of BDF1 mice by cis-diamminedichloroplatinum (II) and its derivatives. *J Pharm Sci* 79:875–80.

Oswald CB, Chaney SG, Hall IH. 1990b. Inhibition of nucleic acid synthesis in P388 lymphocytic leukemia cells in culture by cis-platinum derivatives. *Biomed Biochim Acta* 49:579–87.

Otto S, Bhattacharyya KK, Jefcoate CR. 1992. Polycyclic aromatic hydrocarbon metabolism in rat adrenal, ovary, and testis microsomes is catalyzed by the same novel cytochrome P450 (P450RAP). *Endocrinology* 131:3067–3076.

Parkinson A, Ogilvie BW. 2008. Biotransformation of xenobiotics. In *Casarett and Doull's Toxicology: The Basic Science of Poisons.*, ed. CD Klassen, pp. 131–160. The McGraw-Hill Companies publishing, New York.

Pawson T, Nash P. 2000. Protein-protein interactions define specificity in signal transduction. *Genes Dev* 14:1027–1047.

Pinto N, Ludeman SM, Dolan ME. 2009. Drug focus: Pharmacogenetic studies related to cyclophosphamide-based therapy. *Pharmacogenomics* 10:1897–1903.

Plowchalk DR, Mattison DR. 1991. Phosphoramide mustard is responsible for the ovarian toxicity of cyclophosphamide. *Toxicol Appl Pharmacol* 107:472–481.

National Toxicology Program. 1989. NTP Teach, no. 362.

Rajapaksa KS, Cannady EA, Sipes IG et al. 2007a. Involvement of CYP 2E1 enzyme in ovotoxicity caused by 4-vinylcyclohexene and its metabolites. *Toxicol Appl Pharmacol* 221:215–221.

Rajapaksa KS, Sipes IG, Hoyer PB. 2007b. Involvement of microsomal epoxide hydrolase enzyme in ovotoxicity caused by 7,12-dimethylbenz[a]anthracene. *Toxicol Sci* 96:327–334.

Rappaport SM, Fraser DA. 1977. Air sampling and analysis in a rubber vulcanization area. *Am Ind Hyg Assoc J* 38:205–210.

Rauen HM, Norpoth K. 1968. A volatile alkylating agent in the exhaled air following the administration of Endoxan. *Klinische Wochenschrift* 46:272–275.

Reddy P, Adhikari D, Zheng W et al. 2009. PDK1 signaling in oocytes controls reproductive aging and lifespan by manipulating the survival of primordial follicles. *Hum Mol Genet* 18:2813–2824.

Reddy P, Shen L, Ren C et al. 2005. Activation of Akt (PKB) and suppression of FKHRL1 in mouse and rat oocytes by stem cell factor during follicular activation and development. *Dev Biol* 281:160–170.

Reddy P, Zheng W, Liu K. 2010. Mechanisms maintaining the dormancy and survival of mammalian primordial follicles. *Trends Endo Metab* 21:96–103.

Reinke LA, Moyer MJ. 1985. p-Nitrophenol hydroxylation. A microsomal oxidation which is highly inducible by ethanol. *Drug Metab Disp* 13:548–552.

Rincon M, Whitmarsh A, Yang DD et al. 1998. The JNK pathway regulates the in vivo deletion of immature CD4(+)CD8(+) thymocytes. *J Exp Med* 188:1817–1830.

Roskoski R Jr. 2005. Structure and regulation of Kit protein-tyrosine kinase—The stem cell factor receptor. *Biochem Biophys Res Commun* 338:1307–1315.

Satoh M, Kashihara N, Fujimoto S et al. 2003. A novel free radical scavenger, edarabone, protects against cisplatin-induced acute renal damage in vitro and in vivo. *J Pharmacol Exp Ther* 305:1183–1190.

Schmitt E, Paquet C, Beauchemin M et al. 2004. Bcl-xES, a BH4- and BH2-containing antiapoptotic protein, delays Bax oligomer formation and binds Apaf-1, blocking procaspase-9 activation. *Oncogene* 23:3915–3931.

Shimada T. 2006. Xenobiotic-metabolizing enzymes involved in activation and detoxification of carcinogenic polycyclic aromatic hydrocarbons. *Drug Metab Pharm* 21:257–276.

Shimada T, Fujii-Kuriyama Y. 2004. Metabolic activation of polycyclic aromatic hydrocarbons to carcinogens by cytochromes P450 1A1 and 1B1. *Cancer Sci* 95:1–6.

Shimada T, Sugie A, Shindo M et al. 2003. Tissue-specific induction of cytochromes P450 1A1 and 1B1 by polycyclic aromatic hydrocarbons and polychlorinated biphenyls in engineered C57BL/6J mice of arylhydrocarbon receptor gene. *Toxicol Appl Pharmacol* 187:1–10.

Shiromizu K, Mattison DR. 1985. Murine oocyte destruction following intraovarian treatment with 3-methylcholanthrene or 7,12-dimethylbenz(a)anthracene: protection by alpha-naphthoflavone. *Teratog Carcinog Mutagen* 5:463–472.

Shulman-Roskes EM, Noe DA, Gamcsik MP et al. 1998. The partitioning of phosphoramide mustard and its aziridinium ions among alkylation and P-N bond hydrolysis reactions. *J Med Chem* 41:515–529.

Siegel R, Naishadham D, Jemal A. 2012. Cancer statistics, 2012. *CA Canc J Clinic* 62:10–29.

Sims P, Grover PL. 1974. Epoxides in polycyclic aromatic hydrocarbon metabolism and carcinogenesis. *Adv Cancer Res* 20:165–274.

Sobinoff AP, Mahony M, Nixon B et al. 2011. Understanding the Villain: DMBA-induced preantral ovotoxicity involves selective follicular destruction and primordial follicle activation through PI3K/Akt and mTOR signaling. *Toxicol Sci* 123:563–575.

Springer LN, Flaws JA, Sipes IG et al. 1996a. Follicular mechanisms associated with 4-vinylcyclohexene diepoxide-induced ovotoxicity in rats. *Reprod Toxicol* 10:137–143.

Springer LN, McAsey ME, Flaws JA et al. 1996b. Involvement of apoptosis in 4-vinylcyclohexene diepoxide-induced ovotoxicity in rats. *Toxicol Appl Pharmacol* 139:394–401.

Struck RF, Alberts DS, Horne K et al. 1987. Plasma pharmacokinetics of cyclophosphamide and its cytotoxic metabolites after intravenous versus oral administration in a randomized, crossover trial. *Cancer Res* 47:2723–2726.

Tsai-Turton M, Nakamura BN, Luderer U. 2007. Induction of apoptosis by 9,10-dimethyl-1,2-benzanthracene in cultured preovulatory rat follicles is preceded by a rise in reactive oxygen species and is prevented by glutathione. *Biol Reprod* 77:442–451.

Vahakangas K, Rajaniemi H, Pelkonen O. 1985. Ovarian toxicity of cigarette smoke exposure during pregnancy in mice. *Toxicol Letts* 25:75–80.

Wallace WH, Shalet SM, Crowne EC et al. 1989. Gonadal dysfunction due to cis-platinum. *Med Ped Oncol* 17:409–413.

Weiss NS. 1996. Cancer in relation to occupational exposure to trichloroethylene. *Occup Environ Med* 53:1–5.

Weitzman M, Gortmaker S, Sobol A. 1992. Maternal smoking and behavior problems of children. *Pediatrics* 90:342–349.

Whitmarsh AJ, Davis RJ. 1996. Transcription factor AP-1 regulation by mitogen-activated protein kinase signal transduction pathways. *J Mol Med* 74:589–607.

Wu KL, Berger T. 2007. Trichloroethylene metabolism in the rat ovary reduces oocyte fertilizability. *Chem Biol Interact* 170:20–30.

Wu KL, Berger T. 2008. Reduction in rat oocyte fertilizability mediated by S-(1, 2-dichlorovinyl)-L-cysteine: a trichloroethylene metabolite produced by the glutathione conjugation pathway. *Bull Env Contam Toxicol* 81:490–493.

Wu C, Schaum J. 2000. Exposure assessment of trichloroethylene. *Environ Health Perspect* 108 Suppl 2:359–363.

Xia Z, Dickens M, Raingeaud J et al. 1995. Opposing effects of ERK and JNK-p38 MAP kinases on apoptosis. *Science* 270:1326–1331.

Xu C, Huang MT, Shen G et al. 2006. Inhibition of 7,12-dimethylbenz(a)anthracene-induced skin tumorigenesis in C57BL/6 mice by sulforaphane is mediated by nuclear factor E2-related factor 2. *Cancer Res* 66:8293–8296.

Zanke BW, Boudreau K, Rubie E et al. 1996. The stress-activated protein kinase pathway mediates cell death following injury induced by cis-platinum, UV irradiation or heat. *Curr Biol* 6:606–613.

3 Brain as a Target for Environmental Toxicants That Alter Ovarian Function

Ralph L. Cooper and Jerome M. Goldman

CONTENTS

3.1 INTRODUCTION

In the female reproductive system, hormonal relationships among the ovaries, pituitary, and brain function in an orchestrated manner in order to ensure an orderly maturation of oocytes for fertilization. Steroid feedback from the ovaries to the brain induces coordinated activity within multiple neuronal pathways that collectively serve to provide a hormonal signal to the pituitary, stimulating the midcycle surge of luteinizing hormone (LH). In turn, this surge functions to synchronize the timing of ovulation with the behavioral changes associated with successful reproduction. In this chapter, we review the literature demonstrating that many environmental chemicals have the potential to interfere with the molecular events controlling the normal development and adult function of the reproductive system. As the rat is the primary test animal for toxicological research, our focus is on this species.

The rat is typical of many spontaneous ovulators in that the generation of the LH surge results from the sequential feedback of ovarian estrogen and progesterone on the brain and pituitary. Figure 3.1 depicts the hypothalamic–pituitary–ovarian axis (HPO) emphasizing the many central nervous system (CNS) pathways involved in this process. The focus of the figure is the gonadotropin releasing hormone (GnRH) neurons that reside in discrete hypothalamic nuclei and represent the final common path controlling LH and follicle stimulating hormone (FSH) release and

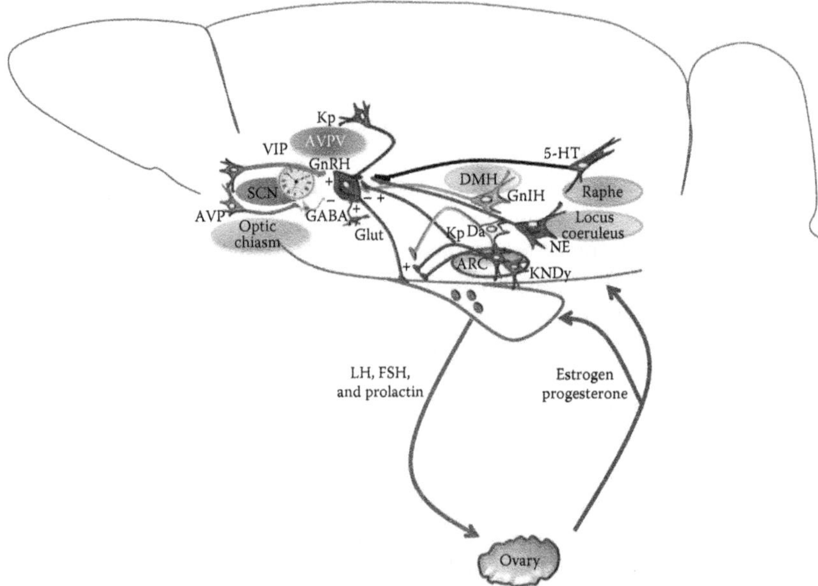

FIGURE 3.1 The brain–pituitary–gonadal axis. Gonadotropin-releasing hormone (GnRH) neurons located in the rostral hypothalamus represent the final common signal regulating pituitary LH and FSH secretion. These neurons are under both stimulatory and inhibitory regulation by other neuronal pathways impinging upon the GnRH neurons; many of the neurons in these pathways contain estrogen and progesterone receptors and are thus sensitive to the positive and negative feedback effects of the ovarian steroids. In addition to the influence of the ovarian hormones, the GnRH cells are regulated by input from the suprachiasmatic nucleus that relay diurnal signals to the GnRH neurons. The pituitary is also sensitive to ovarian hormone influences. Abbreviations: AVP, Arginine vasopressin; Kp, kisspeptin; VIP, vasoactive intestinal peptide; GABA, gamma amino butyric acid; Glut, glutamate; DA, dopamine; NE, norepinephrine; 5-HT, 5-hydroxytryptamine; KNDy, kisspeptin, neurokinin B, dynorphin; GnIH, gonadotropin-inhibiting hormone; SCN, suprachiasmatic nucleus; AVPV, anteroventralperiventricular nucleus; ARC, arcuate nucleus; DMH, dorsomedial hypothalamic nucleus.

subsequently ovarian function. Many of the neuronal pathways afferent to the GnRH neuron contain estrogen and progesterone receptors (PRs); thus, they are sensitive to environmental compounds that interfere with the transactivational effects of the ovarian hormones. In addition, these afferent systems offer additional molecular target sites for environmental chemicals as the synthesis and release of the neurochemical signals contained in the different neurons and their postsynaptic receptors may be altered following exposure to toxicants.

In this chapter, we first discuss the ovarian cycle of the rat in order to familiarize the reader the well-understood timing of the neuroendocrine events preceding ovulation. This is followed by a discussion of the location and function of the estrogen and PRs in the brain. Although this is by no means a comprehensive review, it should provide the reader with an understanding of the role that different hypothalamic nuclei play in the regulation of reproductive function. We then discuss the evidence that there are environmental toxicants that adversely impact ovarian function by targeting specific molecular targets in the brain. The identification of these molecular targets provides the basis for constructing a toxicity pathway responsible for the loss of reproductive function. This type of information is important for rational decisions about the potential impact of a substance on human health, as it can provide a mode of action of a chemical and permit some degree of extrapolation from the rat to the human.

3.2 NEUROENDOCRINE CONTROL OF OVARIAN FUNCTION

3.2.1 Rat Ovarian Cycle

The female rat, like the female human, is a spontaneous ovulator. After puberty, rats display rhythmic 4–5 day estrous cycles which can be divided into three separate segments: a period of diestrus (lasting 2–3 days), proestrus (1 day), and estrus (1 or 2 days). Each segment is readily identified by observing changes in vaginal cytology that occur in response to the fluctuating levels of ovarian steroids in the blood (Figure 3.2) (Butcher et al., 1974; Cooper et al., 1986). The period of vaginal diestrus is associated with follicular growth, a process dependent on the tonic stimulation by the pituitary gonadotropins, primarily FSH. Throughout the animal's reproductive lifespan, there is continuous turnover of ovarian follicles which rise from the pool of primordial follicles, a few of which are destined to mature into ovulatory follicles, while the vast majority undergoes atresia at some stage of their maturation. The dormant primordial follicles are recruited into the growing follicle pool in a continuous manner, whereas increases in circulating FSH during each reproductive cycle recruit a cohort of antral follicles (McGee and Hsueh, 2000). Follicular growth is accompanied by the secretion of estradiol, which increases in the serum late in diestrus, reaching peak values around noon on vaginal proestrus. The rise in estradiol is followed by a sharp increase in serum progesterone on the afternoon of vaginal proestrus, at which time the mature preovulatory follicle becomes the target site for the dramatic increase in pituitary LH secretion (i.e., the preovulatory surge of LH). Ovulation occurs approximately 10–12 h after this surge.

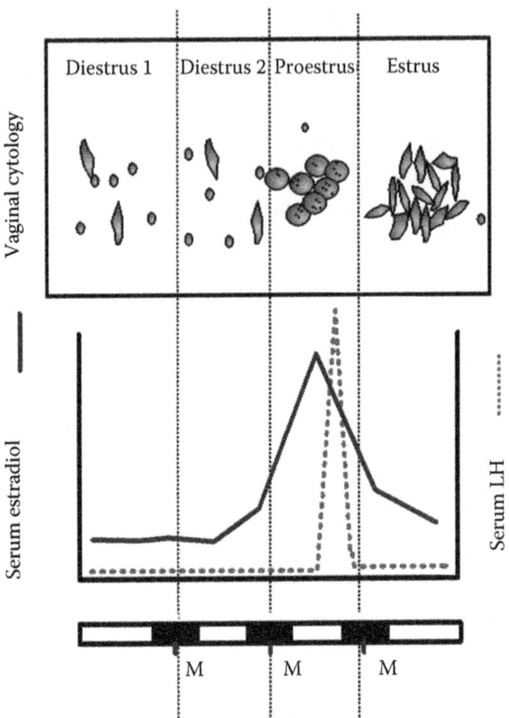

FIGURE 3.2 The rat estrous cycle. The young adult female rat displays regular 4- or 5-day ovarian cycles if they are housed in under conditions of 10 Light:14 h dark or 12 h light:12 h dark (bottom panel). Staging of the ovarian cycle is readily accomplished by observing the vaginal smear (top panels). The cell type present in the smear on vaginal proestrus (round, nucleated epithelial cells generally present in clusters) reflects the increasing levels of ovarian estrogen (lower panel, solid line) beginning on vaginal diestrus 2 and peaking on vaginal proestrus. As estrogen concentrations drop on vaginal estrus, the epithelial cells become flattened and jagged. Following vaginal estrus, the smear has increasing numbers of leukocytes typical of diestrus I and diestrus II. The LH surge occurs on the afternoon of vaginal proestrus usually peaking just prior to lights out. Sexual receptivity in the female is generally restricted to the dark hours between the day of proestrus and estrus. Ovulation occurs in the early morning hours of vaginal estrus. Bottom bars represent daylight and dark periods. M = midnight.

The release of LH is under the control of the decapeptide GnRH. The cell bodies of the neurons containing GnRH are located primarily in the rostral hypothalamus and project to the median eminence region (immediately above the pituitary stalk). The release of a GnRH is dependent upon two major neuroendocrine factors: the positive feedback actions of estrogen and a neural signal generated by the 24-h neural clock (Levine, 1997; Williams and Kriegsfeld, 2012). The elevated E2 levels of the preovulatory period provide a permissive signal for the release of the GnRH surge, whereas the daily neural signal most likely dictates the timing and form of this GnRH secretory event (Levine, 1997). The net result is the release of a

GnRH surge into the hypophyseal portal vessels, which is timed to evoke gonadotropin surges, and hence ovulation. Thus, the synergistic feedback effects of ovarian estrogen and progesterone on the CNS serve to synchronize the physiological events responsible for ovulation with the behavior of the female, maximizing the chances that fertilization will occur.

After rupture of the follicle and discharge of the ovum, the follicle cells enlarge, LH stimulates the granulosa cells to luteinize to form the corpus luteum (CL), and steroid hormone production favors progesterone over estrogen. Importantly, the female is sexually receptive during the intervening hours on the evening of vaginal proestrus. In the rat, maintenance of the CL is under the influence of twice-daily surges of prolactin released from the anterior pituitary. These prolactin surges are initiated as a result of the vaginal–cervical stimulation that occurs during mating. If mating does not occur, twice-daily diurnal surges do not take place, and the CL undergoes atresia. It should be noted that the endocrine support of the CL shows considerable species variation. In some species, including humans, LH and then human chorionic gonadotropin (hCG), not prolactin, maintain the CL.

3.2.2 Estrogen and Progesterone Action on the Brain: Synchronizing Behavior with Ovulation

The patterns of estradiol and progesterone secretion during an ovarian cycle are known to modify brain and pituitary function, again synchronizing the behavioral changes and endocrine events associated with sexual receptivity and ovulation. Both genomic and nongenomic mechanisms (i.e., involving nuclear vs. membrane estrogen and PRs) have been identified as part of the underlying mechanisms coordinating this complex series of events. Within an ovarian cycle, the rising blood estradiol concentration that occurs during diestrus is obligatory to the generation of the GnRH-induced LH surge. In the rat, the effects of estradiol are coupled with circadian changes, ensuring that the onset of the late-afternoon LH surge and ovulation are coincident with the increase in sexual receptivity displayed on the evening of vaginal proestrus.

Within the brain, the rising estradiol concentration acts at the genomic level to bring about a series of changes within the neuronal networks regulating the release of GnRH. Two isoforms of evolutionarily conserved estrogen receptors, ERα and ERβ, are produced from separate genes located on different chromosomes. Work by the laboratories of Korach (Couse and Korach, 1999) and Herbison (Wintermantel et al., 2006) has investigated the estrogen receptors associated with the positive feedback of estradiol using ERα and ERβ knockout mice models. These studies revealed that estrogen-positive feedback was normal in ERβKO mice, but absent in ERαKO mice (Wintermantel et al., 2006). The key role of the ERα receptor was further demonstrated in ovariectomized mice. In this model, the expression of the proto-oncogene c-fos in GnRH neurons and the induction of an LH surge were evaluated following treatment with selective ERα and ERβ agonists. The ERα agonist generated a normal positive feedback [i.e., increased number of GnRH neurons expressing c-fos and an LH surge (Wintermantel et al., 2006)], whereas the ERβ agonist was unable to initiate c-fos expression in GnRH neurons or generate an LH surge (Herbison, 2008).

The pattern of estrogen and progesterone secretion has well-characterized actions on the hypothalamic structures involved in the regulation of GnRH–LH secretion and sexual receptivity. Estrogen alters the expression of a number of intracellular, transcriptional regulators in target hypothalamic neurons, which are subsequently functionally involved in the initiation of the GnRH surge. In this regard, the estrogen-induced expression of the PR is critical to normal reproductive function. This increase in PRs within the rostral hypothalamus, especially the anteroventral periventricular nucleus (AVPV), is required for the activation and amplification of GnRH pulses (Levine and Ramirez, 1980) and LH surges (Krey et al., 1973; Ogawa et al., 1994). Ablation of the AVPV will eliminate the LH surge, demonstrating that this hypothalamic nucleus is an indispensable part of the timing mechanism for the surge (Weigand and Teresawa, 1982). The time course and concentration of estradiol necessary for the induction of PR mRNA (Hagihara et al., 1992; Simerly et al., 1996) and receptor protein (MacLusky and McEwen, 1980) in the AVPV necessary to induce an LH surge have been well characterized using ovariectomized rats, with the peak levels of message occurring within 4–8 h and maximum protein levels within 24 h. More recently, the role of AVPV neuronal networks that regulate GnRH activity has been further elucidated (see discussion later).

Estrogen and progesterone regulate sexual behavior in a manner similar to that described previously for LH. However, the neuronal substrate most frequently associated with behavioral changes is the ventromedial nucleus (VMN) of the hypothalamus. The increase in estrogen activates estrogen receptors (ER) within the VMN, which in turn alters the expression of a number of transcription factors that affect the expression of a number of hypothalamic genes. In the VMN, estrogen causes an increase in PR mRNA levels in the VMN followed by enhanced PR synthesis. A strong correlation exists between the estrogen-induced increase in PR-binding sites in the VMN and the expression of female reproductive behavior in rats. Lesions of the VMN, or placement of antisense oligonucleotides to the PR (Mani et al., 1994), block lordosis behavior, and the application of estrogen or progesterone to this region of the hypothalamus will enhance lordosis.

A final point to be made about the activation of the PR is that, in addition to the activation of sexual receptivity, progesterone serves to downregulate the PR and PR-dependent responses, thus becoming inhibitory to any further effects of continued progesterone stimulation. This refractory period has been termed "sequential inhibition" (Powers and Moreines, 1976), a change in behavior that appears to be related to progesterone-induced changes in gene expression and progesterone-dependent alterations in protein synthesis (Parsons and McEwen, 1981).

3.2.3 Steroid Hormone Source and Synthesis over the Ovarian Cycle

3.2.3.1 Ovarian Steroidogenesis

In response to the gonadotropin stimulation over the ovarian cycle, estradiol, estrone, and progesterone are all generated within the same pathway that involves cooperation between the follicular theca and the granulosa cell compartments. Under the influence of LH, the production of sex steroids in the theca cells begins with the translocation of cholesterol across the outer membrane of a mitochondrion to the inner membrane. This is a rate-limiting process that involves the participation of two principal factors, steroidogenic acute regulatory protein (StAR) and the high-affinity cholesterol-binding translocator protein (TSPO, previously termed the peripheral benzodiazepine receptor). The movement from outer to the inner mitochondrial membrane is initiated by a complex of proteins that also includes a cAMP-dependent protein kinase, a TSPO-associated protein (PAP7), and a voltage-dependent anion channel protein (VDAC) that spans multiple times across the outer membrane, regulating the passage of ions and small molecules (Midzak et al., 2011).

In the inner membrane, cholesterol is converted to pregnenolone by an enzymatic (P450scc, or CYP11A1) side-chain cleavage (Figure 3.3). This conversion involves steps generating two short-lived intermediates, 22R-hydroxycholesterol and (20,22)R-dihydroxycholesterol. Pregnenolone can then enter one of two

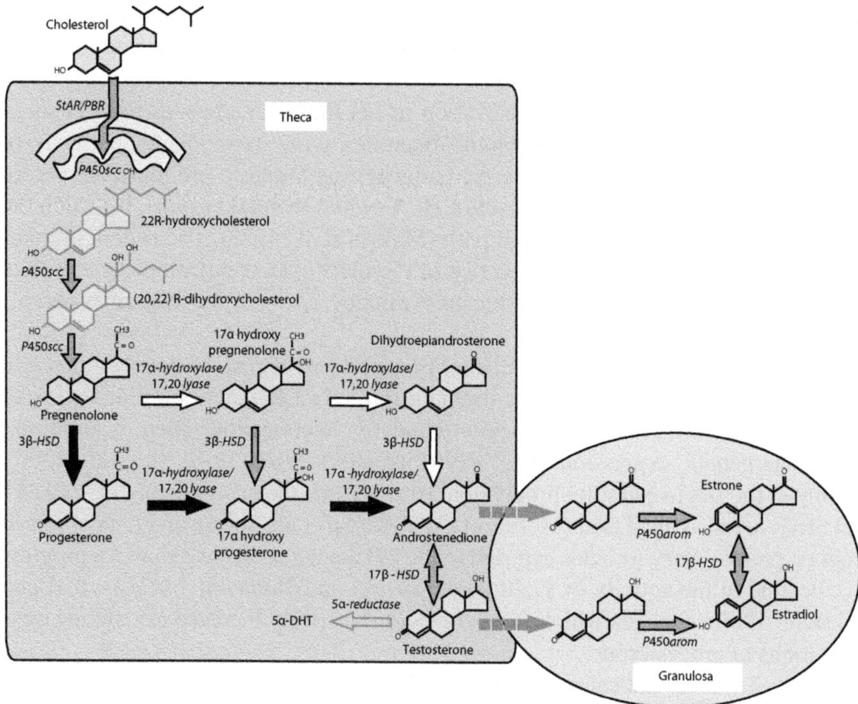

FIGURE 3.3 The steroidogenic pathway, depicting the initial transport of cholesterol from the outer to the inner mitochondrial membrane, with short-lived intermediates 22R-hydroxycholesterol and (20,22)R-dihydroxycholesterol preceding the synthesis of pregnenolone. The pathway diverges into delta 4 (black arrows) and delta 5 (white arrows) directions, and species preferences exist for each path (see text). After their formation in thecal cells, androstenedione and testosterone enter granulosa cells for conversion to estrone or estradiol. Abbreviations: StAR, steroidogenic acute regulatory protein; PBR, peripheral benzodiazepine receptor (translocator protein); P450scc, cytochrome P450 side-chain cleavage (CYP11A1); 3β-HSD, 3β-hydroxysteroid dehydrogenase; 17β-HSD, 17β-hydroxysteroid dehydrogenase; 17α-hydroxylase/17,20 lyase (CYP17); P450arom, cytochrome P450 aromatase (CYP19); 5α-DHT, 5α-dihydrotestosterone.

pathways, Δ4 or Δ5, toward formation of the androgen androstenedione. In the Δ4 direction, the enzyme 3β-hydroxysteroid dehydrogenase (3β-HSD) converts pregnenolone to progesterone, whereas the Δ5 path begins with a pregnenolone conversion to 17α-hydroxypregnenolone. The selected pathway is species-dependent and is related to the substrate preferences of the 17,20 lyase. In humans, the preferred substrate is 17α-hydroxypregnenolone, while in rodents it is 17α-hydroxyprogesterone (Brock and Waterman, 1999). Chickens, ferrets, mares, and some macaques will also direct pregnenolone in a Δ4 direction, while in addition to humans, rabbits, dogs, and cows prefer the Δ5 pathway (Kintner and Mead, 1983; Fortune, 1986; Weusten et al., 1987, 1990). In ovarian follicles, the generated androstenedione from both Δ4 and Δ5 pathways can be converted to testosterone by the action of 17β-hydroxysteroid dehydrogenase (17β-HSD), or it can enter the granulosa cells where it is aromatized to estrone by P450 aromatase (CYP19). Similarly, testosterone transported from theca to granulosa cells is aromatized to estradiol also by the action of CYP19. Estradiol and the weaker estrone may be interconverted one from the other by the action of 17β-HSD.

During the cycle, the marked elevation in LH that characterizes the LH surge has been found to have an impact on the dynamics of the steroidogenic pathway. In hamster preovulatory follicles, the Δ5 pathway was found to predominate before and up to 2 h after exposure *in vitro* to LH. A switch then takes place in which the Δ4 direction becomes the principal path (Makris et al., 1983). The rodent preovulatory period is characterized by a rise in circulating concentrations of estradiol beginning on diestrus II, continuing to a midday apex on the day of proestrus (Figure 3.2).

As these concentrations then decline, progesterone begins a late-afternoon rise around the time of the surge. This dramatic surge in LH induces a remodeling of follicular granulosa cells as they begin to undergo luteinization. There is an inhibition in the genetic expression of CYP19 (Fitzpatrick et al., 1997; Su et al., 2006), leading to the fall in estradiol production. At this time, the expressions of CYP11A1 and StAR are also increased (McRae et al., 2005; Su et al., 2006), and data obtained from rat preovulatory follicles exposed to the LH analog hCG have shown a progressive decline in the activity of 17,20 lyase (Suzuki and Tamaoki, 1983; Tsafriri and Eckstein, 1986), changes which *in vivo* would effectively increase circulating concentrations of progesterone.

Figure 3.3 also indicates that within the theca cells, 5α-dihydrotestosterone (5α-DHT) can also be generated from testosterone. Although 5α-DHT is primarily present in human male prostate glands, some expression of 5α-reductase is seen in normal ovaries, and the catalyzed conversion of testosterone to DHT is markedly increased in polycystic ovary syndrome (Jakimiuk et al., 1999; Magoffin, 2006). In fact, hyperandrogenism from excess theca cell production is the major marker of the condition in women.

3.2.3.2 Extra-Ovarian Synthesis of Sex Steroids

Although the ovaries serve as a principal source of estrogen and progesterone, sex steroid synthesis is present in a number of organs. The adrenal cortex is known to produce significant amounts of steroids. During the rat estrous cycle, concentrations of progesterone obtained from cannulated adrenal and ovarian veins have been found to be comparable, while over a portion of estrus and diestrus adrenal production even exceeds that from the ovaries (Shaikh and Shaikh, 1975).

The brain is now known to be a site for widespread steroidogenesis that participates in a variety of functions. The Purkinje cell, a key cerebellar neuron, actively produces progesterone in the neonate (Ukena et al., 1998, 1999) and is believed to be involved in promoting cerebellar neuronal growth and synaptogenesis. Neonatal Purkinje cells also express P450 aromatase (Sakamoto et al., 2003), suggesting that estradiol is also important in cerebellar development during this time. In addition, neurons in the hippocampus have been found to express enzymes for both P450 side-chain cleavage (P450scc) and 3β-HSD (Kimoto et al., 2001), indicating the presence of progesterone production. The authors speculate that the presence of neurosteroids there could serve as a mediator in mechanisms of neuronal excitability.

Glial cells have been established as an important source of neurosteroid production. P450scc and 3β-HSD activity is present in both oligodendrocytes and astrocytes (Zwain and Yen, 1999). A responsive increase in astrocytic progesterone synthesis by rising estradiol levels over the rat estrous cycle has raised the possibility that this effect has a functional role in generation of the LH surge. In this regard, astrocytes express membrane estrogen receptors (Azcoitia et al., 1999; Pawlak et al., 2005) that, upon estradiol binding, initiate a rapid release of calcium stores (Chaban et al., 2004) and progesterone synthesis within minutes (Micevych et al., 2007). Estradiol also induces the expression of hypothalamic PRs (Chappell and Levine, 2000), enhancing the impact of the increase in progesterone production.

In an ovariectomized, estrogen-primed rat model, estradiol, provided by either subcutaneous injection or capsular implant, is able to stimulate a modest surge of LH a few days later. A suppression of progesterone synthesis in these females by blocking the conversion of pregnenolone to progesterone with the 3β-HSD inhibitor trilostane eliminated the rise in LH, whereas the surge was not affected by adrenalectomy (Micevych et al., 2003). The data suggest that while progesterone is necessary for the emergence of an LH surge in these animals, the surge can be independent of an adrenal source of progesterone.

3.3 DISRUPTION OF OVARIAN FUNCTION THROUGH TOXICANT-INDUCED CHANGES IN CNS CONTROL OF OVARIAN FUNCTION

The range of environmental and man-made chemicals that have the potential to adversely impact the neuroendocrine control of ovarian function is only now beginning to be known. In separate portions of this section, we will discuss research that describes the adverse effects of neuroendocrine toxicants. First, we review the evidence that endocrine disrupting chemicals (EDCs) can impact the developmental organization of the hypothalamus (i.e., the organizational effect of EDCs). Although there are some identified species differences, the developing CNS is clearly sensitive to the effects of endogenous androgens and estrogens. Therefore, it is not surprising that this process is susceptible to the impact of environmental agents possessing estrogenic or other inherent activity that can modify the series of molecular events underlying sexual differentiation of the brain.

The developmental studies will be followed by a discussion of the evidence that chemicals targeting one or more central neuronal networks can impair reproductive performance and fertility in the adult (i.e., activational effects). This will include an evaluation of studies examining those central neural pathways considered critical to the control of GnRH secretion. Two case studies will be presented, demonstrating how an increased understanding of the neuroendocrine factors governing ovulation in the adult can be used to identify molecular targets and the cascade of molecular events leading to a disruption in the female's reproductive system (i.e., the toxicity pathway).

3.3.1 Effect of Environmental Toxicants on Sexual Differentiation of the Brain

3.3.1.1 Steroid Hormones and Environmental Estrogens

In vertebrates, sex steroid hormones play two critical roles over the lifespan of the animal. During the fetal or perinatal period, phenotypical sex is determined. In mammals, the developing brain is essentially female unless there is exposure to testosterone sometime during gestation or the early perinatal period (McCarthy and Arnold, 2011, for review). In genetic males, the embryonic testis synthesizes and releases testosterone, which acts throughout the body to masculinize the external genitalia and to modify the development of several brain structures. In the rat and other laboratory species, these structures are masculinized as a result of early testosterone exposure. However, in most laboratory animals, masculinization of the brain requires the conversion of testosterone to estradiol within neural tissues (both glia and neurons) (McCarthy and Arnold, 2011), a process regulated by the presence of aromatase (CYP19) in selected regions of the CNS. The net result of the sexually distinct hormonal exposure during gestation results in a number of chemical and structural changes that sets apart the male and female brains. Because of these differences, the female pituitary ovarian axis matures and is capable of maintaining functional ovarian cycles, pregnancy and lactation.

If one administers exogenous steroids, such as testosterone propionate, to the genotypic female rodent within the first week of postnatal life, her neuroendocrine system will differentiate phenotypically male (i.e., her brain is masculinized), as the administered testosterone enters the developing brain and is aromatized to estrogen. Exogenous estrogens (i.e., estradiol, ethinyl estradiol, or diethylstilbestrol [DES]) administered perinatally to the genetic female will also masculinize the brain (Gorski, 1985). In adulthood, these "masculinized" females (1) do not ovulate, (2) have polyfollicular ovaries, (3) display persistent vaginal estrus, (4) do not show positive feedback to gonadal hormones (i.e., an ovulatory surge of LH cannot be stimulated), and (5) exhibit sexual behavior at a rate more typical of that observed in the genetic male.

A similar set of endocrine events underlies the masculinization of the primate brain (Thornton et al., 2009), and presumably the human brain. However, in primates, it is believed that testosterone and dihydrotestosterone (DHT), a nonaromatizable metabolite, confer the masculinizing properties of testosterone exposure. It may be that exposure to endogenous estrogens may still impact the developing primate brain as the human CNS is also reported to synthesize estradiol via aromatase (MacLusky et al., 1987; Azcoitia et al., 2011). Furthermore, DHT can itself be metabolized to 5α-androstane-3α,17β-diol (3a-diol) or 5a-androstane-3b,17β-diol (3β-diol), which seem preferentially to bind ERβ (Handa et al., 2009). Moreover, it is also now clear that the fetal rodent brain is itself capable of synthesizing androgens independent of testicular generation (e.g., Konkle and McCarthy, 2011), findings that are altering our understanding of the differentiation process. Thus, species differences notwithstanding, the basic research demonstrate a clear sensitivity of the developing brain to hormonal exposure and place the brain as a target for endocrine disruptors possessing estrogenic, androgenic, and aromatase properties. As a result, it is not surprising that there have been a growing number of studies investigating the potential adverse effects of environmental chemicals.

A number of xenoestrogens, including Kepone (chlordecone) (Gellert, 1978), methoxychlor (Gray et al., 1989), and zearalenone (Kumagai and Shimizu, 1982), have been shown to "masculinize" female rats. Investigations in the neonatal rat also indicate that analogs of the banned pesticide dichlorodiphenyltrichloroethane (DDT) other than methoxychlor, i.e., 1-(o-chlorophenyl)-10-(p-chlorophenyl-222-trichloro-ethane (o,p′-DDT), may also have estrogenic activity at the neuroendocrine level. Heinrichs et al. (1971) found that rats given o,p′-DDT as neonates exhibited advanced puberty (vaginal opening), persistent vaginal estrus after a period of normal cycling, follicular cysts, and a reduction in the number of corpora lutea (anovulation) (Bulger and Kupfer, 1985).

Recent studies have focused on a group of so-called environmental estrogens [e.g., Genistein, BPA (bisphenol A), alkylphenol polyethoxylates] and evaluated more closely the impact that gestational exposure to these EDCs may have on a number of brain and pituitary parameters. These include the identification of agents that disrupt ovarian cyclicity in the adult offspring (Rubin et al., 2001) following gestational/lactational exposure and changes in the neuroanatomical correlates of those hypothalamic structures associated with the maintenance of the LH surge and ovarian function in test species (Faber and Hughes, 1991). Of interest, these studies have begun to correlate the functional changes observed in adulthood with morphological and neurochemical changes detected in specific sexually differentiated brain regions of the treated offspring. For example, the rat's anterior hypothalamus/preoptic region has two sexually dimorphic nuclei. The sexually dimorphic nucleus of the preoptic area (SDN-POA) has more neurons and is larger in males than in females, and the AVPV, which in females is larger and has a higher cell density. The disparities in size have been associated with differences in estrogen-sensitive apoptotic genes in these two regions. Compared to that in females, the SDN-POA of postnatal male rats exhibits a higher expression of the anti-apoptotic gene Bcl-2 and a lower expression of the pro-apoptotic gene Bax, suggesting increased cell death (and a smaller size) in the female SDN-POA. This sex difference is hypothesized to be the result of the male brain being exposed to the perinatal increase in serum testosterone and its subsequent metabolism to estradiol. In contrast, the AVPV of the postnatal female has a greater expression of Bcl-2 and a lower expression of Bax, a finding consistent with the greater size of this nucleus in the female's hypothalamus (Tsukahara, 2009). As with the SDN-POA, exposure to an aromatizable androgen will masculinize (i.e., reduce) the AVPV of the genetic female. As stated earlier, this nucleus is key to the regulation of the ovulatory surge of LH and compared to the male, the AVPV has a greater number of kisspeptin (discussed further in Section 3.3.2) and dopamine (DA)-containing neurons.

Given the sensitivity of the SDN and AVPV to aromatizable androgens or environmental estrogens, it is not surprising that perinatal or gestational exposure to environmental estrogens has been reported to alter the size and/or function of both. For example, Faber and Hughes (1991) reported that high doses of the phytoestrogen genistein or the fungal product zearalenone to the dam were able to increase the size of the SDN of the female offspring when examined in the adulthood. The magnitude of these changes was similar to that observed with DES exposure. Others have reported alterations in the female phenotype in the AVPV following exposure to environmental estrogens such as BPA. In mice, Rubin et al. (2001) reported that subcutaneous administration of BPA delivered via a minipump induced changes in the AVPV similar to those reported to occur after estrogen exposure. This consisted of reduced AVPV size and a reduction in staining for tyrosine hydroxylase (TH, the rate-limiting enzyme for DA synthesis), in essence masculinizing the AVPV. These authors also evaluated open-field behavior in the offspring and reported that the BPA treatment eliminated the sex differences typically observed between male and female control animals. Patisaul et al. (2006) reported a decrease in TH in the AVPV following subcutaneous exposure twice daily to either BPA or genistein on postnatal days 1 and 2. These investigators employed 17β-estradiol as a positive control, which completely masculinized the AVPV. The effects in control females were then greater than for males, with estrogen significantly decreasing TH immunoreactivity to male-like levels. BPA and genistein had minimal effect on overall TH immunoreactivity. However, Patisaul et al. (2006) also reported that the female AVPV had more than twice as many cells that expressed immunoactivity for *both* TH and ERα. When just the cells that co-expressed TH and ERα were examined, they found a significant reduction in the females treated with estradiol, BPA, and genistein. As noted earlier for the SDN-POA, BPA has also been reported to alter sexually dimorphic structures in the rat. In summary, these studies indicate that phytoestrogens and xenoestrogens can impact maturation of those hypothalamic regions known to be critical to normal reproductive function in the female.

3.3.1.2 Sexual Differentiation and Nonsteroidal Chemicals

Interestingly, exposure to agents other than those with steroidogenic activity has also been shown to influence sexual differentiation of the brain, although these chemicals have been studied less systematically. Serotonergic and catecholaminergic agents, when given alone and/or in combination with testosterone or estrogen, have been reported to influence the volume of the SDN-POA (see Dohler [1991] for review). The masculinizing effects of androgens on the female brain can be partially blocked by neuroactive drugs, such as reserpine and chlorpromazine, while pentobarbital and phenobarbital provide more complete protection against the influence of testosterone (Arai and Gorski, 1968). The mechanisms by which such interactions occur remain to be elucidated, but these observations suggest that other mechanisms involved in sexual differentiation of the CNS may render this process susceptible to disruption by environmental compounds that do not necessarily possess steroidogenic activity.

Serotonin is known to exert trophic effects within the CNS during development (Lauder, 1983). Interestingly, both stimulation and inhibition of serotonin synthesis have profound effects on development and differentiation of sexually dimorphic nuclei (Handa et al., 1986). Dohler (1991) reported that NE receptor activation augmented the masculinizing effects of testosterone in male and female neonates. At the very least, these data imply that serotonergic and adrenergic input may play an important role during differentiation of the SDN-POA.

The work of McCarthy (2008) has shed light on how compounds other than aromatizable androgens and estrogens can alter sexual differentiation of the brain. In brief, depending on the brain structure (AVPV, SDN, POA, VMN, arcuate, bed nucleus of the stria terminalis, hippocampus, or amygdala), aromatized estrogen initiates a series of distinct molecular events that result in the final phenotype for that structure. In this regard, many of the downstream molecular events involve changes in neurotransmitter and other signaling pathways that can be modified by different pharmaceutical treatments and thus interfere with the normal estrogen-induced changes typically present in the male. Conversely, chemicals that induce or impair these molecular events in the female brain have the potential to modify the female phenotype. For example, differentiation of the SDN/POA by estradiol involves an upregulation of the cyclooxygenase genes *COX1* and *COX2* to increase prostaglandin synthesis, eventually resulting in an increase of AMPA glutamate receptors in that region of the male brain. This process can be impaired by treatment with *COX2* inhibitors such as indomethacin (Wright and McCarthy, 2009). In the arcuate nucleus, estradiol upregulates glutamic acid decarboxylase (GAD), and the resultant GABA production ultimately differentiates neighboring astrocytes (Schwarz and McCarthy, 2006). It is a process potentially susceptible to inhibition by a GABA agonist or antagonist.

3.3.1.3 Tuberoinfundibular Dopaminergic Pathway

Certain aspects of neuroendocrine function appear to be modified via nonsteroidogenic mechanisms after birth. For example, it appears that early postnatal exposure to prolactin may be important for the normal hypothalamic regulation of prolactin at puberty and in the adult. Prolactin is present in the milk of lactating rats and, when ingested by the pups, can pass through the gut and enter the systemic circulation. Shyr et al. (1986) found that suppression of prolactin levels in the mother's milk by administration of a DA receptor agonist (bromocriptine) on postnatal days 2–5 (but not days 9–12) resulted in very low prolactin levels in the blood of neonates during treatment. However, when measured between days 30 and 35, the concentration and turnover of DA within the tuberoinfundibular tract were depressed, thereby elevating serum prolactin. Importantly, regular postpubertal ovarian cycles were absent in the hyperprolactinemic females until day 60. Shyr et al. (1986) also reported that when tested *in vitro*, the lactotrophs from the pituitaries of hyperprolactinemic animals were unresponsive to DA regulation and tended to secrete more prolactin in response to thyrotropin-releasing hormone (TRH) stimulation (Shah et al., 1988).

The dependence of this effect on prolactin exposure was supported by the observation that these alterations could be reversed if the mother was treated with ovine prolactin at the time bromocriptine was administered.

Experimentally induced hyperprolactinemia in the weanling rat can advance the onset of puberty. Advis and Ojeda (1978) showed that induction of hyperprolactinemia by exposing pups to a DA receptor blocker beginning on postnatal day 22 will significantly advance puberty, as indicated by vaginal opening. However, after puberty there were disturbances noted in the ovarian cycles of these animals. These results raise the possibility that one function of milk-derived prolactin in the neonate involves maturation of the inhibitory DA control over prolactin secretion, and that disruption of this process may have longlasting consequences.

The tuberoinfundibular dopaminergic pathway is known to be involved in the regulation of prolactin secretion under a variety of conditions. Since prolactin plays a key role in the initiation and maintenance of pregnancy in the rat, it is not surprising that inhibition of prolactin release following treatment with bromocriptine can disrupt pregnancy (Cummings et al., 1991). Although, there are several pharmaceutical agents that mimic endogenous DA, we know of no such environmental agents with similar effects. However, it is possible that the loss of pregnancy following carbon tetrachloride exposure (Narotsky and Kavlock, 1995) may reflect a disruption of CNS regulation of the pituitary and so affect the hormonal support for the pregnancy.

Exposing the weanling rat to certain pesticides has been shown to delay the onset of puberty in the rat. For example, we found that lindane (gamma hexachlorohexane) caused a dose-dependent delay in vaginal opening when treatment was initiated on day 21 (Cooper et al., 1989). Lindane is a well-known neurotoxicant that will induce seizure activity as a result of its effect on the chloride ion channels associated with the $GABA_A$ receptor. Lindane inhibits the influx of the chloride ion into the cell and thus leads to depolarization. Initially, it appeared that these effects were a result of an "anti-estrogenic" action of lindane, because in related experiments with prepubertal rats this compound inhibited the estrogen-induced increase in uterine weight. A more recent series of binding studies showed that lindane did not bind to the estrogen receptor *in vitro*, nor did it alter the induction of PRs in response to estrogen stimulation (Laws et al., 1994). This lack of effect on the estrogen receptor suggests that lindane's influence on puberty in the female rat is likely related to its effect on $GABA_A$ receptor function, and that interference with the action of the chloride ion channel at this time may influence hypothalamic–pituitary activity.

In summary, sexual differentiation is affected by a variety of environmental compounds, and although much of the research has focused on those compounds reported to have steroidogenic activity, it may yet be premature to assume that other nonsteroidal compounds are without effect on sexual differentiation of the brain.

3.3.2 Effect of Environmental Toxicants on Hypothalamic–Pituitary Control of Gonadal Function in the Adult

The preceding sections demonstrate the complex involvement of the CNS in reproductive function, as the brain must respond to ovarian hormonal shifts, diurnal factors, and a myriad of other influences that control ovulation. There are a number of papers in the peer-reviewed literature that attest to the significance of different central mechanisms involved in the regulation of the LH surge and behavior (steroid hormones, steroid hormone receptors, neurotransmitters, and neuropeptides, etc.). Thus, from a toxicological perspective, the adult brain has a number of molecular targets for different classes of pharmaceuticals and environmental chemicals. As many of those targets are a functional component of the neuroendocrine axis controlling ovarian function, chemically induced alterations in this important endocrine axis would ultimately impact ovarian function. For example, many pharmaceuticals are designed to enhance or interfere with GABA-ergic, monoaminergic (serotonin and catecholamines), cholinergic, opioidergic, and other neuropeptide neurotransmission. Similarly, many pesticides are formulated on their ability to interfere with CNS function (i.e., cholinesterase inhibitors, ion channel disruptors). Still other environmental chemicals are known to possess estrogenic or antiandrogenic properties and thus have the potential to modify normal feedback of ovarian hormones on brain–pituitary function and consequently gonadotropin secretion.

Chemicals that affect noradrenergic transmission have long been known to have adverse effects on the endocrine regulation of ovarian function. Over 60 years ago, Sawyer and colleagues (1947, 1949) used the adrenergic blocking agent, dibenamine, to suppress ovulation in both rabbits and rats. Using ovariectomized rats, Simpkins et al. (1979) reported that 6-hydroxydopamine introduced near GnRH cell bodies resulted in a depletion of norepinephrine (NE), blocking a steroid-induced LH surge. A similar effect on the surge was seen in ovariectomized (OVX), steroid-primed rats with the formamidine pesticides, chlordimeform and amitraz, both α-noradrenergic receptor antagonists (Goldman et al., 1991; Goldman and Cooper, 1993).

Noradrenergic fibers reaching the area of GnRH neurons extend from cell bodies located in the brainstem. In the nerve terminals of these axons, NE is converted from DA by dopamine-β-hydroxylase (DβH), which requires a copper cofactor for its activity. It appears that this noradrenergic input acts as a permissive factor for GnRH neuronal activity, providing a necessary tone in this area for other processes to proceed. An amplification or suppression in this tone will disrupt the mechanisms of GnRH secretion (Herbison, 1997). Dithiocarbamates are members of a chemical class of pesticides whose members act as metal chelators (e.g., Sørensen and Andersen, 1989; Tandon et al., 1990). They have been used as insecticides, fungicides, miticides, or microbicides, and at least one dithiocarbamate has been employed in wastewater treatment to enhance the precipitation of metals (Matlock et al., 2002). A number of studies have demonstrated that dithiocarbamates, including thiram (tetramethylthiuram disulfide), sodium dimethyldithiocarbamate, and metam sodium (sodium *N*-methyldithiocarbamate), are able to suppress DβH activity in the brain and decrease NE synthesis, thereby elevating its DA precursor (e.g., Maj and Vetulani, 1969; Przewlocka et al., 1975). In estradiol-primed prepubertal OVX rats, an injection of diethyldithiocarbamate diminished both NE synthesis and mRNA for the pro-GnRH precursor in addition to decreasing GnRH secretion *in vitro* (Kim et al., 1994). Moreover, a single presurge administration of dimethyldithiocarbmate given to OVX estradiol-and progesterone-primed rats, showed similar dose relationships (Figure 3.4) among a decline in hypothalamic NE,

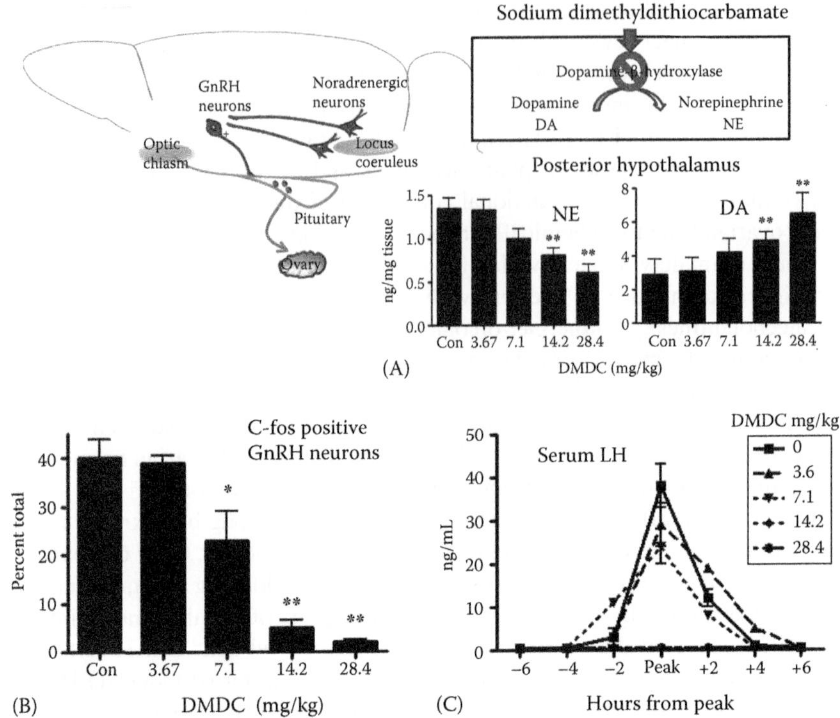

FIGURE 3.4 Toxicity pathway showing the effects in female rats on hypothalamic catecholamines, GnRH neuronal activation, and the LH surge following a single administration of increasing concentrations of the dithiocarbamate pesticide sodium dimethyldithiocarbamate (DMDC). This pesticide blocks the conversion (A) of the neurotransmitter dopamine (DA) to norepinephrine (NE) by chelating the copper cofactor necessary for the activity of the enzyme dopamine-β-hydroxylase. The effect decreased the percentage of activated GnRH neurons indicated by immunostaining for the proto-oncogene c-fos (B) in the GnRH nuclei. In turn, this decline is paralleled by a dose-related suppression in the LH surge (C). (Redrawn from Goldman, J.M. et al., *Toxicol. Sci.*, 104, 107, 2008. With permission.)

a suppression in the LH surge, and an effect on GnRH neuronal activation, the latter represented by a progressive decline in the percentage of c-fos-positive GnRH neurons (Goldman et al., 2008).

Figure 3.4 provides a summary of the toxicity pathways associated with the disruption of normal ovarian function in the female rat following exposure to chemicals known to alter catecholamine synthesis and/or receptor activation. This toxicity pathway starts with the molecular perturbation, in this case either a disruption in NE synthesis or a blockcade of the αNE receptor (such as the case with the formamidine pesticide chlordimeform, Goldman et al., 1993) is followed by alterations/delays in the ovulatory surge of LH, delayed ovulation, compromised oocyte viability, impaired embryo development, and reduced litter size (Cooper et al., 1994).

Ovaries also receive noradrenergic neural input, with evidence in both rodents and primates of *de novo* NE synthesis (Morimoto et al., 1982; Ben-Jonathan et al., 1984;

Dees et al., 1995; Ricu et al., 2008) that has been implicated in follicular maturation and steroidogenesis (Aguado and Ojeda, 1984; Kannisto et al., 1985; Greiner et al., 2008). This would then expand target sites for an exposure to the dithiocarbamates. In fact, a unilateral micro-injection of dimethyldithiocarbamate under the rat ovarian bursal membrane on the day of proestrus caused a dose-related suppression of oocyte release from the exposed ovary (Goldman et al., 1997). Using this type of intrabursal administration, a similar effect on oocyte retrieval was found with the noradrenergic neurotoxin *N*-(2-chloro-ethyl)-*N*-ethyl-2-bromobenzylamine (DSP4) (Goldman et al., 1996).

Whereas there is an accumulation of evidence linking noradrenergic neurotransmitter alterations to the adverse reproductive effects of various environmental toxicants, analogous data implicating targeted GABAergic mechanisms are predominantly limited to pharmacological insult. During development, GABA has been identified as one of the factors regulating the migratory rate of GnRH neurons from the olfactory placode to their final destination in the hypothalamus (Tobet et al., 1996; Wray, 2010). The application of the $GABA_A$ receptor agonist muscimol to explants of the embryonic olfactory placode was able to decrease the rate of GnRH neuronal migration (Fueshko et al., 1998). Such alterations in the temporal patterning of neuronal migration are known to have marked reproductive consequences. Probably, the best example is Kallman's syndrome, an inherited condition in humans tied to an X-linked mutation of the KAL1 gene that is expressed in the developing olfactory bulb. Individuals are anosmic and GnRH neuronal migration is impaired, affecting the ability to secrete GnRH. Hypogonadotropic hypogonadism is present, with a failure to complete a pubertal transition to sexual maturity.

Recent data in young adult rats suggest that on the day of proestrus synaptic GABAergic terminals on GnRH neurons decline while the excitatory influence of glutamatergic terminal appositions increases, diminishing the inhibitory input (Khan et al., 2010) to these neurons. The pentobarbital barbiturate, Nembutal, was employed in a number of early studies to block the LH surge when administered during a sensitive proestrous window of time (e.g., Everett and Sawyer, 1950; Sawyer et al., 1955). This effect is likely attributable to pentobarbital's ability to bind to GABA receptors and open $GABA_A$ receptor channels (Mercado and Czajkowski, 2008), which would preclude the emergence of a presurge disinhibition of GABA input. An increase in brain concentrations of GABA in response to the GABA-transaminase inhibitors, 4-amino-5-hexynoic acid and amino-oxyacetic acid, will also block the LH surge and ovulation by preventing the metabolic conversion of GABA to succinic semialdehyde (Donoso and Banzan, 1986). Muscimol and another GABA agonist baclofen have both been found with increasing doses to block the surge in OVX rats primed with estradiol and progesterone (Adler and Crowley, 1986). Neither drug significantly affected LH secretion in females given GnRH. Both appeared to decrease hypothalamic NE concentrations and turnover rate over the course of several hours, suggesting that GABA was acting to modulate noradrenergic mechanisms involved in GnRH secretion.

Beyond these pharmacological interventions, there is limited evidence showing that environmental toxicants able to target the GABA receptor will adversely affect the neuroendocrine control of the LH surge. Synthetic pyrethroid derivatives of natural pyrethrins found in the chrysanthemum have high insecticidal and low mammalian toxicity. Among other effects, they are able to modulate GABA-activated chloride channels (Narahashi, 1991), but there are little available data to suggest that either type I (e.g., allethrin, pyrethrin, permethrin) or type II pyrethroids (e.g., deltamethrin, fenvalerate, cyhalothrin) will significantly affect central regulation of the LH surge. This may be at least partly attributable to an interaction between inhibitory GABAergic and excitatory glutamatergic neurons, as pyrethroids have also been shown to act on sodium and calcium channels of the presynaptic glutamatergic neurons (Soderlund and Bloomquist, 1989; Hossain et al., 2008).

Whereas GnRH represents the final common pathway from the brain, its secretion into pituitary portal vessels is regulated by a variety of neuroendocrine factors. As discussed previously, it has long been apparent that the rising concentration of estradiol during the ovarian cycle feeds back to the hypothalamus, providing a stimulus for GnRH neuronal secretion. Experimental data from OVX, estradiol-primed mice with knockout deletions of one or the other of ERα and ERβ genes demonstrated that estrogen-positive feedback promoting GnRH neuronal activation and the LH surge appeared unaffected in ERβKO-mutant mice, but absent in those lacking ERα (Wintermantel et al., 2006). GnRH neurons express ERβ, but not ERα (Herbison and Pape, 2001) or PRs (Fox et al., 1990), so sex steroid feedback underlying the hypothalamic mechanisms for GnRH secretion likely employed a secondary cell type, either neuronal or glial. Working with mice in which ERα was specifically deleted from neurons, Wintermantel and colleagues (2006) determined that this feedback involved a neuronal intermediate.

A number of separate, but interconnected, studies revealed the identity of this intermediate. Two concurrently published reports described families with members that exhibited a hypogonadotropic hypogonadism that corresponded to the presence of mutations in the orphan receptor GPR54 (de Roux et al., 2003; Seminara et al., 2003). The natural ligand for GPR54 was discovered to be a group of neuropeptides termed kisspeptins (Kotani et al., 2001; Ohtaki et al., 2001), and it was also found that approximately 75% of GnRH neurons were positive for these receptors (Irwig et al., 2005), now renamed Kiss1r. Kisspeptin-containing nerve cells located in the AVPV, adjacent to the third ventricle, possess ERα and PR and send axonal projections to GnRH neurons. In this linkage between ovarian estradiol feedback to the brain and the secretion of GnRH, it now appears that kisspeptins play an important role in pubertal maturation (Clarkson et al., 2010) and are the most powerful endogenous stimulus to GnRH. Injections of ~1 fmol into the mouse lateral ventricle were reported to elicit a large and rapid release of gonadotropins (Gottsch et al., 2004).

In rodents, kisspeptin (kiss1) neuronal cell bodies are located in two areas of the hypothalamus, the previously mentioned AVPV and the arcuate nucleus, just dorsal to the median eminence. In these females, these neurons now appear to subserve different functions in each area. In the AVPV, estradiol provides positive feedback to the kiss1 neurons, which participate in the generation of the LH surge (Adachi et al., 2007). In the arcuate nucleus, kisspeptin coexists in neurons containing the inhibitory opioid peptide dynorphin and the tachykinin neurokinin B (KNDy neurons). Estradiol feedback here is negative (Smith et al., 2005), and these neurons are now believed to be involved in the regulation of pulsatile GnRH secretion.

There are only a few studies that have focused on alterations in kisspeptin-related endpoints in response to toxicant exposure, and those have employed neonatal exposures to estrogenic chemicals. In female rats, early treatments with BPA (commercially used in the production of plastics and epoxy resins) have been reported to decrease prepubertal expression of the KiSS-1 gene (Navarro et al., 2009) and decrease postpubertal kisspeptin fiber density (Patisaul et al., 2009). A similar postpubertal decrease in AVPV fiber density was present in response to neonatal exposures to estradiol benzoate and the phytoestrogen genistein (Bateman and Patisaul, 2008). Estradiol treatment significantly advanced vaginal opening and caused a prompt increase in the number of acyclic animals. Genistein caused a small advancement, and these females showed a significant decline in cycling by postpubertal week 6.

3.3.3 Adrenal Influences on the Hypothalamic–Pituitary–Ovarian Axis

In addition to ovarian-derived progesterone, the adrenal cortex contributes a significant portion of the serum progesterone over the cycle (Shaikh and Shaikh, 1975), and the adrenal hormones have a well-identified influence on ovarian function and female reproduction. In the intact female, significant fluctuations in adrenal-derived progesterone contribute to normal neuroendocrine function. In contrast, prolonged, or abnormally timed, increases in adrenal corticosterone or progesterone have been shown to impair the positive feedback essential for the ovulatory surge of LH. In this regard, toxicant exposure may influence the activity of the hypothalamic–pituitary–adrenal axis (HPA) in at least two ways. One is through a toxicant-induced stress resulting from exposure to the noxious properties of a test chemical. The other is a specific chemically induced activation or inhibition of the HPA. The former is often accompanied by some indication of systemic toxicity, and any disruption of ovarian cyclicity is generally identified as secondary to the systemic toxicity. In contrast, there are toxicants and pharmaceuticals that do interact at the molecular level to alter HPA activity. As such, this effect can, in turn, modify the hypothalamic–pituitary positive feedback mechanism regulating the LH surge.

As discussed previously, estradiol and progesterone have long been known to play coordinate roles in the generation of the LH surge (Mann and Barraclough, 1973). In a female rat exhibiting a normal 4-day estrous cycle, estradiol begins to rise on diestrus day 2, reaching a midday apex on the following day of proestrus. This increase serves to increase the responsiveness of the hypothalamic mechanisms that promote the secretion of GnRH into the portal vessels and the subsequent surge of LH on the afternoon of proestrus. One outcome of such an increase in estradiol is the previously mentioned augmentation in PRs within the positive feedback sites of the hypothalamus. At the same time, there occurs an estrogen-induced increase in the astrocytic production of progesterone within the hypothalamus (Micevych et al., 2003; Kuo and Micevych, 2012). However, this CNS production of progesterone alone does not appear able to act with estradiol to generate the marked synergistic augmentation in LH typically seen in the intact, cycling rat. The magnitude of the LH surge peak in rats that were OVX and adrenalectomized was quite modest and markedly smaller than the peak height seen in intact, cycling females (Micevych et al., 2003),

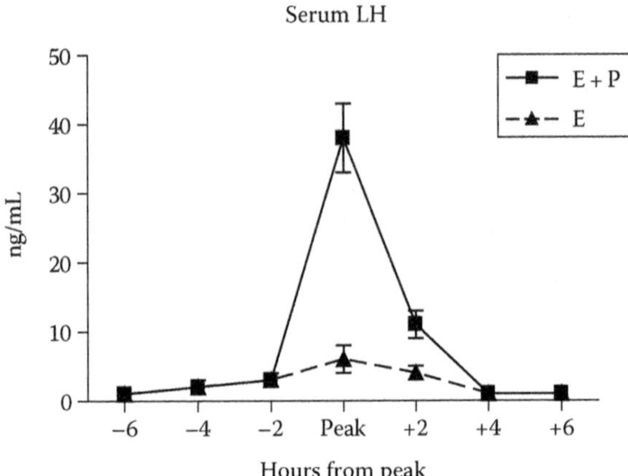

FIGURE 3.5 Augmentation of the LH surge by progesterone. Ovariectomized rats were pretreated with estradiol (3 μg/kg s.c.) three days prior to sampling. Progesterone (2.5 mg/kg) was administered immediately before sampling by tail vein puncture. Concentrations are indicated in ng/mL ± SEM.

which can rise as much as 40–60-fold above baseline concentrations. In contrast, the typical LH surge can be mimicked in an OVX female by priming her with estradiol for 3 days followed by an injection of progesterone (Figure 3.5). This synergistic action of progesterone and estradiol has been well characterized in rodents (e.g., Caligaris et al., 1968; Brown-Grant and Naftolin, 1972; Banks and Freeman, 1978, 1980) and nonhuman primates (e.g., Terasawa et al., 1984) and has been identified in women. In fact, Odell and Swerdloff (1968) found that a progestin injection in postmenopausal women previously treated with ethinyl estradiol could induce a surge-like elevation in circulating LH in samples taken 24 h later.

In contrast to the augmentation in the surge by a progesterone exposure that immediately precedes the rise in LH, a longer exposure is essentially inhibitory to the surge (e.g., Caligaris et al., 1971; Banks and Freeman, 1978, 1980; Prilusky et al., 1984). Such extended treatment will cause a downregulation by progesterone of its own receptors, which appears to be a factor underlying the suppressive effect on LH (Turgeon and Waring, 2000). This influence of progesterone is the basis for the action of many oral contraceptives. Furthermore, increased levels of progesterone during a woman's pregnancy, secreted first from the ovaries and subsequently from the placenta, prevent the appearance of a surge and ovulation over that time. Finally, it is noteworthy that treatment with progestins also lowers serum gonadotropins and testosterone production in men (e.g., Amory, 2004). Similarly, extended exposure to corticosterone also impairs normal HPG function. Repeated exposures to corticosterone will decrease the amplitude and clearly suppress the LH surge, whereas a single dose of corticosterone on the day of the expected surge in the estrogen-primed rat is without effect (Goldman et al., 1991).

The observation that adrenal corticosterone and progesterone can either increase or decrease the amplitude of the LH surge depending on the duration of exposure prompted our laboratory to evaluate the effect of the chlorotriazine herbicide atrazine on adrenal hormone secretion to determine whether or not this important neuroendocrine axis is affected by atrazine or its metabolites in the male (Laws et al., 2009) and female (Fraites et al., 2009; Pruett et al., 2009) rat. These studies demonstrated that atrazine and an equimolar dose of the intermediate metabolite desisopropylatrazine (DIA) induced a rapid and dose-dependent increase in plasma ACTH and subsequently corticosterone and progesterone (Fraites et al., 2009, Figure 3.6). The metabolite diaminochlorotriazine (DACT) had only a minimal effect on these hormones after a single dose, but did not alter them after four days of exposure. The atrazine-induced change in the adrenal hormones did not appear to result from a generalized gastrointestinal discomfort via vagal afferent signaling, but it is likely that acute exposure to ATR and DIA activated the HPA axis through a yet undefined central mechanism (Fraites et al., 2009).

In a recent study, we evaluated the possibility that the atrazine-induced changes in adrenal hormone progesterone and corticosterone secretion can contribute to alterations in LH secretion. It is well recognized that the chlorotriazines will suppress the LH surge following exposures lasting a minimum of three days (Cooper et al., 2000, 2007; McMillan et al., 2004). We reasoned that a repeated increase in adrenal

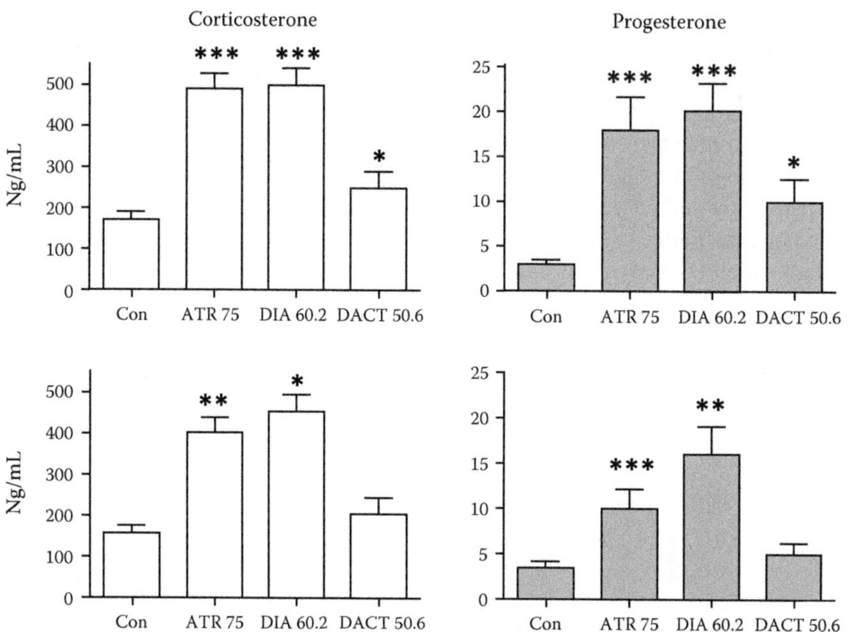

FIGURE 3.6 Effect of atrazine, desisopropylatrazine (DIA), or diamino-s-chlorotriazine (DACT) on serum corticosterone (left two panels) and progesterone (right two panels) following one (top panels) or four (bottom panels) treatment(s). Data were collected from regular 4-day cycling females 15 min after gavage. Rats were killed by decapitation. A consistent increase in both steroids was observed with atrazine and DIA, but to a lesser extent following DACT. (Based on Fraites, M.J.P. et al., *Toxicol. Sci.*, 112, 88, 2009.)

progesterone exposure induced by atrazine would interfere with the positive feedback of estrogen and progesterone on the LH surge during vaginal proestrus because repeated exposures to progesterone would *downregulate* the central PRs that are key to progesterone's synergistic effect on LH. Although such an effect of atrazine on hypothalamic or pituitary PRs has not yet been established, a downregulation of uterine PRs was reported in the ovariectomized female rat treated with atrazine (Tennant et al., 1994). In contrast, we also reasoned that a single dose of atrazine in the estrogen-primed ovariectomized rat would *increase* LH secretion because the atrazine-induced increase in progesterone would act in the same way as exogenous progesterone. That such is the case is shown in Figure 3.7, where a single dose of atrazine led to a significant increase in the estrogen-induced LH peak and the area under the curve (Goldman et al., SOT, 2013). Figure 3.7 also shows that the commonly employed four day exposure decreased the amount of LH release relative to the estrogen-only treatment. These data strongly suggest that changes in adrenal hormone secretion do ultimately influence LH secretion and may play a critical part of the toxicity pathway responsible for the identified effect of atrazine on female reproductive function, a pathway that starts with enhanced HPA activity (likely through a central effect on ACTH secretion), an increase in adrenal progesterone secretion and a downregulation of the PR. This sequence offers the most parsimonious explanation of the data reported for atrazine. The extent to which other environmental agents may induce similar changes in the HPA remains to be determined. The evaluation of environmental chemicals does not typically include measurements of the adrenal hormones, although adrenal histopathology is available from regulatory studies using extended treatment periods such as the 28 and 90 day protocols and multigenerational tests. It may be prudent to consider an alteration in adrenal hormone secretion as a component of a chemical's reproductive toxicity pathway, should both adrenal histopathology and altered ovarian function are identified. Figure 3.8 depicts some of the potential points of interaction between the HPA and the pituitary–gonadal axis through which HPA toxicants can impact pituitary ovarian function.

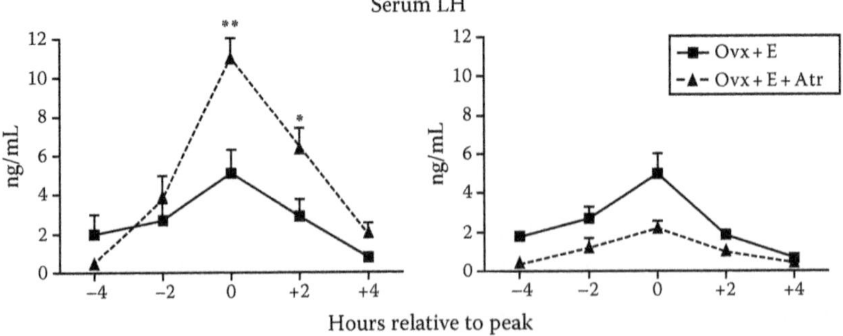

FIGURE 3.7 Effect of one or four daily atrazine treatments on serum LH. A clear statistically significant increase in serum LH was observed following a single dose of the herbicide (100 mg/kg adminstered at 1300 h). However, the opposite was observed following 4 days of exposure as atrazine abolished the LH peak.

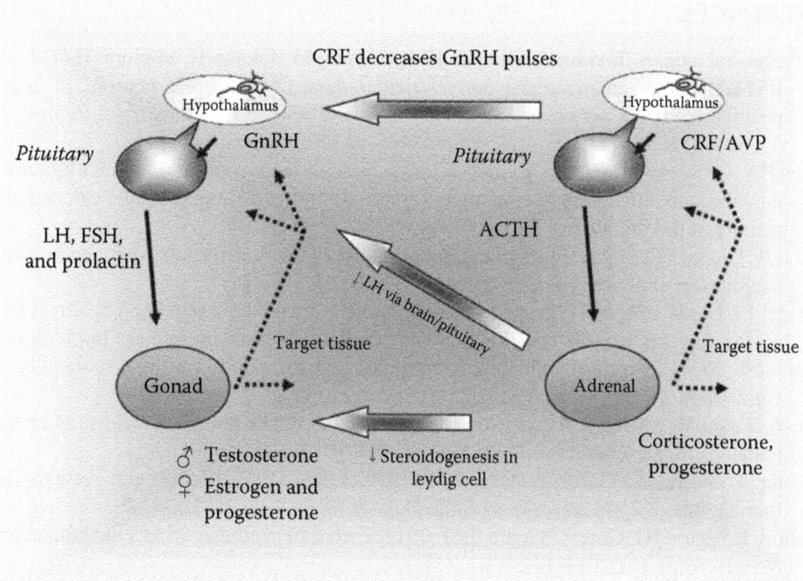

FIGURE 3.8 **(See color insert.)** Schematic depicting several points of interaction between the HPA and the HPG. Activation of the adrenal axis has been shown to inhibit GnRH as a result of CRF-induced changes in GnRH, adrenal steroid actions on the CNS and/or pituitary, and by effects of corticosterone on steroidogenesis within the gonads.

3.4 SUMMARY

The studies discussed in this chapter identify a variety of molecular targets within the brain that are susceptible to environment toxicants as a result of a disruption of the molecular processes involved in the normal control of this neuroendocrine axis. Environmental estrogens, anti-androgens, and pesticides that possess neurotransmitter properties have the potential to disrupt the central control of reproduction. These effects have been identified in the developing animal as well as the adult. We have also shown that the complexity of the CNS's involvement in pituitary–ovarian function can be dissected and studied rationally by identifying through the identification of the molecular targets of the test chemical. As a result, the different toxicity pathways associated with disruption of ovarian cycling provide important information in the risk assessment process as they serve to clarify the science behind different risk assessment decisions.

Disclaimer: The research described in this book chapter has been reviewed by the National Health and Environmental Effects Research Laboratory, U.S. Environmental Protection Agency, and approved for publication. Approval does not signify that the contents necessarily reflect the views and policies of the Agency, nor does the mention of trade names of commercial products constitute endorsement or recommendation for use.

REFERENCES

Adachi, S, Yamada, S, Takatsu, Y, Matsui, H, Kinoshita, M, Takase, K, Sugiura, H et al. 2007. Involvement of anteroventral periventricular metastin/kisspeptin neurons in estrogen positive feedback action on luteinizing hormone release in female rats. *Reprod. Dev.* 53: 367–378.

Adler, BA, Crowley, WR. 1986. Evidence for gamma-aminobutyric acid modulation of ovarian hormonal effects on luteinizing hormone secretion and hypothalamic catecholamine activity in the female rat. *Endocrinology* 118: 91–97.

Advis, JP, Ojeda, SR. 1978. Hyperprolactinemia-induced precocious puberty in the female rat: ovarian site of action. *Endocrinology* 103: 924–935.

Aguado, Ll, Ojeda, SR. 1984. Prepubertal ovarian function is finely regulated by direct adrenergic influence. Role of noradrenergic innervation. *Endocrinology* 114: 1845–1853.

Amory, JK. 2004. Testosterone/progestin regimens: a realistic option for male contraception? *Curr. Opin. Investig. Drugs* 5: 1025–1030.

Arai, Y, Gorski, RA. 1968. Critical exposure time for androgenization of the developing hypothalamus in the female rat. *Endocrinology* 82: 1010–1014.

Azcoitia, I, Sierra, A, Garcia-Segura, LM. 1999. Localization of estrogen receptor beta-immunoreactivity in astrocytes of the adult rat brain. *Glia* 26: 260–267.

Azcoitia, I, Yague, JG, Garcia-Segura, LM. 2011. Estradiol synthesis within the human brain. *Neuroscience* 191: 139–147.

Banks, JA, Freeman, ME. 1978. The temporal requirement of progesterone on proestrus for extinction of the estrogen-induced daily signal controlling luteinizing hormone release in the rat. *Endocrinology* 102: 426–432.

Banks, JA, Freeman, ME. 1980. Inhibition of the daily LH release mechanism by progesterone acting at the hypothalamus. *Biol. Reprod.* 22: 217–222.

Bateman, HL, Patisaul, HB. 2008. Disrupted female reproductive physiology following neonatal exposure to phytoestrogens or estrogen specific ligands is associated with decreased GnRH activation and kisspeptin fiber density in the hypothalamus. *Neurotoxicology* 29: 988–997.

Ben-Jonathan, N, Arbogast, LA, Rhoades, TA, Bahr, JM. 1984. Norepinephrine in the rat ovary: ontogeny and de novo synthesis. *Endocrinology* 115: 1426–1431.

Brock, BJ, Waterman, MR. 1999. Biochemical differences between rat and human cytochrome P450c17 support the different steroidogenic needs of these two species. *Biochemistry* 38: 1598–1606.

Brown-Grant, K, Naftolin, F. 1972. Facilitation of LH secretion in the female rat by progesterone. *J. Endocrinol.* 53: 37–46.

Bulger, WH, Kupfer, D. 1985. Estrogenic activity of pesticides and xenobiotics on uterus and male reproductive tract. In: Thomas, JA, Korach, KS, eds. *Endocrine Toxicology*. New York: Raven Press. pp. 1–33.

Butcher, RL, Collins, WE, Fugo, NW. 1974. Plasma concentration of LH, FSH, prolactin, progesterone and estradiol-17β throughout the 4-day estrous cycle of the rat. *Endocrinology* 94: 1704–1708.

Caligaris, L, Astrada, JJ, Taleisnik, S. 1968. Stimulating and inhibiting effects of progesterone on the release of luteinizing hormone. *Acta Endocrinol. (Copenh.)* 59: 177–185.

Caligaris, L, Astrada, JJ, Taleisnik, S. 1971. Biphasic effect of progesterone on the release of gonadotropin in rats. *Endocrinology* 89: 331–337.

Chaban, VV, Lakhter, AJ, Micevych, P. 2004. A membrane estrogen receptor mediates intracellular calcium release in astrocytes. *Endocrinology* 145: 3788–3795.

Chappell, PE, Levine, JE. 2000. Simulation of gonadotropin-releasing hormone surges by estrogen. I. Role of hypothalamic progesterone receptors. *Endocrinology* 141: 1477–1485.

Clarkson, J, Han, S-K, Liu, X, Lee, K, Herbison, AE. 2010. Neurobiological mechanisms underlying kisspeptin activation of gonadotropin-releasing hormone (GnRH) neurons at puberty. *Mol. Cell. Endocrinol.* 324: 45–50.

Cooper, RL, Barrett, MA, Goldman, JM, Rehnberg, GL, McElroy, WK, Stoker, TE. 1994. Pregnancy alterations following xenobiotic-induced delays in ovulation in the female rat. *Fund. Appl. Toxicol.* 22: 474–480.

Cooper, RL, Chadwick, RW, Rehnberg, GL, Goldman, JM, Booth, KC, Hein, JF, McElroy, WK. 1989. Effect of lindane on hormonal control of reproductive function in the female rat. *Toxicol. Appl. Pharmacol.* 99: 384–394.

Cooper, RL, Goldman, JM, Rehnberg, GL. 1986. Neuroendocrine control of reproductive function in the aging female rodent. *J. Am. Geriatr. Soc.* 34: 735–751.

Cooper, RL, Laws, SC, Das, PC, Narotsky, MC, Goldman, JM, Tyrey, L., Stoker, TE. 2007. Atrazine and reproductive function: mode and mechanism of action studies. *Birth Defects Res. B Dev. Reprod. Toxicol.* 80: 98–112.

Cooper, RL, Stoker, TE, Tyrey, L, Goldman, JM, McElroy, WK. 2000. Atrazine disrupts the hypothalamic control of pituitary-ovarian function. *Toxicol. Sci.* 53: 297–307.

Couse, JF, Korach, KS. 1999. Estrogen receptor null mice: what we have learned and where will they lead us? *Endocr. Rev.* 20: 358–417.

Cummings, AM, Perreault, SD, Harris, ST. 1991. Use of bromoergocryptine in the validation of protocols for the assessment of mechanisms of early pregnancy loss in the rat. *Fund. Appl. Toxicol.* 17: 563–574.

Faber, KA, Hughes, CL Jr. 1991. The effect of neonatal exposure to DES, genistein, and zearalenone on pituitary responsiveness and SDN-POA volume in the castrated adult rat. *Biol. Reprod.* 45: 649–653.

Fitzpatrick, SL, Carlone, DL, Robker, RL, Richards, JS. 1997. Expression of aromatase in the ovary: down-regulation of mRNA by the ovulatory luteinizing hormone surge. *Steroids* 62: 197–206.

Fortune, JE. 1986. Bovine theca and granulose cells interact to promote androgen production. *Biol. Reprod.* 35: 292–299.

Dees, WL, Hiney, JK, Schultea, TD, Mayerhofer, A, Danilchik, M, Dissen, GA, Ojeda, SR. 1995. The primate ovary contains a population of catecholaminergic neuron-like cells expressing nerve growth factor receptors. *Endocrinology* 136: 5760–5768.

Dohler, KD. 1991. The pre-and postnatal influence of hormones and neurotransmitters on sexual differentiation of the mammalian hypothalamus. *Int. Rev. Cytol.* 131: 1–58.

Donoso, AO, Banzan, AM. 1986. Blockade of the LH surge and ovulation by GABA-T inhibitory drugs that increase brain GABA levels in rats. *Psychoneuroendocrinology* 11: 429–435.

Everett, JW, Sawyer, CH. 1950. A 24-hour periodicity in the "LH-release apparatus" of female rats, disclosed by barbiturate sedation. *Endocrinology* 47: 198–218.

Fox, SR, Harlan, RE, Shivers, BD, Pfaff, DW. 1990. Chemical characterization of neuroendocrine targets for progesterone in the female rat brain and pituitary. *Neuroendocrinology* 51: 276–283.

Fraites, MJP, Cooper, RL, Buckalew, A, Jayaraman, S, Mills, L, Laws, SC. 2009. Characterization of the hypothalamic-pituitary-adrenal axis response to atrazine and metabolites in the female rat. *Toxicol. Sci.* 112: 88–99.

Fueshko, SM, Key, S, Wray, S. 1998. GABA inhibits migration of luteinizing hormone-releasing hormone neurons in embryonic olfactory explants. *J. Neurosci.* 18: 2560–2569.

Gellert, RJ. 1978. Kepone, Mirex, Dieldrin, and Aldrin: estrogenic activity and the induction of persistent vaginal estrus and anovulation in rats following neonatal treatment. *Environ. Res.* 16: 131–138.

Goldman, JM, Cooper, RL. 1993. Assessment of toxicant-induced alterations in the luteinizing hormone control of ovulation in the rat. In: Heindel, JJ, Chapin, RE, eds. *Female Reproductive Toxicology. Methods in Toxicology*. Vol. 3B. San Diego, CA: Academic Press, pp. 79–91.

Goldman, JM, Cooper, RL, Edwards, TL, Rehnberg, GL, McElroy, WK, Hein, JF. 1991. Suppression of the luteinizing hormone surge by chlordimeform in ovariectomized, steroid-primed female rats. *Pharmacol. Toxicol.* 68: 131–136.

Goldman, JM, Davis, LK, Murr, AS, Cooper, RL. 2013. Bidirectional impact of atrazine-induced elevations in progesterone (P4) on the LH surge in the ovariectomized (OVX), estradiol (E2)-primed rat. To be presented at the 52nd annual meeting, Society of Toxicology, San Antonio, TX.

Goldman, JM, Murr, AS, Buckalew, AR, Cooper, RL. 2008. Suppression of the steroid-primed luteinizing hormone surge in the female rat by sodium dimethyldithiocarbamate: relationship to hypothalamic catecholamines and GnRH neuronal activation. *Toxicol. Sci.* 104: 107–112.

Goldman, JM, Parrish, MB, Cooper, RL, McElroy, WK. 1997. Blockade of ovulation in the rat by systemic and ovarian intrabursal administration of the fungicide sodium dimethyldithiocarbamate. *Reprod. Toxicol.* 11: 185–190.

Goldman, JM, Stoker, TE, Cooper, RL. 1996. Suppression of oocyte release in rats by local administration of the noradrenergic neurotoxin DSP4. *J. Reprod. Fertil.* 106: 275–283.

Goldman, JM, Stoker, TE, Perreault, SD, Cooper, RL, Crider, MA. 1993. Influence of the formamidine pesticide chlordimeform on ovulation in the female hamster: dissociable shifts in the luteinizing hormone surge and oocyte release. *Toxicol. Appl. Pharmacol.* 121: 279–290.

Gorski, RA. 1985. Sexual dimorphisms of the brain. *J. Animal Science.* 61: 38–61.

Gottsch, ML, Cunningham, MJ, Smith, JT, Popa, SM, Acohido, BV, Crowley, WF, Seminara, S, Clifton, DK, Steiner, RA. 2004. A role for kisspeptins in the regulation of gonadotropin secretion in the mouse. *Endocrinology* 145: 4073–4077.

Gray, LE, Ostby, J, Ferrell, J, Rehnberg, G, Linder, R, Cooper, R, Goldman, J, Slott, V, Laskey, J. 1989. A dose-response analysis of methoxychlor-induced reproductive development and function in the rat. *Fund. Appl. Toxicol.* 12: 92–108.

Greiner, M, Paredes, A, Rey-Ares, V, Saller, S, Mayerhofer, A, Lara, HE. 2008. Catecholamine uptake, storage, and regulated release by ovarian granulosa cells. *Endocrinology* 149: 4988–4996.

Hagihara, K, Hirata, S, Osada, T, Hirai, M, Kato, J. 1992. Distribution of cells containing progesterone receptor mRNA in the female rat di- and telencephalon: an in situ hybridization study. *Mol. Brain Res.* 14: 239–249.

Handa, RJ, Hines, M, Schoonmaker, JN, Shryne, JE, Gorski, RA. 1986. Evidence that serotonin is involved in the sexually dimorphic development of the preoptic area in the rat brain. *Develop. Brian Res.* 30: 278–282.

Handa, RJ, Weiser, MJ, Zuloaga, DG. 2009. A role for the androgen metabolite, 5alpha-androstane- 3beta,17beta-diol, in modulating oestrogen receptor beta-mediated regulation of hormonal stress reactivity. *J. Neuroendocrinol.* 21: 351–358.

Heinrichs, WL, Gellert, RJ, Bakke, JL, Lawrence, NL. 1971. DDT administered to neonatal rats induces persistent estrus syndrome. *Science* 173: 642–643.

Herbison, AE. 1997. Noradrenergic regulation of cyclic GnRH secretion. *Rev. Reprod.* 2: 1–6.

Herbison, AE. 2008. Estrogen positive feedback to gonadotropin-releasing hormone (GnRH) neurons in the rodent: the case for the rostral periventricular area of the third ventricle (RP3V). *Brain Res. Rev.* 57: 277–287.

Herbison, AE, Pape, JR. 2001. New evidence for estrogen receptors in gonadotropin-releasing hormone neurons. *Front. Neuroendocrinol.* 22: 292–308.

Hossain, MM, Suzuki, T, Unno, T, Komori, S, Kobayashi, H. 2008. Differential presynaptic actions of pyrethroid insecticides on glutamatergic and GABAergic neurons in the hippocampus. *Toxicology* 243: 155–163.

Irwig, MS, Fraley, GS, Smith, JT, Acohido, BV, Popa, SM, Cunningham, MJ, Gottsch, ML, Clifton, DK, Steiner, RA. 2004. Kisspeptin activation of gonadotropin releasing hormone neurons and regulation of KiSS-1 mRNA in the male rat. *Neuroendocrinology* 80: 264–272.

Jakimiuk, AJ, Weitsman, SR, Magoffin, DAJ. 1999. 5α-reductase activity in women with polycystic ovary syndrome. *Clin. Endocrinol. Metab.* 84: 2414–2418.

Kannisto, P, Owman, Ch, Walles, B. 1985. Involvement of local adrenergic receptors in the process of ovulation in gonadotropin-primed immature rats. *J. Reprod. Fertil.* 75: 357–362.

Khan, M, De Sevilla, L, Mahesh, VB, Brann, DW. 2010. Enhanced glutamatergic and decreased GABAergic synaptic appositions to GnRH neurons on proestrus in the rat: modulatory effect of aging. *PLoS ONE* 5(4): e10172. doi:10.1371/journal.pone.0010172.

Kim, K, Lee, BJ, Cho, BN, Kang, SS, Choi, WS, Park, SD, Lee, CC, Cho, WK, Wuttke, W. 1994. Blockade of noradrenergic neurotransmission with diethyldithiocarbamic acid decreases the mRNA level of gonadotropin-releasing hormone in the hypothalamus of ovariectomized, steroid-treated pre-pubertal rats. *Neuroendocrinology* 59: 539–544.

Kimoto, T, Tsurugizawa, T, Ohta, Y, Makino, J, Tamura, Ho, Hojo, Y, Takata, N, Kawato, S. 2001. Neurosteroid synthesis by cytochrome p450-containing systems localized in the rat brain hippocampal neurons: N-methyl-D-aspartate and calcium-dependent synthesis. *Endocrinology* 142: 3578–3589.

Kintner, PJ, Mead, RA. 1983. Steroid metabolism in the corpus luteum of the ferret. *Biol. Reprod.* 29: 1121–1127.

Konkle, AT, McCarthy, MM. 2011. Developmental time course of estradiol, testosterone, and dihydrotestosterone levels in discrete regions of male and female rat brain. *Endocrinology* 152: 223–235.

Kotani, M, Detheux, M, Vandenbogaerde, A, Communi, D, Vanderwinden, J-M, Le Poul, E, Brezillon, S. et al. 2001. The metastasis suppressor gene KiSS-1 encodes kisspeptins, the natural ligands for the orphan G protein-coupled receptor GPR54. *J. Biol. Chem.* 276: 34631–34636.

Krey, LC, Tyrey, L, Everett, JW. 1973. The estrogen-induced advance in the cyclic LH surge in the rat: dependency on ovarian progesterone secretion. *Endocrinology* 93: 385–390.

Kumagai, S, Shimizu, T. 1982. Neonatal exposure to zearalenone causes persistent anovulatory estrus in the rat. *Arch. Toxicol.* 50: 279–286.

Kuo, J, Micevych, P. 2012. Neurosteroids, trigger of the LH surge. *J. Steroid Biochem. Mol. Biol.* 131: 57–65.

Lauder, JM. 1983. Hormonal and humoral influences on brain development. *Psychoneuroendocrinology* 8: 121–155.

Laws, SC, Carey, SA, Hart, DW, Cooper, RL. 1994. Lindane does not alter the estrogen receptor or the estrogen-dependent induction of progesterone receptors in sexually immature or ovariectomized adult rats. *Toxicology* 92: 127–142.

Laws, SC, Hotchkiss, M, Ferrell, J, Jayaraman, S, Mills, L, Modic, W, Tinfo, N, Fraites, M, Stoker, T, Cooper, R. 2009. Chlorotriazine herbicides and metabolites activate an ACTH-dependent release of corticosterone in male wistar rats. *Toxicol. Sci.* 112: 78–87.

Levine, JE. 1997. New concepts of the neuroendocrine regulation of gonadotropin surges in rats. *Biol. Reprod.* 56: 293–302.

Levine, JE, Ramirez, VD. 1980. In vivo release of luteinizing hormone-releasing hormone estimated with push-pull cannulae from the mediobasal hypothalamic of ovariectomized, steroid-primed rats. *Endocrinology* 107: 1782–1790.

MacLusky, NJ, Clark, AS, Naftolin, F, Goldman-Rakic, PS. 1987. Estrogen formation in the mammalian brain: possible role of aromatase in sexual differentiation of the hippocampus and neocortex. *Steroids* 50: 459–474.

MacLusky, NJ, McEwen, BS. 1980. Progestin receptors in rat brain: distribution and properties of cytoplasmic progestin-binding sites. *Endocrinology* 106: 192–202.

Magoffin, DA. 2006. Ovarian enzyme activities in women with polycystic ovary syndrome. *Fertil. Steril.* 86(Suppl. 1): S9–S11.

Maj, J, Vetulani, J. 1969. Effect of some N,N-disubstituted dithiocarbamates on catecholamines level in rat brain. *Biochem. Pharmacol.* 18: 2045–2047.

Makris, A, Olsen, D, Ryan, KJ. 1983. Significance of the delta 5 and delta 4 steroidogenic pathways in the hamster. *Steroids* 42: 641–651.

Mani, SJ, Blaustein, JD, Allen, JMC, Law, SW, Omalley, BW, Clark, JH. 1994. Inhibition of rat sexual behavior by antisense oligonucleotides to the progesterone receptor. *Endocrinology* 135: 1409–1414.

Mann, DR, Barraclough, CA. 1973. Role of estrogen and progesterone in facilitating LH release in 4-day cyclic rats. *Endocrinology* 93: 694–699.

Matlock, MM, Henke, KR, Atwood, DA. 2002. Effectiveness of commercial reagents for heavy metal removal from water with new insights for future chelate designs. *J. Haz. Mat.* B92: 129–142.

McCarthy, MM. 2008. Estradiol and the developing brain. *Physiol. Rev.* 88: 91–134.

McCarthy, MM, Arnold, AP. 2011. Reframing sexual differentiation of the brain. *Nat. Neurosci.* June; 14(6): 677–683.

McGee, EA, Hsueh, AJW. 2000. Initial and cyclic recruitment of ovarian follicles. *Endocrine Rev.* 21: 200–214.

McMillin, TS, Andersen, ME, Nagahara, A, Lund, TD, Pak, T, Handa, RJ, Hanneman, WH. 2004. Evidence that atrazine and diaminochlorotriazine inhibit the estrogen/progesterone induced surge of luteinizing hormone in female Sprague-Dawley rats without changing estrogen receptor action. *Toxicol. Sci.* 79: 278–286.

McRae, RS, Johnston, HM, Mihm, M, O'Shaughnessy, PJ. 2005. Changes in mouse granulosa cell gene expression during early luteinization. *Endocrinology* 146: 309–317.

Mercado, J, Czajkowski, C. 2008. {gamma}-aminobutyric acid (GABA) and pentobarbital induce different conformational rearrangements in the GABAA receptor {alpha}1 and {beta}2 pre-M1 regions. *J. Biol. Chem.* 283: 15250–15257.

Micevych, PE, Chaban, V, Ogi, J, Lakhter, A, Lu, JKH, Sinchak, K. 2007. Estradiol stimulates progesterone synthesis in hypothalamic astrocyte cultures. *Endocrinology* 148: 782–789.

Micevych, P, Sinchak, K, Mills, RH, Tao, L, LaPolt, P, Lu, JK. 2003. The luteinizing hormone surge is preceded by an estrogen-induced increase of hypothalamic progesterone in ovariectomized and adrenalectomized rats. *Neuroendocrinology* 78: 29–35.

Midzak, A, Rone, M, Aghazadeh, Y, Culty, M, Papadopoulos, V. 2011. Mitochondrial protein import and the genesis of steriodogenic mitochondria. *Mol. Cell Endocrinol.* 336: 70–79.

Morimoto, K, Okamura, H, Tanaka, C. 1982. Developmental and periovulatory changes of ovarian norepinephrine in the rat. *Am. J. Obstet. Gynecol.* 143: 389–392.

Narahashi, T. 1991. Transmitter-activated ion channels as the target of chemical agents. *Adv. Exp. Med. Biol.* 287: 61–73.

Narotsky, MG, Kavlock, RJ. 1995. A multidisciplinary approach to toxicological screening: II. Developmental toxicity. *J. Toxicol. Environ. Health.* 45: 145–171.

Navarro, VM, Sanchez-Garrido, MA, Castellano, JM, Roa, J, Garcia-Gallano, D, Pineda, R, Aguilar, E, Pinilla, L, Tena-Sempere, M. 2009. Persistent impairment of hypothalamic KiSS-1 system after exposures to estrogenic compounds at critical periods of brain sex differentiation. *Endocrinology* 150: 2359–2367.

Odell, WD, Swerdloff, RS. 1968. Progestogen-induced luteinizing and follicle-stimulating hormone surge in postmenopausal women: a simulated ovary peak. *Proc. Natl. Acad. Sci.* 61: 529–536.

Ogawa, S, Olazabal, UE, Parhar, IS, Pfaff, DW. 1994. Effects of intrahypothalamic administration of antisense DNA for progesterone receptor mRNA on reproductive behavior and progesterone receptor immunoreactivity in female rat. *J. Neurosci.* 14: 1766–1774.

Ohtaki, T, Shintani, Y, Honda, S, Matsumoto, H, Hori, A, Kanehashi, K, Terao, Y et al. 2011. Metastasis suppressor gene KiSS-1 encodes peptide ligand of a G-protein-coupled receptor. *Nature* 411: 613–617.

Parsons, B, McEwen, B. 1981. Sequential inhibition of sexual behavior by progesterone is prevented by a protein synthesis inhibitor and is not causally related to decreased levels of hypothalamic progestin receptors in the female rat. *J. Neurosci.* 1: 527–531.

Patisaul, HB, Fortino, AE, Polston, EK. 2006. Neonatal genistein or bisphenol-A exposure alters sexual differentiation of the AVPV. *Neurotoxicol. Teratol.* 28: 111–118.

Patisaul, HB, Todd, KL, Mickens, JA, Adewale, HB. 2009. Impact of neonatal exposure to the Eα agonist PPT, bisphenol-A or phytoestrogens on hypothalamic kisspeptin fiber density in male and female rats. *Neurotoxicology* 30: 350–357.

Pawlak, J, Karolczak, M, Krust, A, Chambon, P, Beyer, C. 2005. Estrogen receptor-alpha is associated with the plasma membrane of astrocytes and coupled to the MAP/Src-kinase pathway. *Glia* 50: 270–275.

Powers, JB, Moreines, J. 1976. Progesterone: examination of its postulated inhibitory actions on lordosis during the rat estrous cycle. *Physiol. Behav.* 17: 492–498.

Prilusky, J, Vermouth, NT, Deis, RP. 1984. A dual modulatory effect of progesterone on the LHRH-induced LH release. *J. Steroid. Biochem.* 21: 107–110.

Pruett, SB, Fan, R, Zheng, Q, Schwab, C. 2009. Patterns of immunotoxicity associated with chronic as compared to acute exposure to chemical or physical stressors and their relevance with regard to the role of stress and with regard to immunotoxicity testing. *Toxicol. Sci.* 10: 265–275.

Przewlocka, B, Sarnek, J, Szmigielski, A, Niewiadomska, A. 1975. The effect of some dithiocarbamic acids on dopamine-β-hydroxylase and catecholamines level in rat's brain. *Pol. J. Pharmacol. Pharm.* 27: 555–559.

Ricu, M, Paredes, A, Greiner, M, Ojeda, SR, Lara, NE. 2008. Functional development of the ovarian noradrenergic innervations. *Endocrinology* 149: 50–56.

de Roux, N, Genin, E, Carel, J-C, Matsuda, F, Chaussain, J-L, Milgrom, E. 2003. Hypogonadotropic hypogonadism due to loss of function of the KiSS1-derived peptide receptor GPR54. *Proc. Natl. Acad. Sci.* 100: 10972–10976.

Rubin, BS, Murray, MK, Damassa, DA, King, JC, Soto, AM. 2001. Perinatal exposure to low doses of bisphenol-A affects body weight, patterns of estrous cyclicity and plasma LH levels. *Environ. Health Perspect.* 109: 675–680.

Sakamoto, H, Mezaki, Y, Shikimi, H, Ukena, K, Tsutsui, K. 2003. Dendritic growth and spine formation in response to estrogen in the developing Purkinje cell. *Endocrinology* 144: 4466–4477.

Sawyer, CH, Critchlow, BV, Barraclough, CA. 1955. Mechanism of blockade of pituitary activation in the rat by morphine, atropine and barbiturates. *Endocrinology* 57: 345–354.

Sawyer, CH, Everett, JW, Markee, JE. 1949. A neural factor in the mechanism by which estrogen induces the release of luteinizing hormone in the rat. *Endocrinology* 44: 218–233.

Sawyer, CH, Markee, JE, Hollingshead, WH. 1947. Inhibition of ovulation in the rabbit by the adrenergic-blocking agent dibenamine. *Endocrinology* 41: 395–402.

Schwarz, JM, McCarthy, MM. 2006. The role of neonatal NMDA receptor activation in defeminization and masculinization of sex behavior in the rat. *Horm. Behav.* 54: 662–668.

Seminara, S, Messager, S, Chatzidaki, EE, Thresher, RR, Acierno, JS, Shagoury, JK, Bo-Abbas, Y et al. 2003. The GPR54 gene as a regulator of puberty. *N.E. J. Med.* 349: 1614–1627.

Shah, GV, Shyr, SW, Grosvenor, CE, Crowley, WR. 1988. Hyperprolactinemia after neonatal prolactin (PRL) deficiency in rats: Evidence for altered anterior pituitary regulation of PRL secretion. *Endocrinology* 122: 1883–1889.

Shaikh, AA, Shaikh, SA. 1975. Adrenal and ovarian steroid secretion in the rat estrous cycle temporally related to gonadotropins and steroid levels found in peripheral plasma. *Endocrinology* 96: 37–44.

Shyr, SW, Crowley, WR, Grosvenor, CE. 1986. Effect of neonatal prolactin deficiency on prepubertal tuberoinfundibular and tuberohypophyseal dopaminergic neuronal activity. *Endocrinology* 119: 1217–1221.

Simerly, RB, Carr, AM, Zee, MC, Lorang, D. 1996. Ovarian steroid regulation of estrogen and progesterone receptor messenger ribonucleic acid in the anteroventral periventricular nucleus of the rat. *J. Neuroendocrinol.* 8: 45–56.

Simpkins, JW, Advis, JP, Hodson, CA, Meites, J. 1979. Blockade of steroid-induced luteinizing hormone release by selective depletion of anterior hypothalamic norepinephrine activity. *Endocrinology* 104: 506–509.

Smith, JT, Cunningham, MJ, Rissman, EF, Clifton, DK, Steiner, RA. 2005. Regulation of Kiss1 gene expression in the brain of the female mouse. *Endocrinology* 146: 3686–3692.

Soderlund, DM, Bloomquist, JR. 1989. Neurotoxic actions of pyrethroid insecticides. *Ann. Rev. Entomol.* 34: 77–96.

Sørensen, JA, Andersen, O. 1989. Effects of diethyldithiocarbamate and tetraethylthiuram disulfide on zinc metabolism in mice. *Pharmacol. Toxicol.* 65: 209–213.

Su, Y-Q, Nyegaard, M, Overgaard, MT, Qiao, J, Giudice, LC. 2006. Participation of mitogen-activated protein kinase in luteinizing hormone-induced differential regulation of steriodogenesis and steriodogenic gene expression in mural and cumulus granulosa cells of mouse preovulatory follicles. *Biol. Reprod.* 75: 859–867.

Suzuki, K, Tamaoki, B. 1983. Acute decrease by human chorionic gonadotropin of the activity of preovulatory ovarian 17 alpha-hydroxylase and C-17-C-20 lyase is due to decrease of microsomal cytochrome P-450 through de novo synthesis of ribonucleic acid and protein. *Endocrinology* 113: 1985–1991.

Tandon, SK, Hashimi, NS, Kachru, DN. 1990. The lead-chelating effects of substituted dithiocarbamates. *Biomed. Environ. Sci.* 3: 299–305.

Terasawa, E, Yeoman, RR, Schultz, NJ. 1984. Factors influencing the progesterone-induced luteinizing hormone surge in rhesus monkeys: diurnal influence and time interval after estrogen. *Biol. Reprod.* 31: 732–741.

Tennant, MK, Hill, DS, Elridge, JC, Wetzel, LT, Breckenridge, CB, Stevens, JT. 1994. Possible antiestrogenic properties of cholro-s-triazines in rat uterus. *J. Toxicol. Environ. Hlth.* 43: 183–196.

Thornton, J, Zehr, JL, Loose, MD. 2009. Effects of prenatal androgens on rhesus monkeys: a model system to explore the organizational hypothesis in primates. *Horm. Behav.* 55: 633–645.

Tobet, SA, Chickering, TW, King, JC, Stopa, EG, Kim, K, Kuo-Leblank, V, Schwarting, GA. 1996. Expression of γ-aminobutyric acid and gonadotropin-releasing hormone during neuronal migration through the olfactory system. *Endocrinology* 137: 5415–5420.

Tsafriri, A, Eckstein, B. 1986. Changes in follicular steriodogenic enzymes following the preovulatory surge of gonadotropins and experimentally-induced atresia. *Biol. Reprod.* 34: 783–787.

Tsukahara, S. 2009. Sex differences and the roles of sex steroids in apoptosis of sexually dimorphic nuclei of the preoptic area in postnatal rats. *J. Neuroendocrinol.* 21: 370–376.

Turgeon, JL, Waring, DW. 2000. Progesterone regulation of the progesterone receptor in rat gonadotropes. *Endocrinology* 141: 3422–3429.

Ukena, K, Kohchi, C, Tsutsui, K. 1999. Expression and activity of 3b-hydroxysteroid dehydrogenase/Δ5-Δ4-isomerase in the rat Purkinje neuron during neonatal life. *Endocrinology* 140: 805–813.

Ukena, K, Usui, M, Kohchi, C, Tsutsui, K. 1998. Cytochrome P450 side-chain cleavage enzyme in the cerebellar Purkinje neuron and its neonatal change in rats. *Endocirnology* 139: 137–147.

Weigand, SJ, Teresawa, E. 1982. Discrete lesions reveal functional heterogeneity of suprachiasmatic structures in the female rat. *Neuroendocrinology* 34: 395–404.

Weusten, JJ, Smals, AG, Hofman, JA, Kloppenborg, PWC, Benraad, TJ. 1987. Early time sequence in pregnenolone metabolism to testosterone in homogenates of human and rat testis. *Endocrinology* 120: 1909–1913.

Weusten, JJ, van der Wouw, MP, Smals, AG, Hofman, JA, Kloppenborg, PWC, Benraad, TJ. 1990. Differential metabolism of pregnenolone by testicular homogenates of human and two species of macaques. Lack of synthesis of the human sex pheromone precursor 5,16-androstadien-3beta-ol in nonhuman primates. *Horm. Metab. Res.* 22: 619–621.

Williams, WP, Kriegsfeld, LJ. 2012. Circadian control of neuroendocrine circuits regulating female reproductive function. *Front. Endocrinol.* 3: 1–14.

Wintermantel, TM, Campbell, RE, Porteous, R, Bock, D, Grone, HJ, Todman, MG, Korach, KS, Greiner, E, Rerez, CA, Schutz, G, Herbison, AE. 2006. Definition of estrogen receptor pathway critical for estrogen positive feedback to gonadotropin-releasing hormone neurons and fertility. *Neuron* 52: 271–280.

Wray, S. 2010. From nose to brain: development of gonadotropin-releasing hormone-1 neurons. *J. Neuroendocrinology* 22: 743–753.

Wright, CL, McCarthy, MM. 2009. Prostaglandin E2-induced masculinization of brain and Behavior requires protein kinase A, AMPA/kainate and metabotropic glutamate receptor signaling. *J. Neurosci.* 29: 13274–13282.

Zwain, IH, Yen, SSC. 1999. Neurosteroidogenesis in astrocytes, oligodendrocytes, and neurons of cerebral cortex of rat brain. *Endocrinology* 140: 3843–3852.

4 Xenobiotic-Induced Oxidative Stress

Ulrike Luderer

CONTENTS

4.1 REACTIVE OXYGEN SPECIES AND OXIDATIVE STRESS

Reactive oxygen (ROS) and nitrogen (RNS) species, such as superoxide anion radical (SO), hydrogen peroxide (H_2O_2), hydroxyl radical, nitric oxide, peroxynitrite, and others (Figure 4.1), are formed during normal cellular processes and as a result of exposure to toxicants and other stressors. ROS are formed during oxidative phosphorylation as a result of leakage of electrons through the inner mitochondrial membrane. ROS are also formed during steroid synthesis in the ovary and other steroidogenic tissues, as a result of uncoupling of electron transfer from substrate hydroxylation by mitochondrial cytochrome P450 enzymes, producing SO (Hall 1994, Hanukoglu 2006). ROS and RNS play important roles in normal physiology as signaling molecules, but due to their high reactivity, free radical ROS/RNS can damage cellular macromolecules and are, therefore, tightly regulated. Ovulation is an example of a critical ovarian process, which is regulated by ROS. Ovarian levels of ROS rise

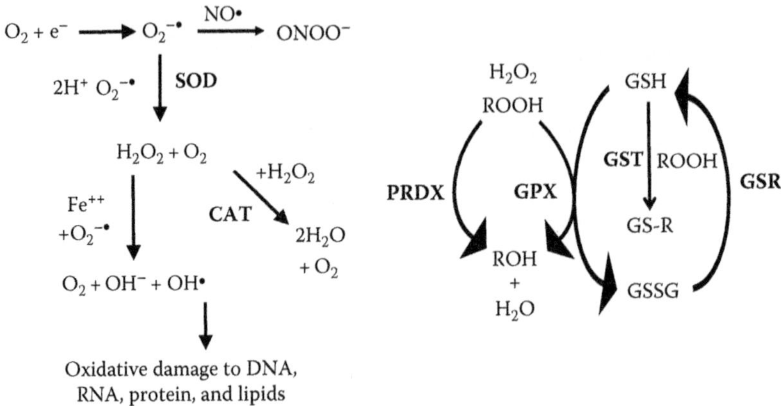

FIGURE 4.1 Reactive oxygen species (ROS) generation and detoxification. ROS are formed by the sequential addition of electrons to molecular oxygen, forming superoxide anion radical ($O_2^{-\bullet}$), H_2O_2, and hydroxyl radical. Peroxynitrite ($ONOO^-$) is formed when superoxide anion radical reacts with nitric oxide (NO). Key antioxidant enzymes (in bold) and the reactions they catalyze are shown. Abbreviations: CAT, catalase; GPX, glutathione peroxidase; GSR, glutathione reductase; GST, glutathione-S-transferase; PRDX, peroxiredoxin; SOD, superoxide dismutase. GPXs and GSTs require glutathione (GSH) as a cofactor, and GSH can also scavenge free radicals through direct chemical reactions. GSR reduces the oxidized form of GSH (GSSG, glutathione disulfide).

and antioxidant levels fall transiently after the preovulatory gonadotropin surge, and treatment with antioxidants inhibits ovulation (Laloraya et al. 1988, Miyazaki et al. 1991, Sato et al. 1992, Shkolnik et al. 2011). There are numerous redox (reduction/oxidation) elements in cells, such as redox-sensitive cysteine residues in proteins, which function in cell signaling, macromolecular trafficking, and regulation of physiological processes. These elements are components of redox circuits and networks, which are controlled by two thiol-containing systems, thioredoxins (TXN) and glutathione (GSH) (Jones 2008). These systems are not in thermodynamic equilibrium with one another, and each system exists in separate cytosolic, mitochondrial, and other subcellular compartments (Go and Jones 2008, Hansen et al. 2006). While oxidative stress was previously defined as oxidative damage to lipids, proteins, and nucleic acids by free radicals, the "redox hypothesis" expands the definition of oxidative stress to include disruption of intracellular redox circuits (Jones 2008).

4.2 ANTIOXIDANT DEFENSES IN THE OVARY

Antioxidant defenses are abundant in cells and include antioxidant enzymes and radical scavenging chemicals (Figure 4.1). Vitamins E (tocopherols) and C (ascorbate) directly react with free radicals to detoxify them. Ascorbate is present at millimolar concentrations in ovarian cells and at 50–200 μM in human follicular fluid (Luck et al. 1995, Zreik et al. 1999). Ascorbate is concentrated in granulosa cells, theca cells, luteal cells, and oocytes, and its uptake and release are hormonally regulated (Aten et al. 1992, Behrman et al. 1996, Luck et al. 1995, Musicki et al. 1996,

Zreik et al. 1999). Vitamin A levels increase in the rat ovary during follicular development and increase further during luteal regression (Aten et al. 1992). Levels of the vitamin A precursor β-carotene and α-tocopherol increase in bovine corpora lutea with increasing progesterone levels (Hanukoglu 2006), and luteal regression in the rat is associated with increased ovarian vitamin E levels (Aten et al. 1992).

The cysteine-containing tripeptide GSH is another key antioxidant, which is present in cells at millimolar concentrations. GSH can scavenge free radicals directly and can reduce peroxides as a cofactor for GSH peroxidases (GPXs), cycling between its reduced and oxidized, disulfide (GSSG) forms. The enzyme GSSG reductase (GSR), which requires NADPH as an electron donor, ensures that the GSH/GSSG redox potential is generally maintained in a highly reduced state. GSH is covalently linked to electrophilic chemicals by the glutathione-*S*-transferase (GST) enzymes, which aids in the detoxification and excretion of toxicants (Hayes and Pulford 1995). Emerging evidence suggests that *S*-glutathionylation of proteins is also catalyzed by GSTs, while the deglutathionylation is catalyzed by glutaredoxins (GRXs; cytosolic GRX1 and mitochondrial GRX2) (Anathy et al. 2012). Glutathionylation is an important mechanism for the regulation of protein activity (Jones 2008, Anathy et al. 2012). Ovarian GSH concentrations increase during equine chorionic gonadotropin (eCG)-stimulated follicular development in the rat due to increased protein levels of the subunits of glutamate cysteine ligase (GCL), the rate-limiting enzyme in GSH synthesis, and resulting in increased GCL enzymatic activity (Aten et al. 1992, Tsai-Turton and Luderer 2005). GSH synthesis is upregulated in ovarian follicles and granulosa cells by the combined actions of follicle-stimulating hormone (FSH) and estradiol to increase mRNA and protein levels of the modifier (GCLM) and the catalytic (GCLC) subunit of GCL (Hoang et al. 2009, Tsai-Turton and Luderer 2006).

TXNs (cytosolic TXN and mitochondrial TXN2) are small proteins with a dithiol motif that allows them to reduce disulfide bonds on other proteins; during this process, the thiols on the TXN form a disulfide, which is reduced by the action of TXN reductases (TXNRD) in the presence of NADPH (Murphy 2012). Peroxiredoxins (PRDXs), which reduce H_2O_2 and allyl peroxides (Figure 4.1), are among the important proteins that are reduced by TXNs (Murphy 2012). Expression of *Txn*2 and *Prdx3*, both localized to the mitochondria, decline with aging in the mouse ovary, concomitant with increased oxidative damage to cellular macromolecules (Lim and Luderer 2011).

Other antioxidant systems directly detoxify SO and H_2O_2. Superoxide dismutases (SOD) catalyze the dismutation of SO to H_2O_2 and oxygen (Figure 4.1). There are three main forms of SOD, copper–zinc SOD (SOD1, Cu-Zn-SOD) in cytosol; manganese SOD (SOD2, Mn-SOD) in mitochondria, and extracellular SOD (SOD3). Catalase (CAT), GPXs, PRDXs, and some GSTs can convert H_2O_2 to water (Figure 4.1). In the ovary, mRNA expression of *Sod2* and *Sod3*, but not *Sod1*, GPX, or catalase, increased during eCG-stimulated follicular development (Tilly and Tilly 1995). The eCG-induced increase in *Sod2* mRNA was localized primarily to the theca interna cells of growing follicles (Sasaki et al. 1994). *Sod2* expression in the theca interna was further increased and granulosa cell expression also increased after ovulatory human CG treatment (Sasaki et al. 1994). Activity and protein levels of SOD1, SOD2, and SOD3 were all highest in follicular fluid of small bovine antral follicles and declined with increasing antral follicle size; protein expression of the three SODs was observed in oocytes and mural granulosa cells, but only SOD3 and SOD2 were detected in cumulus cells and none of these varied with antral follicle size in the bovine (Combelles et al. 2010). Total antioxidant capacity increased, while catalase protein expression and H_2O_2 decreased as bovine antral follicle size increased (Gupta et al. 2011). SOD and catalase activities were highest at the time of peak luteal progesterone production in the bovine ovary (Hanukoglu 2006).

4.3 EVIDENCE FOR XENOBIOTIC-INDUCED OXIDATIVE STRESS IN OVARIAN FOLLICLE TOXICITY

4.3.1 Antioxidant Depletion

Studies showing that antioxidant depletion induces follicular atresia and that antioxidant supplementation inhibits follicular atresia provide evidence that oxidative stress plays a role in initiating follicular atresia. Biochemical depletion of GSH *in vivo* by treatment with two doses of 5 mmol/kg buthionine sulfoximine (BSO, a specific inhibitor of GCL) administered 12 h apart, decreased ovarian GSH concentrations by more than 50% and significantly increased the percentage of atretic antral follicles in adult rat ovaries whether treatment was initiated on proestrus or estrus (Lopez and Luderer 2004). Culture of small and large antral rat follicles without gonadotropin is known to cause apoptosis, while culture with FSH inhibits apoptosis (Chun et al. 1994, 1996). As noted previously, gonadotropin treatment increases ovarian expression of antioxidant genes *in vivo* and in cultured follicles. Treatment with the antioxidants ascorbate, SOD, catalase, or *N*-acetylcysteine inhibited apoptosis, measured by DNA laddering on gel electrophoresis, in cultured large antral rat follicles as effectively as FSH (Tilly and Tilly 1995). When large antral rat follicles were cultured without gonadotropin support, ROS generation increased in a time-dependent manner, while FSH treatment increased follicular GSH levels and inhibited ROS generation (Tsai-Turton and Luderer 2006). Importantly, the rise in ROS preceded increases in indicators of apoptosis (TUNEL and caspase three activation in granulosa cells). When GSH was depleted using BSO in the presence of FSH, there was a significant increase in granulosa cell apoptosis, assessed by TUNEL and activated caspase three immunostaining, and supplementation with a cell-permeable form of GSH prevented this increase in apoptosis (Tsai-Turton and Luderer 2006). Taken together, these studies provide strong evidence that at least some of the antiapoptotic effects of FSH in antral follicles are mediated by upregulation of antioxidant gene expression and that increased ROS production may be an initiating event in antral follicle atresia. The following sections discuss evidence that ROS production mediates the induction of apoptosis by various toxicants in ovarian follicles.

4.3.2 Polycyclic Aromatic Hydrocarbons

Polycyclic aromatic hydrocarbons (PAHs) are ubiquitous environmental pollutants produced during the incomplete combustion of organic materials. Sources of exposure include particulate matter air pollution, tobacco smoke, and grilled foods.

The PAHs benzo[a]pyrene (BaP), 9,10-dimethyl-1,2-benzanthracene (DMBA), and 3-methylcholanthrene (3-MC) destroy primordial and primary follicles in peripubertal mice and rats after both single high doses (Mattison 1979, Mattison and Thorgeirsson 1979, Mattison et al. 1980) and repeated low doses (Borman et al. 2000). Mice are more sensitive than rats to the primordial follicle toxicity of PAHs (Borman et al. 2000, Mattison 1979). Exposure to cigarette smoke, a major source of PAHs, depletes primordial follicles in mice (Tuttle et al. 2009). Primordial follicles in human ovarian explants are also sensitive to destruction by DMBA (Matikainen et al. 2001). In addition to destroying small follicles, 3-MC targets secondary follicles in rats (Borman et al. 2000), and DMBA destroys antral follicles, apparently targeting the granulosa cells (Mattison 1980). Experiments using cultured large antral rat follicles showed that DMBA induced granulosa cell apoptosis in a concentration-dependent manner, with increased protein levels of the proapoptotic protein BAX by 24 h and increased levels of activated caspase 3 and oligonucleosomal DNA fragmentation after 48 h of culture with ≥1 μM DMBA (Tsai-Turton et al. 2007b). Follicular ROS levels, assessed using dichlorofluorescein fluorescence, increased by 12 h, suggesting that this might be the signal initiating apoptosis. The latter conclusion is supported by the observations that supplementation of GSH protected against DMBA-induced apoptosis, while GSH depletion using BSO, an inhibitor of GCL, potentiated DMBA-induced apoptosis (Tsai-Turton et al. 2007b). In contrast, supplementation with the antioxidants butylated hydroxytoluene or dithiothreitol did not protect against DMBA-induced apoptosis (Tsai-Turton et al. 2007b). Therefore, additional studies are needed to clarify the role of ROS in the initiation of apoptosis in antral follicles by DMBA. Thus far, no studies have examined the role of oxidative stress in follicular atresia induced by *in vivo* treatment with PAHs. One study suggested that oxidative stress, as measured by increased protein levels of heat shock protein 25 and decreased SOD2 protein levels, plays a role in the depletion of ovarian follicles by *in vivo* exposure to tobacco smoke, which contains dozens of PAHs. However, this study did not find any effects of tobacco smoke exposure on markers of oxidative protein and DNA damage, and GSH concentrations (Gannon et al. 2012).

4.3.3 Ionizing Radiation

Women who have been treated for cancer with ionizing radiation to the pelvis frequently develop temporary amenorrhea or premature ovarian failure (Lo Presti et al. 2004, Meirow and Nugent 2001). Permanent ovarian failure more commonly occurs with higher doses of radiation and in older women. Ionizing radiation destroys follicles at all stages of development, from primordial to antral follicles in rodents and humans (Hanoux et al. 2007, Jarrell et al. 1987, Kim and Lee 2000, Meirow and Nugent 2001). Destruction of primordial follicles decreases the ovarian reserve, which advances the age of ovarian senescence (menopause in humans) (Kerr et al. 2012). Mathematical models have been used to predict that the estimated dose of ionizing radiation required to destroy half of the primordial follicles in young women is less than 2 Gray (Wallace et al. 1989, 2003). Destruction of later stages of follicular development causes temporary cessation of cycling, but cycles resume once less mature follicles have grown to the ovulatory stage.

In addition to direct ionizations of DNA, exposure of cells to ionizing radiation leads to the generation of ROS due to indirect ionization of water molecules (Spitz et al. 2004, Wiseman and Halliwell 1996), and there is evidence that the toxic effects of ionizing radiation on ovarian follicles are mediated by ROS. Degeneration of primordial and primary follicles was observed as early as 2 h after gamma irradiation of postnatal day 21 mice with a dose of 8.3 Gray (Kim and Lee 2000, Lee et al. 2000). Pretreatment with 100 μg of the antioxidant melatonin significantly protected against radiation-induced primordial follicle destruction at all time points, while 10 μg was less protective; beneficial effects of melatonin were less consistent for primary and larger, growing follicles (Kim and Lee 2000). Rapid, sustained increases in ROS occurred in human COV434 granulosa cells within 30 min after 1 or 5 Gray gamma irradiation, followed by apoptotic death at 6 h (Cortés-Wanstreet et al. 2009). Stable overexpression of one or both subunits of the rate-limiting enzyme in GSH synthesis, *Gclc* and *Gclm*, increased GSH synthesis, prevented the radiation-induced rise in ROS, and prevented apoptotic death of the cells (Cortés-Wanstreet et al. 2009). Taken together, the available data support a role for ROS in initiating apoptosis in granulosa cells and ovarian follicles, but detailed understanding of the mechanisms awaits further study.

4.3.4 Cyclophosphamide

Treatment of women for cancer and autoimmune diseases with alkylating antineoplastic drugs, similar to treatment with ionizing radiation, can cause temporary amenorrhea or premature ovarian failure, consistent with destruction of large, growing follicles and of primordial follicles, respectively (Byrne 1999, Chemaitilly et al. 2006, Howell and Shalet 1998, Meirow and Nugent 2001, Nicosia et al. 1985). Even if menstrual cycles resume, women may subsequently undergo early menopause due to partial depletion of the primordial follicle pool. The cancer therapeutic action of alkylating agents such as cyclophosphamide (CP) results from their ability to alkylate DNA of cancer cells. Unfortunately, DNA damage to nontarget cells may play a role in many of their side effects. CP destroys follicles at all stages of development in rodents and humans (Davis and Maronpot 1996, Jarrell et al. 1987, Kumar et al. 1972, Plowchalk and Mattison 1991, Shiromizu et al. 1984, Warne et al. 1973). Mice are much more sensitive than rats to the primordial follicle toxicity of CP (Meirow et al. 1999, Shiromizu et al. 1984), but rats are highly sensitive to destruction of secondary and antral follicles by CP (Davis and Heindel 1998).

CP requires metabolic activation to exert its anticancer activity, undergoing oxidation by cytochrome P450 enzymes to 4-hydroxycyclophosphamide, which undergoes ring-opening to aldophosphamide, which spontaneously decomposes to phosphoramide mustard (PM) (Chang et al. 1993, Dirven et al. 1994, Gamcsik et al. 1999). PM is thought to be the active metabolite of CP, in terms of both its anticancer activity and its ovarian toxicity (Gamcsik et al. 1999, Plowchalk and Mattison 1991). Treatment of cultured neonatal mouse and rat ovaries, which are enriched in primordial follicles, with PM-depleted primordial follicles at concentrations ≥3 and 30 μM, respectively (Desmeules and Devine 2006, Petrillo et al. 2011). Depletion of primordial follicles by PM did not involve caspase activation (Desmeules and

Devine 2006). However, immunostaining for phosphorylated histone H2AFX, a marker of double-stranded DNA breaks, was increased in oocytes of primordial follicles at concentrations that caused follicle depletion and at time points prior to the onset of follicle degeneration, suggesting that the DNA strand breaks initiate follicular destruction (Petrillo et al. 2011). Double-stranded DNA breaks can be caused by oxidative DNA lesions (Lloyd et al. 1998); however, direct evidence for oxidative DNA damage in primordial follicles by PM is lacking.

As noted previously, secondary and antral follicles are targeted by *in vivo* dosing with CP in adult rats. A single i.p. dose as low as 50 mg/kg significantly increased the percentage of secondary and antral follicles that displayed apoptotic granulosa cells by TUNEL, activated caspase-9 immunostaining, and activated caspase-3 immunostaining 24 h later (Devine et al. 2012, Lopez and Luderer 2004). These data are consistent with caspase-dependent apoptosis of granulosa cells driving the CP-induced destruction of secondary and antral follicles, unlike the absence of caspase involvement in the destruction of primordial follicles described earlier (Desmeules and Devine 2006). The COV434 human granulosa cell tumor line has been used as a model to study the mechanisms by which CP induces apoptosis in steroidogenically active granulosa cells (Tsai-Turton et al. 2007a). These experiments utilized a preactivated form of CP, 4–hydroperoxycyclophosphamide (4HC), which spontaneously decomposes in solution to 4-hydroxycyclophosphamide (Flowers et al. 2000, Gamcsik et al. 1999). Treatment with 4HC (1–50 μM) caused a rapid (within the first 2 h), concentration-dependent decrease in GSH concentrations and increase in ROS measured by dichlorofluorescein fluorescence, followed at 12 and 24 h by oxidative DNA damage measured by 8–hydroxy-2′–deoxyguanosine (8-OHdG) immunofluorescence, activation of caspase-3, and DNA fragmentation measured by TUNEL (Tsai-Turton et al. 2007a). Supplementation with glutathione ethyl ester, a cell-permeable form of GSH, or with the antioxidants ascorbate or dithiothreitol protected against the induction of apoptosis by 4HC, while depletion of GSH with BSO enhanced the induction of apoptosis by 4HC (Tsai-Turton et al. 2007a). These data show that the early rise in ROS is a key event initiating the induction of apoptosis in granulosa cells by 4HC.

4.3.5 Methoxychlor

The organochlorine insecticide, methoxychlor, was used as a more rapidly metabolized alternative to DDT; it has been banned in the United States since 2002 (http://www.epa.gov/oppsrrd1/REDs/methoxychlor_red.htm). *In vivo* administration of methoxychlor for 20 days at doses ≥32 mg/kg in adult mice resulted in atresia of antral follicles, but not smaller follicles (Borgeest et al. 2002). Similar doses and treatment duration with methoxychlor also increased ovarian concentrations of H_2O_2, as well as ovarian immunostaining for 8–OHdG and nitrotyrosine, which are markers of oxidative DNA damage and oxidative protein damage, respectively (Gupta et al. 2006b). These increases in oxidative damage markers were associated with decreased ovarian enzymatic activity and mRNA levels of SOD1, catalase, and GPX (Gupta et al. 2006b). Treatment of cultured antral follicles with methoxychlor (1–100 μg/mL) decreased follicle growth and increased histological evidence of atresia in a concentration- and time-dependent manner (Gupta et al. 2006a). The mRNA levels of GPX and catalase increased in the 100 μg/mL group at 48 h of culture, prior to the earliest evidence of decreased growth, while expression of *Sod1*, *Gpx*, and catalase were significantly decreased by all doses at 96 h, when marked growth inhibition was evident (Gupta et al. 2006a). Cotreatment with the GSH precursor and antioxidant, *N*-acetylcysteine, prevented the effects of methoxychlor on follicle growth, atresia, and antioxidant gene expression (Gupta et al. 2006a). Taken together, these findings support a role for oxidative stress in mediating methoxychlor-induced antral follicle atresia.

In contrast to lack of effects of methoxychlor treatment on small follicles in the adult mouse ovary, Sobinoff et al. found that methoxychlor treatment of neonatal mice for 7 days with 100 mg/kg/day, but not with 50 mg/kg/day, decreased primordial follicle numbers while increasing activating and primary follicle numbers (Sobinoff et al. 2010). These findings suggest that methoxychlor treatment of neonatal mice accelerated primordial follicle activation, and microarray analysis showed that methoxychlor treatment upregulated signaling pathways associated with follicular growth and development, including the PI3K/Akt pathway (Sobinoff et al. 2010). When PND four mouse ovaries were cultured with methoxychlor for 96 h, ovarian oxidative DNA damage, assessed by 8-hydroxy-2′-deoxyguanosine immunostaining, was increased (Sobinoff et al. 2010). The authors speculated that increased ROS generated as a result of methoxychlor metabolism perturbed cysteine oxidation, which increased PI3K/Akt signaling.

4.3.6 Phthalates

Phthalate esters are used to impart flexibility to plastics and are ubiquitous environmental pollutants. Mono(2-ethylhexyl) phthalate (MEHP) is the active metabolite of one of the most commonly used plasticizers, di(2–ethylhexyl) phthalate (DEHP), and both of these compounds have been shown to inhibit follicle growth in cultured antral mouse follicles (Wang et al. 2012a,b). Inhibition of growth by MEHP was preceded by increased expression of the proapoptotic gene *Bax* and decreased expression of the antiapoptotic gene *Bcl2*, as well as of several cell cycle regulatory genes (Wang et al. 2012b). ROS were measured in cultured antral follicles using an assay kit that utilizes the oxidation-sensitive fluorophore, dichlorofluorescein (Wang et al. 2012a,b). A concentration of DEHP (10 μg/mL) that inhibited follicle growth increased ROS at 24, 48, 72, and 96 h of culture, while MEHP at ≥1 μg/mL concentration-dependently increased ROS production at 96 h (Wang et al. 2012a,b). Protection against growth inhibition by both compounds was afforded by treatment with the GSH precursor and antioxidant, *N*–acetylcysteine (NAC). NAC also prevented the changes in apoptosis-related and cell cycle regulatory genes caused by MEHP (Wang et al. 2012b). These very recent findings add phthalate to the growing list of antral follicle toxicants, which appear to initiate apoptosis via an ROS-dependent pathway.

4.3.7 Chromium

The heavy metal chromium (Cr) is used in various industrial applications, including electroplating, leather tanning, wood preservatives, and steel alloys

(Keegan et al. 2008). In addition to occupational exposures, pollution resulting from such processes, as well as naturally occurring Cr, can contaminate drinking water supplies, potentially exposing the general population. Cr exists in several oxidation states, of which CrIII is the most stable. CrVI is a known carcinogen; it is rapidly reduced to CrIII *in vivo* by ascorbate, GSH, and cysteine, but during reduction reactive Cr species and ROS are generated (O'Brien et al. 2003). Exposure to Cr via drinking water decreased sperm counts and antioxidant activities, while increasing H_2O_2 concentration, in the semen of male monkeys, suggesting a role for oxidative stress in its reproductive toxicity (Subramanian et al. 2006).

Treatment of adult mice with Cr in drinking water caused follicular atresia (Murthy et al. 1996). The effects of Cr have been studied in a rat model of lactational exposure; lactating female rats were administered 200 mg/L potassium dichromate with or without 500 mg/L ascorbate in the drinking water from the day of birth until their pups were weaned at postnatal day (PND) 21 (Banu et al. 2008). Primordial and primary follicle numbers in the female offspring exposed to Cr via the milk were significantly decreased at PND 21, 45, and 65, while follicle numbers were not decreased in female offspring whose mothers were given Cr plus ascorbate (Banu et al. 2008). Secondary and antral follicle numbers were decreased in the Cr group at PND 21 and 45, but these follicle numbers recovered by PND 65 (Banu et al. 2008). Serum estradiol, testosterone, and progesterone concentrations were decreased at all time points, and FSH was increased at PND 21 and 45 in the Cr groups, and again ascorbate was protective (Banu et al. 2008). In rat granulosa cells, 10 μM potassium dichromate for 12 and 24 h induced apoptosis, as measured by TUNEL and cleavage of caspase-3 and PARP; induction of apoptosis was prevented by coadministration of a caspase inhibitor (Banu et al. 2011). In addition, translocation of proapoptotic BCL-2 family proteins BAX and BAD and of activated p53 from cytosol to the mitochondria, translocation of cytochrome c from mitochondria to cytosol, and decreased protein levels of antiapoptotic BCL-2 family members BCL-2 and BCL-XL were observed in Cr-treated cells, suggesting activation of the mitochondrial apoptotic pathway (Banu et al. 2011). In another study by the same group, 10 μM Cr also inhibited proliferation and induced cell cycle arrest in cultured rat granulosa cells (Stanley et al. 2011). Pretreatment with 1 mM ascorbate for 24 h mitigated all of these effects of Cr treatment (Banu et al. 2011, Stanley et al. 2011). While the protective effect of ascorbate is consistent with a role for oxidative stress in mediating the ovarian toxicity of Cr, it may simply reflect beneficial effects of reducing CrVI to CrIII. The interpretation is further complicated by evidence that ascorbate may be a pro-oxidant in the presence of Cr. More direct evidence for a role of oxidative stress in Cr-induced ovarian toxicity comes from a recent study in which female rats were continuously exposed to 200 mg/L Cr in the drinking water from GD9 to PND 65, first via treatment of their mothers during pregnancy and lactation and after weaning directly via the drinking water (Samuel et al. 2012). Concentrations of malondialdehyde, an indicator of lipid peroxidation, and H_2O_2 were measured in the ovaries at various ages from birth to PND 65 and were found to be significantly increased compared to controls that received drinking water without Cr (Samuel et al. 2012).

4.4 EVIDENCE FOR XENOBIOTIC-INDUCED OXIDATIVE STRESS IN OOCYTE TOXICITY

A recent study indicates that exposures to toxicants that do not result in destruction of the ovarian follicle may have long-lasting effects on the quality of the oocyte contained within that follicle. *In vivo* treatment of neonatal mice from PND 4 to 10 with the industrial chemical metabolite vinylcyclohexene diepoxide, methoxychlor, or the oxidant menadione dose-dependently decreased oocyte quality as measured by *in vitro* sperm binding and fusion to zona pellucida–free oocytes collected at 6 weeks of age (Sobinoff et al. 2010). Treatment of cultured superovulated oocytes from 6–8-week-old mice with vinylcyclohexene diepoxide, the ovotoxic methoxychlor metabolite 2,2-bis-(p-hydroxyphenyl)-1,1,1–trichloroethane, or menadione at concentrations from 0–25 μM concentration-dependently induced lipid peroxidation in oocytes as measured by BODIPY immunofluorescence (Sobinoff et al. 2010). Taken together, these results are consistent with the possibility that these three agents cause persistent abnormalities of oocyte quality due to lipid peroxidation of the oocyte plasma membrane.

Additional evidence for adverse effects of oxidative stress on oocyte quality comes from observations that oocytes collected for assisted reproduction from older women show signs of oxidative stress and are less likely to result in a successful pregnancy than oocytes from younger women. ROS increased with patient age in follicular fluid obtained at oocyte collection for *in vitro fertilization* (IVF) (Wiener-Megnazi et al. 2004). Follicular fluid levels of ROS were inversely correlated with the quality of ovulated oocytes and/or embryos in IVF patients (Das et al. 2006, Wiener-Megnazi et al. 2004). In human IVF patients, follicular fluid activities of the antioxidant enzymes, GSTs and catalase, declined with age, but SOD activity increased (Carbone et al. 2003). In another study of human IVF patients, SOD enzymatic activity and protein levels of SOD1 in cumulus cells surrounding ovulated oocytes decreased significantly with age, and lower levels of SOD activity were associated with unsuccessful IVF outcomes (Huang et al. 2006). Similarly, protein and mRNA levels of SOD1, SOD2, and catalase were lower, and percentages of cells with morphologically abnormal mitochondria were higher in cultured granulosa cells collected from 38- to 42-year-old IVF patients compared to those collected from 27- to 32-year-old IVF patients (Tatone et al. 2006).

Poor oocyte quality occurs in a mouse model of GSH deficiency, the *Gclm* null mouse, which has oocyte GSH concentrations that are less than 20% of wild-type levels (Nakamura et al. 2011). *Gclm* null females have small litters due to early preimplantation embryo mortality *in vivo*, with only about 10% of embryos surviving to the blastocyst stage at 3.5 days post coitum. Abnormal zygote development is evident at 0.5 days post coitum, with a significant decrease in the percentage of zygotes having two pronuclei and an increase in zygotes having only one pronucleus relative to zygotes from *Gclm+/+* females. The decreased formation of the second, male pronucleus confirms the importance of oocyte GSH in this process, which was first shown in studies using BSO to biochemically deplete oocyte GSH (Calvin et al. 1986, Perreault et al. 1988, Sutovsky and Schatten 1997). *In vitro* fertilization and embryo culture studies showed similar rates of progression to the 2-cell stage, but severely decreased progression to the blastocyst stage in embryos derived from oocytes of *Gclm–/–* mice compared to those from oocytes of *Gclm+/+* mice (Nakamura et al. 2011). At least some of these defects are likely due to increased oxidative stress during early development due to low GSH concentrations in the oocyte, as *de novo* GSH synthesis does not normally occur in the embryo until the blastocyst stage (Gardiner and Reed 1995a,b, Stover et al. 2000).

4.5 EVIDENCE FOR XENOBIOTIC-INDUCED OXIDATIVE STRESS IN FETAL OVARY TOXICITY

4.5.1 Polycyclic Aromatic Hydrocarbons

In addition to being toxic to the postnatal ovary, several studies have shown that prenatal exposure to PAHs destroys germ cells in the developing ovary. Treatment of pregnant mice from gestational day (GD) 7–16 with 10, 40, or 160 mg/kg/day BaP by oral gavage caused dose-dependent decrements in fertility of the F1 female offspring (MacKenzie and Angevine 1981). Ovarian histology showed that ovaries in the high-dose groups were essentially devoid of follicles. A role for ROS in mediating the transplacental ovarian toxicity of BaP is supported by a recent study, which showed that female embryos deficient in GSH synthesis due to deletion of the modifier subunit of the rate-limiting enzyme in its synthesis (*Gclm*) were more sensitive to the destruction of ovarian germ cells by prenatal exposure to BaP (Lim et al. 2012). In that study, pregnant *Gclm+/–* dams were treated with 0, 2, or 10 mg/kg/day BaP from GD7-16. F1 *Gclm–/–* female offspring exposed to BaP prenatally had significantly greater decrements in fertility and in ovarian follicle numbers than did their wild-type littermates (Lim et al. 2012). Previous work has shown that embryos constitutively express prostaglandin-endoperoxide synthase 1 and 2, that prostaglandin-endoperoxide synthases can bioactivate BaP to free radical intermediates that initiate ROS formation, that gestational treatment with BaP increases embryonic oxidative protein and DNA damage, and that antioxidants are protective against teratogenesis caused by BaP (Parman and Wells 2002, Wells et al. 2009, Winn and Wells 1997). Although these previous studies did not examine developmental toxicity to the ovary, the findings of increased sensitivity of GSH-deficient female embryos to transplacental ovarian toxicity of BaP provide further support for a role for oxidative stress in the developmental toxicity of BaP.

4.5.2 Ionizing Radiation

Exposure to 1.5 Gray ionizing radiation caused double-stranded DNA breaks, measured using phosphorylated histone H2AFX immunostaining, in oogonia of cultured human fetal ovary pieces (weeks 6–10 of gestation) and GD 12.5 mouse ovary treated *in vivo* or *in vitro* (Guerquin et al. 2009). At 1 h after irradiation, the number of phosphorylated histone H2AFX foci was similar in fetal testes and gonads, but the number of foci declined more rapidly thereafter in mouse ovaries than in testes, consistent with faster DNA repair in ovaries (Guerquin et al. 2009). Doses of 1.5 Gray and above induced germ cell apoptosis and significantly depleted ovarian germ cells by more than 50% in cultured human and mouse fetal ovaries by 48 h after irradiation. Induction of apoptosis in human and murine oogonia did not involve p53 or p63 (Guerquin et al. 2009). These results contrast with those for fetal testes, where germ cell apoptosis was induced at lower doses and induction of germ cell apoptosis involved p53 activation (Guerquin et al. 2009, Lambrot et al. 2007). Although there is no direct evidence for oxidative stress playing a role in ionizing radiation-induced fetal ovary toxicity, it is well known that exposure to ionizing radiation acutely increases ROS levels by water hydrolysis (Spitz et al. 2004, Wiseman and Halliwell 1996) and causes persistent increases in mitochondrial ROS production (Kim et al. 2006). Future studies should, therefore, examine the effects of ionizing radiation on fetal ovary ROS production and test the protective effects of antioxidants.

4.6 CONCLUSIONS

In the past decade, the importance of ROS and oxidative stress in ovarian toxicity and in normal female reproduction has been increasingly recognized. Endogenous ROS serve important functions as signaling molecules, for example, during ovulation, and have been implicated in the decline in ovarian function that occurs with normal aging. Accumulating evidence supports a role for ROS in initiating apoptosis in antral follicles upon exposure to diverse toxicants and ionizing radiation. Although less attention has been focused on the roles of ROS in primordial and primary follicle atresia, there is evidence that antioxidants are protective against primordial follicle destruction by a few agents, suggesting that ROS may play a role in these smaller follicles as well. Recently, oxidative stress in the oocyte caused by doses of toxicants that do not result in follicular atresia has been implicated in causing persistently decreased oocyte quality. Recent studies also suggest a possible role for oxidative stress in mediating fetal ovary toxicity. Future studies should aim to clarify the mechanisms by which ROS and oxidative stress damage follicles and ovarian germ cells, leading to atresia or altered function. In addition, studies are needed that test the ability of *in vivo* treatment with antioxidants to mitigate adverse effects of ovarian toxicants.

REFERENCES

Anathy, V., Roberson, E. C., Guala, A. S., Godburn, K. E., Budd, R. C., and Janssen-Heininger, Y. M. W. (2012) Redox-based regulation of apoptosis: *S*-glutathionylation as a regulatory mechanism to control cell death. *Antiox. Redox Signal.*, 16, 496–505.

Aten, R. F., Duarte, K. M., and Behrman, H. R. (1992) Regulation of ovarian antioxidant vitamins, reduced glutathione, and lipid peroxidation by luteinizing hormone and prostaglandin f_{2alpha}. *Biol. Reprod.*, 46, 401–407.

Banu, S. K., Samuel, J. B., Arosh, J. A., Burghardt, R. C., and Aruldhas, M. M. (2008) Lactational exposure to hexavalent chromium delays puberty by impairing ovarian development, steroidogenesis, and pituitary hormone synthesis in developing wistar rats. *Toxicol. Appl. Pharmacol.*, 232, 180–189.

Banu, S. K., Stanley, J. A., Lee, J., Stephen, S. D., Arosh, J. A., Hoyer, P. B., and Burghardt, R. C. (2011) Hexavalent chromium-induced apoptosis of granulosa cells involves selective sub-cellular translocation of bcl-2 members, ERK1/2 and p53. *Toxicol. Appl. Pharmacol.*, 251, 253–266.

Behrman, H. R., Preston, S. L., Aten, R. F., Rinaudo, P., and Zreik, T. G. (1996) Hormone induction of ascorbic acid transport in immature granulosa cells. *Endocrinology*, 137, 4316–4321.

Borgeest, C., Symonds, D. A., Mayer, L. P., Hoyer, P. B., and Flaws, J. A. (2002) Methoxychlor may cause ovarian follicular atresia and proliferation of the ovarian surface epithelium in the mouse. *Toxicol. Sci.*, 68, 473–478.

Borman, S. M., Christian, P. J., Sipes, I. G., and Hoyer, P. B. (2000) Ovotoxicity in female fischer rats and b6 mice induced by low-dose exposure to three polycyclic aromatic hydrocarbons: Comparison through calculation of an ovotoxic index. *Toxicol. Appl. Pharmacol.*, 167, 191–198.

Byrne, J. (1999) Long-term genetic and reproductive effects of ionizing radiation and chemotherapeutic agents on cancer patients and their offspring. *Teratology*, 59, 210–215.

Calvin, H. I., Grosshans, K., and Blake, E. J. (1986) Estimation and manipulation of glutathione levels in prepuberal mouse ovaries and ova: Relevance to sperm nucleus transformation in the fertilized egg. *Gamete Res.*, 14, 265–275.

Carbone, M. C., Tatone, C., Monache, S. D. et al. (2003) Antioxidant enzymatic defences in human follicular fluid: Characterization and age-dependent changes. *Mol. Hum. Reprod.*, 9, 639–643.

Chang, T. K., Weber, G. F., Crespi, C. L., and Waxman, D. J. (1993) Differential activation of cyclophosphamide and ifosphamide by cytochromes P-450 2B and 3A in human liver microsomes. *Cancer Res.*, 53, 5629–5637.

Chemaitilly, W., Mertens, A. C., Mitby, P. et al. (2006) Acute ovarian failure in the childhood cancer survivor study. *J. Clin. Endocrinol. Metab.*, 91, 1723–1728.

Chun, S.-Y., Billig, H., Tilly, J. L., Furuta, I., Tsafriri, A., and Hsueh, A. J. W. (1994) Gonadotropin suppression of apoptosis in cultured preovulatory follicles: Mediatory role of endogenous insulin-like growth factor I. *Endocrinology*, 135, 1845–1853.

Chun, S. Y., Eisenhauer, K. M., Minami, S., Billig, H., Perlas, E., and Hsueh, A. J. (1996) Hormonal regulation of apoptosis in early antral follicles: follicle-stimulating hormone as a major survival factor. *Endocrinology*, 137, 1447–1456.

Combelles, C. M. H., Holick, E. A., Paolella, L. J., Walker, D. C., and Wu, Q. (2010) Profiling of superoxide dismutase isoenzymes in compartments of the developing bovine antral follicles. *Reproduction*, 139, 871–881.

Cortés-Wanstreet, M. M., Giedzinski, E., Limoli, C. L., and Luderer, U. (2009) Overexpression of glutamate cysteine ligase protects human cov434 granulosa tumor cells against oxidative and γ-radiation-induced cell death. *Mutagenesis*, 24, 211–224.

Das, S., Chattopadhyay, R., Ghosh, S. et al. (2006) Reactive oxygen species level in follicular fluid—Embryo quality marker in IVF? *Hum. Reprod.*, 21, 2403–2407.

Davis, B. J. and Heindel, J. J. (1998) Ovarian toxicants: Multiple mechanisms of action. In Korach, K. S. (Ed.) *Reproductive and Developmental Toxicology*. New York, Marcel Dekker, Inc.

Davis, B. J. and Maronpot, R. R. (1996) Chemically associated toxicity and carcinogenicity of the ovary. In Huff, J., Boyd, J., and Barrett, J. C. (Eds.) *Cellular and Molecular Mechanisms of Hormonal Carcinogenesis: Environmental Influences*. New York, Wiley-Liss.

Desmeules, P. and Devine, P. J. (2006) Characterizing the ovotoxicity of cyclophosphamide metabolites on cultured mouse ovaries. *Toxicol. Sci.*, 90, 500–509.

Devine, P. J., Perreault, S. D., and Luderer, U. (2012) Roles of reactive oxygen species and antioxidants in ovarian toxicity. *Biol. Reprod.*, 86, 1–10.

Dirven, H. A. A. M., van Ommen, B., and van Bladeren, P. J. (1994) Involvement of human glutathione S-transferase isoenzymes in the conjugation of cyclophosphamide metabolites with glutathione. *Cancer Res.*, 54, 6215–6220.

Flowers, J., Ludeman, S. M., Gamcsik, M. P. et al. (2000) Evidence for a role of chloroethylaziridine in the cytotoxicity of cyclophosphamide. *Cancer Chemother. Pharmacol.*, 45, 335–344.

Gamcsik, M. P., Dolan, M. E., Andersson, B. S., and Murray, D. (1999) Mechanisms of resistance to the toxicity of cyclophosphamide. *Curr. Pharmaceut. Design*, 5, 587–605.

Gannon, A. M., Stämpfli, M. R., and Foster, W. G. (2012) Cigarette smoke exposure leads to follicle loss via an alternative ovarian cell death pathway in a mouse model. *Toxicol. Sci.*, 125, 274–284.

Gardiner, C. S. and Reed, D. J. (1995a) Glutathione redox cycle-driven recovery of reduced glutathione after oxidation by tertiary-butyl hydroperoxide in preimplantation mouse embryos. *Arch. Biochem. Biophys.*, 321, 6–12.

Gardiner, C. S. and Reed, D. J. (1995b) Synthesis of glutathione in the preimplantation mouse embryo. *Arch. Biochem. Biophys.*, 318, 30–36.

Go, Y. M. and Jones, D. P. (2008) Redox compartmentalization in eukaryotic cells. *Biochim. Biophys. Acta*, 1780, 1273–1290.

Guerquin, M.-J., Duquenne, C., Coffigny, H. et al. (2009) Sex-specific differences in fetal germ cell apoptosis induced by ionizing radiation. *Hum. Reprod.*, 24, 670–678.

Gupta, A., Choi, A., Yu, H.Y., Czerniak, S.M., Holick, E.A., Paolella, L.J., Agarwal, A., and Combelles, C.M.H. (2011) Fluctuations in total antioxidant capacity, catalase activity, and hydrogen peroxide levels of follicular fluid during bovine folliculogenesis. *Reprod. Fertil. Dev.*, 23, 673–680.

Gupta, R. K., Miller, K. P., Babus, J. K., and Flaws, J. A. (2006a) Methoxychlor inhibits growth and induces atresia of antral follicles through an oxidative stress pathway. *Toxicol. Sci.*, 93, 382–389.

Gupta, R. K., Schuh, R. A., Fiskum, G., and Flaws, J. A. (2006b) Methoxychlor causes mitochondrial dysfunction and oxidative damage in the mouse ovary. *Toxicol. Appl. Pharmacol.*, 216, 436–445.

Hall, P. F. (1994) Testicular steroid synthesis: Organization and regulation. In Knobil, E. and Neill, J. (eds.) *The Physiology of Reproduction*, 2nd edn. New York, Raven Press, Ltd.

Hanoux, V., Pairault, C., Bakalska, M., Habert, R., and Livera, G. (2007) Caspase-2 involvement during ionizing radiation-induced oocyte death in the mouse ovary. *Cell Death Differ.*, 14, 671–681.

Hansen, J. M., Go, Y.-M., and Jones, D. P. (2006) Nuclear and mitochondrial compartmentation of oxidative stress and redox signaling. *Annu. Rev. Pharmacol. Toxicol.*, 46, 215–234.

Hanukoglu, I. (2006) Antioxidant protective mechanisms against reactive oxygen species (ROS) generated by mitochondrial P450 systems in steroidogenic cells. *Drug Metab. Rev.*, 38, 171–196.

Hayes, J. D. and Pulford, D. J. (1995) The glutathione-*S*-transferase supergene family: Regulation of GST and the contribution of the isoenzymes to cancer chemoprevention and drug resistance. *Crit. Rev. Biochem. Mol. Biol.*, 30, 445–600.

Hoang, Y. D., Nakamura, B. N., and Luderer, U. (2009) Follicle-stimulating hormone and estradiol interact to stimulate glutathione synthesis in rat ovarian follicles and granulosa cells. *Biol. Reprod.*, 81, 636–646.

Howell, S. and Shalet, S. (1998) Gonadal damage from chemotherapy and radiotherapy. *Endocrinol. Metab. Clin. North Am.*, 27, 927–943.

Huang, T.-T., Naeemuddin, M., Elchuri, S. et al. (2006) Genetic modifiers of the phenotype of mice deficient in mitochondrial superoxide dismutase. *Hum. Mol. Genet.*, 15, 1187–1194.

Jarrell, J., Young Lai, E. V., Barr, R., McMahon, A., Belbeck, L., and O'Connell, G. (1987) Ovarian toxicity of cyclophosphamide alone and in combination with ovarian irradiation in the rat. *Cancer Res.*, 47, 2340–2343.

Jones, D. P. (2008) Radical-free biology of oxidative stress. *Am. J. Physiol.*, 295, C849–C868.
Keegan, G. M., Learmonth, I. D., and Case, C. P. (2008) A systematic comparison of the actual, potential, and theoretical health effects of cobalt and chromium exposures from industry and surgical implants. *Crit. Rev. Toxicol.*, 38, 645–674.
Kerr, J. B., Borgan, L., Myers, M. et al. (2012) The primordial follicle reserve is not renewed after chemical or γ-irradiation mediated depletion. *Reproduction*, 143, 469–476.
Kim, G. J., Fiskum, G., and Morgan, W. F. (2006) A role for mitochondrial dysfunction in perpetuating radiation-induced genomic instability. *Cancer Res.*, 66, 10377–10383.
Kim, J. K. and Lee, C. J. (2000) Effect of exogenous melatonin on the ovarian follicles in g-irradiated mouse. *Mutat. Res.*, 449, 33–39.
Kumar, R., Biggart, J. D., McEvoy, J., and McGeown, M. G. (1972) Cyclophosphamide and reproductive function. *Lancet*, June 3, 1212–1214.
Laloraya, M., Kumar, P. G., and Laloraya, M. M. (1988) Changes in the levels of superoxide anion radical and superoxide dismutase during the estrous cycle of rattus norvegicus and induction of superoxide dismutase in rat ovary by lutropin. *Biochem. Biophys. Res. Commun.*, 157, 146–153.
Lambrot, R., Coffigny, H., Pairault, C. et al. (2007) High radiosensitivity of germ cells in human male fetus. *J. Clin. Endocrinol. Metab.*, 92, 2632–2639.
Lee, C. J., Park, H. H., Do, B. R., Yoon, Y. D., and Kim, J. K. (2000) Natural and radiation-induced degeneration of the primordial and primary follicles in the mouse ovary. *Anim. Reprod. Sci.*, 59, 109–117.
Lim, J., Lawson, G. W., Nakamura, B. N. et al. (2012) Glutathione-deficient mice have increased sensitivity to transplacental benzo[a]pyrene-induced premature ovarian failure and ovarian tumorigenesis. *Cancer Res.*, 73, 1–10.
Lim, J. and Luderer, U. (2011) Oxidative damage increases and antioxidant gene expression decreases with aging in the mouse ovary. *Biol. Reprod.*, 84, 775–782.
Lloyd, D. R., Carmichael, P. L., and Phillips, D. H. (1998) Comparison of the formation of 8-hydroxy-2′-deoxyguanosine and single- and double-strand breaks in dna mediated by fenton reactions. *Chem. Res. Toxicol.*, 11, 420–427.
Lo Presti, A., Ruvulo, G., Gancitano, R. A., and Cittadini, E. (2004) Ovarian function following radiation and chemotherapy for cancer. *Eur. J. Obstet. Gynecol. Reprod. Biol.*, 113, S33–S40.
Lopez, S. G. and Luderer, U. (2004) Effects of cyclophosphamide and buthionine sulfoximine on ovarian glutathione and apoptosis. *Free Radic. Biol. Med.*, 36, 1366–1377.
Luck, M. R., Jeyaseelan, I., and Scholes, R. A. (1995) Minireview: Ascorbic acid and fertility. *Biol. Reprod.*, 52, 262–266.
MacKenzie, K. M. and Angevine, D. M. (1981) Infertility in mice exposed in utero to benzo(a) pyrene. *Biol. Reprod.*, 24, 183–191.
Matikainen, T., Perez, G. I., Jurisicova, A. et al. (2001) Aromatic hydrocarbon receptor-driven bax gene expression is required for premature ovarian failure caused by biohazardous environmental chemicals. *Nat. Genet.*, 28, 355–360.
Mattison, D. R. (1979) Difference in sensitivity of rat and mouse primordial oocytes to destruction by polycyclic aromatic hydrocarbons. *Chem. Biol. Interact.*, 28, 133–137.
Mattison, D. R. (1980) Morphology of oocyte and follicle destruction by polycyclic aromatic hydrocarbons in mice. *Toxicol. Appl. Pharmacol.*, 53, 249–259.
Mattison, D. R. and Thorgeirsson, S. S. (1979) Ovarian aryl hydrocarbon hydroxylase activity and primordial oocyte toxicity of polycyclic aromatic hydrocarbons in mice. *Cancer Res.*, 39, 3471–3475.
Mattison, D. R., White, N. B., and Nightingale, M. R. (1980) The effect of benzo(a)pyrene on fertility, primordial oocyte number, and ovarian response to pregnant mare's serum gonadotropin. *Pediatr. Pharmacol.*, 1, 143–151.

Meirow, D., Lewis, H., Nugent, D., and Epstein, M. (1999) Subclinical depletion of primordial follicular reserve in mice treated with cyclophosphamide: Clinical importance and proposed accurate investigative Tool. *Hum. Reprod.*, 14, 1903–1907.

Meirow, D. and Nugent, D. (2001) The effects of radiotherapy and chemotherapy on female reproduction. *Hum. Reprod. Update*, 7, 535–543.

Miyazaki, T., Sueoka, K., Dharmarajan, A. M., Atlas, S. J., Bulkley, G. B., and Wallach, E. E. (1991) Effect of inhibition of oxygen free radical on ovulation and progesterone production by the in vitro perfused rabbit ovary. *J. Reprod. Fertil.*, 91, 207–212.

Murphy, M. P. (2012) Mitochondrial thiols in antioxidant protection and redox signaling: distinct roles for glutathionylation and other thiol modifications. *Antiox. Redox Signal.*, 16, 476–495.

Murthy, R. C., Junaid, M., and Saxena, D. K. (1996) Ovarian dysfunction in mice following chromium (VI) exposure. *Toxicol. Lett.*, 89, 147–154.

Musicki, B., Kodaman, P. H., Aten, R. F., and Behrman, H. R. (1996) Endocrine regulation of ascorbic acid transport and secretion in luteal cells. *Biol. Reprod.*, 54, 399–406.

Nakamura, B. N., Fielder, T. J., Hoang, Y. D. et al. (2011) Lack of maternal glutamate cysteine ligase modifier subunit (*Gclm*) decreases oocyte glutathione concentrations and disrupts preimplantation development in mice. *Endocrinology*, 152, 2806–2815.

Nicosia, S. V., Matus-Riley, M., and Meadows, A. T. (1985) Gonadal effects of cancer therapy in girls. *Cancer*, 55, 2364–2372.

O'Brien, T. J., Ceryak, S., and Patierno, S. R. (2003) Complexities of chromium carcinogenesis: Role of cellular response, repair, and recovery mechanisms. *Mutat. Res.*, 533, 3–36.

Parman, T. and Wells, P. G. (2002) Embryonic prostaglandin H synthase-2 (PHS-2) expression and benzo[*a*]pyrene teratogenicity in PHS-2 knockout mice. *FASEB J.*, 16, 1001–1009.

Perreault, S. D., Barbee, R. R., and Slott, V. L. (1988) Importance of glutathione in the acquisition and maintenance of sperm nuclear decondensing activity in maturing hamster oocytes. *Dev. Biol.*, 125, 181–186.

Petrillo, S. K., Desmeules, P., Truong, T.-Q., and Devine, P. J. (2011) Detection of DNA damage in oocytes of small ovarian follicles following phosphoramide mustard exposures of cultured rodent ovaries *in Vitro. Toxicol. Appl. Pharmacol.*, 253, 84–102.

Plowchalk, D. R. and Mattison, D. R. (1991) Phosphoramide mustard is responsible for the ovarian toxicity of cyclophosphamide. *Toxicol. Appl. Pharmacol.*, 107, 472–481.

Samuel, J. B., Stanley, J. A., Sekar, P., Princess, R. A., Sebastian, M. S., and Aruldhas, M. M. (2012) Persistent hexavalent chromium exposure impaired the pubertal development and ovarian histoarchitecture in wistar rat offspring. *Environ. Toxicol.*, DOI: 10.1002/tox.21810.

Sasaki, J., Sato, E. F., Nomura, T. et al. (1994) Detection of manganese superoxide dismutase mrna in the theca interna cells of rat ovary during the ovulatory process by in situ hybridization. *Histochemistry*, 102, 173–176.

Sato, E. F., Kobuchi, H., Edashige, K. et al. (1992) Dynamic aspects of ovarian superoxide dismutase isozymes during the ovulatory process in the rat. *FEBS Lett.*, 303, 121–125.

Shiromizu, K., Thorgeirsson, S. S., and Mattison, D. R. (1984) Effect of cyclophosphamide on oocyte and follicle number in sprague-dawley rats, C57BL/6N and DBA/2N mice. *Pediatr. Pharmacol.*, 4, 213–221.

Shkolnik, K., Tadmor, A., Ben-Dor, S., Nevo, N., Galiani, D., and Dekel, N. (2011) Reactive oxygen species are indispensable in ovulation. *Proc. Natl. Acad. Sci. USA*, 108, 1462–1467.

Sobinoff, A. P., Pye, V., Nixon, B., Roman, S. D., and McLaughlin, E. A. (2010) Adding insult to injury: effects of xenobiotic-induced preantral ovotoxicity on ovarian development and oocyte fusibility. *Toxicol. Sci.*, 118, 653–666.

Spitz, D. R., Azzam, E. I., Li, J. J., and Gius, D. (2004) Metabolic oxidation/reduction reactions and cellular response to ionizing radiation: A unifying concept in stress response biology. *Cancer Metastasis Rev.*, 23, 311–322.

Stanley, J. A., Lee, J., Nithy, T. K., Arosh, J. A., Burghardt, R. C., and Banu, S. K. (2011) Chromium-VI arrests cell cycle and decreases granulosa cell proliferation by down-regulating cyclin-dependent kinases (CDK) and up-regulating CDK-inhibitors. *Reprod. Toxicol.*, 32(1), 112–123.

Stover, S. K., Gushansky, G. A., Salmen, J. J., and Gardiner, C. S. (2000) Regulation of γ-glutamate cysteine ligase expression by oxidative stress in the mouse preimplantation embryo. *Toxicol. Appl. Pharmacol.*, 168, 153–159.

Subramanian, S., Rajendiran, G., Sekhar, P., Gowri, C., Govindarajulu, P., and Aruldhas, M. M. (2006) Reproductive toxicity of chromium in adult bonnet monkeys (*Macaca radiata* Geoffrey). Reversible oxidative stress in the semen. *Toxicol. Appl. Pharmacol.*, 215, 237–249.

Sutovsky, P. and Schatten, G. (1997) Depletion of glutathione during bovine oocyte maturation reversibly blocks the decondensation of the male pronucleus and pronuclear apposition during fertilization. *Biol. Reprod.*, 56, 1503–1512.

Tatone, C., Carbone, M. C., Falone, S. et al. (2006) Age-dependent changes in the expression of superoxide dismutases and catalase are associated with ultrastructural modifications in human granulosa cells. *Mol. Reprod. Dev.*, 12, 655–660.

Tilly, J. L. and Tilly, K. I. (1995) Inhibitors of oxidative stress mimic the ability of follicle-stimulating hormone to suppress apoptosis in cultured rat ovarian follicles. *Endocrinology*, 136, 242–252.

Tsai-Turton, M. and Luderer, U. (2005) Gonadotropin regulation of glutamate cysteine ligase catalytic and modifier subunit expression in the rat ovary is subunit and follicle stage-specific. *Am. J. Physiol.*, 289, E391–E402.

Tsai-Turton, M. and Luderer, U. (2006) Opposing effects of glutathione depletion and FSH on reactive oxygen species and apoptosis in cultured preovulatory rat follicles. *Endocrinology*, 147, 1224–1236.

Tsai-Turton, M., Luong, B. T., Tan, Y., and Luderer, U. (2007a) Cyclophosphamide-induced apoptosis in cov434 human granulosa cells involves oxidative stress and glutathione depletion. *Toxicol. Sci.*, 98, 216–230.

Tsai-Turton, M., Nakamura, B. N., and Luderer, U. (2007b) Induction of apoptosis by 9,10-dimethyl–1,2–benzanthracene (DMBA) in cultured preovulatory rat follicles is preceded by a rise in reactive oxygen species and is prevented by glutathione. *Biol. Reprod.*, 77, 442–451.

Tuttle, A. M., Stampfli, M., and Foster, W. G. (2009) Cigarette smoke causes follicle loss in mice ovaries at concentrations representative of human exposure. *Hum. Reprod.*, 24, 1452–1459.

Wallace, W. H. B., Shalet, S. M., Hendry, J. H., Morris-Jone, P. H., and Gattamaneni, H. R. (1989) Ovarian failure following abdominal irradiation in childhood: The radiosensitivity of the human oocyte. *Br. J. Radiol.*, 62, 995–998.

Wallace, W. H. B., Thomson, A. B., and Kelsey, T. W. (2003) The radiosensitivity of the human oocyte. *Hum. Reprod.*, 18, 117–121.

Wang, W., Craig, Z. R., Basavarajappa, M. S., Gupta, R. K., and Flaws, J. A. (2012a) Di(w-ehtylhexyl) phthalate inhibits growth of mouse ovarian antral follicles through an oxidative stress pathway. *Toxicol. Appl. Pharmacol.*, 258, 288–295.

Wang, W., Craig, Z. R., Basavarajappa, M. S., Hafner, K. S., and Flaws, J. A. (2012b) Mono (2-ethylhexyl) phthalate induces oxidative stress and inhibits growth of mouse antral follicles. *Biol. Reprod.*, 87(6), 152. DOI: 10.1095/biolreprod.112.102467.

Warne, G. L., Fairley, K. F., Hobbs, J. B., and Martin, F. I. R. (1973) Cyclophosphamide-induced ovarian failure. *N. Engl. J. Med.*, 289, 1159–1162.

Wells, P. G., McCallum, G. P., Chen, C. S. et al. (2009) Oxidative stress in developmental origins of disease: teratogenesis, neurodevelopmental deficits, and cancer. *Toxicol. Sci.*, 108, 4–18.

Wiener-Megnazi, Z., Vardi, L., Lissak, A. et al. (2004) Oxidative stress indices in follicular fluid as measured by the thermochemi-luminescence assay correlate with outcome parameters in in vitro fertilization. *Fertil. Steril.*, 82(Suppl 3), 1171–1176.

Winn, L. M. and Wells, P. G. (1997) Evidence for embryonic prostaglandin H synthase catalyzed bioactivation and reactive oxygen species-mediated oxidation of cellular macromolecules in pheytoin and benzo[a]pyrene teratogenesis. *Free Radic. Biol. Med.*, 22, 607–621.

Wiseman, H. and Halliwell, B. (1996) Damage to DNA by reactive oxygen and nitrogen species: Role in inflammatory disease and progression to cancer. *Biochem. J.*, 313, 17–29.

Zreik, T. G., Kodaman, P. H., Jones, E. E., Olive, D. L., and Behrman, H. R. (1999) Identification and characterization of an ascorbic acid transporter in human granulosa-lutein cells. *Mol. Hum. Reprod.*, 5, 299–302.

5 Ovotoxicity in Small Preantral Follicles

Patricia B. Hoyer and Connie J. Mark-Kappeler

CONTENTS

5.1 FOLLICULAR DEVELOPMENT

Development and maturation of oocytes occur within ovarian follicles. Successful ovulation requires appropriate follicular development, during which the follicle has passed through a number of distinct developmental stages (Hirshfield, 1991). Throughout the life of a mammalian female preceding each ovarian cycle, some follicles are selected to develop to maturity for ovulation and potential fertilization. The most immature stage of ovarian follicular development is termed primordial. This is the stage at which follicles first appear in the ovary of a developing female fetus. Development of a primordial (25 μm diameter) to an ovulatory follicle involves transitions through several stages as a pre-antral follicle (25–250 μm diameter; primordial, primary, small growing, large growing) and later as an antral follicle (>250 μm diameter; early antral and pre-ovulatory). The stages of follicular development toward ovulation involve a continuum of events, each providing further maturation of the follicular cells (Figure 5.1; Hoyer and Devine, 2001). Upon receipt of an as yet unknown signal for development, the primordial follicle is activated and becomes a primary follicle. As the follicle develops, there is proliferation of the granulosa cells surrounding the oocyte, and acquisition of a layer of theca interna cells surrounding the granulosa layer. Follicles progress from the primary stage to the growing stage when multiple layers of granulosa cells have formed around the

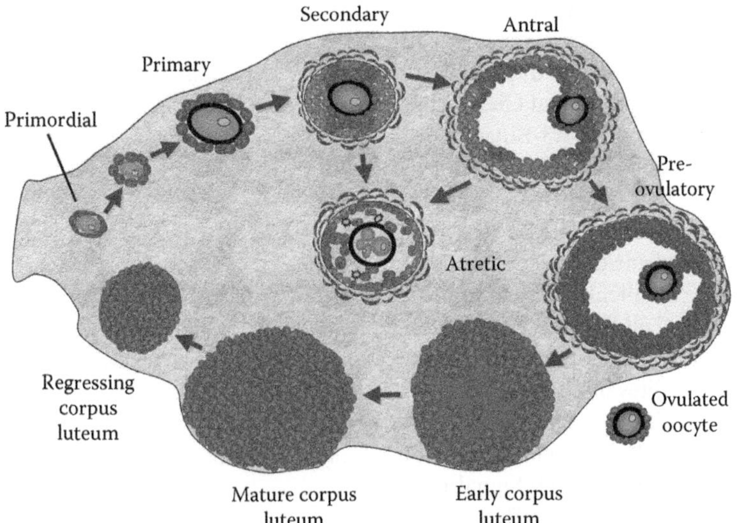

FIGURE 5.1 Development of ovarian follicles. Primordial follicles are activated to grow and develop from primary through secondary and antral stages of follicular development until ovulation. Most follicles degenerate by the process of atresia before reaching the ovulatory stage. Those follicles which do ovulate luteinize to become corpora lutea, which support pregnancy if fertilization occurs. (From Hoyer, P.B. and Devine, P.J., Endocrinology and toxicology: The female reproductive system, In *Handbook of Toxicology*, 2nd edn., eds. M.J. Derelanko and M.A. Hollinger, CRC Press, Boca Raton, FL, 2001. With permission from CRC Press.)

oocyte. When the follicle develops sufficiently, an antrum (fluid-filled space) develops within the granulosa cell layer. The antral follicle continues to grow, and at its most mature stage prior to ovulation is known as a Graaffian (pre-ovulatory) follicle. Resumption of meiosis in the oocyte occurs only at the time of impending ovulation. The exact mechanism for selection of a follicle for ovulation is not well understood, but is believed to be under intra-ovarian control (Richards, 1980).

5.1.1 Fetal Development

Because of the nature of fetal development of ovarian follicles, women are born with a set number of oocytes, which are not regenerated later in life. During fetal development, primordial germ cells that are formed invade the indifferent gonad and undergo rapid hyperplasia. By 1 month of embryonic life, primordial germ cells (oogonia) have become established in the genital ridge, and are proliferating by mitosis (Hoyer and Devine, 2001). During the period of mitotic proliferation of germ cells, somatic cells and supporting connective tissue develop and gradually become interspersed among the oogonia (Hoyer, 1997, 2005). Oogonia develop into oocytes in synchronous waves, once they stop dividing and enter into the first meiotic division. During this period, oocytes grow slowly and proceed to the diplotene stage of the meiotic prophase. The oocyte does not fully complete the first meiotic division at that time but becomes arrested until ovulation, if this should occur. Therefore, the number of oocytes at the time of birth is finite, and comprises the total germ cell pool available to a female throughout her life. Around the time of birth, small individual oocytes within the ovary become surrounded by a few flattened somatic cells (pregranulosa cells), and a basement membrane to form primordial follicles. Association of the granulosa cells with the oocyte at all times is critical for maintenance of viability, and follicle growth and development (Buccione et al., 1990).

5.1.2 Primordial Follicles

Primordial follicles consist of a small oocyte surrounded by a single layer of fusiform-shaped granulosa cells. The small oocyte contained in these follicles is arrested in prophase of the first meiotic division, is nondividing as follicles develop, and does not resume meiotic division until just prior to ovulation. Primordial follicles provide the pool for recruitment of developing follicles; therefore, they are a fundamental reproductive unit within the ovary. In humans, 1–2 pre-ovulatory follicles develop approximately every 28 days, whereas in rats 6–12 follicles develop every 4–5 days (Richards, 1980). The primordial follicles from which pre-ovulatory follicles develop are mainly located near the ovarian cortex and represent the pool for recruitment. Regular waves of the onset of development of primordial follicles are a continuous process from birth, until ovarian senescence occurs (Richards, 1980).

5.1.3 Primary Follicles

Some primordial follicles leave the quiescent state as soon as they are formed, and some are dormant for months or years. The first morphological sign of oocyte growth in primordial follicles is alteration of surrounding squamous (flattened) granulosa cells into cuboidal-shaped cells (follicular activation; Hirshfield, 1991). Once the follicle makes the transition from primordial to primary, other structural changes occur such as development of the zona pellucida, and acquisition of the theca layer. The zona pellucida is composed of a glycoprotein matrix to provide protection for the oocyte as well as to provide attachments for the specialized inner layer of granulosa cells, known as cumulus cells. At this stage, another layer of specialized somatic cells begin to proliferate and form a shell outside the basement membrane enclosing the oocyte and granulosa cell layer. These cells appear in concentric rings surrounding the follicle and are designated theca interna cells. Theca cells provide two important functions: (1) attachment of arterioles for the development of an independent blood supply and (2) secretion of progestins and androgens to regulate follicle development (Hirshfield, 1991).

5.1.4 Growing and Antral Follicles

The oocyte contained in a growing follicle has a large, spherical nucleus (germinal vesicle) that grows in proportion to the growth of the oocyte, and the somatic cells continue to proliferate and form a second layer around the oocyte. As the growing follicle continues to develop, the layers of granulosa cells surrounding the oocyte increase rapidly to reach follicular diameters of up to 250 μm. Gap junctions are formed between individual cells in the granulosa cell layer to facilitate intercellular transport of nutrients and metabolites to the oocyte (Hoyer, 1997). Collectively, primordial, primary, and growing follicles are <250 μm in diameter and are referred to as pre-antral follicles, with primordial and primary being considered small pre-antral follicles. As follicular growth continues, an antrum begins to form within the granulosa cell layer, and this fluid-filled cavity enlarges as the final stages of follicular development are reached. At that point, the follicle begins to come under an expanded set of autocrine, paracrine, and endocrine signals. The number of follicles that reach the antral stage is quite small. In women, usually only one follicle per menstrual cycle is chosen as the dominant follicle destined for ovulation.

5.1.5 Atresia

Throughout the reproductive life span of a female, the total number of primordial follicles selected to develop for ovulation is small compared to the total population. Instead, the vast majority are lost to attrition in various stages of development by a process called atresia. Ovarian content of oocytes is dynamic and fluctuates with age. The total number of oocytes peaks during embryonic development. In humans, the peak number of oocytes ever present, about seven million, occurs at 5 months' gestation, at birth the number has dropped to two million, 250,000–400,000 at puberty, and no functional oocytes remain at menopause (Hirshfield, 1991; Hoyer, 1997). During the lifetime of a woman, ovulation only accounts for 400–600 oocytes. Therefore, >99.9% of the primordial follicles a female is born with are lost by atresia at various stages of development.

5.2 CONSEQUENCES OF FOLLICULAR DESTRUCTION

5.2.1 Follicle-Specific Effects

For chemicals that destroy ovarian follicles, the stage of development at which the follicle is targeted affects the impact that exposure to the chemical will have on ovarian function (Hoyer and Sipes, 1996; Devine and Hoyer, 2005). Damage to large-growing or antral follicles can disrupt ovarian cyclicity by affecting steroid production and ovulation. Chemicals which selectively damage large-growing or antral follicles only temporarily interrupt ovarian cyclicity, because these follicles can be replaced by recruitment from the greater pool of primordial follicles. Thus, these chemicals are likely to produce a readily reversible form of infertility that is manifest as disrupted cyclicity relatively soon after exposure. In contrast, chemicals that extensively destroy oocytes contained in small pre-antral (primordial and primary) follicles can cause permanent infertility and premature ovarian failure (POF) (early menopause in women) since once a primordial follicle is destroyed, it cannot be replaced. Selective destruction of oocytes contained in primordial follicles may have a delayed effect on reproduction until such a time that recruitment for the number of growing and antral follicles can no longer be supported (Hooser et al., 1994; Mayer et al., 2002).

Although direct destruction of ovarian small pre-antral follicles may not immediately alter circulating hormone levels, the long-term result is disruption of negative feedback at the level of the hypothalamus and pituitary in response to loss of ovarian hormone regulation. Follicle stimulating hormone (FSH) produced in the anterior pituitary regulates follicular development, and is under a negative feedback regulation of release by ovarian hormones, such as estrogen, progesterone, and inhibin (Hadley and Levine, 2007). A primary effect at the ovarian level might cause a delayed disruption of this regulatory axis with FSH levels increasing due to loss of negative feedback from ovarian hormones. In a long-term study, female B6C3F1 mice were treated with the occupational chemical, 4-vinylcyclohexene (VCH), for 30 days (age 28–58 days) and then observed for 1 year (Hooser et al., 1994; Table 5.1). Although a greater than 90% loss of oocytes in small pre-antral follicles was measured at the end of 30 days of dosing, FSH levels in VCH-treated animals were only first observed to be increased above control animals at 240 days. Therefore, ovarian changes preceded the rise in circulating FSH levels. Also at 240 days, vaginal cytology still displayed evidence of ovarian cyclicity in VCH-treated mice. However, by 360 days (from the onset of dosing), unlike control animals, complete ovarian failure had resulted in VCH-treated mice, as determined by increased circulating levels of FSH, lack of cyclicity, the complete absence of ovarian follicular or luteal structures, and marked ovarian atrophy. Another study in Fischer 344 rats followed the consequences of 30 days of dosing with the diepoxide metabolite of VCH, 4-vinylcyclohexene diepoxide (VCD), for up to a year after the onset of VCD dosing (d360; Mayer et al., 2002). Following the end of dosing (d30), relative to controls, only 31% of primordial follicles remained. However, circulating FSH levels were only first elevated above control at the d120 time point, and ovarian failure was not observed until d360. Thus, the results in rats were similar to those in mice. From these studies, it was, therefore, concluded that the ovarian failure that occurs

TABLE 5.1
Long-Term Effects of 30d Dosing of Female B6C3F1 Mice with VCH[a,b]

Day[c]	Small Follicles (% Control)	Serum FSH (% above Control)	Estrous Cyclicity[d]
30	11*	30	Yes
120	3*	50	Yes
240	<1*	130*	Yes
360	0*	160*	No*

[a] Summarized from Hooser et al. (1994). With permission from Annual Review of Pharmacology and Toxicology.
[b] Data expressed as % control mice.
[c] Day after onset of dosing (30d).
[d] Determined by vaginal cytology.
* Different from control mice, $p < 0.05$.

long after cessation of dosing with VCH or VCD is an indirect consequence resulting from extensive depletion of small, pre-antral follicles.

5.2.2 Menopause

Ultimately, if the ovary is depleted of primordial follicles, ovarian failure occurs. Ovarian failure (menopause in women) is associated with the cessation of ovarian cyclicity. The average age of menopause in the United States is 51, and this is a direct consequence of depletion of the follicular reserve. Menopause has been associated with a variety of health problems in women. These include increases in osteoporosis, cardiovascular disease, colorectal cancer, depression, and Alzheimer's disease (Christensen et al., 1980; Paganini-Hill and Henderson, 1994; Sowers and LaPietra, 1995; Dhar, 2001; Marjoribanks et al., 2012). Additionally, in laboratory animals, POF is associated in the long term with an increased incidence of ovarian neoplasms (Hoyer and Sipes, 1996). A variety of environmental factors have been highly correlated with early menopause in women (Everson et al., 1986; Cooper et al., 1995; Sadeu et al., 2010; Gannon et al., 2012). Therefore, as a woman ages, her overall health is significantly affected by the onset of menopause, and this can be further impacted by environmental factors to which she has been exposed. Because of these health risks, the subject of this chapter is chemicals that have the potential to cause POF (early menopause) by destruction of ovarian small pre-antral follicles.

5.3 OVOTOXICITY IN SMALL PRE-ANTRAL FOLLICLES

5.3.1 Ionizing Radiation

Rapidly dividing primordial germ cells and oogonia present during fetal development in all species are highly sensitive to destruction (Dobson and Felton, 1983). Destruction of oocytes contained in ovarian primordial follicles can be caused by a variety of environmental chemicals (Mark-Kappeler et al., 2011a). Additionally, exposure to irradiation is known to also produce rapid destruction of oocytes contained in primordial follicles, followed by increased follicular atresia, stromal hypertrophy, and loss of ovarian weight (Dobson and Felton, 1983; Mierow et al., 2010; Aktas et al., 2012; Kerr et al., 2012). In animal studies, Mattison and Schulman (1980) noted that prenatal exposure to ionizing radiation also affects the number of oocytes and reproductive capacity of female offspring. More recently, it was shown in prepubertal female mice that exposure to irradiation caused degeneration of ovarian primordial and primary follicles by causing apoptosis in granulosa cells, oocytes, or both (Lee et al., 2000). These effects are suspected in humans because of reports of amenorrhea and sterility in women undergoing therapeutic irradiation (Chapman, 1983; Damewood and Grochow, 1986; Blumenfeld, 2012).

5.3.2 Chemotherapeutic Agents

A number of chemical agents have the potential to cause POF in women who have undergone chemotherapy for cancer (Mierow et al., 2010; Blumenfeld, 2012). Some of these include alkylating agents (cyclophosphamide [CPA], busulfan, chlorambucil, procarbazine, melphalan, chloromethamine), platinum agents (cisplatin, carboplatin), antibiotics (doxorubicin (DXR), bleomycin), toxoids (docetaxel, paclitaxel), plant alkaloids (vincristine, vinblastine), and antimtabolites (methotrexate, 5-fluorouracil, mercaptopurine; Blumenfeld, 2012). Because of the diversity of types of compounds, their mechanisms of action are likely to be quite varied. However, a common effect appears to be the result of damage/destruction of primordial follicles (Morgan et al., 2012). Recently, it has been demonstrated that circulating levels of anti-mullerian hormone (AMH, produced in the ovary) can provide an estimate of ovarian follicular reserve in girls undergoing cancer treatment (Brougham et al., 2012). Clinically, this can provide a reliable method to monitor the extent of gonotoxicity and ultimate potential for reversal of those effects during the course of therapy.

Since their early use as anti-neoplastic drugs, alkylating agents have been associated with ovarian failure. Animal studies have extensively confirmed this effect by observing follicle destruction caused by CPA. CPA significantly reduced the number of primordial and antral follicles in C57BL/6N and DBA/2N mice and Sprague Dawley (SD) rats, respectively (Shiromizu et al., 1984; Plowchalk and Mattison, 1991). CPA is a precursor for the active form of the drug that must be bioactivated (mostly by the liver) to have anti-cancer effects (Brock, 1967; Anderson et al., 1995). The active metabolites include 4-hydroxy-CPA, aldophosphamide, and phosphoramide mustard.

The relevance of chemotherapeutic-induced follicle loss to subsequent fertility has been a topic of great interest. One recent study assessed the effect of calorie restriction on CPA-induced primordial follicle loss in SD rats (Xiang et al., 2012). The results indicated that calorie restriction can increase the primordial follicle reserve and protect against CPA-induced ovotoxicity. Whether primordial follicle loss can be reversed by ovarian replenishment of that follicle pool was addressed (Kerr et al., 2012). Following *in vivo* exposure of mice to DXR, trichostatin A, or ionizing radiation, no evidence of follicular renewal was seen. Thus, these studies have emphasized the irreversibility of primordial follicle loss following the various therapies used to treat cancer.

Recent reports have addressed the potential for reversal or prevention of the ovotoxic effects of ionizing radiation or chemotherapeutic agents on ovarian primordial follicles. In one study, DXR was cultured with human ovarian cortical tissue (*in vitro*) or injected into SCID mice that had received a xenograph of human ovarian cortical tissue (Soleimani et al., 2011). Extensive damage to primordial follicles in the form of DNA strand breaks was observed in both systems and follicle survival rate was limited. Another study assessing DNA strand breaks investigated the effect of phosphoramide mustard on neonatal mouse ovaries in culture (Petrillo et al., 2011). This report concluded that this type of damage can be detected at lower concentrations than those that cause follicular loss. Conversely, in studies of *in vitro* incubation of cultured neonatal mouse ovaries with metabolites of CPA, extensive loss of primordial follicles was seen on day 8 of culture following a 2 day initial exposure (Desmeules and Devine, 2006). Therefore, there may be some mechanism of DNA repair within the ovary that responds to limited xenobiotic exposure.

In a 5–6 week study in Balb/c mice, CPA destroyed primordial follicles but left larger follicles and ovulation, mating and pregnancy rates intact (Meirow et al., 1999). In contrast, in a study in rats, it was shown that a single injection of CPA caused damage in growing and antral follicles, but spared an effect on primordial follicles, because cyclicity was disrupted within a week of this exposure, but had been restored within 2 weeks of the one-time exposure (Jarrell et al., 1991). Therefore, the impact of CPA on ovarian follicles may be species-dependent.

Collectively, from the research in animal studies, it appears that POF in women treated for cancer with chemo- or radiotherapeutic approaches is likely to be via destruction of primordial follicles.

5.3.3 Polycyclic Aromatic Hydrocarbons

Many animal studies have demonstrated ovotoxic effects of polycyclic aromatic hydrocarbons (PAHs). These chemicals are widely distributed in the environment because they are contained in cigarette smoke, automobile exhaust, and various other combustion processes (Mark-Kappeler et al., 2011a). Cigarette smoke contains high levels of the PAHs such as 9:10-dimethyl-1:2-benzanthracene (DMBA), benzo[a]pyrene (BaP), and 3-methylcholanthrene (3-MC; Mattison and Thorgeirsson, 1978; Vahakangas et al., 1985; Sobinoff et al., 2012). Krarup (1967, 1969) reported that DMBA depletes oocytes and produces ovarian tumors in mice. Subsequently, these effects have also been reported in a number of studies for 3-MC and BaP. Oocyte destruction was shown to occur in response to these three chemicals in mice and rats (Mattison, 1979; Borman et al., 2000; Mark-Kappeler et al., 2011a).

Several studies have demonstrated that mice are more susceptible to ovotoxicity from PAHs than rats (Mattison, 1979; Borman et al., 2000). Oocyte destruction in primordial and primary follicles was observed in mice treated with DMBA, BaP, and 3-MC (Mattison and Thorgeirsson, 1979). The relative toxicities for primordial follicles were DMBA > 3MC > BaP. Furthermore, a direct relationship between the dose of PAHs and destruction of primordial follicles has been shown in the mouse ovary. Daily oral exposure during pregnancy in mice between 7 and 16 days of gestation with high doses of BaP also caused complete sterility of the female offspring (Mackenzie and Angevine, 1981). Pregnant mice exposed to a lower dose (10 mg BaP/kg) gave birth to offspring with severely compromised fertility. In both studies, the litters of exposed mothers were smaller in number and size, compared with controls.

PAHs are not directly ovotoxic but require metabolic activation to reactive metabolites. Ovarian enzymes involved in the biotransformation (i.e., aryl hydrocarbon hydroxylase and epoxide hydrolase) of PAHs have been identified in mice and rats (Mattison et al., 1983), monkeys (Bengtsson and Mattison, 1989), and humans (Bengtsson et al., 1988). Therefore, oocyte destruction by PAHs may involve distribution of the parent compound to the ovary where ovarian enzymes metabolize the compound to reactive intermediates (Mattison et al., 1983).

5.3.4 Occupational Chemicals

5.3.4.1 1,3-Butadiene

1,3-Butadiene (BD) is an industrial compound used in the synthesis of polymers, resins, and plastics (International Agency for Research on Cancer, IARC, 1986). BD is also released as a by-product from the production of plastics, and is found in automobile exhaust, gasoline vapors, and cigarette smoke (NTP, 1984). BD and the related olefins, isoprene and styrene, are also released during the manufacture of synthetic rubber and thermoplastic resins and the estimated annual occupational exposure of U.S. employees has been estimated to be 3,700–1,000,000 people (IARC, 1986). These chemicals have also been reported in cigarette smoke and automobile exhaust. Chronic animal inhalation studies have shown that carcinogenesis caused by BD is higher in mice than rats. At lower doses, female mice exposed daily by inhalation for up to 2 years exhibited ovarian atrophy, granulosa cell hyperplasia, and benign and malignant granulosa cell tumors (Melnick et al., 1990). Thus, ovarian effects of BD appear to occur at lower concentrations than are required to produce effects in other tissues. Because of the possibility of epoxidation of these BD-related compounds, they have the potential to be ovotoxic and carcinogenic. Epoxide metabolites of BD were used in one study in female B6C3F1 mice dosed daily for 30 days. 1,3-butadiene monoepoxide (BMO, 1.43 mmol/kg) depleted small follicles by 98% and growing follicles by 87% compared with control animals (Doerr et al., 1995). At 0.14 mmol/kg another metabolite, 1,3-butadiene diepoxide (BDE) depleted small follicles by 85% and growing follicles by 63%. The findings supported that a diepoxide formed in the metabolism of BD is more potent at inducing follicle loss than BD itself. Additionally, isoprene was reported to be ovotoxic, whereas styrene and its monoepoxide did not reduce mouse ovarian follicle numbers (Doerr et al., 1995). The results of these studies demonstrated direct ovarian targeting of the ovary by the diepoxide of BD, and provided evidence that this is the ovotoxic form of the chemical. Therefore, based on animal studies, ovotoxicity with BD is considered a sensitive end point, which serves as an estimate of non-cancer risk assessment by regulatory agencies (Kirman and Grant, 2012).

5.3.4.2 4-Vinylcyclohexene

VCH is a dimer of 1,3-BD which forms spontaneously in the manufacture of BD (Keller et al., 1997). VCH is also used as an intermediate in the manufacture of flame retardants and plasticizers, as well as a solvent in the manufacture of VCD. Exposure to VCH is likely to be in the occupational and/or industrial setting. Workers could potentially be exposed to VCH during the production of 1,3-BD-based rubber, rubber vulcanization in the manufacture of shoe soles, tires, and other rubber products, as well as in the manufacture of flame retardants and insecticides. However, production policies in these venues have mandated that these chemical processes are performed in closed vessels. Thus, human exposure to VCH is limited, with the exception of accidental spills and leaks (IARC, 1994). Nonetheless, air concentrations of VCH have been measured in the workplace. For instance, levels of 0.03–0.21 mg/m^3 were measured in an Italian shoe plant, levels of 0–0.003 mg/m^3 were measured in an Italian tire factory, and levels of 0.24–0.43 mg/m^3 were measured in an American tire curing room (Rappaport and Fraser, 1977; IARC, 1994). After these short-term air concentration studies, the American Conference of Industrial Hygienists in 1992 established 0.4 mg/m^3 as a threshold value for VCH exposure in an 8 h period. Currently, there are no epidemiological studies to relate human exposures to adverse reproductive effects. However, in animal studies, ovarian damage caused by VCH and its related epoxide metabolites has been demonstrated by a variety of exposure routes, including dermal, oral, inhalation, and intraperitoneal injection (NTP, 1989; Smith et al., 1990; Grizzle et al., 1994; Bevan et al., 1996).

The occupational chemical, VCH, and its diepoxide metabolite, VCD, have been well characterized for their ability to cause selective loss of primordial and primary ovarian follicles in B6C3F1 mice and F344 rats (Smith et al., 1990; Flaws et al., 1994a,b; Springer et al., 1996a; Kao et al., 1999). This effect has more recently also been observed in SD rats (Kodama et al., 2009). The selective loss of primordial and primary follicles has been induced in postnatal day (pnd) 4 rats, in rats that were immature at the onset of dosing (age d28), and in adult rats (age d58; Flaws et al., 1994b; Devine et al., 2002). But, the studies have mostly characterized this follicle loss in d28 rats. Earlier structure–activity studies determined that the diepoxide metabolite, VCD, is the bioactive, ovotoxic form for inducing follicle loss in both mice and rats (Smith et al., 1990, Doerr et al., 1995).

5.3.4.3 2-Bromopropane

A more recently identified ovarian toxicant is 2-bromopropane (2BP, Boekelheide et al., 2004). Concern was raised over the toxicity of this chemical in 1996 due to adverse reproductive problems in workers in a Korean factory (Kim et al., 1996). Subsequent clinical investigations in Korea as well as experimental research in animals demonstrated adverse effects on hematopoiesis and the reproductive system in both males and females, in humans and rats (Park et al., 1997; Takeuchi et al., 1997). 2BP has been used as a cleaning agent, an intermediate for various chemical syntheses, and a replacement for chlorofluorocarbons. Because of the concerns raised in the Korean factory, 2BP use has been limited to some extent in the United States. However, it is also a contaminant of 1-bromopropane, which is widely used as a solvent for the manufacture of a variety of chemicals in the industrial setting (NTP, 2002). Human exposures, therefore, would predominantly occur in industrial settings, and could be through either dermal contact or inhalation. Further, the similarity of effects observed in humans and in experimental animals provides greater credibility to 2BP-induced reproductive effects. There is evidence that male and female germ cells are the ultimate targets of 2BP. Reduced numbers of early stages of spermatogonia (stage 1) were determined to be the initial morphological alteration in response to a single subcutaneous injection of 1355 mg/kg 2BP administered to rats (Omura et al., 1999). Similarly, Yu et al. (1999) demonstrated that primordial follicles of rats were the first ovarian follicle stage to be affected by a single 8 h inhalation exposure to 3000 ppm 2BP. Additionally, loss of ovarian follicles of all types was seen in female offspring of Sprague Dawley rats when mothers were exposed during gestation and lactation (Kang et al., 2002). To date, neither the mechanism nor the cellular or molecular target by which 2BP induces germ cell loss has been elucidated.

5.3.5 Other Ovotoxic Agents

Early observations on ovarian damage caused by a variety of other chemicals have been made. However, detailed characterization of the ovarian effects of these specific agents does not appear in the literature. The alkylating agents 1,4-di(methanesulfonoxy)-butane (Myleran), trimethylenemelamine (TEM), and isopropyl methanesulfonate (IMS) have been shown to destroy oocytes in small follicles in SECXC57BL/F1 mice following a single i.p. injection (Generoso et al., 1971). Daily oral administration of nitrofurazone over 2 years caused ovarian lesions including development of benign mixed tumors and granulosa cell tumors in mice (Kari et al., 1989). In addition to the chemicals discussed so far, Dobson and Felton (1983) reported a variety of other compounds that were capable of producing significant primordial follicle loss in mice. These chemicals included methyl and ethyl methanesulfonate, and urethane. Additionally, of a number of fungal toxins and antibiotics, procarbazine HCl and 4-nitroquinoline-1-oxide were observed to be ovotoxic. Finally, dibromochloropropane, urethane, *N*-ethyl-*N*-nitrosourea, and bleomycin demonstrated primordial follicle killing, with bleomycin being the most potent. In general, all of these ovotoxic chemicals are also known to possess mutagenic–carcinogenic effects. Thus, these studies have further provided a correlation between ovotoxicity and subsequent development of tumorigenesis. How these two events are linked is not clearly understood at this time.

The polychlorinated biphenyl compound, 3,3,4,4-tetrachlorobephenyl (TCB), has been shown to be teratogenic in the mouse and embryolethal in the rat, as well as having transplacental ovarian toxicity in the mouse (Ronnback, 1991). Follicles in all stages of development were reduced 40%–50% in female offspring at 28d of age when mice were exposed *in utero* on day 13 of gestation. Interestingly, during a 5 month period of testing, this extent of follicular damage did not adversely affect reproductive function in these offspring. Furthermore, the chlorinated organic chemical hexachlorobenzene has been shown to cause destruction of primordial follicles in cynomolgus monkeys at doses that did not produce evidence of systemic or hepatic effects (Jarrell et al., 1993).

5.4 MECHANISMS OF OVOTOXICITY

How ovotoxic effects of environmental chemicals are produced in primordial follicles is generally not well understood, but might be due to one of several possible mechanisms. Oocyte destruction can result from a toxic chemical directly impairing oocyte viability. Conversely, because oocytes at all stages of follicular development are surrounded by granulosa cells, these mechanisms might also be indirect, involving alterations within the granulosa cell, which compromise its ability to maintain viability within the oocyte (Buccione et al., 1990). Environmental chemicals might cause follicle loss by accelerating the overall rate of atresia by apoptosis or autophagy, normal mechanisms by which the majority of follicles degenerate during development. On the other hand, recently, there has been growing attention to the possibility that xenobiotic effects on small pre-antral follicles result from unregulated activation of primordial follicles.

5.4.1 Follicular Targeting

In determining the mechanisms involved in ovotoxicity, it is firstly important to determine whether selective or distinct follicular populations are targeted. In studies investigating the mechanism(s) by which VCD is ovotoxic, rats were dosed daily for 30 days. Morphological evaluation of ovaries from control and treated rats revealed that significant loss of small follicles had occurred in follicles in the primordial, primary, and secondary stages (Flaws et al., 1994a; Figure 5.2). However, at a shorter time of dosing, reduced numbers of only primordial and primary follicles were seen on day 15, yet the number of secondary follicles was unchanged. Thus, these findings supported that primordial and primary follicles are directly targeted by VCD and that the loss of secondary follicles seen on day 30 was the result of fewer primordial and primary follicles from which to recruit.

5.4.2 Cell Death

The ultimate event associated with follicular destruction is cell death. This is the natural fate of the majority of ovarian follicles because only a select few follicles that develop will ever become ovulated (Hirshfield, 1991). This process, called atresia, can occur in follicles in all stages of development and can be morphologically distinguished from healthy follicles. Follicular atresia in rats has been shown to occur via a mechanism of physiological cell death, apoptosis (Tilly et al., 1991). Apoptosis is used by many tissues to delete unwanted cells by a noninflammatory mechanism (Wyllie et al., 1980). Apoptosis is generally associated with signaling events leading to genomic degradation. Therefore, this form of cell death is physiological and likely to go undetected by the organism. This is in distinct contrast to cell death by necrosis, which usually occurs in response to injury, and which elicits an inflammatory response in the surrounding tissue. Apoptosis and necrosis can be distinguished by morphological criteria, and the most reliable distinction between apoptotic and necrotic mechanisms of cell death still resides in morphological evaluation at the ultrastructural level (Payne et al., 1995).

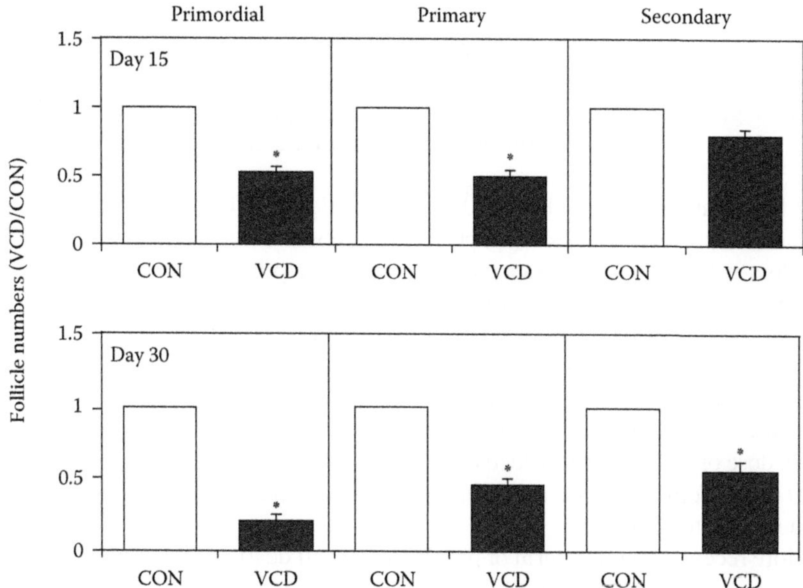

FIGURE 5.2 Reductions of small follicle numbers by repeated dosing with 4-vinylcyclohexene diepoxide. Female Fischer 344 rats (age d28) were dosed daily with vehicle control (open bars) or VCD (80 mg/kg, i.p., closed bars) for 15d or 30d. Ovaries were collected and processed for histological counting of primordial, primary, and secondary follicles. $*p < 0.05$ different from control (n=5 per group). (From *Rep. Toxicol.*, 8, Flaws, J.A., Doerr, J.K., Sipes, I.G., and Hoyer, P.B., Destruction of preantral follicles in adult rats by 4-vinyl-1-cyclohexene diepoxide, 509–514, Copyright 1994, with permission from Elsevier.)

In distinguishing between necrosis and apoptosis as types of cell death, the ovotoxic effects of three PAHs, DMBA, 3-methylcholanthrene (3-MC), and benzo[a]pyrene (BP), were described as morphological changes in primordial follicles more consistent with necrosis (Mattison, 1980). These effects were observed in mice following administration of a single dose. The changes caused by 3-MC and BaP were seen in the absence of visible effects in the associated granulosa cells. However, DMBA produced more visible toxicity by destroying oocytes and follicles more extensively and disrupting ovarian architecture. Ultrastructural evidence consistent with increased atresia (apoptosis) in small pre-antral follicles has also been reported. 3-MC produced a destruction of oocytes in mice that resembled the physiological process of atresia (Gulyas and Mattison, 1979). This was also observed in ovaries collected from rats dosed daily for 10 days with the occupational chemical VCD (Mayer et al., 2002). Under these conditions, there was no evidence of necrosis, such as cellular swelling or infiltration of macrophages in ovaries from treated rats.

In other studies investigating ovotoxicity in rats and mice, morphological evidence consistent with both types of cell death has been reported. Ovaries collected from mice exposed to a relatively high dose of CPA (500 mg/kg) demonstrated necrotic damage in oocytes contained in primordial follicles (Swartz and Mattison, 1985;

Plowchalk and Mattison, 1992). This effect was specific for the oocyte because surrounding granulosa cells appeared unchanged. Conversely, atretic changes in primordial follicles were reported at lower doses (100 mg/kg). Taken together, these results suggest that mild cellular damage can induce physiological cell death, apoptosis; whereas, more severe damage results in passive cell death, necrosis (Corcoran et al., 1994).

It has been determined that VCD-induced follicle loss is also by acceleration of the natural process of atresia (apoptosis). One observation that VCD-induced follicle loss is the result of interactions with the atretic process came from a study in which the effect of a single dose of VCD in rats was evaluated (Borman et al., 1999). Twenty four hours following a single dose, there was an increase in percentage of healthy-appearing ovarian primary follicles, relative to those measured in animals given vehicle control. The importance of this observation was evident 15 days later. Compared with controls, there were more primary follicles in animals treated with a single dose of VCD. This provided evidence that whereas repeated daily dosing with VCD causes follicle loss via acceleration of atresia, a single dose may protect against the normal rate of atresia.

More recently, another form of physiological cell death, autophagy, has become the focus of increased attention as regards a mechanism distinct from apoptosis for physiological deletion of unwanted cells (Mizushima and Levine, 2010). Autophagy is a process by which cytoplasmic components and organelles are degraded by the lysosome. It is thought to have conserved roles in cellular differentiation and development. It can also provide a response to environmental cues. Autophagy has further been proposed as a mechanism involved in establishment of the ovarian primordial follicle pool in mice (Gawriluk et al., 2011). Autophagy can be distinguished from apoptosis by ultrastructural evaluation as well as upregulation of specific genes. Whereas apoptosis is associated with an increase in such markers as caspase 3 and TUNEL staining, autophagy results in increased expression of a cohort of specific genes including Becn1, and Atg7, Beclin-1, LC3, (Gawriluk et al., 2011; Gannon et al., 2012). A recent study in mice concluded that cigarette smoke exposure causes primordial follicle death by autophagy as opposed to apoptosis (Gannon et al., 2012). This finding provides intriguing rationale for reinvestigation of the mechanism(s) of cell death caused by other ovotoxic chemicals.

5.4.3 Follicular Activation

There is also more recent interest in the concept that ovotoxic chemicals do not directly kill primordial follicles, rather initiate uncontrolled primordial follicle activation, accompanied by follicular atresia. Support for this concept has been demonstrated by several different approaches. Genetically altered mice in which signaling pathway genes (FOXO3 and p27) have been deleted have been shown to undergo POF as a result of unregulated primordial follicle activation (Castrillon et al., 2003; Rajareddy et al., 2007). In one study, *in vitro* inhibition of PI3kinase prevented VCD-induced loss of primordial, but not primary follicles in ovaries cultured from neonatal Fischer 344 rats (Keating et al., 2009). Further, microarray analyses of ovaries from neonatal Swiss mice exposed *in vitro* to the PAHs, benzo[*a*]pyrene (BaP) and DMBA, or other ovotoxic chemicals (VCD, methoxychlor, menadione) have identified that some of the groups of genes that are affected are associated with follicle growth, cell cycle progression, and cell death (Sobinoff et al., 2010, 2011, 2012). It will be interesting to see whether other xenobiotics that are ovotoxic to primordial follicles also utilize this mechanism.

5.4.4 Sites of Cellular Damage

Intracellular molecular sites targeted by ovotoxic chemicals have not been extensively identified. Compounds known to contain epoxide moieties (or which are capable of bioactivation by epoxidation) have been shown to affect ovarian function in laboratory animals. Many of these compounds lead to induction of ovarian tumors following long-term exposures. These carcinogens include 1,3-BD and its derivatives (Miller and Boorman, 1990; Mehlman and Legator, 1991) and VCH and its derivatives (NTP, 1986, 1989; Collins et al., 1987; Chhabra et al., 1990).

5.4.4.1 DNA Damage

The ability of epoxides to produce DNA adducts and induce sister chromatin exchanges has also demonstrated effects at the molecular level (Hoyer and Sipes, 1996). However, whether DNA damage is the event that initiates ovotoxicity has not been determined for these chemicals. Several recent studies have reported that DNA damage in the form of DNA double-strand breaks can be caused by the chemotherapeutic agents doxorubicin (DXR) or phosphoramide mustard (Petrillo et al., 2011; Soleimani et al., 2011). Additionally, DNA adduction of BaP was detected in ovaries up to 28 days following a single exposure in rats (Ramesh et al., 2010). Thus, a mechanism involving direct DNA damage by ovotoxicants is gaining support.

5.4.4.2 Gene Expression

Several studies related to ovotoxicity caused by the PAHs have demonstrated that follicle loss is via alterations in genes associated with apoptosis. This involves enhanced expression of the pro-apoptotic gene, Bax, in cultured neonatal mouse ovaries (Matikainen et al., 2001). Further, ovaries from Bax-deficient mice were resistant to DMBA-induced ovotoxicity. An involvement of the arylhydrocarbon receptor (AhR) in this process was also demonstrated as inhibitors of AhR activity and AhR-deficient mouse ovaries were resistant to DMBA-induced apoptosis (Matikainen et al., 2001; Juriscova et al., 2007).

In other studies, characterization of the impact of ovotoxic chemicals on gene expression has been conducted using rats exposed to VCD. Changes in intracellular pathways associated with apoptosis have been measured in follicles undergoing VCD-induced follicle loss, thereby providing additional support that ovotoxicity is via apoptosis. Elevated levels of mRNA encoding the cell death enhancer gene, *bax* (elevated in apoptosis), were measured in isolated fractions of small preantral follicles collected from VCD-dosed rats (Springer et al., 1996b). This effect was specific for the small follicles targeted by VCD, and was not seen in large pre-antral follicles or hepatocytes (nontarget tissues). One study using a microarray analysis compared the effect of *in vivo* versus *in vitro* exposures to identify common genes whose expression was affected by VCD (Fernandez et al., 2008). Of 33 genes affected by VCD in small follicles collected from dosed rats, and 25 genes affected in the *in vitro* cultures, 14 of the affected genes were common to both systems. Interestingly, following collection of isolated follicles from VCD-dosed rats, only seven genes in the larger pre-antral follicle fraction (not targeted by VCD) were affected by VCD. None of those genes were affected in the target populations. This further underscored the selectivity of VCD for small pre-antral (primordial and primary) follicles.

5.4.4.3 Cell Signaling

It has been proposed that plasma membrane damage is more highly correlated with ovotoxicity than DNA damage (Dobson and Felton, 1983). This observation was supported by comparing alkylating properties with genetic activity in a variety of epoxide-containing chemicals (Turchi et al., 1981). Thus, the cellular event(s) initiated directly by ovotoxic chemicals may be at the level of proteins involved in signaling pathways or regulatory mechanisms associated with cell death/viability determination, rather than as a direct result of DNA damage. Effects of VCD on intracellular signaling pathways have included responses in members of the Bcl-2 associated family of proto-oncogenes: increased expression of pro-apoptotic Bad; translocation of Bclx-L from mitochondria to the cytosol; increased ratio of Bax/Bclx-L on the mitochondrial membrane; leakage of cytochrome C from mitochondria to the cytosol; and increased expression and activation of the caspase cascade involving the executioner protease, caspase-3 (Hu et al., 2001a,b). Additionally, it has been demonstrated that pro-apoptotic members of the MAPK kinase family are also activated in VCD-induced apoptosis (Hu et al., 2002).

In evaluating the effects of VCD on gene expression in primordial and primary follicles in rats, one gene of particular interest was decreased under both conditions of *in vivo* and *in vitro* exposure at a time point in which VCD-induced follicle loss was seen. That gene was the cell survival gene, c-kit, which is expressed as a tyrosine kinase receptor on the plasma membrane of the oocyte. Follow-up studies have demonstrated that an early initiating event caused by VCD (prior to changes in gene expression or follicle loss) is the inhibition of autophosphorylation of c-kit (Mark-Kappeler et al., 2011b; Kappeler and Hoyer, 2012 Figure 5.3). This results in inhibited activation of downstream PI3K signaling pathway events within the oocyte (Keating et al., 2009, 2011). This supports that the oocyte membrane is the direct cellular target of VCD, and that VCD directly interacts with c-kit to inhibit its intracellular signal for survival (Mark-Kappeler et al., 2011b; Kappeler and Hoyer, 2012). This event appears to be specific for c-kit because *in vitro* supplementation with its ligand, Kit Ligand, attenuated VCD-induced ovotoxicity, whereas the addition of five other growth factors associated with primordial follicle survival or activation had no effect (Mark-Kappeler et al., 2011b). Whether other ovotoxic chemicals also directly affect follicle survival via interactions with growth factor pathways will be interesting to determine.

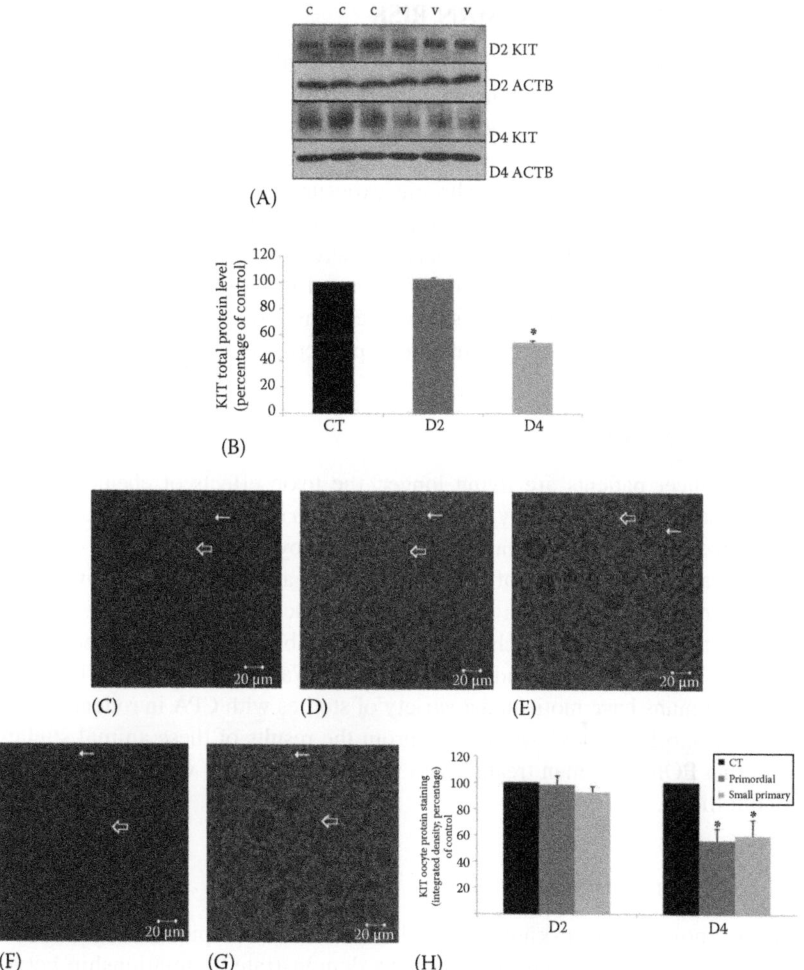

FIGURE 5.3 (See color insert.) Effect of VCD on KIT protein staining. PND4 F344 rat ovaries were cultured with vehicle control or 30 μM VCD for 2 or 4 days and processed for Western blotting or immunofluorescence staining with confocal microscopy. (A) Western blotting for KIT or beta-actin (ACTB) protein on Day 2 and Day 4 of VCD exposure (c, control; v, VCD). (B) Quantification of KIT protein staining with normalization to ACTB. (C–G) Representative images for immunofluorescence staining of KIT protein on Day 4 are shown. Cy-5 red staining (anti-KIT antibody) for control-treated ovary (C) and VCD-treated ovary, and genomic DNA (green YOYO1 stain) overlay (F) for control-treated ovary (D), immunonegative control (E), and VCD-treated ovary (G) at 40× magnification. Thin arrows indicate primordial follicles; thick arrows indicate small primary follicles; bar = 20 μm. (H) Quantification of oocyte pericytoplasmic KIT protein staining on Day 2 and Day 4 of VCD exposure. Values are percentage of control; n = 3. *$p < 0.05$. By either method, oocyte plasma membrane staining was reduced by VCD on Day 4 of incubation, relative to control. (From Keating, A.F., Fernandez, S.M., Sen, N., Mark-Kappeler, C.J., Sipes, I.G., and Hoyer, P.B., Inhibition of PI3K signaling pathway members by the ovotoxicant 4-vinylcyclohexene diepoxide, *Biol. Rep.*, 84, 743–751, 2011. With permission from Society for the Study of Reproduction.)

5.5 PREDICTION OF HUMAN RISK

The level of exposure to an environmental chemical required to produce ovarian damage is of particular importance. It is under rare, accidental circumstances that large groups of individuals are acutely exposed to toxic levels of reproductive toxicants, and the effects of these exposures can usually be detected and evaluated. However, the possible effects of chronic exposure to low levels of reproductive toxicants are more difficult to determine because of the potential for additive or cumulative effects that might be produced. Therefore, fertility problems produced by environmental exposures may go unrecognized for years, but might manifest as early menopause, and/or still later as the development of ovarian cancer. Thus, it is these potential types of exposures that are of particular concern.

5.5.1 Chemotherapy

Now that cancer patients are living longer, the toxic effects of chemotherapeutic drugs on the health and quality of life of these survivors have become important issues. Since the beginning of antineoplastic therapy to treat a variety of diseases and malignancies, the ability of chemotherapeutic agents to produce ovarian failure has been documented. This effect has been described in patients being treated with CPA, nitrogen mustard, chlorambucil, or vinblastine (Sobrinho et al., 1971; Chapman, 1983; Damewood and Grochow, 1986; Wayne et al., 2002). These observations in humans have motivated a variety of studies with CPA in rodents to better elucidate its mechanism of ovotoxicity. From the results of these animal studies, it appears that POF in women treated with CPA is likely to be via destruction of primordial follicles.

5.5.2 Cigarette Smoking

Cigarette smoke is a well-known reproductive toxicant. Epidemiological studies conducted over the past four decades have demonstrated a relationship between smoking and impaired fertility. One study reported that rates of pregnancy were reduced to 57% in heavy smokers and 75% in light smokers when compared with nonsmokers. Furthermore, smokers required 1 year longer to conceive than did nonsmokers (Baird and Wilcox, 1985). Additionally, smoking is known to impair a successful outcome in women undergoing assisted reproductive technologies (IVF; Soares et al., 2007). Women smokers have also been reported to experience a diminished ovarian reserve and a 1–4 year earlier age at the onset of menopause (Jick et al., 1977; El-Nemr et al., 1998). Thus, a significant amount of data exists to demonstrate a relationship between smoking and an impact on ovarian function.

Cigarette smoke is a complex mixture of alkaloids (nicotine), PAHs, nitroso compounds, aromatic amines, and protein pyrolysates, many of which are carcinogenic (Stedman, 1968). Smoking women have been shown to have significantly decreased follicular levels of estradiol, compared with nonsmokers (VanVoorhis et al., 1992). Furthermore, extracts of cigarette smoke significantly decreased estradiol secretion by human granulosa cells in culture (Barbieri et al., 1986). Thus, these effects may relate to the infertility associated with cigarette smoking. However, because of the logical association between early menopause and oocyte destruction, some of the effects of cigarette smoke on fertility are likely to be due to destruction of primordial follicles as has been reported by PAHs in animal studies (Mattison and Thorgeirsson, 1979). Of additional concern is the finding in animal studies that exposure of mice *in utero* to cigarette smoke resulted in a reduced number of ovarian primordial follicles in female offspring (Vahakangas et al., 1985).

5.5.3 Mode of Exposure

The level of exposure to an environmental chemical required to produce ovarian damage is of particular importance. The possible effects of chronic exposure to low levels of reproductive toxicants may go unrecognized for years, due to the potential for additive or cumulative effects that might be produced. Because of their insidious nature, these types of exposures can cause "silent" damage and are of the most concern. This is particularly important when the target cells are of a nonrenewing type (ovarian follicles).

Several studies have addressed the issue of toxicity as a function of the dosing regimen in mice. Primordial follicle destruction is known to result from dosing of mice and rats with the widely studied PAHs (DMBA, 3-MC, BaP), contaminants in cigarette smoke and automobile exhaust. Because these chemicals destroy primordial follicles in laboratory animals, it is likely that they contribute to the early menopause seen in women smokers. Earlier studies examined the ovotoxic effects of these PAHs in mice caused by a single, high-dose exposure. The extent of primordial follicle loss following this high-dose exposure to DMBA, BaP, and 3-MC in mice was reported to be 50% within 1–2 days (Mattison and Thorgeirsson, 1979). Interestingly, significant oocyte destruction was demonstrated following a single high dose of BaP (100 mg/kg), whereas the same level of oocyte loss was observed with a low dose (10 mg/kg) given daily for 10 days (Mattison and Nightingale, 1980; Mattison et al., 1983). This observation provided support for a cumulative ovotoxic effect of chronic exposures to low doses. Because repeated low-dose exposure is a more likely source of toxicity in women, another study was undertaken to evaluate the effects of lower doses of these chemicals. Female mice were exposed repeatedly to doses of the PAHs, sufficient to cause 50% loss of primordial follicles after 15 days of daily dosing (Borman et al., 2000). Calculating an ovotoxic index using the doses required to cause 50% follicle destruction in both studies, it was determined that relative to a single high-dose exposure, repeated low-dose exposure was more ovotoxic by a 250 (DMBA), 120 (3-MC), or 2 (BaP) times greater extent (Table 5.2; Borman et al., 2000). Thus, these results demonstrate that animal studies designed to more closely mimic human types of exposures may reveal surprising and disturbing insights as to realistic risk. Taken together, the reports related to mechanisms of cell death during ovotoxicity suggest that dose and duration of exposure impact the outcome. This provides further rationale for designing animal studies using low-dose, repeated exposure to more closely mimic the nature of human exposures.

TABLE 5.2
Comparison of the OI (ED_{50}, mmol/kg × Days of Dosing) for a Single, High-Dose (1×) Versus Repeated Low Doses (15×) in B6 Mice

	15 × OI	1 × OI[a]
DMBA	0.0012	0.3100
3-MC	0.0030	0.3000
BaP	0.1800	0.3200

Source: Borman, S.M. et al., *Toxicol. Appl. Pharmacol.*, 167, 191, 2000. With permission.

Note: Lowest OI = Greatest Toxicity.

[a] 80 mg/kg; Mattison and Thorgeirsson (1979).

5.6 SUMMARY AND CONCLUSIONS

In summary, environmental chemicals that impact ovarian function can directly disrupt endocrine balance by decreasing production of ovarian hormones, and interfering with ovulation. These effects are rather immediate, target large antral follicles, and can be reversed once there is no longer exposure to the chemical. On the other hand, ovarian function can be impaired by exposure to chemicals that destroy small pre-antral follicles. This produces an indirect disruption of endocrine balance, once hormonal feedback mechanisms have been affected. The manifestation of this type of ovarian toxicity is delayed until irreversible ovarian failure (menopause) has occurred. This specific type of ovotoxicity is of particular concern in women because of the health risks known to be associated with menopause. Future research will undoubtedly continue to be aimed at understanding specific mechanisms of ovotoxicity, and improving our ability to predict human risk from the wide variety of exposures to these chemicals in the environment.

ACKNOWLEDGMENT

Supported by R01ES09246 (to PBH) and Center Grant P30ES06694.

REFERENCES

Anderson, D., Bishop, J.B., Garner, R.C., Ostrodky-Wegman, P., and Selby, P.B. 1995. Cyclophosphamide: Review of its mutagenicity for an assessment of potential of germ cell risks. *Mutation Research* 330:115.

Aktas, C., Kanter, M., and Kocak, Z. 2012. Antiapoptotic and proliferative activity of curcumin on ovarian follicles in mice exposed to whole body radiation. *Toxicology and Industrial Health* 28:852–863.

Baird, D.D. and Wilcox, A.J. 1985. Cigarette smoking associated with delayed conception. *Journal of the American Medical Association* 253:2979–2983.

Barbieri, R.L., McShane, P.M., and Ryan, K.J. 1986. Constituents of cigarette smoke inhibit human granulosa cell aromatase. *Fertility and Sterility* 46:232–236.

Bengtsson, M., Hamberger, L., and Rydstrom, J. 1988. Metabolism of 7,12- dimethylbenz(a) anthracene by different types of cells in the human ovary. *Xenobiotica* 18:1255–1270.

Bengtsson, M. and Mattison, D.R. 1989. Gonadotropin-dependent metabolism of 7,12-dimethylbenz(a)anthracene in the ovary of rhesus monkey. *Biochemical Pharmacology* 38:1869–1872.

Bevan, C., Stadler, J.C., Elliot, G.S., Frame, S.R., Baldwin, J.K., Leung, H.W., Moran, E., and Panepinto, A.S. 1996. Subchronic toxicity of 4-vinylcyclohexene in rats and mice by inhalation exposure. *Fundamentals in Applied Toxicology* 32:1–10.

Blumenfeld, Z. 2012. Chemotherapy and fertility. *Best Practices and Research in Clinical Obstetrics and Gynecology* 26:379–390.

Boekelheide, K., Darney, S.P., Daston, G.P., David, R.M., Luderer, U., Olshen, A.F., Sanderson, W.T., Willhite, C.C., Woskie, S. 2004. NTP-CERHR Expert panel report on the reproductive and developmental toxicity of 2-bromopropane. *Reprod. Toxicol.* 18:189–217.

Borman, S.M., Christian, P.J., Sipes, I.G., and Hoyer, P.B. 2000. Ovotoxicity in female Fischer rats and B6 mice induced by low-dose exposure to three polycyclic aromatic hydrocarbons: Comparison through calculation of an ovotoxic index. *Toxicology and Applied Pharmacology* 167:191–198.

Borman, S.M., VanDePol, B.J., Kao, S.W., Thompson, K.E., Sipes, I.G., and Hoyer, P.B. 1999. A single dose of the ovotoxicant 4-vinylcyclohexene diepoxide is protective in rat primary ovarian follicles. *Toxicology and Applied Pharmacology* 158:244–252.

Brock, N. 1967. Pharmacologic characterization of cyclophosphamide (NSC-26271) and cyclophosphamide metabolites. *Cancer Chemotherapy Reports* 51:315–325.

Brougham, M.F., Crofton, P.M., Johnson, E.J., Evans, N., Anderson, R.A., and Wallace, W.H. 2012. Anti-mullerian hormone is a marker of gonadotoxicity in pre- and postpubertal girls treated for cancer: A prospective study. *Journal of Clinical Endocrinology and Metabolism* 97:2059–2067.

Buccione, R., Schroeder, A.S., and Eppig, J.J. 1990. Interactions between somatic cells and germ cells throughout mammalian oogenesis. *Biology of Reproduction* 43:543–547.

Castrillon, D.H., Miao, L., Kollipara, R., Horner, J.W., and DePinho, R.A. 2003. Suppression of ovarian follicle activation in mice by the transcription factor Foxo3a. *Science* 301:215–218.

Chapman, R.M. 1983. Gonadal injury resulting from chemotherapy. *American Journal of Industrial Medicine* 4:149–161.

Chhabra, R.S., Huff, J., Haseman, J., Jokinen, M.P., and Hetjnancek, M. 1990. Dermal toxicity and carcinogenicity of 4-vinyl-1-cyclohexene diepoxide in Fischer rats and B6C3F1 mice. *Fundamental and Applied Toxicology* 14:752–763.

Christensen, C., Christensen, M.S., McNair, P.L., Hagen, C., Stocklund, K.E., and Transbol, I. 1980. Prevention of early postmenopausal bone loss: Controlled 2-year study in 315 normal females. *European Journal of Clinical Investigations* 10:273–279.

Collins, J.J., Motali, R.J., and Manus, A.G. 1987. Toxicological evaluation of 4-vinylcyclohexene. II. Induction of ovarian tumors in female B6C3F1 mice by chronic oral administration of 4-vinylcyclohexene. *Journal of Toxicology and Environmental Health* 21:507–524.

Cooper, G.S., Baird, D.D., Hulka, B.S., Weinberg, C.R., Savitz, D.A., and Hughes, C.L. 1995. Follicle stimulating hormone concentrations in relation to active and passive smoking. *Obstetrics and Gynecology* 85:407–411.

Corcoran, G.B., Fix, L., Jones, D.P., Moslen, M.T., Oberhammer, F.A., and Buttyan, R. 1994. Apoptosis: Molecular control points in toxicology. *Toxicology and Applied Pharmacology* 128:169–181.

Damewood, M.D. and Grochow, L.B. 1986. Prospects for fertility after chemotherapy or radiation for neoplastic disease. *Fertility and Sterility* 45:443–459.

Desmeules, P. and Devine, P.J. 2006. Characterizing the ovotoxicity of cyclophosphamide metabolites on cultured mouse ovaries. *Toxicological Sciences* 90:500–509.

Devine, P.J. and Hoyer, P.B. 2005. Ovotoxic environmental chemicals: Indirect endocrine disruptors. In *Endocrine Disruptors: Effects on Male and Female Reproductive Systems*, 2nd edn., ed. R. Naz, pp. 67–100. Boca Raton, FL: CRC Press.

Devine, P.J., Sipes, I.G., Skinner, M.K., and Hoyer, P.B. 2002. Characterization of a rat in vitro ovarian culture system to study the ovarian toxicant 4-vinylcyclohexene diepoxide. *Toxicology and Applied Pharmacology* 184:107–115.

Dhar, H.L. 2001. Gender, aging, health and society. *Journal of the Association of Physicians in India* 49:1012–1020.

Dobson, R.L. and Felton, J.S. 1983. Female germ cell loss from radiation and chemical exposures. *American Journal of Industrial Medicine* 4:175–190.

Doerr, J.K., Hooser, S.B., Smith, B.J., and Sipes, I.G. 1995. Ovarian toxicity of 4-vinylcyclohexene and related olefins in B6C3F1 mice: Role of diepoxides. *Chemical Research in Toxicology* 8:963–969.

El-Nemir, A., Al-Shawaf, T., Sabatini, L., Wilson, C., Lower, A.M., and Grudzinskas, J.G. 1998. Effect of smoking on ovarian reserve and ovarian stimulation in in vitro fertilization and embryo transfer. *Human Reproduction* 13:2192–2198.

Everson, R.B., Sandler, D.P., Wilcox, A.J., Schreinemachhers, D., Shore, D.L., and Weinberg, C. 1986. Effect of passive exposure to smoking on age at natural menopause. *British Medical Journal* 293:792.

Fernandez, S.M., Keating, A.F., Christian, P.J., Sen, N., Hoying, J.B., Brooks, H.L., and Hoyer, P.B. 2008. Involvement of the KIT/KITL signaling pathway in 4-vinylcyclohexene diepoxide-induced ovarian follicle loss in rats. *Biology of Reproduction* 79:318–327.

Flaws, J.A., Doerr, J.K., Sipes, I.G., and Hoyer, P.B. 1994a. Destruction of preantral follicles in adult rats by 4-vinyl-1-cyclohexene diepoxide. *Reproductive Toxicology* 8:509–514.

Flaws, J.A., Salyers, K.L., Sipes, I.G., and Hoyer, P.B. 1994b. Reduced ability of rat pre- antral ovarian follicles to metabolize 4-vinyl-1-cyclohexene diepoxide in vitro. *Toxicology and Applied Pharmacology* 126:286–294.

Gannon, A.M., Stampfi, M.R., and Foster, W.G. 2012. Cigarette smoke exposure leads to follicle loss via an alternative ovarian cell death pathway in a mouse model. *Toxicological Sciences* 125:274–284.

Gawriluk, T.R., Hale, A.N., Flaws, J.A., Dillon, C.P., Green, D.R., and Rucker, E.B. 2011. Autophagy is a cell survival program for female germ cells in the murine ovary. *Reproduction* 141:759–765.

Generoso, W.M., Stout, S.K., and Huff, S.W. 1971. Effects of alkylating chemicals on reproductive capacity of adult female mice. *Mutation Research/Fundamental and Molecular Mechanisms of Mutagenesis* 13:172–184.

Grizzle, T.B., George, J.D., Fail, P.A., Seely, J.C., and Heindel, J.J. 1994. Reproductive effects of 4-vinylcyclohexene in Swiss mice assessed by a continuous breeding protocol. *Fundamentals in Applied Toxicology* 22:122–129.

Gulyas, B.J. and Mattison, D.R. 1979. Degeneration of mouse oocytes in response to polycyclic aromatic hydrocarbons. *Anatomical Record* 193:863–882.

Hadley, M.E. and Levine, J.E. 2007. *Endocrinology*, 6th edn. Upper Saddle River, NJ: Pearson Prentice Hall.

Hirshfield, A.N. 1991. Development of follicles in the mammalian ovary. *Internal Reviews in Cytology* 124:43–101.

Hooser, S.B., Douds, D.A., DeMerell, D.G., Hoyer, P.B., and Sipes, I.G. 1994. Long term ovarian and hormonal alterations due to the ovotoxin, 4-vinylcyclohexene. *Reproductive Toxicology* 8:315–323.

Hoyer, P.B. 1997. Female reproductive toxicology—Introduction and overview. In *Comprehensive Toxicology*, Vol. 10, eds. I.G. Sipes, C.A. McQueen, and J.A. Gandolfi. Oxford, England, U.K.: Elsevier Pub.

Hoyer, P.B. 2005. Damage to ovarian development and function. *Cell Tissue Research* 322:99–106.

Hoyer, P.B. and Devine, P.J. 2001. Endocrinology and toxicology: The female reproductive system. In *Handbook of Toxicology*, 2nd edn., eds. M.J. Derelanko and M.A. Hollinger. Boca Raton, FL: CRC Press.

Hoyer, P.B. and Sipes, I.G. 1996. Assessment of follicle destruction in chemical-induced ovarian toxicity. *Annual Reviews in Pharmacology Toxicology* 36:307–331.

Hu, X.M., Christian, P.J., Sipes, I.G., and Hoyer, P.B. 2001a. Expression and redistribution of cellular bad, bax and bcl-xl protein is associated with VCD-induced ovotoxicity in rats. *Biology of Reproduction* 65:1489–1495.

Hu, X.M., Christian, P.J., Thompson, K.E., Sipes, I.G., and Hoyer, P.B. 2001b. Apoptosis induced in rats by 4-vinylcyclohexene diepoxide is associated with activation of the Caspase cascades. *Biology of Reproduction* 65:87–93.

Hu, X.M., Flaws, J.A., Sipes, I.G., and Hoyer, P.B. 2002. Activation of mitogen-activated protein kinases and AP-1 transcription factor in ovotoxicity induced by 4-vinylcyclohexene diepoxide in rats. *Biology of Reproduction* 67:718–724.

International Agency for Research on Cancer (IARC), World Health Organization. 1986. 1,3-Butadiene. *IARC Monographs on the Evaluation of Carcinogenic Risks to Humans* 39:155.

International Agency for Research on Cancer (IARC), World Health Organization. 1994. 4-Vinylcyclohexene, 4-vinylcyclohexene diepoxide. *IARC Monographs on the Evaluation of Carcinogenic Risks to Humans* 60:17–20.

Jarrell, J.F., Bodo, L., Young Lai, E.V., Barr, R.D., and O'Connell, G.J. 1991. The short-term reproductive toxicity of cyclophosphamide in the female rat. *Reproductive Toxicology* 5:481–485.

Jarrell, J.F., McMahon, A., Villeneuve, D., Franklin, C., Singh, A., Valli, V.E., and Bartlett, S. 1993. Hexachlorobenzene toxicity in the monkey primordial germ cell without induced porphyria. *Reproductive Toxicology* 7:41–47.

Jick, H., Porter, J., and Morrison, A.S. 1977. Relation between smoking and age of natural menopause. *Lancet* 1:1354–1355.

Juriscova, A., Taniuchi, A., Li, H. et al. 2007. Maternal exposure to polycyclic aromatic hydrocarbons diminishes murine ovarian reserve via induction of Harakiri. *Journal of Clinical Investigation* 117:3971–3978.

Kang, K.S., Li, G.X., Che, J.H., and Lee, Y.S. 2002. Impairment of male rat reproductive function in F1 offspring from dams exposed to 2-bromopropane during gestation and lactation. *Reproductive Toxicology* 16:151–159.

Kao, S.W., Sipes, I.G., and Hoyer, P.B. 1999. Early effects of ovotoxicity induced by 4-vinylcyclohexene diepoxide in rats and mice. *Reproductive Toxicology* 13:67–75.

Kappeler, C.J. and Hoyer, P.B. 2012. 4-Vinylcyclohexene diepoxide: A model chemical for ovotoxicity. *Systems Biology in Reproductive Medicine* 58:57–62.

Kari, F.W., Huff, J.E., Leininger, J., Haseman, J.K., and Eustis, S.L. 1989. Toxicity and carcinogenicity of nitrofurazone in F344/N rats and B6C3F1 mice. *Food Chemical Toxicology* 27:129–137.

Keating, A.F., Fernandez, S.M., Sen, N., Mark-Kappeler, C.J., Sipes, I.G., and Hoyer, P.B. 2011. Inhibition of PI3K signaling pathway members by the ovotoxicant 4-vinylcyclohexene diepoxide. *Biology of Reproduction* 84:743–751.

Keating, A.F., Mark, C.J., Sen, N., Sipes, I.G., and Hoyer, P.B. 2009. Effect of phosphatidyl inositol-3-kinase inhibition on ovotoxicity caused by 4-vinylyclohexene diepoxide and 7,12-dimethylbenz[a]anthracene in neonatal rat ovaries. *Toxicology and Applied Pharmacology* 241:127–134.

Keller, D.A., Carpenter, S.C., Cagen, S.Z., and Reitman, F.A. 1997. In vitro metabolism of 4-vinylcyclohexene in rat and mouse liver, lung, and ovary. *Toxicology and Applied Pharmacology* 144:36–44.

Kerr, J.B., Brogan, L., Myers, M., Hutt, K.J., Mladnovska, T., Ricardo, S., Hamza, K., Scott, C.L., Strasser, A., and Findlay, J.K. 2012. The primordial follicle reserve is not renewed after chemical or γ-irradiation mediated depletion. *Reproduction* 143:469–476.

Kim, Y., Jung, K., Hwang, T. et al. 1996. Hematopoietic and reproductive hazards of Korean electronic workers exposed to solvents containing 2-bromopropane. *Scandinavian Journal of Work Environmental Health* 22:387–391.

Kirman, C.R. and Grant, R.L. 2012. Quantitative human health risk assessment for 1,3 butadiene based upon ovarian effects in rodents. *Regulatory and Toxicology Pharmacology* 62:371–384.

Kodama, T., Yoshida, J., Miwa, T., Hasegawa, D., and Masuyama, T. 2009. Collaborative work on evaluation of ovarian toxicity. 4) effects of fertility study of 4-vinylcyclohexene diepoxide in female rats. *Journal of Toxicological Sciences* 34(Suppl 1):SP59–SP63.

Krarup, T. 1967. 9:10-Dimethyl-1:2-benzantracene induced ovarian tumors in mice. *Acta Pathologica Microbiologica Scandinavica* 70:241–248.

Krarup, T. 1969. Oocyte destruction and ovarian tumorigenesis after direct application of a chemical carcinogen (9:10-dimethyl-1:2-benzanthrene) to the mouse ovary. *International Journal of Cancer* 4:61–75.

Lee, C.J., Park, H.H., Do, B.R., Yoon, Y., and Kim, J.K. 2000. Natural and radiation-induced degeneration of primordial and primary follicles in mouse ovary. *Animal Reproduction Science* 59:109–117.

Mackenzie, K.M. and Angevine, D.M. 1981. Infertility in mice exposed in utero to benzo(a) pyrene. *Biology of Reproduction* 24:183–191.

Marjoribanks, J., Farquhar, C., Roberts, H., and Lethaby, A. 2012. Long-term hormone therapy for perimenopausal and postmenopausal women. *Cochrane Database of Systematic Reviews* July 11, 7i:CD004143.

Mark-Kappeler, C.J., Hoyer, P.B., and Devine, P.J. 2011a. Xenobiotic effects on ovarian preantral follicles. *Biology of Reproduction* 85:871–883.

Mark-Kappeler, C.J., Sen, N., Lukefahr, A., McKee, L., Sipes, I.G., Konhilas, J., and Hoyer, P.B. 2011b. Inhibition of ovarian KIT phosphorylation by the ovotoxicant 4-vinylcyclohexene diepoxide in rats. *Biology of Reproduction* 85:755–762.

Matikainen, T., Perez, G.I., Jurisicova, A. et al. 2001. Aromatic hydrocarbon receptor-driven Bax gene expression is required for premature ovarian failure caused by biohazardous environmental chemicals. *Nature Genetics* 28:355–360.

Mattison, D.R. 1979. Difference in sensitivity of rat and mouse primordial oocytes to destruction by polycyclic aromatic hydrocarbons. *Chemical-Biological Interactions* 28:133–137.

Mattison, D.R. 1980. Morphology of oocyte and follicle destruction by polycyclic aromatic hydrocarbons in mice. *Toxicology and Applied Pharmacology* 53:249–259.

Mattison, D.R. and Nightingale, M.R. 1980. The biochemical and genetic characteristics of murine ovarian aryl hydrocarbon (Benzo(a)pyrene)hydroxylase activity and its relationship to primordial oocyte destruction by polycyclic aromatic hydrocarbons. *Toxicology and Applied Pharmacology* 56:399–408.

Mattison, D.R. and Schulman, J.D. 1980. How xenobiotic compounds can destroy oocytes. *Contememporary Obstetrics and Gynecology* 15:157.

Mattison, D.R., Shiromizu, K., and Nightingale, M.S. 1983. Oocyte destruction by polycyclic aromatic hydrocarbons. *American Journal of Industrial Medicine* 4:191–202.

Mattison, D.R. and Thorgeirsson, S.S. 1978. Smoking and industrial pollution, and their effects on menopause and ovarian cancer. *Lancet* 1:187–188.

Mattison, D.R. and Thorgeirsson, S.S. 1979. Ovarian aryl hydrocarbon hydroxylase activity and primordial oocyte toxicity of polycyclic aromatic hydrocarbons in mice. *Cancer Research* 39:3471–3475.

Mayer, L.P., Pearsall, N.A., Christian, P.J., Devine, P.J., Payne, C.M., McCuskey, M.K., Marion, S.L., Sipes, I.G., and Hoyer, P.B. 2002. Long-term effects of ovarian follicular depletion in rats by 4-vinylcyclohexene diepoxide. *Reproductive Toxicology* 16:775–781.

Mehlman, M.A. and Legator, M.S. 1991. Dangerous and cancer-causing properties of products and chemicals in the oil refining and petrochemical industry. Part II: Carcinogenicity mutagenicity and developmental toxicity of 1,3-butadiene. *Toxicology and Industrial Health* 7:207–220.

Melnick, R.L., Huff, J., Chou, B.J., and Miller, R.A. 1990. Carcinogenicity of 1,3-butadiene in C57BL/6 X C3HF1 mice at low exposure concentrations. *Cancer Research* 50:6592–6599.

Mierow, D., Biederman, H., Anderson, R.A., and Wallace, W.H. 2010. Toxicity of chemotherapy and radiation on female reproduction. *Clinical Obstetrics Gynecology* 53:727–739.

Mierow, D., Lewis, H., Nugent, D., and Epstein, M. 1999. Subclinical depletion of primordial follicular reserve in mice treated with cyclophosphamide: Clinical importance and proposed accurate investigative tool. *Human Reproduction* 14:1903–1907.

Miller, R.A. and Boorman, G.A. 1990. Morphology of neoplastic lesions induced by 1,3 butadiene in B6C3F1 mice. *Environmental Health Perspectives* 86:37–48.

Mizushima, N. and Levine, B. 2010. Autophagy in mammalian development and differentiation. *Nature Cell Biology* 12:823–830.

Morgan, S., Anderson, R.A., Gourley, C., Wallace, W.H., and Spears, N. 2012. How do chemotherapeutic agents damage the ovary? *Human Reproduction Update* 18:525–535.

National Toxicology Program (NTP). 1984. Toxicology and carcinogenesis studies of 1,3-butadiene (CAS No. 106-99-0) in B6C3F1 mice (Inhalation studies). *NTP Technical Report* 288:1–111.

National Toxicology Program (NTP). 1986. Toxicology and carcinogenesis studies of 4-vinylcyclohexene in F344/N rats and B6C3F1 mice. *NTP Technical Report* 303:1–190.

National Toxicology Program (NTP). 1989. Toxicology and carcinogenesis studies of 4-vinyl-1-cyclohexene diepoxide in F344/N rats and B6C3F1 mice. *NTP Technical Report* 362:1–249.

Omura, M., Romero, Y., Zhao, M., and Inoue, N. 1999. Histopathological evidence that spermatogonia are the target cells of 2-bromopropane. *Toxicology Letters* 104:19–26.

Paganini-Hill, A. and Henderson, V.W. 1994. Estrogen deficiency and risk of Alzheimer's disease in women. *American Journal of Epidemiology* 140:256–261.

Park, J., Kim, Y., Park, D., Choi, K., Park, S., and Moon, Y. 1997. An outbreak of hematopoietic and reproductive disorders due to solvents containing 2-bromopropane in an electronic factory, South Korea: Epidemiological survey. *Journal of Occupational Health* 39:138–143.

Payne, C.M., Bernstein, C., and Bernstein, H. 1995. Apoptosis overview emphasizing the role of oxidative stress, DNA damage and signal-transduction pathways. *Leukemia and Lymphoma* 19:43–93.

Petrillo, S.K., Desmeules, P., Truong, T.Q., and Devine, P.J. 2011. Detection of DNA damage in oocytes of small ovarian follicles following phosphoramide mustard exposures of cultured rodent ovaries in vitro. *Toxicology and Applied Pharmacology* 253:94–102.

Plowchalk, D.R. and Mattison, D.R. 1991. Phosphoramide mustard is responsible for the ovarian toxicity of cylcophosphamide. *Toxicology and Applied Pharmacology* 107:472–481.

Plowchalk, D.R. and Mattison, D.R. 1992. Reproductive toxicity of cyclophosphamide in the C57GBL/6N mouse. 2. Effects on ovarian structure and function. *Reproductive Toxicology* 6:411–421.

Rajareddy, S., Reddy, P., Du, C. et al. 2007. p27^{kip1} (cyclin-dependent kinase inhibitor 1B) controls ovarian development by suppressing follicle endowment and activation and promoting follicle atresia in mice. *Molecular Endocrinology* 21:2189–2202.

Ramesh, A., Archibong, A.E., and Niaz, M.S. 2010. Ovarian susceptibility to benzo[a]pyrene: Tissue burden of metabolites and DNA adducts in F-344 rats. *Journal of Toxicology and Environmental Health* 73:1611–1625.

Rappaport, S.M. and Fraser, D.A. 1977. Air sampling and analysis in a rubber vulcanization area. *American Industrial Hygiene Association Journal* 38:205–210.

Richards, J.S. 1980. Maturation of ovarian follicles: Actions and interactions of pituitary and ovarian hormones on follicular cell differentiation. *Physiological Reviews* 60:51–89.

Ronnback, C. 1991. Effects of 3,3′,4,4′-tetrachlorobiphenyl (TCB) on ovaries of foetal mice. *Pharmacology and Toxicology* 69:340.

Sadeu, J.C., Hughers, C.L., Agarwal, S., and Foster, W.G. 2010. Alcohol, drugs, caffeine, tobacco and environmental contaminant exposure: Reproductive health consequences and clinical implications. *Critical Reviews Toxicology* 40:633–652.

Shiromizu, K., Thorgeirsson, S.S., and Mattison, D.R. 1984. Effect of cyclophosphamide on oocyte and follicle number in Sprague Dawley rats, C57BL/6N and DBA/2N mice. *Pediatric Pharmacology* 4:213–21.

Smith, B.J., Mattison, D.R., and Sipes, I.G. 1990. The role of epoxidation in 4-vinylcyclohexene-induced ovarian toxicity. *Toxicology and Applied Pharmacology* 105:372–381.

Soares, S.R., Simon, C., Remohi, J., and Pellicer, A. 2007. Cigarette smoking affects uterine receptiveness. *Human Reproduction* 22:543–547.

Sobinoff, A.P., Mahony, M., Nixon, B., Roman, S.D., and McLaughlin, E.A. 2011. Understanding the villain: DMBA-induced pre-antral ovotoxicity involves selective follicular destruction and primordial follicle activation through PI3K/Akt and mTOR signaling. *Toxicological Sciences* 123:563–575.

Sobinoff, A.P., Pye, V., Nixon, B., Roman, S.D., and McLaughlin, E.A. 2010. Adding insult to injury: Effects of xenobioitic-induced pre-antral ovotoxicity on ovarian development and oocyte fusibility. *Toxicological Sciences* 118:653–666.

Sobinoff, A.P., Pye, V., Nixon, B., Roman, S.D., and McLaughlin, E.A. 2012. Jumping the gun: Smoking constituent BaP causes premature primordial follicle activation and impairs oocyte fusibility through oxidative stress. *Toxicology and Applied Pharmacology* 260:70–80.

Sobrinho, L.G., Levine, R.A., and DeConti, R.C. 1971. Amenorrhea in patients with Hodgkin's disease treated with antineoplastic agents. *American Journal of Obstetrics and Gynecology* 109:135–139.

Soleimani, R., Heytens, E., Darzynkiewicz, Z., and Oktay, K. 2011. Mechanisms of chemotherapy-induced human ovarian aging: Double strand DNA breaks and microvascular compromise. *Aging (Albany NY)* 3:782–793.

Sowers, M.R. and La Pietra, M.T. 1995. Menopause: Its epidemiology and potential association with chronic diseases. *Epidemiological Reviews* 17:287–302.

Springer, L.N., McAsey, M.E., Flaws, J.A., Tilly, J.L., Sipes, I.G., and Hoyer, P.B. 1996a. Involvement of apoptosis in 4-vinylcyclohexene diepoxide-induced ovotoxicity in rats. *Toxicology and Applied Pharmacology* 139:394–401.

Springer, L.N., Tilly, J.L., Sipes, I.G., and Hoyer, P.B. 1996b. Enhanced expression of bax in small preantral follicles during 4-vinylcyclohexene diepoxide-induced ovotoxicity in the rat. *Toxicology and Applied Pharmacology* 139:402–410.

Stedman, R.L. 1968. The chemical composition of tobacco and tobacco smoke. *Chemical Reviews* 68:153–207.

Swartz, W.J. and Mattison, D.R. 1985. Benzo(a)pyrene inhibits ovulation in C57BL/6N mice. *Anatomical Record* 212:268–276.

Takeuchi, Y., Ichihara, G., and Kamijima, M. 1997. A review of toxicity of 2-bromopropane: Mainly on its reproductive toxicity. *Journal of Occupational Health* 39:191.

Tilly, J.L., Kowalski, K.I., Johnson, A.L., and Hsueh, A.J.W. 1991. Involvement of apoptosis in ovarian follicular atresia and post-ovulatory regression. *Endocrinology* 129:2799–2801.

Turchi, G., Bonatti, S., Citti, L., Gervasi, P.G., and Abbondandolo, A. 1981. Alkylating properties and genetic activity of 4-vinylcyclohexene metabolites and structurally related epoxides. *Mutation Research* 83:419–430.

Vahakangas, K., Rajaniemi, H., and Pelkonen, O. 1985. Ovarian toxicity of cigarette smoke exposure during pregnancy in mice. *Toxicological Letters* 25:75–80.

VanVoorhis, B.J., Syrop, C.H., Hammit, D.H., Dunn, M.S., and Snyder, G.D. 1992. Effects of smoking on ovulation induction for assisted reproductive techniques. *Fertility and Sterility* 58:981–985.

Wayne, G.L., Fairley, K.F., Hobbs, J.B., and Martin, F.I.R. 2002. Cyclophosphamide-induced ovarian failure. *New England Journal of Medicine* 289:1159–1162.

Wyllie, A.H., Kerr, J.F.R., and Currie, A.R. 1980. Cell death: The significance of apoptosis. *Internal Reviews in Cytology* 68:251–306.

Xiang, Y., Xu, J., Li, L., Lin, X., Chen, X., Zhang, X., Fu, Y., and Luo, L. 2012. Calorie restriction increases primordial follicle reserve in mature female chemotherapy-treated rats. *Gene* 493:77–82.

Yu, X.Z., Kamijima, M., Ichihara, G., Li, W., Kitoh, J., Xie, Z., Shibata, E., Hisanaga, N., and Takeuchi, Y. 1999. 2-Bromopropane causes ovarian dysfunction by damaging primordial follicles and their oocytes in female rats. *Toxicology and Applied Pharmacology* 159:185–193.

Part II

Ovotoxic Chemical Classes

6 Ovarian Toxicity Caused by Pesticides

Wei Wang, Patrick Hannon, and Jodi A. Flaws

CONTENTS

6.1 INTRODUCTION

Based on the Environmental Protection Agency (EPA) definition, a pesticide is any substance or mixture of substances intended for preventing, destroying, repelling, or mitigating any pest or intended for use as a plant regulator, defoliant, or desiccant. Pests can be insects, a variety of animals, unwanted plants (weeds), fungi, or microorganisms like bacteria and viruses. Though the term of pesticide is often misunderstood to refer only to insecticides, it also applies to herbicides, fungicides, and various other substances used to control pests. Pesticides have been widely used to prevent crop losses and control disease spread via insects and other pests (Bretveld et al., 2006). Because of the widespread use of pesticides, humans and wildlife are chronically exposed to low levels of pesticide residues through their diet. Furthermore, some pesticides are hard to biodegrade and thus, they readily accumulate in the food chain and environment (Tiemann, 2008). Because pesticides are nonspecific in both the species and the tissues they target, some pesticides that are intended to attack pest nervous systems are also ovarian toxicants in humans and wildlife. For example, the organochlorine pesticide methoxychlor (MXC), a neurotoxicant, has been found to adversely affect various ovarian functions (Gaido et al., 2000; Waters et al., 2001; Zachow and Uzumcu, 2006; Craig et al., 2010; Basavarajappa et al., 2011). Often, pesticide-induced ovarian toxicity can lead to adverse reproductive outcomes. In recent epidemiological studies, exposure to pesticides has been associated with various reproductive dysfunctions in women, such as irregular menstruation, reduced fertility, prolonged time-to-pregnancy, and spontaneous abortion (Smith et al., 1997; Farr et al., 2004; Hanke and Jurewicz, 2004; Idrovo et al., 2005).

Studies have shown that some pesticides can act as endocrine disruptors and affect ovarian function by disturbing hormonal signaling in the body. Specifically, according to the EPA, endocrine-disrupting pesticides are natural or synthetic chemicals that interfere with the production, release, transport, metabolism, binding, action, or elimination of the natural hormones in the body that are responsible for the maintenance of homeostasis and the regulation of developmental processes. In particular, endocrine-disrupting pesticides can bind to and activate various hormone receptors, such as estrogen receptors, thyroid hormone receptors, and androgen receptors, and then mimic the natural hormone's action (agonist action) or block the natural hormone's action (antagonist action). Many pesticides have been identified as endocrine disruptors in humans and wildlife and raise public health concerns because they can mimic, enhance, or inhibit endogenous hormones (Hayes et al., 2006; Kortenkamp, 2007; Mnif et al., 2011).

In females, the ovary is the primary functional organ that is responsible for the differentiation and release of a mature oocyte for fertilization and secretion of important sex steroid hormones, estrogen and progesterone. Estrogen is responsible for the maturation and function of female reproductive organs, while progesterone is critical for pregnancy maintenance. Ovarian function is also strictly controlled by the hypothalamus and pituitary via endogenous hormones. Any pesticide that acts as an endocrine disruptor could potentially harm the ovary and therefore, affect fertility and lead to other dysfunctions in the body. The mechanisms by which pesticides affect ovarian development and function are not fully understood. Because there are many different kinds of pesticides with distinct structures and targets, each pesticide may exert its effects on the ovary via different mechanisms. For example, some pesticides may damage the ovary directly by inducing cytotoxicity in the follicles, the corpora lutea, or the ovarian surface epithelium (OSE), therefore, affecting ovarian development and function and, leading to reduced fertility and premature ovarian failure (Symonds et al., 2006; Armenti et al., 2008; Symonds et al., 2008; Shibayama et al., 2009). In contrast, other pesticides may indirectly impair the development and function of the ovary by disrupting hormonal balance in the hypothalamic–pituitary–ovarian axis (Mahoney and Padmanabhan, 2010; Zorrilla et al., 2010).

This chapter focuses on the effects of pesticides on the ovary by first providing background information on the ovary and then by updating information on the major classes of pesticides that have been shown to affect the ovary. After a description of normal ovarian function, this chapter has been divided into sections on different classes of pesticides, namely organochlorine pesticides (OCP), organophosphate pesticides (OPP), pyrethroids, herbicides, and fungicides. This chapter focuses on these chemicals due to the number of well-documented examples of exposure to them in the environment and their arising public health concerns. OCPs were banned in the 1970s in the United States and replaced by more biodegradable organophosphate and pyrethroids. In addition, the herbicides make up a rapidly growing category of pesticides in use, while fungicides are important in fighting mycotoxins in food.

6.2 NORMAL OVARIAN FUNCTION

In mammals, the follicles are the functional units of the ovary. Before birth, oocytes are closely associated in clusters called germ cell nests. Shortly after birth in rodents, as shown in Figure 6.1, germ cell nests break down via apoptosis and only a small portion of the oocytes becomes surrounded by a single layer of flattened pregranulosa cells to form primordial follicles. Primordial follicles provide the finite pool for recruitment of developing follicles. Some primordial follicles are selected to grow and become primary follicles. At this stage, the flattened pregranulosa cells become cuboidal-shaped cells and the oocytes enlarge. Following the primary stage, the follicles grow to the pre-antral stage, which is characterized by a large oocyte surrounded by multiple layers of granulosa cells. At this stage, another layer of specialized somatic cells begins to proliferate and forms a layer around the granulosa cells. These cells are known as theca cells. In addition, a fluid-filled cavity, called the antrum, begins to form between the granulosa cells. The pre-antral follicles then grow into antral follicles, which contain an oocyte surrounded by several layers of granulosa cells, an antrum, and at least two distinct layers of theca cells. By this stage, the follicle can produce and secrete estrogen and progesterone and it can respond to follicle-stimulating hormone (FSH) secreted from the anterior pituitary. The final stage is the pre-ovulatory stage. Follicles in this stage contain a mature oocyte surrounded by a cumulus layer of granulosa cells, a large antral space, membrana granulosa, and at least two distinct thecal layers. In response to luteinizing hormone (LH) from the anterior pituitary, the pre-ovulatory follicle ruptures and releases an oocyte with a complement of cumulus cells (Son et al., 2011). The ruptured follicle eventually

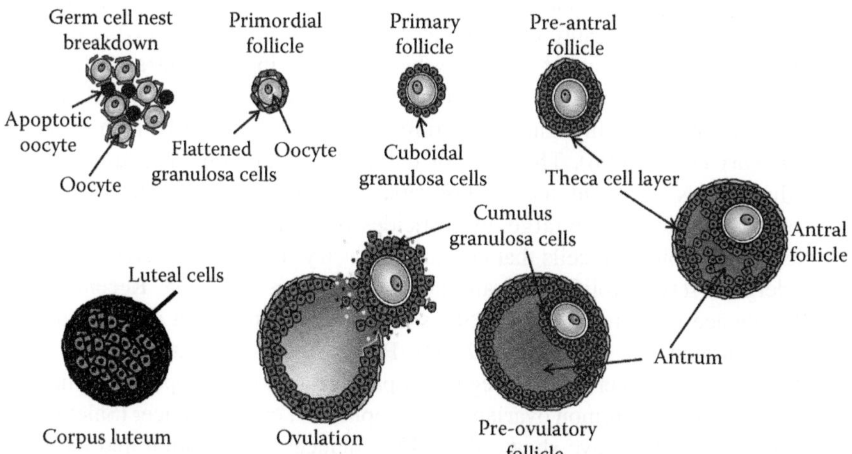

FIGURE 6.1 (See color insert.) Stages of folliculogenesis. This schematic shows the normal developmental stages of ovarian follicles beginning with germ cell nest breakdown around birth, formation of primordial follicles, and the growth of primary follicles, pre-antral, antral follicles, and pre-ovulatory follicles. This schematic also shows ovulation and the formation of the corpus luteum.

undergoes a dramatic transformation into a corpus luteum, which secretes large amounts of progesterone to maintain pregnancy if fertilization occurs (Figure 6.1). This complex process of folliculogenesis is strictly regulated by various signaling molecules in the body. For example, basic fibroblast growth factor, phosphate and tensin homolog (PTEN, a tumor suppressor gene), and anti-mullerian hormone (AMH) are critical to preserve the follicle pool at early stages. In contrast, correct responses to estradiol, FSH, and LH are essential for late stages of folliculogenesis (Barnett et al., 2006; Oktem and Urman, 2010; Son et al., 2011). Any disruptions during the process of folliculogenesis will eventually affect the development and function of the ovary and therefore, impact female reproductive health.

Throughout the reproductive life span of a female, only a very small portion of primordial follicles are selected to develop and ovulate. The vast majority (over 99%) are lost in various stages of development via a process called atresia (Hoyer and Sipes, 1996). Atresia is the process by which ovarian follicles undergo programmed cell death via apoptosis. This process is well controlled by various proliferation regulators and apoptotic factors (Matsuda-Minehata et al., 2006). Studies have shown that environmental toxicants, such as pesticides, can interrupt the expression and activities of factors that regulate atresia and therefore, induce atresia in the ovary (Miller et al., 2005; Basavarajappa et al., 2012). Because the vast majority of ovarian follicles are naturally lost via atresia, any pesticide that hastens this process could potentially cause premature ovarian failure.

Some pesticides can directly damage the ovary, but the specific effects and its implications for female reproductive health depend on the exposure time and the type of follicles targeted by the pesticide. Acute exposure to pesticides that selectively damage large growing or antral follicles only causes temporary disruption of cyclicity by reducing ovarian steroid production and ovulation. This is because the lost follicles can be replaced from the primordial follicle pool if the exposure is removed. Chronic exposure to pesticides, which damage large growing or antral follicles will cause permanent infertility because growing and antral follicles are required for fertility. Exposure to pesticides, which target primordial follicles can cause permanent infertility and premature ovarian failure (early menopause in women) (Farr et al., 2006). This kind of damage is irreversible because once the primordial pool is destroyed, it cannot be replaced (Sobinoff et al., 2010).

Another possible ovarian target of pesticides is the OSE, which is composed of a single layer of epithelial cells that envelop the ovary. The OSE is a dynamic tissue that undergoes serial proliferation and apoptosis during ovulation. Recent experimental evidence indicates that the OSE is an obligate component of the ovulatory process (Murdoch and McDonnel, 2002). Pesticides that target the OSE might impact ovulation. Furthermore, unregulated proliferation and apoptosis in the OSE may lead to the most common ovarian cancer, epithelial ovarian cancer (Salehi et al., 2008). Animal studies have shown that MXC induces proliferation and oxidative DNA damage in the mouse OSE (Symonds et al., 2006, 2008). Epidemiology studies also suggest that herbicide exposure is positively associated with ovarian cancer (Young et al., 2005; Salehi et al., 2008). Thus, it is possible that chronic pesticide exposure may be one of the risk factors for ovarian cancer.

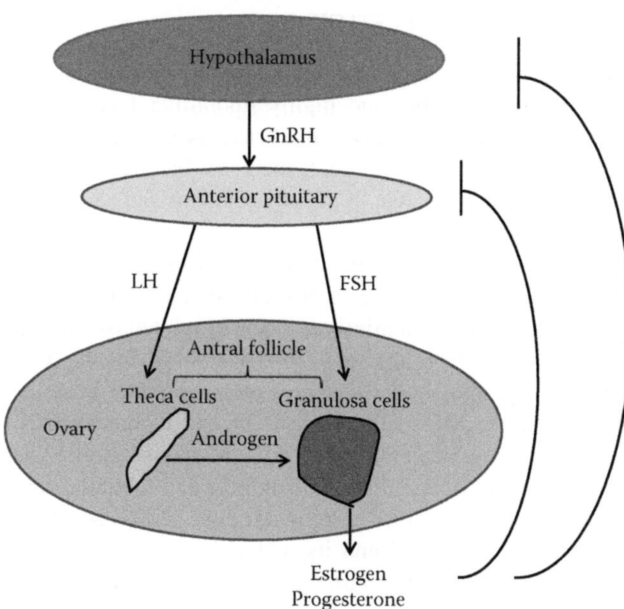

FIGURE 6.2 The hypothalamic–pituitary–ovarian axis. This schematic diagram shows the negative feedback system between the ovary, pituitary, and hypothalamus. Gonadotropin releasing hormone (GnRH) released from the hypothalamus binds to receptors on the gonadotropes in the anterior pituitary and causes the release of follicle-stimulating hormone (FSH) and luteinizing hormone (LH). FSH and LH bind to receptors on the granulosa cells and theca cells in ovarian follicles, and stimulate the production of estrogen and progesterone. These two important steroid hormones feedback negatively to the hypothalamus and the pituitary to stop excessive production of GnRH, FSH, and LH.

Finally, pesticides can impair proper ovarian function and cause fertility problems by disrupting the hormonal balance in the hypothalamic–pituitary–ovarian axis. One of the most important functional roles of the ovary is the production of the steroid hormones, estrogen and progesterone. Estrogens are essential for maintenance of reproduction and cyclicity, while progesterone is critical for maintenance of pregnancy (Christensen et al., 2012). In females, estrogen and progesterone production are strictly controlled by hormones secreted from the hypothalamus and the pituitary via feedback mechanisms (Figure 6.2). The hypothalamus produces and secretes gonadotropin releasing hormone (GnRH), which binds to receptors on the anterior pituitary and stimulates it to secrete FSH and LH. FSH and LH bind to their receptors on the ovary and regulate various critical processes for female reproduction, such as steroidogenesis, folliculogenesis, and ovulation. In turn, estrogen and progesterone feedback to the hypothalamus and the pituitary to regulate GnRH, FSH, and LH, respectively (Christensen et al., 2012). Pesticides with estrogenic activities mimic the ability of endogenous estrogen to negatively feedback to the hypothalamus and the pituitary and inhibit the production and secretion of GnRH, FSH, and LH and therefore, affect ovarian function.

6.3 ORGANOCHLORINE PESTICIDES

OCPs are present in various agricultural and industrial compounds. Organochlorine compounds are chemically stable and highly lipophilic; thus, they have a slow degradation rate, tend to accumulate in lipid-rich tissues, and bioaccumulate up the food chain (Tiemann, 2008). Although their use has been restricted in North America, many banned OCPs persist in the environment and several new OCPs are still being used in the United States.

1,1,1-trichloro-2,2-bis(4-chlorophenyl)ethane (DDT) is an OCP that was banned in the 1970s in the United Sates; however, it is still being used in Mexico to control mosquitoes. Commercial DDT is a mixture of closely related isomers. DDT consists of 80% p, p′-DDT, 15% o,p′DDT, and about 5% 1,1-dichloro-2,2-bis(p-chlorophenyl) ethane (DDE), the major metabolite and breakdown product present in the environment (Wojtowicz et al., 2011). Studies on DDT and its metabolites suggest that DDT is a potential human toxicant because DDT and its metabolite DDE have been consistently found in serum (range: 1.08–1.68 ng/mL) and follicular fluids (0.01–1.11 ng/mL) of women (Jarrell et al., 1993b; Younglai et al., 2002; Meeker et al., 2009). Further, studies suggest that DDT and its metabolites are potential reproductive toxicants. High levels of serum DDE have been associated with early onset of menopause (Akkina et al., 2004), shortened menstrual cyclicity (Ouyang et al., 2005), longer time-to-pregnancy (Axmon et al., 2006; Harley et al., 2008), and development of polycystic ovaries (Dorner et al., 2001; Gotz et al., 2001; Holloway et al., 2007). Further, studies have shown a correlation between high levels of DDE in follicular fluid and failed fertilization in women undergoing *in vitro* fertilization (IVF) procedures (Younglai et al., 2002). In addition, studies have shown that DDT and its metabolites affect steroidogenesis in the ovary in a complex manner. *In vitro* studies using porcine granulosa cells have shown that the effects of DDE on progesterone synthesis depend on dosage. Specifically, at lower doses (10 ng/mL), DDE increases progesterone synthesis (Crellin et al., 1999), while at higher doses (0.3–320 μg/mL), DDE blocks progesterone synthesis (Chedrese and Feyles, 2001). Furthermore, different effects on steroidogenesis have been reported for different isomers of DDT (p,p′- and o,p′-DDT) and its metabolites (p,p′- and o,p′-DDE) in porcine granulosa cells. Specifically, o,p′-DDT and DDE isomers (4–4000 ng/mL) increase estradiol production, but p,p′-DDT does not have the same effect. While DDT isomers and p,p′-DDE (4 μg/mL) decrease progesterone secretion, o,p′-DDE does not do so (Wojtowicz et al., 2007).

The mechanisms by which DDT and/or DDE affect ovarian function are not well known. Some studies suggest that DDT may affect ovarian function by altering the activity of key steroidogenic enzymes because treatment with DDT and/or DDE increases aromatase activity in porcine follicular cells (Wojtowicz et al., 2007) and human granulosa cells (Younglai et al., 2004b). Further, studies on DDE in porcine and Chinese hamster ovary cells showed that DDE decreases progesterone synthesis by suppressing cAMP synthesis (Chedrese and Feyles, 2001) and by decreasing the expression of *Cyp11a1*, which encodes the key rate-limiting enzyme in steroidogenesis (Crellin et al., 2001). Studies done by Younglai et al. showed that DDE, at concentrations that are present in human tissues (100 ng/mL), enhances FSH stimulation of aromatase activity and elevates cytosolic calcium levels and oscillation in cultured human granulosa cells (Younglai et al., 2004a,b). Therefore, it is likely that DDT not only interferes with gonadotropin receptor signaling second messengers such as cAMP but also directly alters enzymatic activity and modulates Ca^{2+}-dependent pathways. *In vitro* studies also show that DDT and DDE exposure affect the secretion levels of oxytocin by altering the expression of its precursor and metabolic enzymes in bovine granulosa cells and luteal cells (Mlynarczuk et al., 2009; Wrobel et al., 2009). Interestingly, studies have shown that DDE, at an environmentally relevant dose range (100–1000 ng/mL), increases the expression of vascular endothelial growth factor and insulin-like growth factor in human ovarian cells and in the rat ovary. It is thought that these changes may lead to altered ovarian function such as that seen in polycystic ovaries and impaired fertility (Holloway et al., 2007).

MXC is another organochlorine pesticide commonly used in the United States as a replacement for DDT. Although the use of MXC as a pesticide was banned in the United States in 2003 (Stuchal et al., 2006), humans and animals are still exposed to MXC through extensive global usage and through imported agricultural products (Basavarajappa et al., 2012). MXC is metabolized predominantly to 1,1,1-trichloro-2-(4-hydroxyphenyl)-2-(4-methoxyphenyl) ethane (MOH) and the bisphenolic compound 1,1,1-trichloro-2,2-bis(4-hydroxyphenyl)ethane (HPTE) by cytochrome p450 enzymes in the body (Stresser and Kupfer, 1998). MXC is considered to be an ovarian toxicant because studies have shown that MXC exposure decreases ovarian weights (Martinez and Swartz, 1991). Further, neonatal MXC exposure (between embryonic day 19 and postnatal day 7) reduces ovulation and fertility, causes premature aging, and alters folliculogenesis by reducing the expression of estrogen receptor beta (ERβ) and by increasing the expression of AMH in pre-antral and early antral follicles (Armenti et al., 2008). AMH is expressed by granulosa cells of the ovary and controls the formation of primary follicles by inhibiting the responsiveness of growing follicles to FSH, thereby preventing excessive follicular recruitment by FSH (Weenen et al., 2004). Early postnatal MXC exposure (postnatal day 3–7) inhibits folliculogenesis and stimulates AMH expression (Uzumcu et al., 2006).

Further, many *in vivo* and *in vitro* studies indicate that MXC and its metabolites inhibit growth and steroidogenesis in antral follicles. For example, studies show that MXC and its metabolites reduce key sex steroid hormone levels by decreasing steroidogenic enzymes and by increasing metabolic enzymes in mouse antral follicles (Craig et al., 2010; Basavarajappa et al., 2011; Craig et al., 2011). Specifically, MOH (10 μg/mL) decreases synthesis of progesterone, androstenedione, testosterone, and estradiol in isolated mouse antral follicles by decreasing the expression of cholesterol side-chain cleavage (*Cyp11a1*), 17α-hydroxylase/17,20-lyase (*Cyp17a1*), and aromatase (*Cyp19a1*), which are key steroidogenic enzymes (Craig et al., 2010). In addition, MXC decreases the expression of 17β-hydroxysteroid dehydrogenase 1 (*Hsd17b1*), Cyp17a1, 3β-hydroxysteroid dehydrogenase 1 (*Hsd3b1*), and steroid acute regulatory protein (*Star*), but increases the expression of the metabolic enzyme cytochrome P450 1b1 (*Cyp1b1*) in mouse antral follicles (Basavarajappa et al., 2011). Similarly, HPTE (1–10 μM) has been shown to reduce FSH-stimulated synthesis of

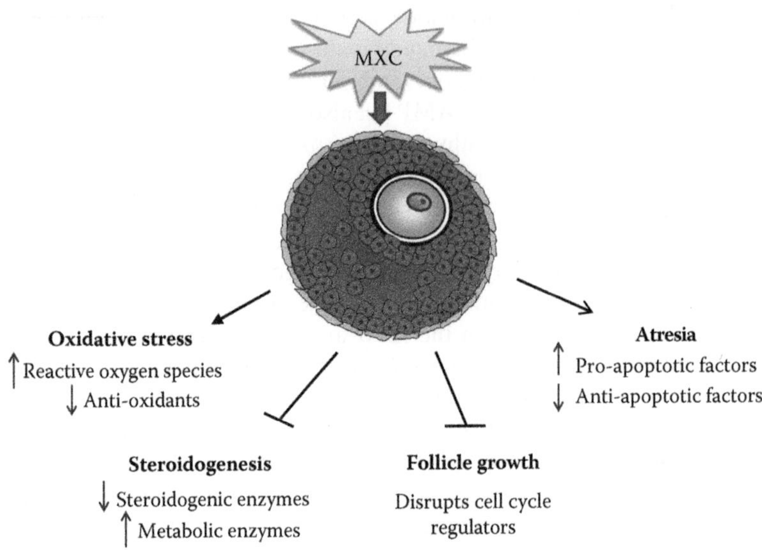

FIGURE 6.3 The ovotoxic effects of methoxychlor (MXC). This schematic diagram summarizes the toxic effects of MXC on antral follicles in the ovary. MXC causes oxidative stress in antral follicles. MXC also inhibits steroidogenesis by inhibiting steroidogenic enzymes and by inducing metabolic enzymes. In addition, MXC suppresses antral follicle growth by disrupting cell cycle regulators and induces atresia by increasing pro-apoptotic factors and by decreasing anti-apoptotic factors.

progesterone and estrogen in cultured rat granulosa cells by decreasing the expression of *Cyp11a1* and *Cyp19a1* (Zachow and Uzumcu, 2006).

Other studies show that MXC inhibits growth and induces atresia (programmed death) of mouse antral follicles. Specifically, MXC inhibits growth of antral follicles and induces atresia by reducing the expression of G1-S phase cell cycle regulators such as cyclin D2 and cyclin-dependent kinase 4, by decreasing the anti-apoptotic factors, B cell lymphoma 2 (*Bcl2*), and increasing the pro-apoptotic factors, Bcl2 associated X protein (*Bax*) (Miller et al., 2005; Gupta et al., 2009). In addition, MXC induces oxidative stress and causes DNA damage in the mouse ovary (Gupta et al., 2006; Symonds et al., 2008). These effects of MXC are summarized in Figure 6.3.

MXC and its metabolites have estrogenic, anti-estrogenic, and anti-androgenic properties depending on the receptor subtype with which it interacts (Gaido et al., 2000; Waters et al., 2001). Studies using transfected cell lines have demonstrated that the active metabolites of MXC are agonists of estrogen receptor alpha (ERα), but antagonists for both ERβ and androgen receptor (AR) (Gaido et al., 2000). Other studies have shown that fetal and neonatal exposure to MXC (20 μg/kg and 100 mg/kg) alters methylation on the promoter region of ERβ and therefore suppresses the expression of ERβ, causing ovarian dysfunction in the rat (Armenti et al., 2008; Zama and Uzumcu, 2009). Studies done by Paulose et al. show that ERα overexpressing antral follicles are more sensitive to toxicity induced by MXC and its metabolites than control antral follicles, suggesting that the disruption in the equilibrium between ERα and ERβ in the ovary may alter the response of the ovary to estrogenic chemicals (Paulose et al., 2011). Furthermore, evidence provided by Basavarajappa et al. suggests that MXC may act through the aryl hydrocarbon receptor pathway to inhibit follicle growth and induce atresia in mouse antral follicles (Basavarajappa et al., 2012).

Lindane (gamma-hexachlorocyclohexane) has been widely used since 1950 as an insecticide to treat food crops and forests and as a pharmaceutical treatment for lice and scabies (U.S. Environmental Protection Agency, 2006). Although the use of lindane in agriculture was banned in the United States in 2002 and banned worldwide in 2009 because of its neurotoxicity, human exposure still is a concern because it persists in the environment and bioaccumulates in the food chain. Recent studies suggest that lindane is an ovarian toxicant. For example, studies in ducks found fewer healthy antral follicles and significantly smaller eggs with thinner eggshells in lindane-treated ducks compared to control ducks (Chakravarty et al., 1986). A study in cockroaches found that low doses of lindane (about 3 μg/g of body mass) act as a juvenile hormone analog by enhancing protein uptake, ovarian growth, and vitellogenesis (yolk protein deposition) onset in ovaries (Goudey-Perriere et al., 2007). Studies also show that lindane exposure inhibits FSH and transforming growth factor beta (TGFβ) stimulated progesterone synthesis by disrupting gap junction formation and decreasing the expression levels of key steroidogenic enzymes (cytochrome P450 side-chain cleavage enzyme and steroidogenic acute regulatory protein) in bovine and rat granulosa cells (Ke et al., 2005; Tiemann, 2008). In contrast, Maranghi et al. reported that prenatal lindane exposure causes earlier vaginal patency and reduces the size of primary oocytes at sexual maturity, but does not affect steroidogenesis (Maranghi et al., 2007). It is likely that some of these effects of prenatal lindane exposure on ovarian development are mediated by an ERβ-dependent pathway (Maranghi et al., 2007).

Endosulfan was another globally used OCP until it was banned due to its acute neurotoxicity, potential for bioaccumulation, and role as an endocrine disruptor (Silva and Gammon, 2009). Endosulfan is considered to be a developmental and reproductive toxicant because of its estrogenic and anti-androgenic properties (Andersen et al., 2002; Varayoud et al., 2008; Silva and Gammon, 2009). Endosulfan is highly toxic to fish. Specifically, studies have shown that endosulfan exposure causes synchronous precocious ovarian development by enhancing the expression of steroidogenic acute regulatory protein and aromatase in the ovary and by decreasing gonadotropin-releasing hormone in juvenile catfish (Chakravarty et al., 1986). Endosulfan also reduces the gonadosomatic index and decreases the hatching rate in zebrafish (Han et al., 2011). Neonatal endosulfan exposure alters post-hatching folliculogenesis and decreases testosterone levels in *Caiman latirostris* (Stoker et al., 2008). In mice, endosulfan exposure (3 mg/kg/day) disrupts estrous cyclicity, decreases ovarian weight, and increases the numbers of atretic follicle (Hiremath and Kaliwal, 2002). Further, studies show that endosulfan exposure significantly increases atretic follicles numbers and malondialdehyde levels, which suggests that endosulfan might induce oxidative stress in the rat ovary (Koc et al., 2009). More recently, Nandi et al. examined the effects of endosulfan on buffalo oocyte viability, maturation, fertilization, and developmental competence *in vitro* and found a dose-dependent decline in viability and the developmental competence rate of oocytes. This suggests that endosulfan blocks *in vitro* oocyte maturation by affecting the oocyte, cumulus cell–mediated action, and hormonal reaction (Nandi et al., 2011).

6.4 ORGANOPHOSPHATE PESTICIDES

OPPs are widely used in agriculture. To date, around 40 OPPs are registered in the United States, with at least 7.3 million pounds being used in agricultural and residential settings (US EPA, 2001). Because they are less chemically stable than OCPs and can be degraded rapidly by hydrolysis by exposure to sunlight, air, and soil, OPPs do not accumulate readily in the environment and thus, they have become an attractive alternative to persistent OCPs. The insecticidal activity of OPP is due to its ability to irreversibly inactivate acetyl cholinesterase, which is critical for nerve function, and to subsequently cause neurotoxicity in insects, humans, and many other animals. Because of their neurotoxicity, OPPs are generally more overtly toxic than the OCPs and are in fact a major culprit in acute accidental poisonings (Klaassen, 1996). A variety of health effects have been correlated with chronic low-dose exposure to OPPs, such as birth defects, childhood brain tumors, and neurobehavioral and neurodevelopmental defects (Colosio et al., 2003; Rauh et al., 2012). Furthermore, OPPs have been known to accumulate in the ovary and to cause ovarian damage (Piao et al., 1997; Koc et al., 2009).

Although the effects of chronic OPP exposure on human neurodevelopment and neurobehavior have been exclusively studied, OPPs also have been shown to damage the ovaries of various species. For example, *in vitro* studies have shown that 24 h malathion exposure (250–900 μM), the most commonly used OPP in residential landscaping and public recreation areas to control mosquitoes in the United States, inhibits early oogenesis in the mouse (Bonilla et al., 2008). Further, malathion (11–33 mg/kg) decreases healthy follicles and increases atretic follicles in rat ovaries. It is likely that these effects are due to an ability of malathion to induce oxidative stress in the ovary because studies show that malathion increases malondialehyde levels in the ovary, an indicator of oxidative stress (Koc et al., 2009). IVF studies using porcine oocytes and sperm have shown that malathion and diazinon (another commonly used OPP) impair IVF and embryo development (Ducolomb et al., 2009). Studies in *Channa punctatus* (Bloch) found that malathion inhibits steroidogenesis by blocking the activities of ovarian delta-hydroxysteroid dehydrogenease and glucose-6-phophate dehydrogenase, leading to the loss of stage II and III oocytes (Inbaraj and Haider, 1988). In similar studies, malathion has been shown to inhibit ovarian steroidogenesis by inhibiting the availability of free cholesterol in the catfish ovary (Singh, 1992).

Trichlorfon, an OPP with comparatively mild side effects and good anthelmintic properties in human therapy, disturbs spindle assembly and chromosome congression in meiosis I and II during *in vitro* maturation of isolated mouse oocytes, suggesting that OPP exposure–induced spindle aberration could lead to human trisomy (Yin et al., 1998). Further studies found that exposure to high concentrations of trichlorfon induce nondisjunction at meiosis I of oogenesis, while lower doses preferentially cause errors in chromosome segregation at meiosis II due to disturbances in spindle function and chromosome congression as well as precocious separation of chromatids prior to anaphase II (Cukurcam et al., 2004). In addition, studies using a pre-antral follicle culture system show that trichlorfon affects follicle cell function, cytokinesis, and chromosome alignment in oocytes (Sun et al., 2008). These studies suggest that alterations in oocyte–follicle cell communication by trichlorfon may compromise normal maturation and chromosome segregation in follicle-enclosed mammalian oocytes. Granulosa cells in the ovary produce acetylcholine and express choline esterases, and both granulosa cells and oocytes express muscarinic acetylcholine receptors, which can be activated by acetylcholine (Fritz et al., 2001; Kang et al., 2003). Thus, trichlorfon may impact oogenesis indirectly by inhibiting the activity of choline esterases and receptors on granulosa cells and oocytes. In turn, this may affect folliculogenesis and oocytes activation *in vitro* (Lawrence and Cuthbertson, 1995; Fritz et al., 2002).

Other OPPs also have been shown to affect the ovary. Studies have shown that exposure to dimethoate for 10 days leads to a significant decrease in ovarian weight, a decrease in the number of estrous cycles, and a decrease in the duration of proestrus, estrus, and metestrus, but an increase in the duration of the diestrous phase and the number of atretic antral follicles in the ovary. Collectively, these data suggest that dimethoate might directly or indirectly affect ovarian function in pubertal mice (Mahadevaswami and Kaliwal, 2002). Monocrotophos also has been found to decrease ovarian weight, disrupt estrous cyclicity, decrease healthy follicle number, and increase atretic follicle number in mice (Rao and Kaliwal, 2002). Chloryrifos reduces *in vitro* maturation and development of buffalo oocytes directly and indirectly by blocking the action of estrogen and FSH (Nandi et al., 2011). Parathion (3–5 mg/kg) has been found to decrease ovarian weight and the number of healthy follicles in the rat ovary (Ducolomb et al., 2009) and to disrupt estrous cyclicity in rats (Asmathbanu and Kaliwal, 1997). Studies in *Biomphalaria glabrata* show that azinpho-methyl causes a decline in reproduction by decreasing egg mass and reducing hatching rate (Kristoff et al., 2011).

6.5 PYRETHRINS AND PYRETHROIDS

Pyrethrins are natural organic compounds derived from the flowers of pyrethrum (*Chrysanthemum cinerariaefolium*) that have been used as insecticides because of their neurotoxicity to insects (Casida, 1980). Since pyrethrins are nonpersistent and biodegradable (i.e., they break down by exposure to sunlight and the atmosphere within 2 days), they are gradually replacing organochlorines and organophosphates and becoming the first choice for use in agriculture and household products (Katsuda, 2012). Based on the chemical structure of pyrethrin, synthetic pyrethroid insecticides were produced that have higher insecticidal potency and stability in the environment than natural pyrethrin. Currently, pyrethroids have become the main active component in commercial household insecticides (Koureas et al., 2012). Pyrethroids and their metabolites have been found to persist in the environment, including soil, aquatic microcosms (Katagi, 2010), sediments (Palmquist et al., 2011), and food products (Hanafi et al., 2010). These compounds also have been detected in human samples such as urine (Babina et al., 2012) and breast milk (Sereda et al., 2009).

The insecticidal actions of pyrethrins and pyrethroids depend on their abilities to bind to and disrupt voltage-gated sodium, calcium, and chloride channels of insect nerves (Soderlund, 2012). In recent years, studies have shown that pyrethroid insecticides also have endocrine disrupting properties and can affect reproduction and sexual development in both males and females (Pine et al., 2008; Jin et al., 2012). In males, developmental pyrethroid exposure impairs testicular development and spermatogenesis in the mouse (Zhang et al., 2010; Wang et al., 2011). *In vivo* and *in vitro* studies have shown that pyrethroid exposure reduces sperm count and motility, causes deformity of the sperm head, increases the count of abnormal sperm, damages sperm DNA, induces aneuploidy, and affects testosterone levels in the mouse testes (Abdallah et al., 2010; Perobelli et al., 2010; Zhao et al., 2011).

In females, numerous studies have shown that pyrethroid exposure leads to reproductive dysfunction. Studies on fenvalerate, one of the most studied pyrethroids, have shown that *in utero* and lactational fenvalerate (40 mg/kg) exposure impairs ovarian development of female rat offspring by reducing the numbers of pre-antral follicles and corpora lutea, resulting in reduced fecundity in female rats (Guerra et al., 2011). Another study done by Fei et al. examined the effects of fenvalerate on follicular development. In that study, the authors found that fenvalerate suppresses follicle growth and decreases the levels of sex steroid hormones such as progesterone, testosterone, and estradiol by reducing the expression of key steroidogenic enzymes, cytochrome P450 side-chain cleavage enzyme, and steroidogenic acute regulatory protein (Fei et al., 2010). Furthermore, Chen et al. found similar effects of fenvalerate on steroid production in rat granulosa cells (Chen et al., 2005). In addition, studies have shown that fenvalerate interferes with calcium homeostasis in the rat ovary and primary cultured human luteinized granulosa cells (He et al., 2004, 2006). Specifically, fenvalerate (31.8 mg/kg) increases serum free calcium levels and total content of calmodulin significantly during estrus, but decreases progesterone levels during diestrus in the rat (He et al., 2004). In another study, He et al. reported that fenvalerate also inhibits FSH-stimulated progesterone production and increases calcium levels in primary cultured human luteinized granulosa cells, suggesting that the effects of fenvalerate on ovarian steroidogenesis may be mediated partly through the calcium signaling pathway (He et al., 2006).

Esfenvalerate, another pyrethroid, has the same components as fenvalerate and has replaced fenvalerate use in the United States because it is less chronically toxic and more powerful due to a higher percentage of one insecticidal isomer. Studies in rats show that prepubertal exposure to esfenvalerate suppresses the afternoon rise of LH and delays puberty (Pine et al., 2008). Studies using rat granulosa cells indicate that bifenthrin, another broad-spectrum synthetic pyrethroid, inhibits the expression of various LH-inducible ovulatory genes and prostaglandin synthesis, suggesting that exposure to bifenthrin may lead to ovulatory dysfunction in females (Liu et al., 2011). Further, studies show that the pyrethroid cypermethrin induces toxicity and reduces progesterone production in primary cultured bovine corpora luteal cells (Gill et al., 2011).

Recently accumulated evidence suggests that pyrethroid pesticides have estrogenic and/or androgenic activities; however, the results of these studies are, in some respects, contradictory and the mechanisms for pyrethroid-induced endocrine disruption still remain unclear. Studies using different *in vitro* methods such as E-Screen assays, estrogen receptor competition binding assays, and pS2 expression assays show that some of pyrethroid pesticides, including cypermethrin, permethrin, deltamethrin, and lambda-cyhalothrin, cause ER-specific agonist responses because their estrogenic effects on MCF-7 cell proliferation can be completely blocked by the ER antagonist, ICI 182.780. Some pyrethroid pesticides, like fenvalerate, induce MCF-7 cell proliferation via ER-independent pathways (Chen et al., 2002; Zhao et al., 2008). In addition, other studies show that some pyrethroids (empenthrin, imiprothrin, and prallethrin) have no anti-estrogenic or anti-androgenic activity (Saito et al., 2000). Du et al. evaluated and compared ER, androgen receptor, and thyroid hormone receptor activities of different pyrethroids and their metabolites using receptor-mediated luciferase reporter gene assays. The data from that study suggest that different pyrethroids and their metabolites might affect the reproductive system by disrupting the function of multiple nuclear hormone receptors (Du et al., 2010). Currently, two standard *in vivo* short-term assays, the uterotrophic assay and Hershberger assay, have been widely used to evaluate potential hormonal activities of pyrethroids. Based on the results of these two *in vivo* assays, permethrin has estrogenic effects in female rats, but anti-androgenic effects in males (Kim et al., 2005b). Tetramethrin (5–800 mg/kg) exerts anti-estogenic effects in female rats (Kim et al., 2005a); however, esfenvalerate (20 mg/kg/day) and fenvalerate (80 mg/kg/day) do not exhibit estrogenic or anti-androgenic effects in rats (Kunimatsu et al., 2002). These results are somewhat contradictory, probably because of the different sensitivity and specificity of *in vitro* and *in vivo* test systems. Therefore, further characterization of the endocrine-disrupting effects of pyrethroids, especially their hormone receptor activities, is required for assessing their potential human health risks.

6.6 HERBICIDES

Insecticides are not the only pesticides known to elicit damage to the ovary. Herbicides, designed to inhibit photosynthesis and eliminate unwanted plant growth, can also adversely affect the ovary. The first generation of herbicides, including sulfuric acid, iron sulfate, copper sulfate, sodium chlorate, and arsenic trioxide, were developed in the 1930s, but were highly toxic and far too nonspecific for the unwanted crop or plant (Gysin and Knusli, 1960; Jager, 1983; Ecobichon, 1996). The second generation of herbicides proved to be more specific, yet were still toxic to mammals (Ecobichon, 1996). Herbicides used today are considered to be less toxic than their predecessors; however, these chemicals still possess many carcinogenic, mutagenic, and teratogenic properties, affecting both human and animal life (Ecobichon, 1996). The extensive variety of herbicide classification groups and the myriad of chemicals within each group may prove to be a concern to ovarian toxicologists, in that toxicities exist within a wide range of acute and chronic exposures with unspecified mechanisms of action.

First introduced in the 1950s, chlorotriazines, such as atrazine, simazine, and cyanazine, were used as broad-spectrum herbicides (Eldridge et al., 1994; U.S. Environmental Protection Agency, 1994). The pesticidal mechanism of action of the chlorotriazines is inhibition of photosynthesis, specifically by prevention of electron transfer at the reducing site of the photosynthesis complex II in the chloroplasts (Gysin and Knusli, 1960). Atrazine, one of the most commonly used herbicides, is applied to control annual grasses and broadleaf weeds. It is estimated that approximately 76 million pounds of atrazine are used annually on corn, sorghum, and sugarcane within the United States, with corn accounting for the greatest amount of use. Of particular concern to human and animal exposure, the major route of atrazine entry into surface water is via erosion and runoff, while leaching or lateral movement through soil or tile drains are secondary routes of exposure. Due to the timing of herbicide application, atrazine levels in aquatic tributaries are at their highest in spring (Withgott, 2002). Atrazine is considered to be a persistent environmental chemical found in soil residues, environmental and drinking water, and crops (Norris and Fong, 1983; Goh, 1993; Gojmerac et al., 1994; Vidacek and Karavidovic, 1994).

Several previous studies implicate atrazine as an endocrine-disrupting chemical with both direct and indirect toxic responses on the ovary. Specifically, atrazine has been shown to act directly on the ovary by altering the normal levels of circulating sex steroid hormones produced by the ovary and by disrupting normal follicular atresia. Atrazine has been shown to indirectly affect the ovary by altering the neuroendocrine control of ovarian function.

Studies have linked atrazine exposure to direct physiological changes in the ovary as well as alterations in the circulating sex steroid hormone levels in mammals. Low-dose exposure of atrazine in female pigs undergoing intensive breeding caused the persistence of corpora lutea and multiple follicular cysts in the ovary (Gojmerac et al., 1996). The same study showed that subacute exposure to atrazine increased serum progesterone and decreased serum 17β-estradiol concentrations at 24 and 48 h before the onset of the next predicted estrus (Gojmerac et al., 1996). Taketa and colleagues (2011) found that subacute oral exposure to atrazine caused a similar increase in serum progesterone levels in female rats (Taketa et al., 2011). This is due to an increase in the levels of steroidogenic factors and a decrease in the levels of luteolytic factors. Further, they showed that atrazine may directly target newly formed corpora lutea to promote steroidogenesis and suppress progesterone catabolism, thus elevating progesterone secretion by the newly formed corpora lutea. Taken together, their findings indicate that atrazine may directly stimulate progesterone secretion by newly formed corpora lutea (Taketa et al., 2011).

Other studies detailing the adverse effects of atrazine on ovarian morphology and hormone production exist. A study with two strains of female rats showed that exposure to both atrazine and simazine, another chlorotriazine herbicide, reduced ovarian and uterine weights and decreased estradiol levels (Eldridge et al., 1994). Furthermore, subchronic exposure to atrazine significantly increased the incidence of multi-oocyte pre-antral follicles and increased the intensity of granulosa cell apoptotic body staining in antral follicles (Juliani et al., 2008). However, the total number of atretic antral follicles did not differ from the control treated females. In the same study, a subacute dose of atrazine caused disorganization of the granulosa cell layer and/or degeneration of the oocyte in pre-antral follicles. The same doses of atrazine also caused a discontinuous zona pellucida in antral follicles that was not seen in atretic antral follicles in the control group (Juliani, 2008). Together, these studies indicate that atrazine exposure can lead to ovarian damage and disrupt the normal circulating levels of key sex steroid hormones necessary for reproductive homeostasis.

Recent studies also suggest that atrazine may directly target the ovary causing atresia (i.e., follicular death via apoptosis). Because the vast majority of follicles are destined to undergo atresia, any chemical that disrupts the balance of apoptosis will have adverse effects on the number of ovarian follicles. Many cellular processes dictate whether a cell will undergo apoptosis or survive, two of which include heat shock proteins and oxidative stress. Atrazine has been shown to alter atresia by altering heat shock proteins and causing oxidative stress. Subacute atrazine exposure was able to induce a change in 90 kDa heat shock protein (HSP90) expression, thus, altering apoptosis in granulosa cells (Juliani, 2008). Following subchronic exposure to atrazine, expression of HSP90 was higher in granulosa cells when compared to the control group; however, no HSP90 expression was detected in the ovaries of rats exposed to subacute treatment of atrazine (Juliani, 2008). This suggests that subchronic exposure to atrazine caused the overexpression of HSP90, which allowed the granulosa cells to adapt and avoid apoptotic induced cell death (Juliani, 2008). Conversely, the more concentrated subacute exposure of atrazine overpowered the ability of the cell to survive, and HSP90 expression was depleted in that treatment group (Juliani, 2008). An additional study observing the effect of atrazine on oxidative stress response, a possible facilitator of follicular atresia, was performed in adult zebrafish. An increase in the accumulation of reactive oxygen species or a decrease in the activities of antioxidant enzymes will favor an apoptotic response in cells. Thus, an elevated oxidative stress response is an indication of ovarian harm via apoptosis. In the zebrafish, fourteen days of exposure to atrazine increased superoxide dismutase (SOD) and catalase (CAT) activity and decreased glutathione activity in the ovary. Surprisingly, the mRNA expression of the enzymes responsible in mediating oxidative stress was unchanged (Jin et al., 2010). Because an increase in SOD and CAT activities contributes to the elimination of reactive oxygen species from the cell, it appears that a compensatory mechanism is in place to alleviate the atrazine-induced oxidative stress response in zebrafish (Jin et al., 2010).

Atrazine also has indirect toxicity on ovarian function by altering the neuroendocrine system (Figure 6.4). Atrazine exposure reportedly increased dopamine and decreased norepinephrine concentrations in the hypothalamus (Cooper, 1998). It also diminished the prolactin and LH surges induced by estrogen, following single or multiple doses of the chemical in ovariectomized rats (Cooper et al., 2000). These studies indicate a disruption of the hypothalamic control of both the hypothalamus and pituitary. Thus, it is hypothesized that atrazine indirectly affects the ovary by altering the neuroendocrine axis in an anti-estrogenic manner, leading to premature reproductive aging.

A common indirect ovarian effect involving atrazine is the ability of the chemical to alter estrous cyclicity (Cooper et al., 1996; Gojmerac et al., 1996; Eldridge et al., 1999). Important for successful mating and often subsequent ovulation, the estrous cycle in animals can be used as an indication of reproductive harm. Toxicants that cause abnormal estrous cyclicity can interfere with the ability of the ovary to ovulate. In a study using pigs, atrazine prolonged the estrous stage, causing a cessation of ovulation which lead to multiple unruptured, cystic follicles

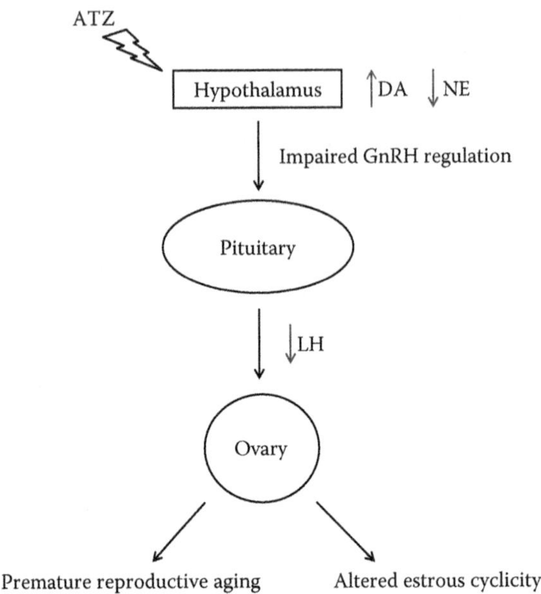

FIGURE 6.4 The ovotoxic effects of atrazine (ATZ). ATZ indirectly targets the ovary by disrupting the hypothalamic control of the neuroendocrine axis, as well documented by Cooper and colleagues (1998 and 2000). Specifically, ATZ increases dopamine (DA) and decreases norepinephrine (NE), leading to impaired gonadotropin releasing hormone (GnRH) release by the hypothalamus. This is followed by decreased luteinizing hormone (LH) secretion and eventually premature reproductive aging and altered estrous cyclicity.

(Gojmerac et al., 1996). In Fischer 344 rats, atrazine exposure caused an extended period of vaginal diestrus, confirming the ability of atrazine to disrupt estrous cyclicity and decreasing the occurrence of successful matings (Simic et al., 1994). Other rat strains, Sprague Dawley and Long-Evans-hooded, exposed to an acute dose of atrazine exhibited abnormal estrous cycles, whereas subchronic exposure to atrazine resulted in an early, age-related termination of cycling, categorized by constant vaginal estrus (Cooper et al., 1996; Eldridge et al., 1999). High doses of atrazine have been shown to cause irregular cycling, repetitive pseudopregnancies, atrophied ovaries, induced anestrus, and prolonged vaginal diestrus (Cooper et al., 1996). Although pseudopregnancy was observed following a dose of atrazine on the day of proestrus, ovulation was unaffected in the study (Cooper et al., 2000). Future studies are necessary for better understanding of the effect of atrazine on estrous cyclicity, be it via a direct effect on ovarian hormone production or rather a direct effect on vaginal cytology.

Atrazine also affects the reproductive health of amphibians of both sexes. Because a major source of exposure to atrazine is via agricultural runoff, it is of additional interest to observe the effects of atrazine on the amphibian population, as amphibians inhabit potential runoff sites. The current literature suggests that atrazine has the ability to both demasculinize, defined as a decrease in male gonadal characteristics, and feminize, defined as a development of ovaries in male amphibians

(Hayes et al., 2011). *Xenopus laevis* (African clawed frog) male tadpoles exposed to atrazine in laboratory studies developed extra gonads and were categorized as hermaphrodites (Hayes et al., 2002). At an environmentally relevant dose, a 30-fold lower dose than the EPA safe drinking water level, 16%–20% of exposed frogs developed up to six gonads, including both testes and ovaries. The hermaphroditic tendencies were hypothesized to be caused by the ability of the chemical to activate aromatase; thus, resulting in a greater production of estrogens than testosterone (Hayes et al., 2002). Interestingly, mortality, growth rate, and external appearance were unchanged after atrazine exposure, and it is currently unknown whether the reproductive abilities of atrazine-induced hermaphroditic frogs are affected (Withgott, 2002). However, some discrepancies exist in the literature because Kloas et al. (2009) were unable to find atrazine-induced hermaphroditic tendencies in the African clawed frog (Kloas et al., 2009). It is hypothesized that the discrepancies between studies could be attributed to population-specific effects of atrazine on gonadal development in *Xenopus laevis* (Du Preez et al., 2009).

Atrazine is also known to cause direct ovarian harm by reducing germ cell numbers and inducing atresia in amphibious populations. A study examining *Xenopus laevis* female tadpoles showed that atrazine induced depletion of primary germ cells by 20% following 48 hours of exposure. Additionally, both primary and secondary oogonia displayed an increase in atresia in response to atrazine (Tavera-Mendoza et al., 2002).

Although atrazine is a widely used and studied ovotoxicant, it is not the only herbicide known to elicit ovarian toxicity. The chlorophenoxy herbicide 2,4-diclorophenoxyacetic acid, commonly referred to as 2,4-D, is used to control the growth of broadleaf and woody plants by disrupting the biological responses to hormones in plants (Munro et al., 1992). This herbicide also accounts for 50% of the defoliant Agent Orange used extensively in the Vietnam War (Ecobichon, 1996). Preliminary ovotoxicity studies using subchronic doses of 2,4-D resulted in decreased ovarian weights in rats (Charles et al., 1996). A more mechanistic study was conducted in pre- and postnatal exposed rats to 2,4-D, examining oxidative stress in the ovary. Exposure to 2,4-D increased oxidative stress and altered enzymatic activity at different ages of development (Pochettino et al., 2011). After cessation of 2,4-D treatment on postnatal day 23, glutathione-S-transferase and CAT activity were decreased and accompanied by an increase in oxidative stress biomarkers, specifically in lipid peroxidation at all-time points and in hydroxyl radical levels and carbonyl groups at selected time points (Pochettino et al., 2011). Pre- and postnatal exposure to 2,4-D appears to cause oxidative stress in the ovary, which potentially could affect ovarian apoptosis and circulating hormone levels. The separate time points used following cessation of exposure to 2,4-D show that the effects of this herbicide fluctuate across different stages of development, and these effects could reflect the responsiveness of ovarian cells to xenobiotics and steroid hormones across development (Pochettino et al., 2011).

The chloracetamide herbicide butachlor is another known disruptor of ovarian function. Butachlor is extensively applied to control weeds in rice fields, and it is a persistent chemical in agricultural soil and water systems (Yu et al., 2003). Butachlor exposure for 30 days had adverse effects on reproductive efficiency and hormone levels in adult zebrafish. Following exposure, butachlor reduced the number of eggs produced/female/day, which complemented a decrease in both plasma estradiol and testosterone levels (Chang et al., 2011). Furthermore, a decrease in estradiol and testosterone is thought to cause a decline in egg quality. It is hypothesized that the decrease in sex steroid levels is attributed to competitive binding of butachlor to steroid-binding proteins which would, in turn, increase the clearance rate of estradiol and testosterone. In male zebrafish, butachlor increased plasma vitellogenin, a lipoprotein precursor of egg yolk proteins synthesized in the liver of female fish in response to estrogens, thus highlighting the potential estrogenic activity of the chemical (Chang et al., 2011).

Though not extensively studied, multiple herbicides including the carbamates chlorpropham and cycloate, the urea derivative chloroxurone, the anilide propanil, and the chlorotriazines simazine and terbutryne cause toxic responses in the ovary. Using low concentrations in freshwater snails, these herbicides delayed the time of egg maturation and increased the amount of nonviable embryos (Kosanke et al., 1988).

In terms of environmental exposure to herbicides, humans and animals are typically exposed to a combination of multiple herbicidal toxicants. Not only is it important to study the effects of individual herbicides, but it is also necessary to evaluate the effects on the ovary of an environmental mixture of herbicides. Herbicidal mixtures used in modern agricultural practices found in California and Iowa have been studied for their toxic effects on the ovary (Heindel et al., 1994). The California mixture contained aldicarb, atrazine, dibromochloropropane, 1,2-dichloropropane, ethylene dibromide, simazine, and ammonium nitrate, whereas the Iowa mixture contained alachlor, atrazine, cyanazine, metolachlor, metribuzin, and ammonium nitrate. Neither mixture reduced fertility, decreased reproductive performance, increased embryo/fetal toxicity, or caused fetal malformations in either mice or rats, even though these mixtures were prepared at 100 times the median level found in groundwater in each of these areas. Though these mixtures at high doses may not elicit a toxic response in the rodent ovary, it should be noted that each individual chemical, on its own, could yield toxic effects in the ovary. In fact, the addition or subtraction of certain herbicidal chemicals may interfere with the interactions of each individual chemical in the mixture, thus triggering different effects. Additionally, chemicals that interfere with the endocrine system often elicit different effects at low doses compared to high doses. Future work on herbicidal mixtures in smaller concentrations would help address some of these concerns.

6.7 FUNGICIDES

Fungicides are another class of pesticides that have been studied in the field of ovarian toxicology. Used extensively in tropical climates and agricultural-based regions, fungicides control fungal infestations of crops. Although many fungicides were predicted to have low toxicity in mammals, studies indicate that 90% of fungicides are carcinogenic in animals. This is problematic because it is estimated that 75 million pounds of fungicides are used agriculturally per year (Ecobichon, 1996). Like the chemicals previously discussed, several classes of fungicides are known to harm ovarian function.

Hexachlorobenzene (HCB) is one example of an ovotoxic fungicide. This chlorinated organic compound is banned due to its known toxic properties, but it is still persistent in the environment and is a chemical by-product of commercial chlorination processes. One particular event that led to its discontinuation occurred in Turkey in the 1950s. An epidemic poisoning of 4000 people resulted in extreme dermal toxicities after the consumption of treated grain products exposed to HCB (Ecobichon, 1996). Despite the ban, HCB is still detected in follicular fluid of females undergoing assisted reproductive technologies (Meeker et al., 2009).

Low levels of HCB exposure cause morphological and functional changes in the ovaries of several animal species (Babineau et al., 1991; Foster et al., 1992, 1993). Chronic administration of HCB resulted in common toxicities, including altered estrous cyclicity, follicular damage in small follicle types, OSE injury, increased atresia in antral follicles, reduced estradiol levels, and reduced number of ova (Babineau et al., 1991; Sims et al., 1991; Bourque et al., 1995; Alvarez et al., 2000). In particular to the rat model, female Wistar rats exposed to a chronic dose of HCB exhibited irregular and abnormal cycling, specifically extended periods of estrus, with an additional loss in the number of ova (Alvarez et al., 2000). Sprague Dawley rats exposed to HCB displayed changes in the smooth endoplasmic reticulum and Golgi complexes, along with prominent free polysomes in granulosa lutein cells (MacPhee et al., 1993). The dilated appearance of the smooth endoplasmic reticulum as a result of hyperactivity leads to the hypothesis that HCB upregulates the synthetic activity of the granulosa lutein cells to produce additional hormones as a compensatory response to HCB toxicity (MacPhee et al., 1993). Strain-specific effects of HCB on altered hormonal status in rats also exist. For instance, exposure to HCB in Wistar rats decreased serum estradiol levels, with progesterone levels remaining unchanged (Alvarez et al., 2000). However, the opposite effect was seen in Sprague Dawley rats treated with HCB, in that the chemical caused an elevation in progesterone levels, but serum estradiol concentrations did not change (Foster et al., 1993).

Aside from the effects seen in rodents, HCB is also known to disrupt antral follicle steroidogenesis in porcine models. HCB alone, as well as exposure to pentachlorobenzene (PeCB), a metabolite of HCB and an intermediate in the manufacturing of other fungicides, target the antral follicle in opposing ways (Gregoraszczuk et al., 2011). Accumulation of the two chemicals in ovarian tissue was seen, and observations suggest that the ovary is capable of metabolizing HCB to PeCB (Gregoraszczuk et al., 2011). Cultured antral follicles exhibited chemical-dependent effects in that HCB decreased testosterone and estradiol secretion, whereas PeCB increased secretion of the two hormones (Gregoraszczuk et al., 2011). This is because HCB exposure caused an increase in cholesterol side-chain cleavage (CYP11) protein expression and a dose-dependent inhibitory effect on cytochrome P450 17α-hydroxylase/17,20-lyase (CYP17), 17β-hydroxysteroid dehydrogenase (17β-HSD), and aromatase (CYP19) protein expression, while causing a dose-dependent stimulatory effect of PeCB exposure on CYP11, CYP17, and CYP19 protein expression (Gregoraszczuk et al., 2011). The varying effects of hormone secretion and steroidogenic protein expression are possibly linked to the degree of chlorination of the two chemicals (Gregoraszczuk et al., 2011).

HCB also causes adverse ovarian effects in primates. The pool of primary follicles appears to be the major target of HCB toxicity in cynomolgus monkeys (Bourque et al., 1995). HCB exposure for 13 weeks caused alterations in follicular structure, characterized by internal lesions, and condensed mitochondria within the ova and follicular cells. Furthermore, ooplasm herniation, follicular cell degeneration, and abnormal gaps between follicular cells were observed in response to HCB exposure. HCB toxicity may be due to an augmentation of lipid peroxidation adversely affecting the cellular membrane leading to impaired permeability. Conversely, other studies suggest that the immature primordial germ cell population is another target of toxicity (Jarrell et al., 1993a). In the Rhesus monkey, both the capability of steroidogenesis and receptivity to gonadotropin stimulation were inhibited in the corpora lutea of HCB-exposed subjects (Iatropoulos et al., 1976). HCB exposure also caused a decline in estrogen levels without decreasing FSH and LH levels (Muuller et al., 1978). Aside from follicular toxicity, HCB has also been shown to elicit a toxic effect on the cellular structure of the OSE in primates. Low doses of HCB caused surface epithelial cell degeneration categorized by tall columnar shape, irregular outline, and numerous lysosomes and vesicles within the cytoplasm. High doses of HCB have been shown to advance the stages of degeneration of the OSE (Babineau et al., 1991).

Belonging to the fungicidal class of imidazole, prochloraz is another extensively studied chemical with links to ovarian toxicity. Prochloraz has been shown to inhibit aromatase activity and subsequently decrease estradiol levels in fish and other vertebrates (Monod et al., 1993; Hinfray et al., 2006; Vinggaard et al., 2006). Other kinetic properties specific to prochloraz include the ability of the chemical to antagonize both the androgen and the estrogen receptors and to agonize the aryl hydrocarbon receptor. This widely used agricultural fungicide acts through multiple mechanisms of action involving interactions with cytochrome P450s and related monooxygenases. The imidazole class of fungicides is designed to inhibit the enzyme 14α-demethylase, a cytochrome P450 isoform significant in ergosterol biosynthesis in fungal cells. In animal species, 14α-demethylase (CYP51) demethylates lanosterol, which is a vital reaction in the biosynthesis of cholesterol. The binding of imidazole to the cytochrome P450 enzyme is fairly nonspecific and thus, these fungicides have the capability to inactivate a broad spectrum of cytochrome P450 enzymes, including those necessary for steroid hormone biosynthesis, such as aromatase (Laignelet et al., 1989).

Prochloraz-induced ovotoxicity results in alterations in the mRNA expression of steroidogenic enzymes and growth factors. In early ovarian development of brown trout, prochloraz was able to reduce estradiol production and increase insulin-like growth factor 1, *Igf1*, mRNA expression (Marca Pereira et al., 2011). The observed effects on IGF signaling may not be via an aromatase-inhibiting mechanism, but rather an antagonism of the androgen receptor. It is further hypothesized that prochloraz may directly or indirectly modify IGF signaling and estradiol production independently, leading to altered ovarian development (Marca Pereira et al., 2011). This anti-androgenic mechanism of action was supported by Vinggaard and colleagues (2006) who showed that pre- and postnatal exposure to prochloraz caused feministic qualities in males, such as nipple retention and decreased weights in bulbourethral glands after birth with an accompanying decrease in testosterone levels *in utero* (Vinggaard et al., 2006). This feminization is due, in part, to diminished steroidogenesis in fetal male rats. Short-term exposure to prochloraz also reduced plasma levels of estradiol and vitellogenin in adult fathead minnows, but interestingly, *Star*, *Cyp19a1*, and *Cyp17* mRNA expression were upregulated in a hypothesized compensatory mechanism in response to steroid hormone inhibition (Skolness et al., 2011). However, this upregulated steroidogenic gene expression compensatory mechanism is not adequate enough to overcome prochloraz toxicity of estradiol inhibition following a longer period (21 days) of exposure (Ankley et al., 2005).

Prochloraz exposure also affects the maturation of the oocyte. There is a strong indication that prochloraz and LH-rich partially purified gonadotropin act in a synergistic manner when co-administered in post-vitellogenic rainbow trout follicles. The combined treatment group had a higher instance of germinal vesicle breakdown when compared to a low concentration of LH-treated follicles (Rime et al., 2010). Additionally, prochloraz and LH treatment produced a higher concentration of 17,20β-dihydroxy-4-pregnen-3-one (17,20βP), the oocyte maturation–inducing steroid in rainbow trout, in media when compared to LH treatment alone (Rime et al., 2010). Synergism aside, prochloraz treatment alone was also able to induce germinal vesicle breakdown and trigger 17,20βP production. Exposure to prochloraz also upregulated genes involved in 17,20βP production, intercellular communication, and pre-ovulatory follicular differentiation. Thus, this fungicide has the ability to act on follicular layers to induce oocyte maturation (Rime et al., 2010).

Vinclozolin, a dicarboximide fungicide, has recently been shown to disrupt normal ovarian function. Vinclozolin antagonizes the androgen receptor in yeast-based assays (Sohoni and Sumpter, 1998). Thus, vinclozolin, like prochloraz, has the potential to create an estrogenic environment by acting as an anti-androgen. These findings were confirmed in a microarray of zebrafish gonads (Martinovi-Weigelt, 2011). Additional findings after exposure to vinclozolin showed that vinclozolin alters activin and fibroblast growth factor signaling. Vinclozolin downregulated MAD homolog 2 (*Smad2*) and upregulated fibroblast growth factor receptor 1 (*Fgfr1*) in a microarray analysis of zebrafish ovaries. The decreased activin expression may interfere with normal regulation and secretion of gonadotropins. Additionally, the increased fibroblast growth factor expression could alter transcriptional targets of the androgen receptor (Martinovi-Weigelt, 2011).

Dithiocarbamates are another widely used class of fungicides known to elicit direct ovarian toxicity. These chemicals have low acute toxicity and high LD50 levels, thus making them a popular fungicide. However, they are known to cause severe carcinogenic and teratogenic effects following chronic exposure (Ecobichon, 1996). Administered in high doses, dithiocarbamates decreased ovarian hypertrophy and altered estrous cyclicity by decreasing the number of cycles and duration of each phase (Mahadevaswami et al., 2000). Furthermore, ovarian follicles are targeted, in that, dithiocarbamates reduce the number of healthy follicles while increasing the number of atretic follicles. This observed increase in follicular atresia may be attributed to a direct effect on the ovary or an indirect effect targeting the hypothalamic–pituitary–ovarian axis (Mahadevaswami et al., 2000). Additional toxicological evidence shows that dithiocarbamates reduce lipid synthesis. These fungicides decreased protein, glycogen, total lipid, phospholipid, and neutral lipid levels in the ovary, which potentially could be caused by tissue damage or increased catabolism of these biomolecules (Mahadevaswami et al., 2000). Important to the field of toxicology, species specificity of certain dithiocarbamates at high doses, namely mancozeb and maneb, exist in which both are teratogenic in rats, but not in mice (Larsson et al., 1976). This evidence outlines the importance of understanding the species-specific effects of not just dithiocarbamates, but all classes of fungicides in regard to ovarian toxicology.

Dithiocarbamates also indirectly target the ovary. In fact, a single dose of thiram given prior to the LH surge during vaginal proestrus delays ovulation (Stoker et al., 1993). Yet, this outcome did not appear to decrease the number of oocytes shed during ovulation. This single dose of thiram, however, was able to significantly reduce the number of live births, despite normal embryonic implantation on gestational day 7 and embryonic stability at gestational day 11. A reduction in embryonic survival was observed on gestational day 20, proving that thiram-induced alteration of the LH surge and subsequent delay in ovulation by 24 h were capable of decreasing the number of live births (Stoker et al., 2001).

Certain chemicals within the conazole class of fungicides have also been shown to be detrimental to ovarian function. Used extensively in agricultural applications as well as a pharmaceutical agent for the treatment of candidiasis, cryptococcosis, and coccidiomycosis, conazoles act as ergosterol inhibitors. Pre- and postnatal exposure to three conazoles (myclobutanil, propiconazole, and triadimefon) led to adverse reproductive outcomes in rats (Rockett et al., 2006). As is often observed, both propiconazole and triadimefon altered normal estrous cyclicity early after the onset of puberty, but cycling resumed normally after 9 weeks postpuberty. Exposure to both myclobutanil and triadimefon delayed the onset of puberty with an additional increase in ovarian weights observed after the course of the study. Myclobutanil exposure was also seen to increase the anogenital distance of the female pups, indicating an androgenic or anti-estrogenic effect. This androgenic/anti-estrogenic hypothesis is also supported by the delay in pubertal onset. Furthermore, previous studies have shown that exposure to anti-estrogens increases ovarian weight, which may provide further support to the hypothesized anti-estrogenic mechanism of action of the conazole fungicides (Rockett et al., 2006).

6.8 CONCLUSIONS

Pesticides have been used in agriculture for decades to prevent crop loss and in daily life to control disease spread via insects or other pests. Humans and wildlife are chronically exposed to low levels of various pesticide residues. This is a concern because many pesticides are known reproductive toxicants. In this chapter, we discussed the ovarian toxicity and the mechanisms of action of some widely used pesticides. Certain pesticides are known to directly disrupt ovarian steroidogenesis, folliculogenesis, and cause atresia, whereas others are known to indirectly affect the ovary by disrupting the hormonal balance of the hypothalamic–pituitary–ovarian axis. However, the underlying ovotoxic mechanisms for the majority of pesticides have yet to be elucidated. In the future, it is important to perform more studies to uncover the mechanisms by which different pesticides affect the female reproductive system. Such studies need to take into account that dose, timing, and duration of exposure are critical for the ability of a pesticide to cause adverse reproductive effects. In addition, we need to broaden our testing scope of potential reproductive hazards to mixtures of different types of compounds, including those pesticides that have not been studied. Finally, we need to investigate the effects of action of multiple commonly used pesticides at environmental concentrations to evaluate the reproductive health risk in humans and wildlife. The ultimate goal of ovarian toxicity studies on pesticides is to understand the effects and the mechanisms of various pesticides on the ovary, so that we may develop ways to treat and prevent the ovotoxicity caused by pesticides.

REFERENCES

Abdallah, F.B., Slima, A.B., Dammak, I., Keskes-Ammar, L., Mallek, Z., 2010. Comparative effects of dimethoate and deltamethrin on reproductive system in male mice. *Andrologia* **42**, 182–186.

Akkina, J., Reif, J., Keefe, T., Bachand, A., 2004. Age at natural menopause and exposure to organochlorine pesticides in Hispanic women. *Journal of Toxicology and Environmental Health. Part A* **67**, 1407–1422.

Alvarez, L., Randi, A., Alvarez, P., Piroli, G., Chamson-Reig, A., Lux-Lantos, V., Pisarev, D.K.D., 2000. Reproductive effects of hexachlorobenzene in female rats. *Journal of Applied Toxicology* **20**, 81–87.

Andersen, H.R., Vinggaard, A.M., Rasmussen, T.H., Gjermandsen, I.M., Bonefeld-Jorgensen, E.C., 2002. Effects of currently used pesticides in assays for estrogenicity, androgenicity, and aromatase activity *in vitro*. *Toxicology and Applied Pharmacology* **179**, 1–12.

Ankley, G.T., Jensen, K.M., Durhan, E.J., Makynen, E.A., Butterworth, B.C., Kahl, M.D., Villeneuve, D.L. et al. 2005. Effects of two fungicides with multiple modes of action on reproductive endocrine function in the fathead minnow (Pimephales promelas). *Toxicological Sciences* **86**, 300–308.

Armenti, A.E., Zama, A.M., Passantino, L., Uzumcu, M., 2008. Developmental methoxychlor exposure affects multiple reproductive parameters and ovarian folliculogenesis and gene expression in adult rats. *Toxicology and Applied Pharmacology* **233**, 286–296.

Asmathbanu, I., Kaliwal, B.B., 1997. Temporal effect of methyl parathion on ovarian compensatory hypertrophy, follicular dynamics and estrous cycle in hemicastrated albino rats. *Journal of Basic and Clinical Physiology and Pharmacology* **8**, 237–254.

Axmon, A., Thulstrup, A.M., Rignell-Hydbom, A., Pedersen, H.S., Zvyezday, V., Ludwicki, J.K., Jonsson, B.A. et al., 2006. Time to pregnancy as a function of male and female serum concentrations of 2,2′4,4′5,5′-hexachlorobiphenyl (CB-153) and 1,1-dichloro-2,2-bis (p-chlorophenyl)-ethylene (p,p′-DDE). *Human Reproduction (Oxford, England)* **21**, 657–665.

Babina, K., Dollard, M., Pilotto, L., Edwards, J.W., 2012. Environmental exposure to organophosphorus and pyrethroid pesticides in South Australian preschool children: A cross sectional study. *Environment International* **48C**, 109–120.

Babineau, K.A., Singh, A., Jarrell, J.F., Villeneuve, D.C., 1991. Surface epithelium of the ovary following oral administration of hexachlorobenzene to the monkey. *Journal of Submicroscopic Cytology and Pathology* **23**, 457–464.

Barnett, K.R., Schilling, C., Greenfeld, C.R., Tomic, D., Flaws, J.A., 2006. Ovarian follicle development and transgenic mouse models. *Human Reproduction Update* **12**, 537–555.

Basavarajappa, M.S., Craig, Z.R., Hernandez-Ochoa, I., Paulose, T., Leslie, T.C., Flaws, J.A., 2011. Methoxychlor reduces estradiol levels by altering steroidogenesis and metabolism in mouse antral follicles *in vitro*. *Toxicology and Applied Pharmacology* **253**, 161–169.

Basavarajappa, M.S., Hernandez-Ochoa, I., Wang, W., Flaws, J.A., 2012. Methoxychlor inhibits growth and induces atresia through the aryl hydrocarbon receptor pathway in mouse ovarian antral follicles. *Reproductive Toxicology* (New York) **34**, 16–21.

Bonilla, E., Hernandez, F., Cortes, L., Mendoza, M., Mejia, J., Carrillo, E., Casas, E., Betancourt, M., 2008. Effects of the insecticides malathion and diazinon on the early oogenesis in mice *in vitro*. *Environmental Toxicology* **23**, 240–245.

Bourque, A.C., Singh, A., Lakhanpal, N., McMahon, A., Foster, W.G., 1995. Ultrastructural changes in ovarian follicles of monkeys administered hexachlorobenzene. *American Journal of Veterinary Research* **56**, 1673–1677.

Bretveld, R.W., Thomas, C.M., Scheepers, P.T., Zielhuis, G.A., Roeleveld, N., 2006. Pesticide exposure: the hormonal function of the female reproductive system disrupted? *Reproductive Biology and Endocrinology: RB&E* **4**, 30.

Casida, J.E., 1980. Pyrethrum flowers and pyrethroid insecticides. *Environmental Health Perspectives* **34**, 189–202.

Chakravarty, S., Mandal, A., Lahiri, P., 1986. Effect of lindane on clutch size and level of egg yolk protein in domestic duck. *Toxicology* **39**, 93–103.

Chang, J., Liu, S., Zhou, S., Wang, M., Zhu, G., 2011. Effects of butachlor on reproduction and hormone levels in adult zebrafish (Danio rerio). *Experimental and Toxicologic Pathology* **65**, 205–209.

Charles, J.M., Cunny, H.C., Wilson, R.D., Bus, J.S., 1996. Comparative subchronic studies on 2,4-dichlorophenoxyacetic acid, amine, and ester in Rats. *Fundamental and Applied Toxicology* **33**, 161–165.

Chedrese, P.J., Feyles, F., 2001. The diverse mechanism of action of dichlorodiphenyldichloroethylene (DDE) and methoxychlor in ovarian cells *in vitro*. *Reproductive Toxicology* (New York) **15**, 693–698.

Chen, J.F., Chen, H.Y., Liu, R., He, J., Song, L., Bian, Q., Xu, L.C. et al., 2005. Effects of fenvalerate on steroidogenesis in cultured rat granulosa cells. *Biomedical and Environmental Sciences: BES* **18**, 108–116.

Chen, H., Xiao, J., Hu, G., Zhou, J., Xiao, H., Wang, X., 2002. Estrogenicity of organophosphorus and pyrethroid pesticides. *Journal of Toxicology and Environmental Health. Part A* **65**, 1419–1435.

Christensen, A., Bentley, G.E., Cabrera, R., Ortega, H.H., Perfito, N., Wu, T.J., Micevych, P., 2012. Hormonal regulation of female reproduction. *Hormone and Metabolic Research* **44**, 587–591.

Colosio, C., Tiramani, M., Maroni, M., 2003. Neurobehavioral effects of pesticides: State of the art. *Neurotoxicology* **24**, 577–591.

Cooper, R.L., Stoker, T.E., Goldman, J.M., Parrish, M.B., Tyrey, L., 1996. Effect of atrazine on ovarian function in the rat. *Reproductive Toxicology* **10**, 257–264.

Cooper, R.l., Stoker T. E, McElroy W. K, Hein J., 1998. Atrazine (ATR) disrupts hypothalamic catecholamines and pituitary function. *Toxicologist* **42**, 160.

Cooper, R.L., Stoker, T.E., Tyrey, L., Goldman, J.M., McElroy, W.K., 2000. Atrazine disrupts the hypothalamic control of pituitary-ovarian function. *Toxicological Sciences* **53**, 297–307.

Craig, Z.R., Leslie, T.C., Hatfield, K.P., Gupta, R.K., Flaws, J.A., 2010. Mono-hydroxy methoxychlor alters levels of key sex steroids and steroidogenic enzymes in cultured mouse antral follicles. *Toxicology and Applied Pharmacology* **249**, 107–113.

Craig, Z.R., Wang, W., Flaws, J.A., 2011. Endocrine-disrupting chemicals in ovarian function: effects on steroidogenesis, metabolism and nuclear receptor signaling. *Reproduction* **142**, 633–646.

Crellin, N.K., Kang, H.G., Swan, C.L., Chedrese, P.J., 2001. Inhibition of basal and stimulated progesterone synthesis by dichlorodiphenyldichloroethylene and methoxychlor in a stable pig granulosa cell line. *Reproduction* **121**, 485–492.

Crellin, N.K., Rodway, M.R., Swan, C.L., Gillio-Meina, C., Chedrese, P.J., 1999. Dichlorodiphenyldichloroethylene potentiates the effect of protein kinase A pathway activators on progesterone synthesis in cultured porcine granulosa cells. *Biology of Reproduction* **61**, 1099–1103.

Cukurcam, S., Sun, F., Betzendahl, I., Adler, I.D., Eichenlaub-Ritter, U., 2004. Trichlorfon predisposes to aneuploidy and interferes with spindle formation in in vitro maturing mouse oocytes. *Mutation Research* **564**, 165–178.

Dorner, G., Gotz, F., Rohde, W., Plagemann, A., Lindner, R., Peters, H., Ghanaati, Z., 2001. Genetic and epigenetic effects on sexual brain organization mediated by sex hormones. *Neuro Endocrinology Letters* **22**, 403–409.

Du, G., Shen, O., Sun, H., Fei, J., Lu, C., Song, L., Xia, Y., Wang, S., Wang, X., 2010. Assessing hormone receptor activities of pyrethroid insecticides and their metabolites in reporter gene assays. *Toxicological Sciences* **116**, 58–66.

Du Preez, L.H., Kunene, N., Hanner, R., Giesy, J.P., Solomon, K.R., Hosmer, A., Van Der Kraak, G.J., 2009. Population-specific incidence of testicular ovarian follicles in Xenopus laevis from South Africa: A potential issue in endocrine testing. *Aquatic Toxicology* **95**, 10–16.

Ducolomb, Y., Casas, E., Valdez, A., Gonzalez, G., Altamirano-Lozano, M., Betancourt, M., 2009. In vitro effect of malathion and diazinon on oocytes fertilization and embryo development in porcine. *Cell Biology and Toxicology* **25**, 623–633.

Ecobichon, D.J., 1996. *Toxic Effects of Pesticides, Casarett and Doull's Toxicology: The Basic Science of Poisons*. McGraw-Hill, New York, pp. 643–689.

Eldridge, J., Fleenor-Heyser, D.G., Extrom, P.C,, Wetzel, L.T., Breckenridge, C.B., Gillis, J.H., Luempert, L.G., Stevens, J.T., 1994. Short-term effects of chlorotriazines on estrus in female Sprague Dawley and Fischer 344 rats. *Journal of Toxicology and Environmental Health* **43,** 155–167.

Eldridge, J.C., Wetzel, L.T., Stevens, J.T., Simpkins, J.W., 1999. The mammary tumor response in triazine-treated female rats: A threshold-mediated interaction with strain and species-specific reproductive senescence. *Steroids* **64**, 672–678.

Farr, S.L., Cai, J., Savitz, D.A., Sandler, D.P., Hoppin, J.A., Cooper, G.S., 2006. Pesticide exposure and timing of menopause: the agricultural health study. *American Journal of Epidemiology* **163**, 731–742.

Farr, S.L., Cooper, G.S., Cai, J., Savitz, D.A., Sandler, D.P., 2004. Pesticide use and menstrual cycle characteristics among premenopausal women in the Agricultural Health Study. *American Journal of Epidemiology* **160**, 1194–1204.

Fei, J., Qu, J.H., Ding, X.L., Xue, K., Lu, C.C., Chen, J.F., Song, L. et al., 2010. Fenvalerate inhibits the growth of primary cultured rat preantral ovarian follicles. *Toxicology* **267**, 1–6.

Foster, W.G., Pentick, J.A., McMahon, A., Lecavalier, P.R., 1992. Ovarian toxicity of hexachlorobenzene (HCB) in the superovulated female rat. *Journal of Biochemical Toxicology* **7**, 1–4.

Foster, W.G., Pentick, J.A., McMahon, A., Lecavalier, P.R., 1993. Body distribution and endocrine toxicity of hexachlorobenzene (HCB) in the female rat. *Journal of Applied Toxicology* **13**, 79–83.

Fritz, S., Grunert, R., Stocco, D.M., Hales, D.B., Mayerhofer, A., 2001. StAR protein is increased by muscarinic receptor activation in human luteinized granulosa cells. *Molecular and Cellular Endocrinology* **171**, 49–51.

Fritz, S., Kunz, L., Dimitrijevic, N., Grunert, R., Heiss, C., Mayerhofer, A., 2002. Muscarinic receptors in human luteinized granulosa cells: Activation blocks gap junctions and induces the transcription factor early growth response factor-1. *The Journal of Clinical Endocrinology and Metabolism* **87**, 1362–1367.

Gaido, K.W., Maness, S.C., McDonnell, D.P., Dehal, S.S., Kupfer, D., Safe, S., 2000. Interaction of methoxychlor and related compounds with estrogen receptor alpha and beta, and androgen receptor: Structure-activity studies. *Molecular Pharmacology* **58**, 852–858.

Gill, S.A., Rizvi, F., Khan, M.Z., Khan, A., 2011. Toxic effects of cypermethrin and methamidophos on bovine corpus luteal cells and progesterone production. *Experimental and Toxicologic Pathology* **63**, 131–135.

Goh, K.S., Weaver D.J., Hsu, J., Richman, S.J., Tran, D., Barry, T.A., 1993. ELISA regulatory application: compliance monitoring of simazine and atrazine in California soils. *Bulletin of Environmental Contamination and Toxicology* **51**, 333–340.

Gojmerac, T., Kartal, B., Curic, S., Zuric, M., Kusevic, S., Cvetnic Z., 1996. Serum biochemical changes associated with cystic ovarian degeneration in pigs after atrazine treatment. *Toxicology Letters* **85**, 9–15.

Gojmerac, T, Kartal, B., Zuric M., Zidar, V., 1994. Use of immunoassay (ELISA) in determination of s-triazine herbicide in drinking water. Vet Stanica **25**, 75–80.

Gotz, F., Thieme, S., Dorner, G., 2001. Female infertility—Effect of perinatal xenoestrogen exposure on reproductive functions in animals and humans. *Folia histochemica et Cytobiologica* **39**(Suppl 2), 40–43.

Goudey-Perriere, F., Lemonnier, F., Bergougnoux, V., Perriere, C., 2007. Low doses of the pesticide lindane induce protein release by the fat body of female cockroach Blaberus craniifer (Dictyoptera). Comparative biochemistry and physiology. *Toxicology and Pharmacology: CBP* **146**, 492–501.

Gregoraszczuk, E., Ptak, A., Rak-Mardya, A., Falandysz, J., 2011. Differential accumulation of HCBz and PeCBz in porcine ovarian follicles and their opposing actions on steroid secretion and CYP11, CYP17, 17β-HSD and CYP19 protein expression—A tissue culture approach. *Reproductive Toxicology* **31**, 494–499.

Guerra, M.T., de Toledo, F.C., Kempinas Wde, G., 2011. *In utero* and lactational exposure to fenvalerate disrupts reproductive function in female rats. *Reproductive Toxicology* **32**, 298–303.

Gupta, R.K., Meachum, S., Hernandez-Ochoa, I., Peretz, J., Yao, H.H., Flaws, J.A., 2009. Methoxychlor inhibits growth of antral follicles by altering cell cycle regulators. *Toxicology and Applied Pharmacology* **240**, 1–7.

Gupta, R.K., Schuh, R.A., Fiskum, G., Flaws, J.A., 2006. Methoxychlor causes mitochondrial dysfunction and oxidative damage in the mouse ovary. *Toxicology and Applied Pharmacology* **216**, 436–445.

Gysin, H., Knusli, E., 1960. *Chemistry and Herbicidal Properties of Triazine Derivatives. Advances in Pest Control* **3**, 289–353.

Han, Z., Jiao, S., Kong, D., Shan, Z., Zhang, X., 2011. Effects of beta-endosulfan on the growth and reproduction of zebrafish (Danio rerio). *Environmental Toxicology and Chemistry* **30**, 2525–2531.

Hanafi, A., Garau, V.L., Caboni, P., Sarais, G., Cabras, P., 2010. Minor crops for export: A case study of boscalid, pyraclostrobin, lufenuron and lambda-cyhalothrin residue levels on green beans and spring onions in Egypt. *Journal of Environmental Science and Health. Part. B, Pesticides, Food Contaminants, and Agricultural Wastes* **45**, 493–500.

Hanke, W., Jurewicz, J., 2004. The risk of adverse reproductive and developmental disorders due to occupational pesticide exposure: An overview of current epidemiological evidence. *International Journal of Occupational Medicine and Environmental Health* **17**, 223–243.

Harley, K.G., Marks, A.R., Bradman, A., Barr, D.B., Eskenazi, B., 2008. DDT exposure, work in agriculture, and time to pregnancy among farm workers in California. *Journal of Occupational Medicine and Environmental Health* **50**, 1335–1342.

Hayes, T.B., Anderson, L.L., Beasley, V.R., de Solla, S.R., Iguchi, T., Ingraham, H., Kestemont, P. et al., 2011. Demasculinization and feminization of male gonads by atrazine: Consistent effects across vertebrate classes. *The Journal of Steroid Biochemistry and Molecular Biology* **127**, 64–73.

Hayes, T.B., Case, P., Chui, S., Chung, D., Haeffele, C., Haston, K., Lee, M. et al., 2006. Pesticide mixtures, endocrine disruption, and amphibian declines: Are we underestimating the impact? *Environmental Health Perspectives* **114**(Suppl 1), 40–50.

Hayes, T.B., Collins, A., Lee, M., Mendoza, M., Noriega, N., Stuart, A.A., Vonk, A., 2002. Hermaphroditic, demasculinized frogs after exposure to the herbicide atrazine at low ecologically relevant doses. *Proceedings of the National Academy of Sciences* **99**, 5476–5480.

He, J., Chen, J.F., Liu, R., Song, L., Chang, H.C., Wang, X.R., 2006. Fenvalerate-induced alterations in calcium homeostasis in rat ovary. *Biomedical and Environmental Sciences* **19**, 15–20.

He, J., Chen, J., Liu, R., Wang, S., Song, L., Chang, H.C., Wang, X., 2004. Alterations of FSH-stimulated progesterone production and calcium homeostasis in primarily cultured human luteinizing-granulosa cells induced by fenvalerate. *Toxicology* **203**, 61–68.

Heindel, J.J., Chapin, R.E., Gulati, D.K., George, J.D., Price, C.J., Marr, M.C., Myers, C.B. et al., 1994. Assessment of the reproductive and developmental toxicity of pesticide/fertilizer mixtures based on confirmed pesticide contamination in California and Iowa groundwater. *Fundamental and Applied Toxicology* **22**, 605–621.

Hinfray, N., Porcher, J.M., Brion, F.O., 2006. Inhibition of rainbow trout (Oncorhynchus mykiss) P450 aromatase activities in brain and ovarian microsomes by various environmental substances. *Comparative Biochemistry and Physiology Part C: Toxicology and Pharmacology* **144**, 252–262.

Hiremath, M.B., Kaliwal, B.B., 2002. Effect of endosulfan on ovarian compensatory hypertrophy in hemicastrated albino mice. *Reproductive Toxicology (New York)* **16**, 783–790.

Holloway, A.C., Petrik, J.J., Younglai, E.V., 2007. Influence of dichlorodiphenylchloroethylene on vascular endothelial growth factor and insulin-like growth factor in human and rat ovarian cells. *Reproductive Toxicology (New York)* **24**, 359–364.

Hoyer, P.B., Sipes, I.G., 1996. Assessment of follicle destruction in chemical-induced ovarian toxicity. *Annual Review of Pharmacology and Toxicology* **36**, 307–331.

Iatropoulos, M.J., Hobson, W., Knauf, V., Adams, H.P., 1976. Morphological effects of hexachlorobenzene toxicity in female rhesus monkeys. *Toxicology and Applied Pharmacology* **37**, 433–444.

Idrovo, A.J., Sanin, L.H., Cole, D., Chavarro, J., Caceres, H., Narvaez, J., Restrepo, M., 2005. Time to first pregnancy among women working in agricultural production. *International Archives of Occupational and Environmental Health* **78**, 493–500.

Inbaraj, R.M., Haider, S., 1988. Effect of malathion and endosulfan on brain acetylcholinesterase and ovarian steroidogenesis of Channa punctatus (Bloch). *Ecotoxicology and Environmental Safety* **16**, 123–128.

Jager, G., 1983. *Herbicides*. Wiley, New York, pp. 322–393.

Jarrell, J.F., McMahon, A., Villeneuve, D., Franklin, C., Singh, A., Valli, V.E., Bartlett, S., 1993a. Hexachlorobenzene toxicity in the monkey primordial germ cell without induced porphyria. *Reproductive Toxicology* **7**, 41–47.

Jarrell, J.F., Villeneuve, D., Franklin, C., Bartlett, S., Wrixon, W., Kohut, J., Zouves, C.G., 1993b. Contamination of human ovarian follicular fluid and serum by chlorinated organic compounds in three Canadian cities. *Canadian Medical Association Journal* **148**, 1321–1327.

Jin, Y., Liu, J., Wang, L., Chen, R., Zhou, C., Yang, Y., Liu, W., Fu, Z., 2012. Permethrin exposure during puberty has the potential to enantioselectively induce reproductive toxicity in mice. *Environment International* **42**, 144–151.

Jin, Y., Zhang, X., Shu, L., Chen, L., Sun, L., Qian, H., Liu, W., Fu, Z., 2010. Oxidative stress response and gene expression with atrazine exposure in adult female zebrafish (Danio rerio). *Chemosphere* **78**, 846–852.

Juliani, C.C., Silva-Zacarin, E.C.M., Santos, D.C., Boer, P.A., 2008. Effects of atrazine on female Wistar rats: Morphological alterations in ovarian follicles and immunocytochemical labeling of 90kDa heat shock protein. *Micron* **39**, 607–616.

Kang, D., Park, J.Y., Han, J., Bae, I.H., Yoon, S.Y., Kang, S.S., Choi, W.S., Hong, S.G., 2003. Acetylcholine induces Ca2+ oscillations via m3/m4 muscarinic receptors in the mouse oocyte. *Pflugers Archiv: European Journal of Physiology* **447**, 321–327.

Katagi, T., 2010. Bioconcentration, bioaccumulation, and metabolism of pesticides in aquatic organisms. *Reviews of Environmental Contamination and Toxicology* **204**, 1–132.

Katsuda, Y., 2012. Progress and future of pyrethroids. *Topics in Current Chemistry* **314**, 1–30.

Ke, F.C., Fang, S.H., Lee, M.T., Sheu, S.Y., Lai, S.Y., Chen, Y.J., Huang, F.L. et al., 2005. Lindane, a gap junction blocker, suppresses FSH and transforming growth factor beta1-induced connexin43 gap junction formation and steroidogenesis in rat granulosa cells. *The Journal of Endocrinology* **184**, 555–566.

Kim, S.S., Kwack, S.J., Lee, R.D., Lim, K.J., Rhee, G.S., Seok, J.H., Kim, B.H. et al., 2005a. Assessment of estrogenic and androgenic activities of tetramethrin in vitro and in vivo assays. *Journal of Toxicology and Environmental Health. Part A* **68**, 2277–2289.

Kim, S.S., Lee, R.D., Lim, K.J., Kwack, S.J., Rhee, G.S., Seok, J.H., Lee, G.S.et al., 2005b. Potential estrogenic and antiandrogenic effects of permethrin in rats. *The Journal of Reproduction and Development* **51**, 201–210.

Klaassen, D.D. (Ed.) 1996. *Casareet and Doull's Toxicology: The Basic Science of Poisons.* McGraw-Hill, New York.

Kloas, W., Lutz, I., Springer, T., Krueger, H., Wolf, J., Holden, L., Hosmer, A., 2009. Does atrazine influence larval development and sexual differentiation in Xenopus laevis? *Toxicological Sciences* **107**, 376–384.

Koc, N.D., Kayhan, F.E., Sesal, C., Muslu, M.N., 2009. Dose-dependent effects of endosulfan and malathion on adult Wistar albino rat ovaries. *Pakistan Journal of Biological Sciences* **12**, 498–503.

Kortenkamp, A., 2007. Ten years of mixing cocktails: A review of combination effects of endocrine-disrupting chemicals. *Environmental Health Perspectives* **115**(Suppl 1), 98–105.

Kosanke, G.J., Schwippert, W.W., Beneke, T.W., 1988. The impairment of mobility and development in freshwater snails (Physa fontinalis and Lymnaea stagnalis) caused by herbicides. *Comparative Biochemistry and Physiology Part C* **90**, 373–379.

Koureas, M., Tsakalof, A., Tsatsakis, A., Hadjichristodoulou, C., 2012. Systematic review of biomonitoring studies to determine the association between exposure to organophosphorus and pyrethroid insecticides and human health outcomes. *Toxicology Letters* **210**, 155–168.

Kristoff, G., Cacciatore, L.C., Guerrero, N.R., Cochon, A.C., 2011. Effects of the organophosphate insecticide azinphos-methyl on the reproduction and cholinesterase activity of Biomphalaria glabrata. *Chemosphere* **84**, 585–591.

Kunimatsu, T., Yamada, T., Ose, K., Sunami, O., Kamita, Y., Okuno, Y., Seki, T., Nakatsuka, I., 2002. Lack of (anti-) androgenic or estrogenic effects of three pyrethroids (esfenvalerate, fenvalerate, and permethrin) in the Hershberger and uterotrophic assays. *Regulatory Toxicology and Pharmacology: RTP* **35**, 227–237.

Laignelet, L., Narbonne, J.F., Lhuguenot, J.C., Riviere, J.L., 1989. Induction and inhibition of rat liver cytochrome(s) P-450 by an imidazole fungicide (prochloraz). *Toxicology* **59**, 271–284.

Larsson, K.S., Arnander, C., Cekanova, E., Kjellberg, M., 1976. Studies of teratogenic effects of the dithiocarbamates maneb, mancozeb, and propineb. *Teratology* **14**, 171–183.

Lawrence, Y.M., Cuthbertson, K.S., 1995. Thapsigargin induces cytoplasmic free Ca2+ oscillations in mouse oocytes. *Cell Calcium* **17**, 154–164.

Liu, J., Yang, Y., Zhang, Y., Liu, W., 2011. Disrupting effects of bifenthrin on ovulatory gene expression and prostaglandin synthesis in rat ovarian granulosa cells. *Toxicology* **282**, 47–55.

MacPhee, I.J., Singh, A., Wright, G.M., Foster, W.G., LeBlanc, N.N., 1993. Ultrastructure of granulosa lutein cells from rats fed hexachlorobenzene. *Histology and Histopathology* **8**, 35–40.

Mahadevaswami, M.P., Jadaramkunti, U.C., Hiremath, M.B., Kaliwal, B.B., 2000. Effect of mancozeb on ovarian compensatory hypertrophy and biochemical constituents in hemicastrated albino rat. *Reproductive Toxicology* **14**, 127–134.

Mahadevaswami, M.P., Kaliwal, B.B., 2002. Effect of dimethoate administration schedules on compensatory ovarian hypertrophy, follicular dynamics, and estrous cycle in hemicastrated mice. *Journal of Basic and Clinical Physiology and Pharmacology* **13**, 225–248.

Mahoney, M.M., Padmanabhan, V., 2010. Developmental programming: Impact of fetal exposure to endocrine-disrupting chemicals on gonadotropin-releasing hormone and estrogen receptor mRNA in sheep hypothalamus. *Toxicology and Applied Pharmacology* **247**, 98–104.

Maranghi, F., Rescia, M., Macri, C., Di Consiglio, E., De Angelis, G., Testai, E., Farini, D. et al., 2007. Lindane may modulate the female reproductive development through the interaction with ER-beta: An *in vivo-in vitro* approach. *Chemico-Biological Interactions* **169**, 1–14.

Marca Pereira, M.L., Eppler, E., Thorpe, K.L., Wheeler, J.R., Burkhardt-Holm, P., 2011. Molecular and cellular effects of chemicals disrupting steroidogenesis during early ovarian development of brown trout (Salmo trutta fario). *Environmental Toxicology*, doi: 10.1002/tox.20786. Epub ahead of print.

Martinez, E.M., Swartz, W.J., 1991. Effects of methoxychlor on the reproductive system of the adult female mouse. 1. Gross and histologic observations. *Reproductive Toxicology (New York)* **5**, 139–147.

Martinovi-Weigelt, D.W., Rong Lin, Villeneuve, D.L., Bencic, D.C., Lazorchak, J., Ankley, G.T., 2011. Gene expression profiling of the androgen receptor antagonists flutamide and vinclozolin in zebrafish (Danio rerio) gonads. *Aquatic Toxicology* **101**, 447–458.

Matsuda-Minehata, F., Inoue, N., Goto, Y., Manabe, N., 2006. The regulation of ovarian granulosa cell death by pro- and anti-apoptotic molecules. *The Journal of Reproduction and Development* **52**, 695–705.

Meeker, J.D., Missmer, S.A., Altshul, L., Vitonis, A.F., Ryan, L., Cramer, D.W., Hauser, R., 2009. Serum and follicular fluid organochlorine concentrations among women undergoing assisted reproduction technologies. *Environmental Health* **8**, 32.

Miller, K.P., Gupta, R.K., Greenfeld, C.R., Babus, J.K., Flaws, J.A., 2005. Methoxychlor directly affects ovarian antral follicle growth and atresia through Bcl-2- and Bax-mediated pathways. *Toxicological Sciences* **88**, 213–221.

Mlynarczuk, J., Wrobel, M.H., Kotwica, J., 2009. The influence of polychlorinated biphenyls (PCBs), dichlorodiphenyltrichloroethane (DDT) and its metabolite-dichlorodiphenyldichloroethylene (DDE) on mRNA expression for NP-I/OT and PGA, involved in oxytocin synthesis in bovine granulosa and luteal cells. *Reproductive Toxicology (New York)* **28**, 354–358.

Mnif, W., Hassine, A.I., Bouaziz, A., Bartegi, A., Thomas, O., Roig, B., 2011. Effect of endocrine disruptor pesticides: A review. *International Journal of Environmental Research and Public Health* **8**, 2265–2303.

Monod, G., De Mones, A.l., Fostier, A., 1993. Inhibition of ovarian microsomal aromatase and follicular oestradiol secretion by imidazole fungicides in Rainbow trout. *Marine Environmental Research* **35**, 153–157.

Munro, I.C., Carlo, G.L., Orr, J.C., Sund, K.G., Wilson, R.M., Kennepohl, E., Lynch, B.S., Jablinske, M., 1992. A comprehensive, integrated review and evaluation of the scientific evidence relating to the safety of the herbicide 2,4-D. *International Journal of Toxicology* **11**, 559–664.

Murdoch, W.J., McDonnel, A.C., 2002. Roles of the ovarian surface epithelium in ovulation and carcinogenesis. *Reproduction (Cambridge, England)* **123**, 743–750.

Muuller, W.F., Hobson, W., Fuller, G.B., Knauf, W., Coulston, F., Korte, F., 1978. Endocrine effects of chlorinated hydrocarbons in rhesus monkeys. *Ecotoxicology and Environmental Safety* **2**, 161–172.

Nandi, S., Gupta, P.S., Roy, S.C., Selvaraju, S., Ravindra, J.P., 2011. Chlorpyrifos and endosulfan affect buffalo oocyte maturation, fertilization, and embryo development in vitro directly and through cumulus cells. *Environmental Toxicology* **26**, 57–67.

Norris, R.F., Fong, J.L., 1983. Localization of atrazine in corn (Zea mays), oat (Avena staiva) and kidney beans (Phaseolus vulgaris) leaf cells. *Weed Sciences* **31**, 664–671.

Oktem, O., Urman, B., 2010. Understanding follicle growth. *Human Reproduction* **25**, 2944–2954.

Ouyang, F., Perry, M.J., Venners, S.A., Chen, C., Wang, B., Yang, F., Fang, Z. et al., 2005. Serum DDT, age at menarche, and abnormal menstrual cycle length. *Occupational and Environmental Medicine* **62**, 878–884.

Palmquist, K., Fairbrother, A., Salatas, J., Guiney, P.D., 2011. Environmental fate of pyrethroids in urban and suburban stream sediments and the appropriateness of Hyalella azteca model in determining ecological risk. *Integrated Environmental Assessment and Management* **7**, 325–335.

Paulose, T., Hernandez-Ochoa, I., Basavarajappa, M.S., Peretz, J., Flaws, J.A., 2011. Increased sensitivity of estrogen receptor alpha overexpressing antral follicles to methoxychlor and its metabolites. *Toxicological Sciences* **120**, 447–459.

Perobelli, J.E., Martinez, M.F., da Silva Franchi, C.A., Fernandez, C.D., de Camargo, J.L., Kempinas Wde, G., 2010. Decreased sperm motility in rats orally exposed to single or mixed pesticides. *Journal of Toxicology and Environmental Health. Part A* **73**, 991–1002.

Piao, F.Y., Xie, X.K., Kitabatake, M., Yamauchi, T., 1997. Transfer of leptophos in hen eggs and tissues of embryonic rats. *The Journal of Toxicological Sciences* **22**, 99–109.

Pine, M.D., Hiney, J.K., Lee, B., Dees, W.L., 2008. The pyrethroid pesticide esfenvalerate suppresses the afternoon rise of luteinizing hormone and delays puberty in female rats. *Environmental Health Perspectives* **116**, 1243–1247.

Pochettino, A.A., Bongiovanni, B., Duffard, R.O., Evangelista de Duffard, A.M.A., 2011. Oxidative stress in ventral prostate, ovary, and breast by 2,4-dichlorophenoxyacetic acid in pre- and postnatal exposed rats. *Environmental Toxicology*, doi: 10.1002/tox.20690. Epub ahead of print.

Rao, R.P., Kaliwal, B.B., 2002. Monocrotophos induced dysfunction on estrous cycle and follicular development in mice. *Industrial Health* **40**, 237–244.

Rauh, V.A., Perera, F.P., Horton, M.K., Whyatt, R.M., Bansal, R., Hao, X., Liu, J. et al., 2012. Brain anomalies in children exposed prenatally to a common organophosphate pesticide. *Proceedings of the National Academy of Sciences of United States* **109**, 7871–7876.

Rime, H., Nguyen, T., Bobe, J., Fostier, A., Monod, G., 2010. Prochloraz-induced oocyte maturation in Rainbow Trout (Oncorhynchus mykiss), a molecular and functional analysis. *Toxicological Sciences* **118**, 61–70.

Rockett, J.C., Narotsky, M.G., Thompson, K.E., Thillainadarajah, I., Blystone, C.R., Goetz, A.K., Ren, H. et al., 2006. Effect of conazole fungicides on reproductive development in the female rat. *Reproductive Toxicology* **22**, 647–658.

Saito, K., Tomigahara, Y., Ohe, N., Isobe, N., Nakatsuka, I., Kaneko, H., 2000. Lack of significant estrogenic or antiestrogenic activity of pyrethroid insecticides in three in vitro assays based on classic estrogen receptor alpha-mediated mechanisms. *Toxicological Sciences* **57**, 54–60.

Salehi, F., Dunfield, L., Phillips, K.P., Krewski, D., Vanderhyden, B.C., 2008. Risk factors for ovarian cancer: An overview with emphasis on hormonal factors. *Journal of Toxicology and Environmental Health. Part B, Critical reviews* **11**, 301–321.

Sereda, B., Bouwman, H., Kylin, H., 2009. Comparing water, bovine milk, and indoor residual spraying as possible sources of DDT and pyrethroid residues in breast milk. *Journal of Toxicology and Environmental Health. Part A* **72**, 842–851.

Shibayama, H., Kotera, T., Shinoda, Y., Hanada, T., Kajihara, T., Ueda, M., Tamura, H. et al., 2009. Collaborative work on evaluation of ovarian toxicity. 14) Two- or four-week repeated-dose studies and fertility study of atrazine in female rats. *The Journal of Toxicological Sciences* **34**(Suppl 1), SP147–SP155.

Silva, M.H., Gammon, D., 2009. An assessment of the developmental, reproductive, and neurotoxicity of endosulfan. *Birth Defects Research. Part B, Developmental and Reproductive Toxicology* **86**, 1–28.

Simic, B., Kniewald, J., Kniewald, Z., 1994. Effects of atrazine on reproductive performance in the rat. *Journal of Applied Toxicology* **14**, 401–404.

Sims, D.E., Singh, A., Donald, A., Jarrell, J., Villeneuve, D.C., 1991. Alteration of primate ovary surface epithelium by exposure to hexachlorobenzene: A quantitative study. *Histol. Histopathol.* **6**, 525–529.

Singh, P.B., 1992. Impact of malathion and gamma-BHC on lipid metabolism in the freshwater female catfish, Heteropneustes fossilis. *Ecotoxicology and Environmental Safety* **23**, 22–32.

Skolness, S.Y., Durhan, E.J., Garcia-Reyero, N., Jensen, K.M., Kahl, M.D., Makynen, E.A., Martinovic-Weigelt, D. et al., 2011. Effects of a short-term exposure to the fungicide prochloraz on endocrine function and gene expression in female fathead minnows (Pimephales promelas). *Aquatic Toxicology* **103**, 170–178.

Smith, E.M., Hammonds-Ehlers, M., Clark, M.K., Kirchner, H.L., Fuortes, L., 1997. Occupational exposures and risk of female infertility. *Journal of Occupational and Environmental Medicine* **39**, 138–147.

Sobinoff, A.P., Pye, V., Nixon, B., Roman, S.D., McLaughlin, E.A., 2010. Adding insult to injury: effects of xenobiotic-induced preantral ovotoxicity on ovarian development and oocyte fusibility. *Toxicological Sciences* **118**, 653–666.

Soderlund, D.M., 2012. Molecular mechanisms of pyrethroid insecticide neurotoxicity: recent advances. *Archives of Toxicology* **86**, 165–181.

Sohoni, P., Sumpter, J.P., 1998. Several environmental oestrogens are also anti-androgens. *Journal of Endocrinology* **158**, 327–339.

Son, W.Y., Das, M., Shalom-Paz, E., Holzer, H., 2011. Mechanisms of follicle selection and development. *Minerva Ginecologica* **63**, 89–102.

Stoker, C., Beldomenico, P.M., Bosquiazzo, V.L., Zayas, M.A., Rey, F., Rodriguez, H., Munoz-de-Toro, M., Luque, E.H., 2008. Developmental exposure to endocrine disruptor chemicals alters follicular dynamics and steroid levels in Caiman latirostris. *General and Comparative Endocrinology* **156**, 603–612.

Stoker, T.E., Goldman, J.M., Cooper, R.L., 1993. The dithiocarbamate fungicide thiram disrupts the hormonal control of ovulation in the female rat. *Reproductive Toxicology* **7**, 211–218.

Stoker, T.E., Goldman, J.M., Cooper, R.L., 2001. Delayed ovulation and pregnancy outcome: Effect of environmental toxicants on the neuroendocrine control of the ovary. *Environmental Toxicology and Pharmacology* **9**, 117–129.

Stresser, D.M., Kupfer, D., 1998. Human cytochrome P450-catalyzed conversion of the proestrogenic pesticide methoxychlor into an estrogen: Role of CYP2C19 and CYP1A2 in o-demethylation. *Drug Metabolism and Disposition: The Biological Fate of Chemicals* **26**, 868–874.

Stuchal, L.D., Kleinow, K.M., Stegeman, J.J., James, M.O., 2006. Demethylation of the pesticide methoxychlor in liver and intestine from untreated, methoxychlor-treated, and 3-methylcholanthrene-treated channel catfish (Ictalurus punctatus): Evidence for roles of CYP1 and CYP3A family isozymes. *Drug Metabolism and Disposition: The Biological Fate of Chemicals* **34**, 932–938.

Sun, F., Betzendahl, I., Van Wemmel, K., Cortvrindt, R., Smitz, J., Pacchierotti, F., Eichenlaub-Ritter, U., 2008. Trichlorfon-induced polyploidy and nondisjunction in mouse oocytes from preantral follicle culture. *Mutation Research* **651**, 114–124.

Symonds, D.A., Merchenthaler, I., Flaws, J.A., 2008. Methoxychlor and estradiol induce oxidative stress DNA damage in the mouse ovarian surface epithelium. *Toxicological Sciences* **105**, 182–187.

Symonds, D.A., Miller, K.P., Tomic, D., Flaws, J.A., 2006. Effect of methoxychlor and estradiol on cytochrome p450 enzymes in the mouse ovarian surface epithelium. *Toxicological Sciences* **89**, 510–514.

Taketa, Y., Yoshida, M., Inoue, K., Takahashi, M., Sakamoto, Y., Watanabe, G., Taya, K., Yamate, J., Nishikawa, A., 2011. Differential stimulation pathways of progesterone secretion from newly formed corpora lutea in rats treated with ethylene glycol monomethyl ether, sulpiride, or atrazine. *Toxicological Sciences* **121**, 267–278.

Tavera-Mendoza, L., Ruby, S., Brousseau, P., Fournier, M., Cyr, D., Marcogliese, D., 2002. Response of the amphibian tadpole Xenopus laevis to atrazine during sexual differentiation of the ovary. *Environmental Toxicology Chemistry* **21**, 1264–1267.

Tiemann, U., 2008. in vivo and in vitro effects of the organochlorine pesticides DDT, TCPM, methoxychlor, and lindane on the female reproductive tract of mammals: A review. *Reproductive Toxicology (New York)* **25**, 316–326.

U.S. Environmental Protection Agency, 2001, Organophosphate Pesticides: Revised Cumulative Risk Assessment.

U.S. Environmental Protection Agency, E., 2006. Addendum to the 2002 lindane reregistration eligibility decision (red) Prevention, Pesticides and Toxic Substances (7508P). EPA 738-k-06-028.

U.S. Environmental Protection Agency, 1994. Atrazine, simazine and cyanazine: Notice of initiation of special review. *Federal Register* **59**, 60412–60443.

Uzumcu, M., Kuhn, P.E., Marano, J.E., Armenti, A.E., Passantino, L., 2006. Early postnatal methoxychlor exposure inhibits folliculogenesis and stimulates anti-Mullerian hormone production in the rat ovary. *The Journal of Endocrinology* **191**, 549–558.

Varayoud, J., Monje, L., Bernhardt, T., Munoz-de-Toro, M., Luque, E.H., Ramos, J.G., 2008. Endosulfan modulates estrogen-dependent genes like a non-uterotrophic dose of 17beta-estradiol. *Reproductive Toxicology (New York)* **26**, 138–145.

Vidacek, Z., D.V.H.S.S.M., Karavidovic, P., 1994. Nitrates, pesticides and heavy metals in the soils and water of the territory drained by the Karasica and Vucica river system, Bizovacke Toplice, Croatia, pp. 211–222.

Vinggaard, A.M., Hass, U.L.L.A., Dalgaard, M.A.J.K., Andersen, H.R., Bonefeld-Jorgensen, E.V.A., Christiansen, S.O.F.I., Laier, P.E.T.E., Poulsen, M.E., 2006. Prochloraz: An imidazole fungicide with multiple mechanisms of action. *International Journal of Andrology* **29**, 186–192.

Wang, H., Wang, S.F., Ning, H., Ji, Y.L., Zhang, C., Zhang, Y., Yu, T. et al., 2011. Maternal cypermethrin exposure during lactation impairs testicular development and spermatogenesis in male mouse offspring. *Environmental Toxicology* **26**, 382–394.

Waters, K.M., Safe, S., Gaido, K.W., 2001. Differential gene expression in response to methoxychlor and estradiol through ERalpha, ERbeta, and AR in reproductive tissues of female mice. *Toxicological Sciences* **63**, 47–56.

Weenen, C., Laven, J.S., Von Bergh, A.R., Cranfield, M., Groome, N.P., Visser, J.A., Kramer, P., Fauser, B.C., Themmen, A.P., 2004. Anti-Mullerian hormone expression pattern in the human ovary: Potential implications for initial and cyclic follicle recruitment. *Molecular Human Reproduction* **10**, 77–83.

Withgott, J., 2002. Ubiquitous herbicide emasculates frogs. *Science* **296**, 447–448.

Wojtowicz, A.K., Honkisz, E., Zieba-Przybylska, D., Milewicz, T., Kajta, M., 2011. Effects of two isomers of DDT and their metabolite DDE on CYP1A1 and AhR function in human placental cells. *Pharmacological Reports: PR* **63**, 1460–1468.

Wojtowicz, A.K., Kajta, M., Gregoraszczuk, E.L., 2007. DDT- and DDE-induced disruption of ovarian steroidogenesis in prepubertal porcine ovarian follicles: A possible interaction with the main steroidogenic enzymes and estrogen receptor beta. *Journal of Physiology and Pharmacology* **58**, 873–885.

Wrobel, M., Mlynarczuk, J., Kotwica, J., 2009. The adverse effect of dichlorodiphenyltrichloroethane (DDT) and its metabolite (DDE) on the secretion of prostaglandins and oxytocin in bovine cultured ovarian and endometrial cells. *Reproductive Toxicology (New York)* **27**, 72–78.

Yin, H., Cukurcam, S., Betzendahl, I., Adler, I.D., Eichenlaub-Ritter, U., 1998. Trichlorfon exposure, spindle aberrations and nondisjunction in mammalian oocytes. *Chromosoma* **107**, 514–522.

Young, H.A., Mills, P.K., Riordan, D.G., Cress, R.D., 2005. Triazine herbicides and epithelial ovarian cancer risk in central California. *Journal of Occupational and Environmental Medicine/American College of Occupational and Environmental Medicine* **47**, 1148–1156.

Younglai, E.V., Foster, W.G., Hughes, E.G., Trim, K., Jarrell, J.F., 2002. Levels of environmental contaminants in human follicular fluid, serum, and seminal plasma of couples undergoing in vitro fertilization. *Archives of Environmental Contamination and Toxicology* **43**, 121–126.

Younglai, E.V., Holloway, A.C., Lim, G.E., Foster, W.G., 2004a. Synergistic effects between FSH and 1,1-dichloro-2,2-bis(P-chlorophenyl)ethylene (P,P′-DDE) on human granulosa cell aromatase activity. *Human Reproduction (Oxford, England)* **19**, 1089–1093.

Younglai, E.V., Kwan, T.K., Kwan, C.Y., Lobb, D.K., Foster, W.G., 2004b. Dichlorodiphenylchloroethylene elevates cytosolic calcium concentrations and oscillations in primary cultures of human granulosa-lutein cells. *Biology of Reproduction* **70**, 1693–1700.

Yu, Y.L., Chen, Y.X., Luo, Y.M., Pan, X.D., He, Y.F., Wong, M.H., 2003. Rapid degradation of butachlor in wheat rhizosphere soil. *Chemosphere* **50**, 771–774.

Zachow, R., Uzumcu, M., 2006. The methoxychlor metabolite, 2,2-bis-(p-hydroxyphenyl)-1,1,1-trichloroethane, inhibits steroidogenesis in rat ovarian granulosa cells *in vitro*. *Reproductive Toxicology (New York)* **22**, 659–665.

Zama, A.M., Uzumcu, M., 2009. Fetal and neonatal exposure to the endocrine disruptor methoxychlor causes epigenetic alterations in adult ovarian genes. *Endocrinology* **150**, 4681–4691.

Zhang, H., Wang, H., Ji, Y.L., Zhang, Y., Yu, T., Ning, H., Zhang, C. et al., 2010. Maternal fenvalerate exposure during pregnancy persistently impairs testicular development and spermatogenesis in male offspring. *Food and Chemical Toxicology* **48**, 1160–1169.

Zhao, X.F., Wang, Q., Ji, Y.L., Wang, H., Liu, P., Zhang, C., Zhang, Y., Xu, D.X., 2011. Fenvalerate induces germ cell apoptosis in mouse testes through the Fas/FasL signaling pathway. *Archives of Toxicology* **85**, 1101–1108.

Zhao, M., Zhang, Y., Liu, W., Xu, C., Wang, L., Gan, J., 2008. Estrogenic activity of lambda-cyhalothrin in the MCF-7 human breast carcinoma cell line. *Environmental Toxicology and Chemistry* **27**, 1194–1200.

Zorrilla, L.M., Gibson, E.K., Stoker, T.E., 2010. The effects of simazine, a chlorotriazine herbicide, on pubertal development in the female Wistar rat. *Reproductive Toxicology (New York)* **29**, 393–400.

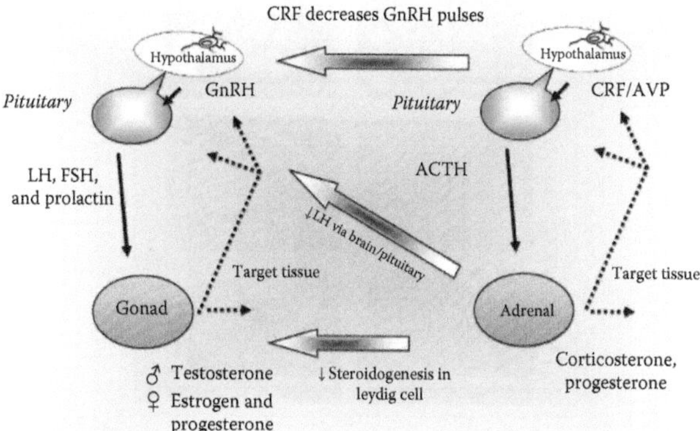

FIGURE 3.8 Schematic depicting several points of interaction between the HPA and the HPG. Activation of the adrenal axis has been shown to inhibit GnRH as a result of CRF-induced changes in GnRH, adrenal steroid actions on the CNS and/or pituitary, and by effects of corticosterone on steroidogenesis within the gonads.

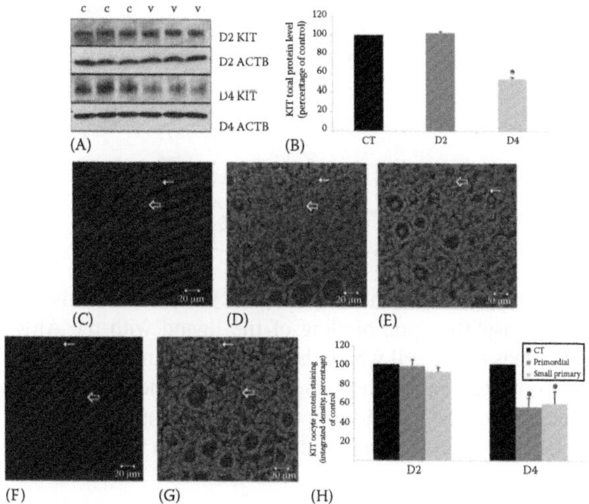

FIGURE 5.3 Effect of VCD on KIT protein staining. PND4 F344 rat ovaries were cultured with vehicle control or 30 μM VCD for 2 or 4 days and processed for Western blotting or immunofluorescence staining with confocal microscopy. (See full caption on page 105.)

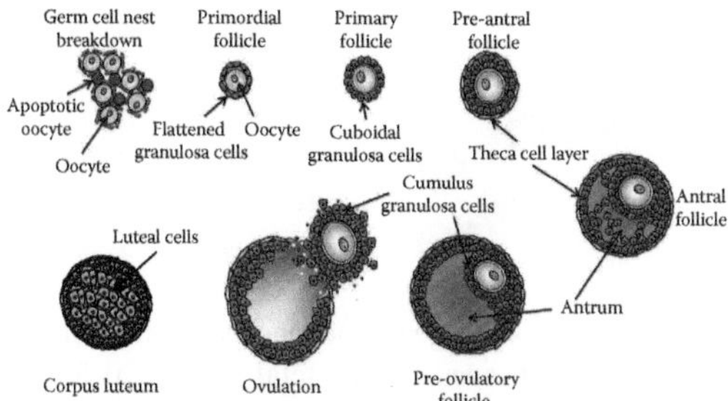

FIGURE 6.1 Stages of folliculogenesis. This schematic shows the normal developmental stages of ovarian follicles beginning with germ cell nest breakdown around birth, formation of primordial follicles, and the growth of primary follicles, pre-antral, antral follicles, and pre-ovulatory follicles. This schematic also shows ovulation and the formation of the corpus luteum.

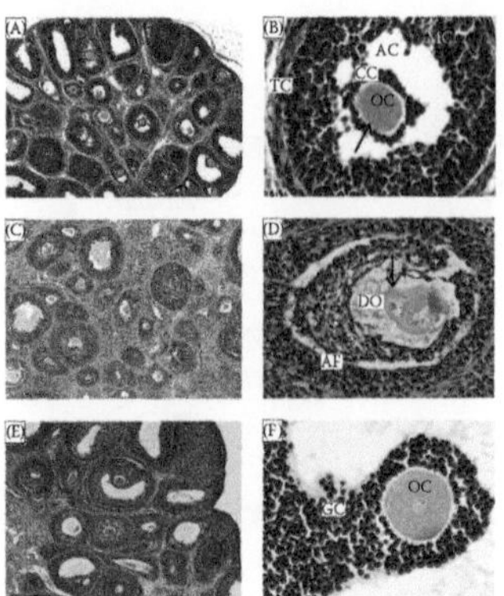

FIGURE 9.1 Histology of the ovary in postnatal day (PND) 21 rats exposed to chromium through mother's milk from PND 1–21. (See full caption on page 201.)

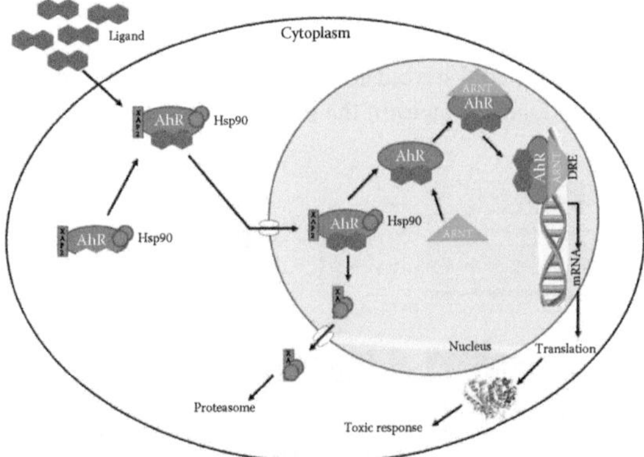

FIGURE 10.1 The aryl hydrocarbon receptor (AhR) is present in the cytoplasm coupled to heat shock protein (hsp90). Upon binding of the ligand with the AhR, the complex is transported to the nucleus of the cell where the receptor–ligand complex binds with the aryl hydrocarbon receptor nuclear transporter protein (ARNT), and hsp90 exits the nucleus to be degraded in the proteasome. The ligand–receptor–ARNT complex then binds with the dioxin response element (DRE) in AhR-regulated genes, resulting in their expression.

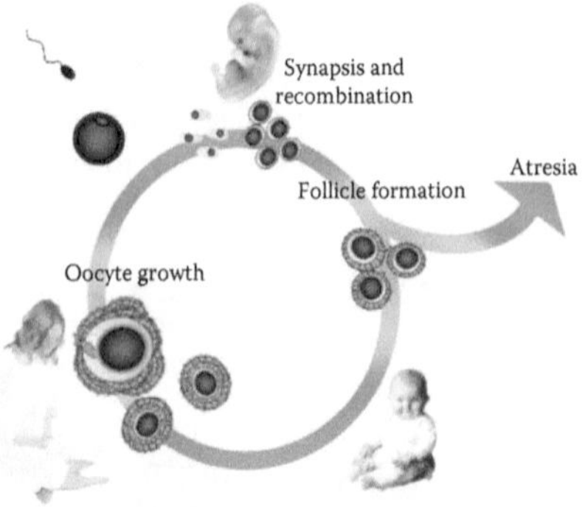

FIGURE 11.1 The three vulnerable stages of oogenesis: (i) the meiotic prophase events of synapsis and recombination, which occur in the fetal ovary; (ii) follicle formation, which occurs during the second trimester of fetal development and is associated with a dramatic loss of oocytes caused by atresia, and (iii) oocyte growth, which occurs in the adult ovary and culminates in the resumption and completion of meiosis I and ovulation of a metaphase II–arrested egg. Figure by Crystal Lawson. (From Hunt, P.A. and Hassold, T.J., *Trends Genet.*, 24(2), 86, 2008. With permission, Figure 1, p. 87).

7 Endocrine Disruptors

Katherine F. Roby

CONTENTS

7.1 ENDOCRINE DISRUPTORS

A role for exogenous factors disrupting reproductive function has been appreciated for some time. However, more recent investigation, in part fueled by a greater public awareness, has heightened the general understanding of the significance the environment plays in our reproductive health as a society.

Endocrine disruptors are exogenous chemicals that interfere with the function of the endocrine system. The U.S. Environmental Protection Agency defines an endocrine disruptor as an exogenous agent that interferes with the synthesis, secretion, transport, binding, action, or elimination of natural hormones in the body that are responsible for the maintenance of normal cell metabolism, reproduction, development, and/or behavior (Kavlock et al., 1996).

It was originally thought that the mechanisms leading to endocrine disruption involved only perturbation of steroid receptors; estrogen, androgen, progesterone, and thyroid hormone receptors. However, it is now clear that the ability of a chemical to disrupt function of the endocrine system may occur through significantly more complex and intertwined mechanisms. For example, it is now understood that the aryl hydrocarbon receptor (AhR) mediates significant endocrine disruption. In addition, endocrine disruption occurs through neurotransmitter pathways, disruption of enzymatic processes, and activation of membrane receptors independent of direct effects on steroid receptors. Any chemical that alters the physiological processes of the endocrine system can be considered an endocrine-disrupting chemical.

The types of chemicals that are considered to be endocrine disruptors are diverse. Endocrine disruptors can be man-made chemicals such as pesticides and plasticizers, natural chemicals found in plants (phytoestrogens), manufactured pharmaceuticals, or hormones. Endocrine disruptors may influence function of the ovary directly, for example, by interfering with ovarian estrogen receptor binding or indirectly via modification of the normal pattern of gonadotropin synthesis and release.

Adding to the array of endocrine-disrupting chemicals and the multiple biological mechanisms for mediating disruption, additional factors play key roles in the potential impact on any endocrine system. Specifically in regard to function of the ovary, the developmental time of exposure to an endocrine disruptor may significantly affect the outcome of that exposure. There appear to be times during development that exhibit greater or lesser sensitivity to exposure by an endocrine disruptor, or exposure at different phases of the reproductive life span may alter the overall impact of exposure. In addition, the impact of a single exposure may differ from the impact of chronic exposure. Further, exposure dose may result in variable impact, for example, a high-dose exposure that may occur with an industrial accident versus a low-level exposure that may occur via contaminated drinking water. Recent study has also demonstrated that exposure to endocrine-disrupting chemicals can affect multiple generations by inducing epigenetic modifications that alter ovarian function and thus reproductive capacity across generations. Significantly adding to this complexity is that any individual's exposure is not to a single possible endocrine disruptor, but exposure is to a mixture of chemicals and this array of exposures likely changes throughout a lifetime. In addition, it has become clear that metabolism of endocrine-disrupting chemicals often results in by-products with greater potency than the parent.

7.2 EXPERIMENTAL APPROACHES

Multiple experimental approaches have been employed both to define what chemicals constitute endocrine disruptors and to define the effects of exposure on ovarian function. The classical laboratory models include use of the rat, although mouse models have gained in use over recent years. Additional models include sheep, pig, and nonhuman primate. Exposure to a single chemical is examined in nearly all cases. Models of exposure include acute exposure and chronic exposure. Exposure may be to a female during gestation, during early postnatal development, prior to puberty, during adulthood, or across the entire life span. Exposure may also be to relatively high doses, to mimic accidental exposure, or to lower doses that approximate basal environmental exposures.

One model commonly used is the immature gonadotropin-stimulated rodent. The immature ovary contains a population of small follicles and is devoid of corpora lutea. Administration of equine chorionic gonadotropin (eCG) initiates the development of a cohort of follicles that will reach the preovulatory stage within approximately 48 h when human chorionic gonadotropin (hCG) is administered, simulating an ovulatory surge, inducing ovulation. Additional models include *in vitro* systems culturing granulosa or theca cells or alternatively, granulosa-luteal cells that are collected at the time of oocyte retrieval in women undergoing IVF-related procedures. Culture of rodent whole follicles has also more recently been employed. Individual follicles can be isolated and maintained *in vitro* where follicle development will proceed.

Following chemical exposure, multiple endpoints may be measured to assess effects on ovarian function and to uncover mechanisms leading to ovarian dysfunction. Typical endpoints include vaginal opening to assess the onset of puberty, vaginal cyclicity to determine characteristics of the estrous cycle and timing of senescence, and ovarian morphology to define parameters of follicle dynamics. Effects of exposure on ovulation may be assessed by counting ova in the oviduct following anticipated ovulation. Measurement of hormones provides key insight as to tissues and mechanisms potentially affected by exposure and typically includes quantitation of ovarian steroids; estradiol, testosterone, androstenedione, progesterone, and hypothalamic and pituitary hormone including GnRH, LH, FSH, and prolactin.

Although this short description does not include all possible laboratory models and endpoints measured, multiple approaches have been used and continue to be used to define chemicals as endocrine disruptors and to uncover the mechanisms whereby a given endocrine disruptor alters ovarian function.

This chapter will highlight the effects of endocrine disruptors with demonstrated impact on ovarian function. Emphasis will be given to endocrine disruptors that function, at least in part, by interaction with the AhR. However, recent studies have provided evidence that multiple compounds function as endocrine disruptors and alter ovarian function through varied mechanisms. A list of recent reviews focused on ovarian endocrine disruptors is provided in Table 7.1.

TABLE 7.1
Recent Reviews Related to Endocrine Disruptors and Ovarian Function

Bhattacharya, P. and Keating, A. F. (2012) Impact of environmental exposures on ovarian function and role of xenobiotic metabolism during ovotoxicity, *Toxicol Appl Pharmacol*, 261:227–235.
Craig, Z. R., Wang, W., and Flaws, J. A. (2011) Endocrine-disrupting chemicals in ovarian function: Effects on steroidogenesis, metabolism and nuclear receptor signaling, *Reproduction*, 142:633–646.
Jefferson, W. N. and Williams, C. J. (2011) Circulating levels of genistein in the neonate, apart from dose and route, predict future adverse female reproductive outcomes, *Reprod Toxicol*, 31:272–279.
Skinner, M. K., Manikkam, M., and Guerrero-Bosagna, C. (2011) Epigenetic transgenerational actions of endocrine disruptors, *Reprod Toxicol*, 31:337–343.
Mark-Kappeler, C. J., Hoyer, P. B., and Devine, P. J. (2011) Xenobiotic effects on ovarian preantral follicles, *Biol Reprod*, 85:871–883.
Dechanet, C., Anahory, T., Mathieu Daude, J. C., Quantin, X., Reyftmann, L., Hamamah, S., Hedon, B., and Dechaud, H. (2011) Effects of cigarette smoking on reproduction, *Hum Reprod Update*, 17:76–95.
Zama, A. M. and Uzumcu, M. (2010) Epigenetic effects of endocrine-disrupting chemicals on female reproduction: An ovarian perspective, *Front Neuroendocrinol*, 31:420–430.
Crain, D. A., Janssen, S. J., Edwards, T. M., Heindel, J., Ho, S. M., Hunt, P., Iguchi, T. et al. (2008) Female reproductive disorders: The roles of endocrine-disrupting compounds and developmental timing, *Fertil Steril*, 90:911–940.
Uzumcu, M. and Zachow, R. (2007) Developmental exposure to environmental endocrine disruptors: Consequences within the ovary and on female reproductive function, *Reprod Toxicol*, 23:337–352.
Guillette, L. J. J. and Moore, B. C. (2006) Environmental contaminants, fertility, and multioocytic follicles: A lesson from wildlife? *Semin Reprod Med*, 24:134–141.
Hombach-Klonisch, S., Pocar, P., Kietz, S., and Klonisch, T. (2005) Molecular actions of polyhalogenated arylhydrocarbons (PAHs) in female reproduction, *Curr Med Chem*, 12:599–616.
Brevini, T., Cillo, F., Antonini, S., and Gandolfi, F. (2005) Effects of endocrine disrupters on the oocytes and embryos of farm animals, *Reprod Domest Anim*, 40:291–299.

7.3 AhR AGONISTS AS OVARIAN ENDOCRINE DISRUPTORS

The AhR is a member of the basic helix-loop-helix–Per-ARNT-Sim (PAS) family of transcriptional regulators that have diverse functions in developmental and physiological processes as well as responses to toxic and hypoxic stimuli. AhR plays an important role in modulating the effects of exposure to toxicants by regulating the expression of several xenobiotic-metabolizing enzymes including the CYP1A1 family of genes. Thus, AhR-agonist binding stimulates metabolism and detoxification of the agonist. An endogenous ligand for the AhR has not been identified. However, a diverse group of exogenous chemicals exhibit AhR-agonist activity, and many have been classified as endocrine disruptors including the halogenated aromatic hydrocarbons (polychlorinated dibenzodioxins (PCDDs), polychlorinated dibenzofurans (PCDFs), and polychlorinated biphenyls (PCBs)) and polycyclic aromatic hydrocarbons (3-methylcholanthrene (MCA), benzo(a)pyrene, benzanthracenes, and benzoflavones). In addition, dietary factors, some also considered to be endocrine disruptors, such as indole-3-carbinol (I3C) and resveratrol, are AhR agonists (Ciolino et al., 1998, 1999, Heath-Pagliuso et al., 1998, Safe, 1990, Singh et al., 2000). The accumulated data demonstrate that AhR agonist–mediated activation plays a significant role in endocrine disruption of ovarian function. Thus, some attention will be given here to the AhR. It is of further interest to note that as the significance of the AhR in endocrine disruption at the level of the ovary has been investigated, evidence has accumulated supporting a role for the AhR in normal ovarian processes. In spite of the recent increased attention given to the AhR, it is important to note that an endogenous high-affinity ligand has yet to be identified.

In regard to control of ovarian function and endocrine disruption, AhR binding has been demonstrated at the hypothalamus, pituitary, and ovary and thus allows for the potential that AhR agonists may ultimately mediate effects on the ovary from multiple tissues.

The hypothalamus and pituitary express AhR (Cao et al., 2011, Hays et al., 2002, Huang et al., 2000, Jablonska et al., 2011a, Kainu et al., 1995, Korkalainen et al., 2005, Petersen et al., 2000, Trewin et al., 2007). AhR messenger RNA (mRNA) and protein have been localized to the posterior and anterior pituitary and the medial basal hypothalamus (Jablonska et al., 2011a). Additional studies have further localized AhR expression to both lactotrophs and gonadotrophs in the rat anterior pituitary (Cao et al., 2011).

The presence of the AhR in the ovary has been demonstrated in multiple species including rats, mice, pigs, humans, and macaques (Baldridge and Hutz, 2007, Benedict et al., 2000, Chaffin et al., 1999, 2000, Davis et al., 2000, Enan et al., 1996b, Gregoraszczuk, 2002, Jablonska et al., 2011a, Khorram et al., 2002, Mattison et al., 1990, Mizuyachi et al., 2002, Sakurada et al., 2011, Wojtowicz et al., 2005, Yamamoto et al., 2004). Ovarian expression has been localized to granulosa, theca, interstitium, corpus luteum, and the oocyte. AhR expression analysis has included mRNA and protein expression and ^{3}H-TCDD binding studies. In addition, the expression of AhR in human fetal ovaries has been described (Yamamoto et al., 2004) and adds to the potential for impact of exposure to an AhR agonist during human fetal ovarian development.

Several studies provide evidence that AhR expression is modulated with the estrous or menstrual cycle. *In situ* hybridization of AhR mRNA in immature rat ovaries demonstrated binding in both granulosa and theca cells with expression occurring in follicles of all developmental stages. The same study collected granulosa from large antral, early antral, and preantral follicles by laser dissection of frozen sections and AhR mRNA levels were assessed by real-time PCR. Expression of AhR mRNA was highest in preantral follicles and lowest in large antral follicles, and expression of β-subunit of inhibin A mRNA inversely correlated with expression of AhR (Sakurada et al., 2011). In another study, AhR mRNA expression levels were assessed by northern blot analysis on each day of the estrous cycle in adult cycling rats. Expression fluctuated with the estrous cycle where mRNA levels were increased on the morning of proestrus compared to the evening of proestrus and the morning of estrus, metestrus, and diestrus (Chaffin et al., 2000). Ovarian cell type–specific expression of AhR was also assessed by RT-PCR in macaque granulosa cells collected from ovaries during controlled ovarian stimulation. AhR message was not detectable in granulosa cells collected just prior to the ovulatory surge and then exhibited biphasic expression with levels increased at 12 h, lower at 24 h, and increased again at 36 h after hCG (Chaffin et al., 1999). The maintenance of AhR expression by primary cell cultures has also provided a model for mechanistic studies. Treatment of rat granulosa cells with FSH and estradiol *in vitro*, each alone and together, decreased AhR mRNA and protein expression and exposure to the agonist β-naphthoflavone decreased granulosal AhR protein levels (Bussmann and Barañao, 2006). Variation in the expression patterns of AhR described may be due to different model systems used across the studies. However, ovarian granulosa and theca cells express AhR and the expression in granulosa cells varies during the cycle and with gonadotropin stimulation. These data indicate that the AhR may be involved in normal ovarian processes but also indicate that specific ovarian cell types may be more vulnerable to exposure to AhR agonists and this vulnerability may vary during the cycle.

This brief description highlights the numerous AhR agonists known to be endocrine disruptors and the expression of AhR in critical tissues regulating ovarian function. As a means to address this complexity and to approach understanding the full range of effects resulting from exposure to AhR agonists, somewhat simplified approaches have been investigated. Researchers have primarily utilized 2,3,7,8-tetrachlorodibenzodioxin (TCDD) (also commonly referred to as dioxin) as an AhR prototypic agonist. In addition, effects of exposure and AhR activation have been generally explored in defined settings, for example, using *in utero* and lactational exposure, single or limited exposure during adulthood, or more chronic exposure.

7.4 TCDD

TCDD is a by-product of combustion, the burning of fossil fuels, and multiple industrial processes including the bleaching of wood pulp in paper mills. TCDD was a contaminant in the defoliant Agent Orange and has on several occasions been inadvertently released in into the environment. TCDD is a potent AhR agonist, an established human carcinogen, and a known endocrine disruptor (Hites, 2011). Significant research has addressed the impact of TCDD exposure on the ovary.

In utero exposure to an endocrine disruptor by nature exposes both the mother and the developing fetus. This may alter the hormonal and nutritional support by the mother to the fetus and, thus, indirectly affect development of the fetal reproductive axis. Alternatively or in addition, exposure at this time may more directly affect the fetus altering the ovarian potential such as limiting the primordial pool or altering the "hard-wiring" of the brain and thus affect regulatory mechanisms controlling later gonadotropin stimulation of the ovary.

Effects of exposure to TCDD during gestation and development of the ovary have been addressed in several studies. A single low dose of TCDD (200 or 800 ng/kg) on day 15 of gestation in Long–Evans–Hooded rats accelerated reproductive maturation of female offspring. Puberty, evidenced by the age of vaginal opening and the first estrus, occurred early in female offspring. In addition, ovarian weight gain, another measure of the attainment of ovarian cyclicity, was accelerated (Kakeyama et al., 2008). In another study, a single dose of TCDD (1 μg/kg) administered on day 15 of gestation in Holtzman rats led to reduced numbers of preantral and antral follicles without an increase in apoptosis (Heimler et al., 1998b). Lack of an effect of *in utero* exposure to TCDD on follicle numbers in offspring has also been reported where a single dose of 1 μg/kg TCDD on day 11, 15, or 18 of gestation in Holtzman rats had no effect on the day of vaginal opening or the numbers of primordial follicles (Flaws et al., 1997). In yet another study, a single dose of TCDD (2.5 μg/kg) administered to pregnant Sprague–Dawley rats on day 15 of gestation had no effect on the compliment of follicles on day 23 of age. However, ovulation in response to eCG and hCG administration was lower in females exposed *in utero* to TCDD (Salisbury and Marcinkiewicz, 2002). Therefore, some discrepancy exists in specific study outcomes in the described studies and the explanation for these differences is not clear. However, overall results indicate exposure to TCDD and presumably, activation of the AhR at critical times during development alters ovarian function in female offspring as evidenced by altered puberty, estradiol production, and ovulatory responsiveness to gonadotropins.

Single exposures to TCDD in the immature rat model have been used to assess more acute effects of TCDD exposure. In some studies, intact animals are used and thus maintain the potential for endogenous cross talk between the hypothalamus–pituitary and ovary. In other studies, hypophysectomized animals are used and, thus, direct effects at the level of the ovary can be measured.

Intact immature rats exposed to a single dose of TCDD (32 μg/kg, day 23 of age) exhibited reduced ovulation following gonadotropin-mediated ovulation induction. In the absence of ovulation, serum estradiol levels were maintained at high levels (Li et al., 1995). The same study found that TCDD elicited a rapid rise in serum gonadotropin within 24 h of treatment and subsequently, LH and FSH levels at the time of the ovulatory surge were reduced (Gao et al., 2001, Li et al., 1995). This altered gonadotropin profile is evidence of endocrine disruption following TCDD exposure. Further studies demonstrated that TCDD altered the responsiveness of the hypothalamus to the positive feedback stimulus of estradiol (Gao et al., 2001) because exogenous estradiol could induce LH and FSH surges and at least partially reverse the ovulation defect in TCDD-treated animals (Petroff et al., 2000). When other AhR agonists such as PCDFs, PCBs, and I3C were used in place of TCDD in the same model, similar results were obtained (Gao et al., 2000, 2002). Even in the face of TCDD-mediated changes in gonadotropins in this intact model, direct effects of TCDD on the ovary are also apparent. COX2 expression in granulosa cells from TCDD-treated rats using the same model was reduced (Mizuyachi et al., 2002), and this may be one mechanism whereby TCDD exposure inhibits ovulation. In a similar study, granulosa cells were harvested from TCDD-treated and control rats 24 and 48 h after eCG and cell cycle analysis was performed. The data demonstrated that the percent of granulosa cells in S-phase after eCG was reduced in TCDD-treated animals, and this was accompanied with reduced granulosal mRNA levels of Cdk2 and cyclin D2 and increased levels of AhR mRNA (Jung et al., 2010). These two studies provide some evidence that TCDD alters gene expression in granulosa cells that may limit follicle growth and ovulation. However, if these effects are strictly independent of TCDD-mediated alterations in hypothalamic–pituitary axis is not clear.

In order to separate effects of TCDD on the ovary from feedback and direct effects on the hypothalamus–pituitary, the immature hypophysectomized gonadotropin-stimulated rat model is often used. Similar to the intact model, the number of ova shed in response to the ovulatory hCG stimulus was reduced when TCDD was administered 24 h before eCG (Li et al., 1995, Petroff et al., 2000, Roby, 2001). Again, this effect was at least partially reversed by the administration of estradiol (Petroff et al., 2000) indicating TCDD was exhibiting antiestrogenic activity directly at the level of the ovary. In similar studies, TCDD altered follicle dynamics, whereby, the numbers of follicles greater than 350 μm in diameter were reduced, and at this time, serum levels of estradiol and granulosal hCG (LH) and FSH binding were reduced. This TCDD-induced dysregulation of follicle development was confirmed because fewer follicles were capable of ovulation in response to hCG (Roby, 2001). Thus, TCDD acting directly on the ovary disrupted the ability of follicles to respond to the stimulatory actions of gonadotropin.

A study carried out by Jablonska et al. (2010) used a complex scheme of *in utero* and lactational exposure to TCDD followed by ovary transplant to address the impact of hypothalamic–pituitary exposure versus ovarian exposure. This study found direct effects of TCDD exposure on the ovary leading to premature senescence and further that the developing ovary was particularly sensitive to the effects of TCDD.

Studies assessing effects of TCDD exposure over a lifetime have also revealed insight as to accumulated impacts of continuous exposure. Two studies have reported similar outcomes when pregnant Sprague–Dawley rats were exposed to TCDD beginning on day 14 of gestation with repeated exposure once per week. These studies using between 1 and 200 ng/kg TCDD (Franczak et al., 2006, Shi et al., 2007) demonstrated delayed vaginal opening, early onset of altered cyclicity, and reduced serum estradiol levels in exposed females. However, no differences in the number or size distribution of follicles were observed in the TCDD-treated animals (Franczak et al., 2006, Shi et al., 2007). It is of interest to note that accelerated aging appears to occur without a change in the complement of ovarian follicles; this implies a central effect of TCDD in altering the progression of aging.

Chronic low-dose exposure to TCDD and activation of the AhR result in reduced estradiol production and acceleration of senescence. The overall response of the ovary to TCDD exposure in the intact rat has now been addressed at the gene expression and proteomic levels. Ovarian gene expression analysis was carried out in whole ovaries following weekly exposure to TCDD (1, 5, 50, or 200 ng/kg/week) for approximately 11 months in Sprague–Dawley rats beginning on day 14 of gestation (Valdez et al., 2009). Interestingly, microarray analysis revealed only a modest number of differentially expressed genes. Results indicated 19 genes of known function were upregulated, while 31 genes of known function were downregulated in ovaries from rats treated with 200 ng/kg/week TCDD compared to controls. Upregulated genes included peroxisomal membrane protein 4, Cyp1B1, lipase, integrin alpha 1, and integrin beta 5. Downregulated genes included 17α-hydroxylase, aquaporin 9, FoxA2, FoxJ1, and GDF-9. Downregulation of 17α-hydroxylase was hypothesized to result in reduced substrate for aromatase and thus account for the reduced serum levels of estradiol found following TCDD exposure in this model (Valdez et al., 2009). Using a similar approach, female Sprague–Dawley rats were administered TCDD (20, 50, or 125 ng/kg) once weekly for 29 weeks after which treatment-related changes in ovarian proteins were assessed by 2D gel electrophoresis and matrix-assisted laser desorption/ionization (MALDI) tandem mass spectrometry. As in previous studies, treated rats had lower serum estradiol levels and ovary weights. Although strict conclusions were not drawn from this study, several proteins were shown to be increased and decreased in the ovaries from TCDD-exposed rats. Upregulated proteins included selenium-binding protein 2, glutathione S-transferase mu type 3, Lrpap1 protein, NADPH, and peptidylprolyl isomerase D, while downregulated proteins included prohibitin and N-ethylmaleimide-sensitive factor (Chen et al., 2009). Although definitive conclusions are not clear from the outcomes of these studies, the data do begin to provide some insight as to potential TCDD–AhR-mediated responses that will be ultimately related to the altered ovarian function following exposure to this endocrine disruptor.

Additional alternative mechanisms have been explored to define the effects of TCDD treatment and AhR activation at the level of the ovary. Previous studies have demonstrated an interaction between the AhR and several circadian clock genes and although poorly understood, circadian clock genes are present in the ovary, they are regulated by gonadotropins and steroids, and can affect steroidogenesis and cell proliferation (Karman and Tischkau, 2006, Nakamura et al., 2010, Ratajczak et al., 2009). Thus, effects of TCDD on ovarian clock genes were examined to determine if TCDD might exert its effects on the ovary, at least in part by altering circadian rhythmicity. TCDD exposure did alter the expression and rhythmicity of the canonical clock genes, brain and muscle ARNT-like 1 (Bmal1) and period circadian protein homolog 2 (Per2) in the ovary. In addition, expression of AhR transcript and protein, which in ovaries from control mice exhibited a circadian pattern of expression, was also altered after TCDD treatment (Tischkau et al., 2011). Thus, AhR activation by TCDD or other agonists may function to disrupt ovarian physiology at least in part via a disruption of normal circadian rhythms.

Primary culture models have been used to extend understanding of the endocrine disruption observed *in vivo* to a cell-specific and mechanistic level. Rat granulosa cells collected from eCG-primed rats and cultured with TCDD exhibited reduced basal estradiol accumulation in the media without altering aromatase expression. When the cultured granulosa cells were treated with FSH, TCDD exposure reduced

FSH-stimulated estradiol secretion and reduced expression of P450scc and aromatase (Dasmahapatra et al., 2000). In contrast, TCDD treatment *in vitro* has no effect on basal or gonadotropin-stimulated steroid production by granulosa cells collected from immature-untreated rats (Son et al., 1999). The lack of effect of TCDD on immature granulosa cells may be a reflection of the developmental state of the granulosa. Most studies have used granulosa or granulosa-luteal cells that have been exposed to gonadotropins *in vivo* and in these studies, TCDD treatment *in vitro* generally exhibits an inhibitory effect on steroidogenesis similar to that observed with *in vivo* exposure.

Culture of whole follicles has demonstrated similar effects of TCDD exposure. The growth of mouse antral follicles *in vitro* was not affected by TCDD; however, steroid production was inhibited. Levels of estradiol, progesterone, androstenedione, and testosterone in the follicle culture medium were all reduced with TCDD treatment. The addition of pregnenolone as a steroidogenic precursor to the cultures restored steroid synthesis indicating that the effect of TCDD in steroidogenesis would be at the level of steroidogenic acute regulatory (StAR) and or P450scc (Karman et al., 2012a). Subsequent follow-up studies demonstrated that treatment of mouse follicles with a low dose of TCDD *in vitro* (1 nM) had a significant effect on steroid enzyme expression. By 96 h of culture, transcript levels for CYP11A1, CYP17A1, HSD17β1, and CYP19A1 were decreased, while HSD3β1 transcript was increased (Karman et al., 2012b). Thus, TCDD acting directly on the granulosa cell can block steroidogenesis at multiple levels within the steroidogenic pathway.

In a variation on the whole follicle culture model, pig granulosa and theca cells were cocultured, and the effects of TCDD were examined. TCDD treatment decreased estradiol secretion in the coculture system. Similar to the mouse whole follicle culture model, addition of precursor 25-OH-cholesterol restored estradiol production. The authors hypothesize that TCDD affects porcine granulosal–thecal steroidogenesis by acting at P450scc and aromatase (Gregoraszczuk, 2002). In another study, the effects of TCDD in combination with prolactin on cultured porcine theca cells were examined. Prolactin is a hormone regulator of ovarian function and treatment of porcine theca cells with prolactin increases steroid production. TCDD treatment alone had no effect on thecal progesterone production but TCDD inhibited prolactin-stimulated progesterone production (Jablonska et al., 2011b). Although not specifically measured, it was hypothesized that TCDD may inhibit expression of the prolactin receptor as previous studies have demonstrated in breast cancer cells (Lu et al., 1996).

The effects of TCDD on granulosa cells and whole follicle cultures are consistent with findings in human granulosa-luteal cells. Progesterone and estradiol production by human granulosa-luteal cells collected from women at the time of oocyte retrieval is reduced and the addition of androgen precursors reversed these effects of TCDD (Enan et al., 1996a,b, Heimler et al., 1998a). Additional studies have indicated that the target of TCDD-mediated inhibition of granulosa-luteal steroidogenesis is Cyp17 (Morán et al., 2003a,b). An alternative or additional mechanism was proposed in a series of experiments where low-dose TCDD (low nanomolar to micromolar) treatment of human granulosa-luteal cells stimulated a rapid and significant increase in inhibin A secretion without altering inhibin B. With increased duration of exposure, even picomolar concentrations of TCDD stimulated increased inhibin A production. It was hypothesized that TCDD may increase inhibin A production as an indirect means to reduce FSH-stimulated estradiol secretion (Ho et al., 2006). Although the described culture studies utilize different models and measure different endpoints, TCDD can directly alter ovarian cell function by modulation of gene expression. Consistent key targets include steroidogenic enzymes.

An additional mechanism whereby TCDD has the potential to modulate steroid production is through regulation of gonadotropin receptor expression. Following *in vivo* exposure to TCDD rat, whole ovary binding of radioiodinated FSH and LH was reduced (Roby, 2001). Analysis of FSH and LH receptor expression *in vitro* in rat granulosa cells yielded similar results. FSH-stimulated FSHR mRNA expression was dose-dependently reduced by TCDD (Hirakawa et al., 2000a,b). Similarly, cAMP-stimulated FSH receptor expression was reduced by TCDD treatment indicating TCDD was acting at a post-cAMP site. Those studies also demonstrated that the rate of transcription of the FSHR and LHR was reduced by TCDD, while mRNA stability of LHR only was affected by TCDD (Hirakawa et al., 2000a,b). Recent studies have also demonstrated interplay between FSH-regulated LH receptor expression and the IGF1 pathway. In rat granulosa cells, FSH-mediated upregulation of LHR is augmented by IGF1. TCDD treatment inhibited both the FSH-stimulated and the FSH+IGF1-stimulated increased LHR expression. In this case, studies revealed that TCDD reduced both the rate of transcription and the half-life of LHR transcripts (Minegishi et al., 2003, 2004).

Genetic disruption of the AhR has provided additional evidence for a role of AhR in normal function of the ovary. AhR-deficient (AhRKO) mice exhibit reduced fertility, reduced numbers of preantral and antral follicles, and reduced ovulation (Baba et al., 2005, Barnett et al., 2007a,b, Benedict et al., 2000, 2003). Follicles from AhRKO ovaries express lower levels of LH and FSH receptor compared to wild type. In addition, CHiP analysis demonstrated a direct interaction of AhR and the FSHR promoter (Barnett et al., 2007). Data from AhRKO mice demonstrate a role for AhR in normal ovarian function; however, these studies also highlight the complexity of the system. For example, several different model systems have demonstrated that TCDD-mediated activation of AhR inhibits estradiol production; however, in the AhRKO mouse, estrogen production is reduced (Hernandez-Ochoa et al., 2010). Several possibilities have been posed to explain these apparent inconsistencies such as varied receptor occupancy, experimental variations, feedback mechanisms, and difference between *in vivo* and *in vitro* systems. It is clear that TCDD exposure and subsequent activation of the AhR disrupts normal ovarian function and at the same time, the absence of the AhR results in altered ovarian function. It is likely a balance of AhR activation occurs with normal ovarian function. Taken together, these findings illustrate the complexity of the system. Further investigation will likely define additional factors influencing AhR-mediated effects in the ovary and may lead to identification of an endogenous ligand with important roles in normal ovarian physiology.

TCDD is an endocrine disruptor altering ovarian function indirectly by altering gonadotropin production and directly at the level of the ovary modulating folliculogenesis. Recent studies have also demonstrated multigenerational effects of TCDD exposure on ovarian competence. Exposure of pregnant female rats during mid-gestation (d8–14) resulted in ovarian deficits seen in three subsequent generations. The transgenerational impact of TCDD was evidence by early onset of puberty and reduced primordial follicle pools in F3 females (Manikkam et al., 2012). Thus, the complete impact of TCDD and other AhR agonists on ovarian function and fertility is yet to be fully understood.

7.5 GENISTEIN

Genistein is a phytoestrogen endocrine disruptor found in a number of plants including soybeans. Genistein exhibits estrogenic activity with significant potency and is also an AhR antagonist. The general consumption of, and thus exposure to, phytoestrogens varies considerably with diet.

Neonatal exposure of mice and rats to genistein results in multi-oocytic follicles that are maintained into adulthood (Cimafranca et al., 2010, Jefferson et al., 2005, 2006b, Losa et al., 2011). Genistein appears to impact the development of follicles during the early postnatal period when primordial follicles are established with the breakdown of oocyte nests. The oocytes from genistein-treated mice retained intercellular bridges several days after the breakdown was complete in control mice. In addition to disrupted nest breakdown, there was significantly less apoptosis of oocytes in genistein-treated animals (Jefferson et al., 2006a). *In vitro* studies where postnatal mouse ovaries were cultured further demonstrated that genistein altered the processes of nest breakdown and primordial follicle assembly (Chen et al., 2007). Studies using mice with disrupted ERα or ERβ indicated that the effects of genistein in altering follicle assembly are dependent on ERβ (Jefferson et al., 2006a). In addition, neonatal treatment of mice with genistein resulted in altered estrous cyclicity during adulthood characterized by increased duration of the estrus phase (Bateman and Patisaul, 2008, Jefferson et al., 2005, Kouki et al., 2003, Nagao et al., 2001, Suzuki et al., 2002).

Several *in vitro* studies have also revealed effects of genistein in altering steroidogenesis. Rat follicles cultured with FSH and genistein exhibited decreased cAMP accumulation and reduced testosterone production; however, estradiol secretion was not altered (Myllymäki et al., 2005). Similarly, genistein treatment of porcine granulosa cells reduced progesterone production (Basini et al., 2010, Nynca and Ciereszko, 2006, Tiemann et al., 2007). In addition, human granulosa-luteal cells exhibited reduced 17β-HSD and aromatase mRNA and activity following treatment with genistein (Rice et al., 2006).

Thus, genistein, a compound that exhibits estrogenic activity and has been considered to be an AhR antagonist, has significant effects in disrupting ovarian function. Data in rodents indicate that the late developing ovary is particularly sensitive to genistein exposure. This characteristic is noteworthy given that genistein and related isoflavones are abundant in soy-based infant formulas.

7.6 BENZO(A)PYRENE

Benzo(a)pyrene (BaP) is a polycyclic aromatic hydrocarbon and is a product of combustion and a component of cigarette smoke. BaP is a well-known ovotoxicant; the rapid and dramatic effects of BaP exposure on the oocyte compliment within the ovary of experimentally treated animals have been described. The ovotoxic effect is thought to largely be the result of the generation of reactive species in the ovary following BaP exposure and the resultant destruction of the primordial and primary follicle pool (Borman et al., 2000, MacKenzie and Angevine, 1981, Mattison et al., 1980, 1983, Shiromizu and Mattison, 1984). BaP is also an AhR agonist and more recent studies have addressed the potential for BaP to function like other AhR agonists as an endocrine disruptor.

Mice administered a single intraperitoneal injection of BaP exhibited reduced ovulation and reduced number and volume of copra lutea. Interestingly, this effect appeared to be transient because ovulation rate and copra lutea number and volume recovered by 2 weeks after BaP administration (Miller et al., 1992, Swartz and Mattison, 1985). Isolated mouse follicles cultured in the presence of BaP exhibited reduced antral follicle development and decreased estradiol output. BaP exposure also decreased production of AMH by preantral and antral follicles but had no effects on progesterone production (Sadeu and Foster, 2011). A similar study culturing rat follicles demonstrated that BaP exposure inhibited follicle growth and cell proliferation and reduced estradiol and AMH production (Neal et al., 2007, 2010).

Several studies in fish have also demonstrated an effect of BaP exposure on the ovary. *In vitro* incubation of flounder ovaries with BaP inhibited CYP17 activity (Rocha Monteiro et al., 2000). In another study, waterborne exposure of killifish resulted in lower CYP19 mRNA expression in the ovary, while CYP19 mRNA levels in the brain increased (Patel et al., 2006).

Like many environmental toxicants and endocrine disruptors, BaP appears to concentrate in follicular fluid. In a comparative study in women that were smokers and undergoing oocyte retrieval, BaP levels were higher in follicular fluid compared to systemic blood. In addition, that study found significantly higher levels of follicular fluid BaP in women who did not conceive compared to women who did (Neal et al., 2007).

Thus, it appears that BaP, a known ovotoxicant, likely also functions as an endocrine disruptor and alters development of growing follicles.

7.7 BISPHENOL A

Bisphenol A (BPA) (2,2-bis(4-hydroxyphenyl)) is a chemical used primarily in the manufacture of polycarbonate plastic, epoxy resins, and as an additive to other plastics (Kang et al., 2006). BPA has been found in serum, follicular fluid, amniotic fluid, fetal serum, and in tissues of men and women of different ages and ethnic groups (Ikezuki et al., 2001, Schönfelder et al., 2002, Tsutsumi, 2005). BPA functions at least in part as a nonsteroidal estrogen disrupting the activity of endogenous estrogens (Matthews et al., 2001). In addition, BPA can bind the AhR (Bonefeld-Jørgensen et al., 2007, Krüger et al., 2008) and thus may also function as an ovarian endocrine disruptor via its AhR-agonist activity.

Initial studies describing bisphenol A–mediated disruption of oocyte meiosis called attention to not only the effect of this compound on reproduction and fertility but importantly heightened awareness of the widespread existence of this toxicant and the unanticipated impact (Hunt et al., 2003). Studies related to understanding the full effects of BPA on the process of oocyte meiosis continue (Muhlhauser et al., 2009, Zhang et al., 2012); however, additional effects of BPA on ovarian function have been uncovered.

When pregnant female mice were exposed to BPA from gestation day 9 to parturition, female pups exhibited abnormal estrous cycles with greater time spent in estrus or metestrus (Markey et al., 2003). In a similar study, exposure to BPA between days 9–16 of gestation was correlated with the presence of ovarian cysts by 18 months of age (Newbold et al., 2009). Higher exposure levels of BPA (100 or 1000 μg/kg/day) beginning day 1 of gestation to postnatal day 7 also revealed a significant ovarian effect including reduced numbers of developing follicles and increased follicular atresia (Signorile et al., 2012). The effects of *in utero* exposure to BPA on the developing ovary were further assessed by gene expression analysis. In this study, a low dose of BPA previously shown to effect meiosis (20 ng/g) was administered beginning on day 11 of gestation and fetal ovaries were collected between 1 and 3.5 days after the start of dosing. It is important to note that this dose of BPA was chosen because similar studies had demonstrated an effect on meiosis (Susiarjo et al., 2007). Gene expression analysis revealed several genes related to mitosis to be dysregulated in BPA-exposed ovaries. The authors hypothesize that an inappropriately and premature cessation of mitosis and entry into meiosis would reduce the primordial follicle pool and limit reproductive potential (Lawson et al., 2011). This understanding that BPA can alter the establishment of the primordial pool at the level of mitosis was a novel finding and extends the impact of BPA from the meiosis-related effects already understood. Ovarian effects in addition to ovotoxicity following BPA exposure during the neonatal period have also been described. Exposure of mice during the first postnatal week resulted in a reduction in the primordial follicle pool and in the numbers of growing follicles, indicating a dysregulation of follicle recruitment (Rodríguez et al., 2010). In addition, similar to studies where exposure was limited to mid-late gestation, neonatal exposure to BPA resulted in the presence of ovarian cysts by 18 months of age (Newbold et al., 2007). More extensive endocrine-disrupting actions of BPA exposure were uncovered in a series of studies carried out in rats. Female rats were exposed to BPA (5–500 μg/kg/day; doses both above and below the LOAEL) on postnatal days 1 through 10, and subsequent effects were measured in adulthood. Hormone analysis on the day of estrus revealed elevated levels of estradiol and testosterone and reduced progesterone levels. In addition, GnRH pulsatility was altered as determined in explant cultures where the inter pulse interval in BPA-exposed rats was reduced. Further, ovarian weight was reduced and histological analysis of the ovaries demonstrated reduced numbers of corpora lutea and antral follicles and increased numbers of atretic follicles. In addition, cystic follicles were present. The number of ova shed in a natural cycle was also reduced in animals exposed to the higher dose (Fernández et al., 2009, 2010). These *in vivo* studies clearly demonstrate the ovotoxic activities of BPA and also indicate that BPA likely functions as an endocrine disruptor at the level of the ovary and hypothalamus.

In vitro studies have addressed direct effects of BPA exposure on steroidogenesis by ovarian cells. BPA treatment inhibited FSH-induced aromatase and estradiol secretion by human granulosa-luteal cells collected at the time of oocyte retrieval (Kwintkiewicz et al., 2010). In addition, the expression of several downstream effectors known to play a role in FSH-mediated control of aromatase expression was examined. SF-1 and GATA4 were decreased in BPA-treated cells although CREB-1 was not. In addition, PPARγ a known inhibitor of aromatase (Fan et al., 2005) was increased in BPA-treated cells and increased PPARγ correlated with reduced aromatase in a dose-dependent manner. The same study showed that BPA reduced DNA synthesis by granulosa-luteal cells but did not induce DNA fragmentation (Kwintkiewicz et al., 2010). It is of interest to note that other endocrine disruptors such as phthalates have been shown to inhibit aromatase expression by activating PPARγ (Lovekamp-Swan et al., 2003, Xu et al., 2010).

Another study has examined the effects of BPA treatment on rat theca-interstitial cells and granulosa cells cultured individually. BPA induced thecal-interstitial testosterone production that was accompanied with increased expression of P45017c, P450scc, and StAR mRNA. In granulosa cell cultures, BPA treatment increased progesterone production and decreased estradiol production. In addition, granulosal StAR and P450scc mRNA were increased, while CYP19 mRNA was decreased (Zhou et al., 2008). Thus, BPA alters the expression of key steroidogenesis-related genes.

Direct effects of BPA on antral follicles have been addressed using the mouse whole follicle culture model. BPA had a significant effect on both follicle growth and steroid production. Treatment of follicles with BPA inhibited follicle growth and inhibited progesterone, dehydroepiandrosterone, androstenedione, estrone, testosterone, and estradiol production. mRNA expression levels of StAR, P450scc, and 3βHSD were inhibited in BPA-treated follicles and there appeared to be reduced CYP19 mRNA levels although effects did not reach statistical significance (Peretz et al., 2011). In another study, follicles from ESR1 overexpressing mice were also used to examine a relationship between BPA activity, ESR1, and follicular growth and atresia (Peretz et al., 2012). As in the previous study, follicles treated with BPA exhibited reduced growth in both wild-type and ESR1 overexpressing follicles and reduced follicle growth was associated with atresia. ESR1 overexpressing follicles were not more sensitive to the effects of BPA when compared to wild-type follicles and replacement of estradiol to the cultures did not affect the BPA-induced follicle growth inhibition. To begin to determine potential BPA-initiated mechanisms of growth inhibition and atresia, the expression of several genes was assessed. BPA treatment *in vitro* induced upregulated Cdk4, Ccne1, and Trp53 expression, whereas it downregulated Ccnd2 expression. In addition, Bax and Bcl2 expression was upregulated correlating with follicular atresia. Because ESR1 overexpression and estradiol replacement did not alter BPA's effects on cell cycle and apoptosis-related gene expression, it appears that the effects of BPA on follicle growth and atresia are independent of estrogen-regulated pathways (Peretz et al., 2012). It would be of interest to more directly examine the potential that AhR may play a role, at least in part, in BPA-mediated impacts at the level of the ovary.

Several studies have investigated an interaction of BPA exposure with ovarian dysfunction in women. Higher levels of serum BPA are associated with women with PCO, regardless of body weight or levels of testosterone and androstenedione (Kandaraki et al., 2011, Tarantino et al., 2012, Takeuchi et al., 2004). In addition, in women undergoing IVF procedures, higher urinary BPA concentrations were found to be associated with decreased number of oocytes retrieved, decreased peak estradiol levels, reduced rates of fertilization, and reduced blastocyst formation (Ehrlich et al., 2012, Mok-Lin et al., 2010).

Separating the impact of BPA as an ovotoxicant and an endocrine disruptor on overall fertility is sometimes difficult. However, recent studies have described the ability of BPA to not only affect the oocyte but also alter ovarian steroidogenesis and, either directly or as a consequence of ovarian effects, alter hypothalamic GnRH secretion. Increasing data further draw an association between BPA and PCOS. Given the widespread presence of BPA in the environment, continued attention to the reproductive significance of BPA exposure is warranted.

7.8 ATRAZINE

Atrazine (2-chloro-4-ethylamino-6-isopropylamino-s-triazine) was introduced in the 1950s as a broad-spectrum herbicide and remains one of the most widely used herbicides in the United States. It has been extensively studied as an endocrine disruptor. Early studies demonstrated that atrazine exposure reduced ovarian weights and serum estradiol levels and resulted in lengthening of the estrous cycle (Eldridge et al., 1994, Wetzel et al., 1994). The ovarian endocrine-disrupting effects of atrazine were confirmed in a study where feeding atrazine (150 mg/kg) to rats over 21 consecutive days altered estrous cycles and a higher dose (300 mg/kg) led to ovarian regression and acyclicity (Cooper et al., 1996). Subsequent studies described a central effect of atrazine in altering GnRH pulse frequency (Cooper et al., 1996, 2000, Das et al., 2000, 2001, Tennant et al., 1994). Thus, atrazine functions as an ovarian endocrine disruptor, at least in part, indirectly but altering gonadotropin inputs to the ovary.

Ovarian endocrine-disrupting effects of atrazine have also been examined using models of gestational exposure. Female offspring of pregnant dams treated with atrazine at high doses (100 mg/kg/day) on days 14–21 of gestation exhibited delayed vaginal opening; however, cyclicity was not altered and the onset of senescence was not different in treated rats (Davis et al., 2011). The ovarian impact of atrazine was more apparent when exposure occurred in adult cycling rats. In one study, adult females were administered atrazine for 14 days and monitored for an additional 14 days. Treated rats exhibited disrupted estrous cycles and reduced ovary weight, and ovaries had reduced numbers of old corpora lutea and completely lacked new corpora lutea; serum estradiol was increased. Analysis of specific mRNAs revealed that AR, ERα, LHR, and sulfatase mRNA were reduced in ovaries from treated rats, while aromatase mRNA levels and aromatase activity were increased (Quignot et al., 2012a). Established atrazine-mediated disruption of ovarian function occurs due to effects at the level of the brain and pituitary and alters LH production. Effects of atrazine demonstrated in the studies described earlier could largely be attributed to altered LH. Additional studies have addressed the potential for direct effects of atrazine on ovarian cells using *in vitro* models.

Similar to observations made *in vivo*, culture of human granulosa-luteal cells with atrazine resulted in increased aromatase activity. It is interesting to note that the same study found that aromatase activity in endometrial stroma was not affected by atrazine indicating a level of specificity toward ovarian type aromatase (Holloway et al., 2008). Culture of primary rat granulosa cells collected from immature rats after eCG administration and treated *in vitro* with atrazine demonstrated a stimulation of aromatase activity and increased estradiol production although increased estradiol production was apparent only when measured for 1 h following 24 h of exposure to atrazine (Tinfo et al., 2011). Granulosa cells collected from immature DES-treated rats exhibited both increased aromatase activity and mRNA levels after atrazine treatment (Quignot et al., 2012b). Atrazine treatment of porcine granulosa cells collected from follicles greater than 5 mm in diameter and irrespective of the day of the cycle inhibited estradiol at low doses (0.1 μM) and increased progesterone at higher doses (10 μM). Changes in steroid production were modest yet statistically different (Basini et al., 2012).

The effects of atrazine exposure on luteal function have also been addressed. Luteal cell hypertrophy was observed in adult rats treated with atrazine (Shibayama et al., 2009); thus, an experiment was designed to assess effects of atrazine on luteal function. A high dose of atrazine (300 mg/kg) was administered to adult cycling rats on proestrus through diestrus when ovaries were collected. Atrazine-treated animals had significantly higher progesterone levels, while no effect on prolactin levels was observed. In addition, newly formed corpora lutea in atrazine-treated animals exhibited higher levels of SR-B1 mRNA and protein. Expression of other steroidogenesis-related factors including StAR, P450scc, and 3βHSD mRNAs was not altered although StAR and 3βHSD protein levels were increased based on density analysis of immunohistochemical-stained sections. Because progesterone was increased with no change in prolactin, the authors hypothesize that atrazine exhibits direct effects on luteal cells (Taketa et al., 2011).

Data from multiple *in vivo* and *in vitro* studies confirm the central effects of atrazine in disrupting the gonadotropin surge and the resultant effects on the ovarian cycle. Additional studies indicate that atrazine can also directly impact ovarian function via effects on both granulosa, through regulation of aromatase expression, and on corpora lutea via impacting progesterone production. Thus, atrazine has the potential to function as a multiple tissue endocrine disruptor ultimately impacting ovarian function and fertility.

7.9 SUMMARY

Endocrine disruptors are natural chemicals such as phytoestrogens, man-made chemicals such as herbicides, chemicals used in the manufacture of products such as plasticizers, and by-products resulting from combustion. Significant data demonstrate that endocrine disruptors alter ovarian function and thus overall fertility. The data described in this review highlight the complexity of how endocrine disrupters can impact ovarian function. In general, the data reveal that the developmental period of exposure, the duration of exposure, the level of exposure, and the specific chemical all play a role in the final potential influence on the ovary. Over the last several years, our understanding of what chemicals constitute ovarian endocrine disruptors has expanded and our understanding of the mechanisms altered by these chemicals impacting the physiological function of the ovary has become more precise. Although significant gains have been met, this new understanding has in many ways revealed gaps in our knowledge. The absolute effects of exposure to endocrine disruptors on the ovary and fertility remain to be fully understood.

REFERENCES

Baba, T., Mimura, J., Nakamura, N., Harada, N., Yamamoto, M., Morohashi, K., and Fujii-Kuriyama, Y. (2005) Intrinsic function of the aryl hydrocarbon (dioxin) receptor as a key factor in female reproduction, *Mol Cell Biol*, 25:10040–10051.

Baldridge, M. G. and Hutz, R. J. (2007) Autoradiographic localization of aromatic hydrocarbon receptor (AHR) in rhesus monkey ovary, *Am J Primatol*, 69:681–691.

Barnett, K. R., Tomic, D., Gupta, R. K., Babus, J. K., Roby, K. F., Terranova, P. F., and Flaws, J. A. (2007a) The aryl hydrocarbon receptor is required for normal gonadotropin responsiveness in the mouse ovary, *Toxicol Appl Pharmacol*, 223:66–72.

Barnett, K. R., Tomic, D., Gupta, R. K., Miller, K. P., Meachum, S., Paulose, T., and Flaws, J. A. (2007b) The aryl hydrocarbon receptor affects mouse ovarian follicle growth via mechanisms involving estradiol regulation and responsiveness, *Biol Reprod*, 76:1062–1070.

Basini, G., Bianchi, F., Bussolati, S., Baioni, L., Ramoni, R., Grolli, S., Conti, V., Bianchi, F., and Grasselli, F. (2012) Atrazine disrupts steroidogenesis, VEGF and NO production in swine granulosa cells, *Ecotoxicol Environ Saf*, 85C:59–63.

Basini, G., Bussolati, S., Santini, S. E., and Grasselli, F. (2010) The impact of the phytooestrogen genistein on swine granulosa cell function, *J Anim Physiol Anim Nutr*, 94:e374–e382.

Bateman, H. L. and Patisaul, H. B. (2008) Disrupted female reproductive physiology following neonatal exposure to phytoestrogens or estrogen specific ligands is associated with decreased GnRH activation and kisspeptin fiber density in the hypothalamus, *Neurotoxicology*, 29:988–997.

Benedict, J. C., Lin, T. M., Loeffler, I. K., Peterson, R. E., and Flaws, J. A. (2000) Physiological role of the aryl hydrocarbon receptor in mouse ovary development, *Toxicol Sci*, 56:382–388.

Benedict, J. C., Miller, K. P., Lin, T. M., Greenfeld, C., Babus, J. K., Peterson, R. E., and Flaws, J. A. (2003) Aryl hydrocarbon receptor regulates growth, but not atresia, of mouse preantral and antral follicles, *Biol Reprod*, 68:1511–1517.

Bonefeld-Jørgensen, E. C., Long, M., Hofmeister, M. V., and Vinggaard, A. M. (2007) Endocrine-disrupting potential of bisphenol A, bisphenol A dimethacrylate, 4-n-nonylphenol, and 4-n-octylphenol *in vitro*: New data and a brief review, *Environ Health Perspect*, 115:69–76.

Borman, S. M., Christian, P. J., Sipes, I. G., and Hoyer, P. B. (2000) Ovotoxicity in female Fischer rats and B6 mice induced by low-dose exposure to three polycyclic aromatic hydrocarbons: Comparison through calculation of an ovotoxic index, *Toxicol Appl Pharmacol*, 176:191–198.

Bussmann, U. A. and Barañao, J. L. (2006) Regulation of aryl hydrocarbon receptor expression in rat granulosa cells, *Biol Reprod*, 75:360–369.

Cao, J., Patisaul, H. B., and Petersen, S. L. (2011) Aryl hydrocarbon receptor activation in lactotropes and gonadotropes interferes with estradiol-dependent and -independent preprolactin, glycoprotein alpha and luteinizing hormone beta gene expression, *Mol Cell Endocrinol*, 333:151–159.

Chaffin, C. L., Stouffer, R. L., and Duffy, D. M. (1999) Gonadotropin and steroid regulation of steroid receptor and aryl hydrocarbon receptor messenger ribonucleic acid in macaque granulosa cells during the periovulatory interval, *Endocrinology*, 140:4753–4760.

Chaffin, C. L., Trewin, A. L., and Hutz, R. J. (2000) Estrous cycle-dependent changes in the expression of aromatic hydrocarbon receptor (AHR) and AHR-nuclear translocator (ARNT) mRNAs in the rat ovary and liver, *Chem Biol Interact*, 124:205–216.

Chen, Y., Jefferson, W. N., Newbold, R. R., Padilla-Banks, E., and Pepling, M. E. (2007) Estradiol, progesterone, and genistein inhibit oocyte nest breakdown and primordial follicle assembly in the neonatal mouse ovary in vitro and *in vivo*, *Endocrinology*, 148:3580–3590.

Chen, X., Ma, X. M., Ma, S. W., Coenraads, P. J., Zhang, C. M., Liu, J., Zhao, L. J., Sun, M., and Tang, N. J. (2009) Proteomic analysis of the rat ovary following chronic low-dose exposure to 2,3,7,8-tetrachlorodibenzo-p-dioxin (TCDD), *J Toxicol Environ Health A*, 72:717–726.

Cimafranca, M. A., Davila, J., Ekman, G. C., Andrews, R. N., Neese, S. L., Peretz, J., Woodling, K. A., Helferich, W. G., Sarkar, J., Flaws, J. A., Schantz, S. L., Doerge, D. R., and Cooke, P. S. (2010) Acute and chronic effects of oral genistein administration in neonatal mice, *Biol Reprod*, 83:114–121.

Ciolino, H. P., Daschner, P. J., Wang, T. T., and Yeh, G. C. (1998) Effect of curcumin on the aryl hydrocarbon receptor and cytochrome P450 1A1 in MCF-7 human breast carcinoma cells, *Biochem Pharmacol*, 56:197–206.

Ciolino, H. P., Daschner, P. J., and Yeh, G. C. (1999) Dietary flavonols quercetin and kaempferol are ligands of the aryl hydrocarbon receptor that affect CYP1A1 transcription differentially, *Biochem J*, 340:715–722.

Cooper, R. L., Stoker, T. E., Goldman, J. M., Parrish, M. B., and Tyrey, L. (1996) Effect of atrazine on ovarian function in the rat, *Reprod Toxicol*, 10:257–264.

Cooper, R. L., Stoker, T. E., Tyrey, L., Goldman, J. M., and McElroy, W. K. (2000) Atrazine disrupts the hypothalamic control of pituitary-ovarian function, *Toxicol Sci*, 53:297–307.

Das, P. C., McElroy, W. K., and Cooper, R. L. (2000) Differential modulation of catecholamines by chlorotriazine herbicides in pheochromocytoma (PC12) cells *in vitro*, *Toxicol Sci*, 56:324–331.

Das, P. C., McElroy, W. K., and Cooper, R. L. (2001) Alteration of catecholamines in pheochromocytoma (PC12) cells in vitro by the metabolites of chlorotriazine herbicide, *Toxicol Sci*, 59:127–137.

Dasmahapatra, A. K., Wimpee, B. A., Trewin, A. L., Wimpee, C. F., Ghorai, J. K., and Hutz, R. J. (2000) Demonstration of 2,3,7,8-tetrachlorodibenzo-p-dioxin attenuation of P450 steroidogenic enzyme mRNAs in rat granulosa cell in vitro by competitive reverse transcriptase-polymerase chain reaction assay, *Mol Cell Endocrinol*, 164:5–18.

Davis, B. J., Mccurdy, E. A., Miller, B. D., Lucier, G. W., and Tritscher, A. M. (2000) Ovarian tumors in rats induced by chronic 2,3,7,8-tetrachlorodibenzo-p-dioxin treatment, *Cancer Res*, 60:5414–5419.

Davis, L. K., Murr, A. S., Best, D. S., Fraites, M. J., Zorrilla, L. M., Narotsky, M. G., Stoker, T. E., Goldman, J. M., and Cooper, R. L. (2011) The effects of prenatal exposure to atrazine on pubertal and postnatal reproductive indices in the female rat, *Reprod Toxicol*, 32:43–51.

Ehrlich, S., Williams, P. L., Missmer, S. A., Flaws, J. A., Ye, X., Calafat, A. M., Petrozza, J. C., Wright, D., and Hauser, R. (2012) Urinary bisphenol A concentrations and early reproductive health outcomes among women undergoing IVF, *Hum Reprod*, 27:3583–3592.

Eldridge, J. C., Fleenor-Heyser, D. G., Extrom, P. C., Wetzel, L. T., Breckenridge, C. B., Gillis, J. H., Luempert, L. G. R., and Stevens, J. T. (1994) Short-term effects of chlorotriazines on estrus in female Sprague-Dawley and Fischer 344 rats, *J Toxicol Environ Health*, 43:155–167.

Enan, E., Lasley, B., Stewart, D., Overstreet, J., and VandeVoort, C. A. (1996a) 2,3,7,8-Tetrachlorodibenzo-p-dioxin (TCDD) modulates function of human luteinized granulosa cells via cAMP signaling and early reduction of glucose transporting activity, *Reprod Toxicol*, 10:191–198.

Enan, E., Moran, F., VandeVoort, C. A., Stewart, D. R., Overstreet, J. W., and Lasley, B. L. (1996b) Mechanism of toxic action of 2,3,7,8-tetrachlorodibenzo-p-dioxin (TCDD) in cultured human luteinized granulosa cells, *Reprod Toxicol*, 10:497–508.

Fan, W., Yanase, T., Morinaga, H., Mu, Y. M., Nomura, M., Okabe, T., Goto, K., Harada, N., and Nawata, H. (2005) Activation of peroxisome proliferator-activated receptor-gamma and retinoid X receptor inhibits aromatase transcription via nuclear factor-kappaB, *Endocrinology*, 146:85–92.

Fernández, M., Bianchi, M., Lux-Lantos, V., and Libertun, C. (2009) Neonatal exposure to bisphenol a alters reproductive parameters and gonadotropin releasing hormone signaling in female rats, *Environ Health Perspect*, 117:757–762.

Fernández, M., Bourguignon, N., Lux-Lantos, V., and Libertun, C. (2010) Neonatal exposure to bisphenol a and reproductive and endocrine alterations resembling the polycystic ovarian syndrome in adult rats, *Environ Health Perspect*, 118:1217–1222.

Flaws, J. A., Sommer, R. J., Silbergeld, E. K., Peterson, R. E., and Hirshfield, A. N. (1997) *In utero* and lactational exposure to 2,3,7,8-tetrachlorodibenzo-p-dioxin (TCDD) induces genital dysmorphogenesis in the female rat, *Toxicol Appl Pharmacol*, 147: 351–362.

Franczak, A., Nynca, A., Valdez, K. E., Mizinga, K. M., and Petroff, B. K. (2006) Effects of acute and chronic exposure to the aryl hydrocarbon receptor agonist 2,3,7,8-tetrachlorodibenzo-p-dioxin on the transition to reproductive senescence in female Sprague-Dawley rats, *Biol Reprod*, 74:125–130.

Gao, X., Mizuyachi, K., Terranova, P. F., and Rozman, K. K. (2001) 2,3,7,8-Tetrachlorodibenzo-p-dioxin decreases responsiveness of the hypothalamus to estradiol as a feedback inducer of preovulatory gonadotropin secretion in the immature gonadotropin-primed rat, *Toxicol Appl Pharmacol*, 179:181–190.

Gao, X., Petroff, B. K., Oluola, O., Georg, G., Terranova, P. F., and Rozman, K. K. (2002) Endocrine disruption by indole-3-carbinol and tamoxifen: Blockage of ovulation, *Toxicol Appl Pharmacol*, 183:179–188.

Gao, X., Terranova, P. F., and Rozman, K. K. (2000) Effects of polychlorinated dibenzofurans, biphenyls, and their mixture with dibenzo-p-dioxins on ovulation in the gonadotropin-primed immature rat: Support for the toxic equivalency concept, *Toxicol Appl Pharmacol*, 163:115–124.

Gregoraszczuk, E. L. (2002) Dioxin exposure and porcine reproductive hormonal activity, *Cad Saude Publica*, 18:453–462.

Hays, L. E., Carpenter, C. D., and Petersen, S. L. (2002) Evidence that GABAergic neurons in the preoptic area of the rat brain are targets of 2,3,7,8-tetrachlorodibenzo-p-dioxin during development, *Environ Health Perspect*, 110:369–376.

Heath-Pagliuso, S., Rogers, W. J., Tullis, K., Seidel, S. D., Cenijn, P. H., Brouwer, A., and Denison, M. S. (1998) Activation of the Ah receptor by tryptophan and tryptophan metabolites, *Biochemistry*, 37:11508–11515.

Heimler, I., Rawlins, R. G., Owen, H., and Hutz, R. J. (1998a) Dioxin perturbs, in a dose- and time-dependent fashion, steroid secretion, and induces apoptosis of human luteinized granulosa cells, *Endocrinology*, 139:4373–4379.

Heimler, I., Trewin, A. L., Chaffin, C. L., Rawlins, R. G., and Hutz, R. J. (1998b) Modulation of ovarian follicle maturation and effects on apoptotic cell death in Holtzman rats exposed to 2,3,7,8-tetrachlordibenzo-p-dioxin (TCDD) *in utero* and lactationally, *Reprod Toxicol*, 12:69–73.

Hernandez-Ochoa, I., Barnett-Ringgold, K. R., Dehlinger, S. L., Gupta, R. K., Leslie, T. C., Roby, K. F., and Flaws, J. A. (2010) The ability of the aryl hydrocarbon receptor to regulate ovarian follicle growth and estradiol biosynthesis in mice depends on stage of sexual maturity, *Biol Reprod*, 83:698–706.

Hirakawa, T., Minegishi, T., Abe, K., Kishi, H., Ibuki, Y., and Miyamoto, K. (2000a) Effect of 2,3,7,8-tetrachlorodibenzo-p-dioxin on the expression of luteinizing hormone receptors during cell differentiation in cultured granulosa cells, *Arch Biochem Biophys*, 15:371–376.

Hirakawa, T., Minegishi, T., Abe, K., Kishi, H., Inoue, K., Ibuki, Y., and Miyamoto, K. (2000b) Effect of 2,3,7,8-tetrachlorodibenzo-p-dioxin on the expression of follicle-stimulating hormone receptors during cell differentiation in cultured granulosa cells, *Endocrinology*, 141:1470–1476.

Hites, R. A. (2011) Dioxins: An overview and history, *Environ Sci Technol*, 45:16–20.

Ho, H. M., Ohshima, K., Watanabe, G., Taya, K., Strawn, E. Y., and Hutz, R. J. (2006) TCDD increases inhibin A production by human luteinized granulosa cells *in vitro*, *J Reprod Dev*, 52:523–528.

Holloway, A. C., Anger, D. A., Crankshaw, D. J., Wu, M., and Foster, W. G. (2008) Atrazine-induced changes in aromatase activity in estrogen sensitive target tissues, *J Appl Toxicol*, 28:260–270.

Huang, P., Rannug, A., Ahlbom, E., Håkansson, H., and Ceccatelli, S. (2000) Effect of 2,3,7,8-tetrachlorodibenzo-p-dioxin on the expression of cytochrome P450 1A1, the aryl hydrocarbon receptor, and the aryl hydrocarbon receptor nuclear translocator in rat brain and pituitary, *Toxicol Appl Pharmacol*, 169:159–167.

Hunt, P. A., Koehler, K. E., Susiarjo, M., Hodges, C. A., Ilagan, A., Voigt, R. C., Thomas, S., Thomas, B. F., and Hassold, T. J. (2003) Bisphenol a exposure causes meiotic aneuploidy in the female mouse, *Curr Biol*, 13:546–553.

Ikezuki, Y., Tsutsumi, O., Takai, Y., Kamei, Y., and Taketani, Y. (2001) Determination of bisphenol A concentrations in human biological fluids reveals significant early prenatal exposure, *Hum Reprod*, 17:2839–2841.

Jablonska, O., Piasecka, J., Ostrowska, M., Sobocinska, N., Wasowska, B., and Ciereszko, R. E. (2011a) The expression of the aryl hydrocarbon receptor in reproductive and neuroendocrine tissues during the estrous cycle in the pig, *Anim Reprod Sci*, 126:221–228.

Jablonska, O., Piasecka, J., Petroff, B. K., Nynca, A., Siawrys, G., Wąsowska, B., Zmijewska, A., Lewczuk, B., and Ciereszko, R. E. (2011b) In vitro effects of 2,3,7,8-tetrachlorodibenzo-p-dioxin (TCDD) on ovarian, pituitary, and pineal function in pigs, *Theriogenology*, 15:921–932.

Jablonska, O., Shi, Z., Valdez, K. E., Ting, A. Y., and Petroff, B. K. (2010) Temporal and anatomical sensitivities to the aryl hydrocarbon receptor agonist 2,3,7,8-tetrachlorodibenzo-p-dioxin leading to premature acyclicity with age in rats, *Int J Androl*, 33:405–412.

Jefferson, W., Newbold, R., Padilla-Banks, E., and Pepling, M. (2006a) Neonatal genistein treatment alters ovarian differentiation in the mouse: Inhibition of oocyte nest breakdown and increased oocyte survival, *Biol Reprod*, 74:161–168.

Jefferson, W. N., Padilla-Banks, E., and Newbold, R. R. (2005) Adverse effects on female development and reproduction in CD-1 mice following neonatal exposure to the phytoestrogen genistein at environmentally relevant doses, *Biol Reprod*, 73:798–806.

Jefferson, W. N., Padilla-Banks, E., and Newbold, R. R. (2006b) Studies of the effects of neonatal exposure to genistein on the developing female reproductive system, *J AOAC Int*, 89:1189–1199.

Jung, N. K., Park, J. Y., Park, J. H., Kim, S. Y., Park, J. K., Chang, W. K., Lee, H. C., Kim, S. W., and Chun, S. Y. (2010) Attenuation of cell cycle progression by 2,3,7,8-tetrachlorodibenzo-p-dioxin eliciting ovulatory blockade in gonadotropin-primed immature rats, *Endocr J*, 57:863–871.

Kainu, T., Gustafsson, J. A., and Pelto-Huikko, M. (1995) The dioxin receptor and its nuclear translocator (Arnt) in the rat brain, *Neuroreport*, 6:2557–2560.

Kakeyama, M., Sone, H., and Tohyama, C. (2008) Perinatal exposure of female rats to 2,3,7,8-tetrachlorodibenzo-p-dioxin induces central precocious puberty in the offspring, *J Endocrinol*, 197:351–358.

Kandaraki, E., Chatzigeorgiou, A., Livadas, S., Palioura, E., Economou, F., Koutsilieris, M., Palimeri, S., Panidis, D., and Diamanti-Kandarakis, E. (2011) Endocrine disruptors and polycystic ovary syndrome (PCOS): Elevated serum levels of bisphenol A in women with PCOS, *J Clin Endocrinol Metab*, 96:E480–E484.

Kang, J. H., Kondo, F., and Katayama, Y. (2006) Human exposure to bisphenol A, *Toxicology*, 226:79–89.

Karman, B. N., Basavarajappa, M. S., Craig, Z. R., and Flaws, J. A. (2012a) 2,3,7,8-Tetrachlorodibenzo-p-dioxin activates the aryl hydrocarbon receptor and alters sex steroid hormone secretion without affecting growth of mouse antral follicles *in vitro*, *Toxicol Appl Pharmacol*, 261:88–96.

Karman, B. N., Basavarajappa, M. S., Hannon, P., and Flaws, J. A. (2012b) Dioxin exposure reduces the steroidogenic capacity of mouse antral follicles mainly at the level of HSD17B1 without altering atresia, *Toxicol Appl Pharmacol*, 264:1–12.

Karman, B. N. and Tischkau, S. A. (2006) Circadian clock gene expression in the ovary: Effects of luteinizing hormone, *Biol Reprod*, 75:624–632.

Kavlock, R. J., Daston, G. P., DeRosa, C., Fenner-Crisp, P., Gray, L. E., Kaattari, S., Lucier, G. et al. (1996) Research needs for the risk assessment of health and environmental effects of endocrine disruptors: A report of the U.S. EPA-sponsored workshop, *Environ Health Perspect*, 104:715–740.

Khorram, O., Garthwaite, M., and Golos, T. (2002) Uterine and ovarian aryl hydrocarbon receptor (AHR) and aryl hydrocarbon receptor nuclear translocator (ARNT) mRNA expression in benign and malignant gynaecological conditions, *Mol Hum Reprod*, 8:75–80.

Korkalainen, M., Lindén, J., Tuomisto, J., and Pohjanvirta, R. (2005) Effect of TCDD on mRNA expression of genes encoding bHLH/PAS proteins in rat hypothalamus, *Toxicology*, 208:1–11.

Kouki, T., Kishitake, M., Okamoto, M., Oosuka, I., Takebe, M., and Yamanouchi, K. (2003) Effects of neonatal treatment with phytoestrogens, genistein and daidzein, on sex difference in female rat brain function: Estrous cycle and lordosis, *Horm Behav*, 44:140–145.

Krüger, T., Long, M., and Bonefeld-Jørgensen, E. C. (2008) Plastic components affect the activation of the aryl hydrocarbon and the androgen receptor, *Toxicology*, 246:112–123.

Kwintkiewicz, J., Nishi, Y., Yanase, T., and Giudice, L. C. (2010) Peroxisome proliferator-activated receptor-gamma mediates bisphenol A inhibition of FSH-stimulated IGF-1, aromatase, and estradiol in human granulosa cells, *Environ Health Perspect*, 118:400–406.

Lawson, C., Gieske, M., Murdoch, B., Ye, P., Li, Y., Hassold, T., and Hunt, P. A. (2011) Gene expression in the fetal mouse ovary is altered by exposure to low doses of bisphenol A, *Biol Reprod*, 84:79–86.

Li, X., Johnson, D., and Rozman, K. (1995) Reproductive effects of 2,3,7,8-tetrachlorodibenzo-p-dioxin (TCDD) in female rats: Ovulation, hormonal regulation and possible mechanism, *Toxicol Appl Pharmacol*, 133:321–327.

Losa, S. M., Todd, K. L., Sullivan, A. W., Cao, J., Mickens, J. A., and Patisaul, H. B. (2011) Neonatal exposure to genistein adversely impacts the ontogeny of hypothalamic kisspeptin signaling pathways and ovarian development in the peripubertal female rat, *Reprod Toxicol*, 31:280–289.

Lovekamp-Swan, T., Jetten, A. M., and Davis, B. J. (2003) Dual activation of PPARalpha and PPARgamma by mono-(2-ethylhexyl) phthalate in rat ovarian granulosa cells, *Mol Cell Endocrinol*, 201:133–141.

Lu, Y., Sun, G., Wang, X., and Safe, S. (1996) Inhibition of prolactin receptor gene expression by 2,3,7,8-tetrachlorodibenzo-p-dioxin in MCF-7 human breast cancer cells, *Arch Biochem Biophys*, 332:35–40.

MacKenzie, K. M. and Angevine, D. M. (1981) Infertility in mice exposed *in utero* to benzo(a) pyrene, *Biol Reprod*, 24:183–191.

Manikkam, M., Guerrero-Bosagna, C., Tracey, R., Haque, M. M., and Skinner, M. K. (2012) Transgenerational actions of environmental compounds on reproductive disease and identification of epigenetic biomarkers of ancestral exposures, *PLoS One*, 7:e31901.

Markey, C. M., Coombs, M. A., Sonnenschein, C., and Soto, A. M. (2003) Mammalian development in a changing environment: Exposure to endocrine disruptors reveals the developmental plasticity of steroid-hormone target organs, *Evol Dev*, 5:67–75.

Matthews, J. B., Twomey, K., and Zacharewski, T. R. (2001) In vitro and in vivo interactions of bisphenol A and its metabolite, bisphenol A glucuronide, with estrogen receptors alpha and beta, *Chem Res Toxicol*, 14:149–157.

Mattison, D. R., Plowchalk, D. R., Meadows, M. J., Al-Juburi, A. Z., Gandy, J., and Malek, A. (1990) Reproductive toxicity: Male and female reproductive systems as targets for chemical injury, *Environ Med*, 72:391–411.

Mattison, D. R., Shiromizu, K., and Nightingale, M. S. (1983) Oocyte destruction by polycyclic aromatic hydrocarbons, *Am J Ind Med*, 4:191–202.

Mattison, D. R., White, N. B., and Nightingale, M. R. (1980) The effect of benzo(a)pyrene on fertility, primordial oocyte number, and ovarian response to pregnant mare's serum gonadotropin, *Pediatr Pharmacol (New York)*, 1:143–151.

Miller, M. M., Plowchalk, D. R., Weitzman, G. A., London, S. N., and Mattison, D. R. (1992) The effect of benzo(a)pyrene on murine ovarian and corpora lutea volumes, *Am J Obstet Gynecol*, 166:1535–1541.

Minegishi, T., Hirakawa, T., Abe, K., Kishi, H., and Miyamoto, K. (2003) Effect of IGF-1 and 2,3,7,8-tetrachlorodibenzo-p-dioxin (TCDD) on the expression of LH receptors during cell differentiation in cultured granulosa cells, *Mol Cell Endocrinol*, 202:123–131.

Minegishi, T., Hirakawa, T., Abe, K., Kishi, H., and Miyamoto, K. (2004) Effect of insulin-like growth factor-1 and 2,3,7,8-tetrachlorodibenzo-p-dioxin on the expression of luteinizing hormone receptors in cultured granulosa cells, *Environ Sci*, 11:57–71.

Mizuyachi, K., Son, D., Rozman, K., and Terranova, P. (2002) Alteration in ovarian gene expression in response to 2,3,7,8-tetrachlorodibenzo-p-dioxin: Reduction of cyclooxygenase-2 in the blockage of ovulation, *Reprod Tox*, 16:299–307.

Mok-Lin, E., Ehrlich, S., Williams, P., Petrozza, J., Wright, D. L., Calafat, A. M., Ye, X., and Hauser, R. (2010) Urinary bisphenol A concentrations and ovarian response among women undergoing IVF, *Int J Androl*, 33:385–393.

Morán, F. M., Lohstroh, P., VandeVoort, C. A., Chen, J., Overstreet, J. W., Conley, A. J., and Lasley, B. L. (2003a) Exogenous steroid substrate modifies the effect of 2,3,7,8-tetrachlorodibenzo-p-dioxin on estradiol production of human luteinized granulosa cells *in vitro*, *Biol Reprod*, 68:244–251.

Morán, F. M., VandeVoort, C. A., Overstreet, J. W., Lasley, B. L., and Conley, A. J. (2003b) Molecular target of endocrine disruption in human luteinizing granulosa cells by 2,3,7,8-tetrachlorodibenzo-p-dioxin: Inhibition of estradiol secretion due to decreased 17alpha-hydroxylase/17,20-lyase cytochrome P450 expression, *Endocrinology*, 144: 467–473.

Muhlhauser, A., Susiarjo, M., Rubio, C., Griswold, J., Gorence, G., Hassold, T., and Hunt, P. A. (2009) Bisphenol A effects on the growing mouse oocyte are influenced by diet, *Biol Reprod*, 80:1066–1071.

Myllymäki, S., Haavisto, T., Vainio, M., Toppari, J., and Paranko, J. (2005) In vitro effects of diethylstilbestrol, genistein, 4-tert-butylphenol, and 4-tert-octylphenol on steroidogenic activity of isolated immature rat ovarian follicles, *Toxicol Appl Pharmacol*, 204:69–80.

Nagao, T., Yoshimura, S., Saito, Y., Nakagomi, M., Usumi, K., and Ono, H. (2001) Reproductive effects in male and female rats of neonatal exposure to genistein, *Reprod Toxicol*, 15:399–411.

Nakamura, T. J., Sellix, M. T., Kudo, T., Nakao, N., Yoshimura, T., Ebihara, S., Colwell, C. S., and Block, G. D. (2010) Influence of the estrous cycle on clock gene expression in reproductive tissues: Effects of fluctuating ovarian steroid hormone levels, *Steroids*, 75:203–212.

Neal, M. S., Mulligan Tuttle, A. M., Casper, R. F., Lagunov, A., and Foster, W. G. (2010) Aryl hydrocarbon receptor antagonists attenuate the deleterious effects of benzo[a]pyrene on isolated rat follicle development, *Reprod Biomed Online*, 21:100–108.

Neal, M. S., Zhu, J., Holloway, A. C., and Foster, W. G. (2007) Follicle growth is inhibited by benzo-[a]-pyrene, at concentrations representative of human exposure, in an isolated rat follicle culture assay, *Hum Reprod*, 22:961–967.

Newbold, R. R., Jefferson, W. N., and Padilla-Banks, E. (2007) Long-term adverse effects of neonatal exposure to bisphenol A on the murine female reproductive tract, *Reprod Toxicol*, 24:253–258.

Newbold, R. R., Jefferson, W. N., and Padilla-Banks, E. (2009) Prenatal exposure to bisphenol a at environmentally relevant doses adversely affects the murine female reproductive tract later in life, *Environ Health Perspect*, 117:879–885.

Nynca, A. and Ciereszko, R. E. (2006) Effect of genistein on steroidogenic response of granulosa cell populations from porcine preovulatory follicles, *Reprod Biol*, 6:31–50.

Patel, M. R., Scheffler, B. E., Wang, L., and Willett, K. L. (2006) Effects of benzo(a)pyrene exposure on killifish (*Fundulus heteroclitus*) aromatase activities and mRNA, *Aquat Toxicol*, 77:267–278.

Peretz, J., Craig, Z. R., and Flaws, J. A. (2012) Bisphenol a inhibits follicle growth and induces atresia in cultured mouse antral follicles independently of the genomic estrogenic pathway, *Biol Reprod*, 87:63.

Peretz, J., Gupta, R. K., Singh, J., Hernández-Ochoa, I., and Flaws, J. A. (2011) Bisphenol A impairs follicle growth, inhibits steroidogenesis, and downregulates rate-limiting enzymes in the estradiol biosynthesis pathway, *Toxicol Sci*, 119:209–217.

Petersen, S. L., Curran, M. A., Marconi, S. A., Carpenter, C. D., Lubbers, L. S., and McAbee, M. D. (2000) Distribution of mRNAs encoding the arylhydrocarbon receptor, arylhydrocarbon receptor nuclear translocator, and arylhydrocarbon receptor nuclear translocator-2 in the rat brain and brainstem, *J Comp Neurol*, 427:428–439.

Petroff, B. K., Gao, X., Rozman, K. K., and Terranova, P. F. (2000) Interaction of estradiol and 2,3,7,8-tetrachlorodibenzo-p-dioxin (TCDD) in an ovulation model: Evidence for systemic potentiation and local ovarian effects, *Reprod Toxicol*, 14:247–255.

Quignot, N., Arnaud, M., Robidel, F., Lecomte, A., Tournier, M., Cren-Olivé, C., Barouki, R., and Lemazurier, E. (2012a) Characterization of endocrine-disrupting chemicals based on hormonal balance disruption in male and female adult rats, *Reprod Toxicol*, 33:339–352.

Quignot, N., Desmots, S., Barouki, R., and Lemazurier, E. (2012b) A comparison of two human cell lines and two rat gonadal cell primary cultures as in vitro screening tools for aromatase modulation, *Toxicol In vitro*, 26:107–118.

Ratajczak, C. K., Boehle, K. L., and Muglia, L. J. (2009) Impaired steroidogenesis and implantation failure in Bmal1–/– mice, *Endocrinology*, 150:1879–1885.

Rice, S., Mason, H. D., and Whitehead, S. A. (2006) Phytoestrogens and their low dose combinations inhibit mRNA expression and activity of aromatase in human granulosa-luteal cells, *J Steroid Biochem Mol Biol*, 101:216–225.

Roby, K. F. (2001) Alterations in follicle development, steroidogenesis, and gonadotropin receptor binding in a model of ovulatory blockade, *Endocrinology*, 142:2328–2335.

Rocha Monteiro, P. R., Reis-Henriques, M. A., and Coimbra, J. (2000) Polycyclic aromatic hydrocarbons inhibit *in vitro* ovarian steroidogenesis in the flounder (*Platichthys flesus* L.), *Aquat Toxicol*, 48:549–559.

Rodríguez, H. A., Santambrosio, N., Santamaría, C. G., Muñoz-de-Toro, M., and Luque, E. H. (2010) Neonatal exposure to bisphenol A reduces the pool of primordial follicles in the rat ovary, *Reprod Toxicol*, 30:550–557.

Sadeu, J. C. and Foster, W. G. (2011) Effect of in vitro exposure to benzo[a]pyrene, a component of cigarette smoke, on folliculogenesis, steroidogenesis and oocyte nuclear maturation, *Reprod Toxicol*, 31:402–408.

Safe, S. (1990) Polychlorinated biphenyls (PCBs), dibenzo-p-dioxins (PCDDs), dibenzofurans (PCDFs), and related compounds: Environmental and mechanistic considerations which support the development of toxic equivalency factors (TEFs), *Crit Rev Toxicol*, 21:51–88.

Sakurada, Y., Sawai, M., Inoue, K., Shirota, M., and Shirota, K. (2011) Comparison of aryl hydrocarbon receptor gene expression in laser dissected granulosa cell layers of immature rat ovaries, *J Vet Med Sci*, 73:923–926.

Salisbury, T. B. and Marcinkiewicz, J. L. (2002) *In utero* and lactational exposure to 2,3,7,8-tetrachlorodibenzo-p-dioxin and 2,3,4,7,8-pentachlorodibenzofuran reduces growth and disrupts reproductive parameters in female rats, *Biol Reprod*, 66:1621–1626.

Schönfelder, G., Wittfoht, W., Hopp, H., Talsness, C. E., Paul, M., and Chahoud, I. (2002) Parent bisphenol A accumulation in the human maternal-fetal-placental unit, *Environ Health Perspect*, 110:A703–A707.

Shi, Z., Valdez, K. E., Ting, A. Y., Franczak, A., Gum, S. L., and Petroff, B. K. (2007) Ovarian endocrine disruption underlies premature reproductive senescence following environmentally relevant chronic exposure to the aryl hydrocarbon receptor agonist 2,3,7,8-tetrachlorodibenzo-p-dioxin, *Biol Reprod*, 76:198–202.

Shibayama, H., Kotera, T., Shinoda, Y., Hanada, T., Kajihara, T., Ueda, M., Tamura, H., Ishibashi, S., Yamashita, Y., and Ochi, S. (2009) Collaborative work on evaluation of ovarian toxicity. 14) Two- or four-week repeated-dose studies and fertility study of atrazine in female rats, *J Toxicol Sci*, 34:SP147–SP155.

Shiromizu, K. and Mattison, D. R. (1984) The effect of intraovarian injection of benzo(a) pyrene on primordial oocyte number and ovarian aryl hydrocarbon [benzo(a)pyrene] hydroxylase activity, *Toxicol Appl Pharmacol*, 76:18–25.

Signorile, P. G., Spugnini, E. P., Citro, G., Viceconte, R., Vincenzi, B., Baldi, F., and Baldi, A. (2012) Endocrine disruptors *in utero* cause ovarian damages linked to endometriosis, *Front Biosci (Elite Ed)*, 4:1724–1730.

Singh, S. U., Casper, R. F., Fritz, P. C., Sukhu, B., Ganss, B., Girard, B. J., Savouret, J. F., and Tenenbaum, H. C. (2000) Inhibition of dioxin effects on bone formation in vitro by a newly described aryl hydrocarbon receptor antagonist, resveratrol, *J Endocrinol*, 167:183–195.

Son, D. S., Ushinohama, K., Gao, X., Taylor, C. C., Roby, K. F., Rozman, K. K., and Terranova, P. F. (1999) 2,3,7,8-Tetrachlorodibenzo-p-dioxin (TCDD) blocks ovulation by a direct action on the ovary without alteration of ovarian steroidogenesis: Lack of a direct effect on ovarian granulosa and thecal-interstitial cell steroidogenesis *in vitro*, *Reprod Toxicol*, 13:521–530.

Susiarjo, M., Hassold, T. J., Freeman, E., and Hunt, P. A. (2007) Bisphenol A exposure *in utero* disrupts early oogenesis in the mouse, *PLoS Genet*, 3:e5.

Suzuki, A., Sugihara, A., Uchida, K., Sato, T., Ohta, Y., Katsu, Y., Watanabe, H., and Iguchi, T. (2002) Developmental effects of perinatal exposure to bisphenol-A and diethylstilbestrol on reproductive organs in female mice, *Reprod Toxicol*, 16:107–116.

Swartz, W. J. and Mattison, D. R. (1985) Benzo(a)pyrene inhibits ovulation in C57BL/6N mice, *Anat Rec*, 212:268–276.

Taketa, Y., Yoshida, M., Inoue, K., Takahashi, M., Sakamoto, Y., Watanabe, G., Taya, K., Yamate, J., and Nishikawa, A. (2011) Differential stimulation pathways of progesterone secretion from newly formed corpora lutea in rats treated with ethylene glycol monomethyl ether, sulpiride, or atrazine, *Toxicol Sci*, 121:267–278.

Takeuchi, T., Tsutsumi, O., Ikezuki, Y., Takai, Y., and Taketani, Y. (2004) Positive relationship between androgen and the endocrine disruptor, bisphenol A, in normal women and women with ovarian dysfunction, *Endocr J*, 51:165–169.

Tarantino, G., Valentino, R., Somma, C. D., D'Esposito, V., Passaretti, F., Pizza, G., Brancato, V., Orio, F., Formisano, P., Colao, A., and Savastano, S. (2012) Bisphenol A in polycystic ovary syndrome and its association with liver-spleen axis, *Clin Endocrinol (Oxf)*, 78:447–453.

Tennant, M. K., Hill, D. S., Eldridge, J. C., Wetzel, L. T., Breckenridge, C. B., and Stevens, J. T. (1994) Chloro-s-triazine antagonism of estrogen action: Limited interaction with estrogen receptor binding, *J Toxicol Environ Health*, 43:197–211.

Tiemann, U., Schneider, F., Vanselow, J., and Tomek, W. (2007) In vitro exposure of porcine granulosa cells to the phytoestrogens genistein and daidzein: Effects on the biosynthesis of reproductive steroid hormones, *Reprod Toxicol*, 24:317–325.

Tinfo, N. S., Hotchkiss, M. G., Buckalew, A. R., Zorrilla, L. M., Cooper, R. L., and Laws, S. C. (2011) Understanding the effects of atrazine on steroidogenesis in rat granulosa and H295R adrenal cortical carcinoma cells, *Reprod Toxicol*, 31:184–193.

Tischkau, S. A., Jaeger, C. D., and Krager, S. L. (2011) Circadian clock disruption in the mouse ovary in response to 2,3,7,8-tetrachlorodibenzo-p-dioxin, *Toxicol Lett*, 201:116–122.

Trewin, A. L., Woller, M. J., Wimpee, B. A., Conley, L. K., Baldridge, M. G., and Hutz, R. J. (2007) Short-term hormone release from adult female rat hypothalamic and pituitary explants is not altered by 2,3,7,8-tetrachlorodibenzo-p-dioxin, *J Reprod Dev*, 53:765–775.

Tsutsumi, O. (2005) Assessment of human contamination of estrogenic endocrine-disrupting chemicals and their risk for human reproduction, *J Steroid Biochem Mol Biol*, 93:325–330.

Valdez, K. E., Shi, Z., Ting, A. Y., and Petroff, B. K. (2009) Effect of chronic exposure to the aryl hydrocarbon receptor agonist 2,3,7,8-tetrachlorodibenzo-p-dioxin in female rats on ovarian gene expression, *Reprod Toxicol*, 28:32–37.

Wetzel, L. T., Luempert, L. G. R., Breckenridge, C. B., Tisdel, M. O., Stevens, J. T., Thakur, A. K., Extrom, P. J., and Eldridge, J. C. (1994) Chronic effects of atrazine on estrus and mammary tumor formation in female Sprague-Dawley and Fischer 344 rats, *J Toxicol Environ Health*, 43:169–182.

Wojtowicz, A., Tomanek, M., Augustowska, K., and Gregoraszczuk, E. L. (2005) Aromatic hydrocarbon receptor (AhR) in the porcine theca and granulosa cells: Effect of TCDD, PCB 126 and PCB 153 on the expression of AhR, *Endocr Regul*, 39:109–118.

Xu, C., Chen, J. A., Qiu, Z., Zhao, Q., Luo, J., Yang, L., Zeng, H., Huang, Y., Zhang, L., Cao, J., and Shu, W. (2010) Ovotoxicity and PPAR-mediated aromatase downregulation in female Sprague-Dawley rats following combined oral exposure to benzo[a]pyrene and di-(2-ethylhexyl) phthalate, *Toxicol Lett*, 199:323–332.

Yamamoto, J., Ihara, K., Nakayama, H., Hikino, S., Satoh, K., Kubo, N., Iida, T., Fujii, Y., and Hara, T. (2004) Characteristic expression of aryl hydrocarbon receptor repressor gene in human tissues: Organ-specific distribution and variable induction patterns in mononuclear cells, *Life Sci*, 74:1039–1049.

Zhang, H. Q., Zhang, X. F., Zhang, L. J., Chao, H. H., Pan, B., Feng, Y. M., Li, L., Sun, X. F., and Shen, W. (2012) Fetal exposure to bisphenol A affects the primordial follicle formation by inhibiting the meiotic progression of oocytes, *Mol Biol Rep*, 39:5651–5657.

Zhou, W., Liu, J., Liao, L., Han, S., and Liu, J. (2008) Effect of bisphenol A on steroid hormone production in rat ovarian theca-interstitial and granulosa cells, *Mol Cell Endocrinol*, 283:12–18.

8 Phthalates

Timothy P. DelValle, Katlyn S. Hafner, and Zelieann R. Craig

CONTENTS

8.1 INTRODUCTION

Phthalate esters, most commonly referred to as phthalates, are a group of chemicals frequently used to impart flexibility and durability to plastics such as polyvinylchloride (PVC) products. Phthalates are ubiquitous chemicals as demonstrated by their presence in a wide variety of industrial and consumer products including medical devices, clothing, enteric coating of medications, food packaging, toys, cosmetics, and building materials among others. Unfortunately, phthalates are not covalently bound to products and are therefore easily released into the environment. Therefore, exposure to humans may occur via oral intake, intravenous infusion, dermal contact, and inhalation (reviewed in Heudorf et al. 2007). Because worldwide use of phthalates has been estimated at 18 billion pounds each year (Blount et al. 2000), the impact of exposure to phthalates on human health has become an important public health issue.

In their parent form, phthalates are dialkyl or alkyl aryl esters of 1,2-benzenedicarboxylic acid; but upon entering the body, the ester linkages may be cleaved by esterases in the gut to produce a wide variety of metabolites. Although dozens of phthalates exist, most toxicological studies have been limited to characterizing di-(2-ethylhexyl) phthalate (DEHP), di-n-butyl phthalate (DBP), diethyl phthalate (DEP), butyl benzyl phthalate (BBP) and their major metabolites mono-(2-ethylhexyl) phthalate (MEHP), monobutyl phthalate (MBP), monoethyl phthalate (MEP), and monobenzyl phthalate (MBzP). Further, many studies have demonstrated that phthalates are endocrine-disrupting chemicals because they disrupt developmental and reproductive processes in male and female rodents (reviewed in Howdeshell et al. 2008;

Lovekamp-Swan and Davis 2003; Lyche et al. 2009). Most importantly, constant daily exposure in humans has been confirmed by various epidemiological studies. For example, the National Health and Nutrition Examination Survey (NHANES) conducted from 1999 to 2000 and 2001 to 2002 reported that the most common phthalate metabolites found in human urine were MEP, MBP, MBzP, and MEHP and that females had the highest levels of MEP, MBP, and MBzP observed (CDC 2005). Furthermore, other studies have detected phthalate metabolites in lactating mother's urine and human breast milk (Hines et al. 2009), maternal plasma and cord blood (Latini et al. 2003; Lin et al. 2008), and human follicular fluid (Krotz et al. 2012).

This chapter reviews current literature describing the reproductive toxicity of phthalates and the findings from mechanistic studies aimed at understanding how phthalate exposure leads to reproductive toxicity. It is important to note that the discussion will concentrate on DEHP, DBP, and their metabolites because most studies have focused on these phthalates. However, we also discuss the few studies describing other phthalates hoping to stimulate further work in this area.

8.2 REPRODUCTIVE TOXICITY

8.2.1 Effects on Steroidogenesis

One of the most notable studies that supported ovarian toxicity by DEHP was conducted by Davis et al. (1994a). In this study, female rats dosed orally with DEHP at 2000 mg/kg/day had significantly longer estrous cycles, impaired ovulation, decreased circulating 17β-estradiol (E_2), and increased follicle-stimulating hormone (FSH) levels. Further, DEHP exposure at 2000 mg/kg for eight consecutive days resulted in decreased E_2 levels, increased progesterone (P_4), decreased luteinizing hormone (LH) surges, and impaired ovulation. Interestingly, pre-ovulatory follicles in DEHP-treated groups were significantly smaller than those from controls after 3 days of exposure due to a smaller granulosa cell area (Davis et al. 1994a). Therefore, the granulosa cell compartment was considered a direct target of the DEHP-induced ovarian toxicity, and impaired E_2 production its primary consequence. Alterations in E_2 production were also reported in a study showing that rats dosed with DEHP at 1500 mg/kg for 10 consecutive days had significantly decreased E_2 levels during estrus compared to untreated rats (Laskey and Berman 1993). Also, rats dosed orally with DEHP (1400 mg/kg) twice a week for 26 weeks had significantly lower serum E_2 and FSH levels, when compared to control animals (Hirosawa et al. 2006). Similarly, another study in rats showed that DEHP (50 and 500 mg/kg/day for 28 days) decreased circulating levels of FSH, testosterone, and E_2, but increased P_4 (Ma et al. 2011). Twenty-day-old rats, dosed with DEHP at 500 mg/kg daily for 10 days, showed both significantly decreased circulating E_2 and P_4 levels, but increased pituitary LH. When granulosa cells obtained from these mice were cultured to evaluate their ability to synthesize steroids, they produced 30% less P_4 in response to FSH and LH (Svechnikova et al. 2007). Interestingly, when 21-day-old rats were exposed to DEHP by inhalation (0, 5, or 25 mg/m^3 for 6 h a day, 5 days a week), no significant effects were seen on serum FSH, LH, or E_2. However, when a similar cohort was analyzed at postnatal day 42, significantly lower levels of serum

E_2 and LH were seen at the 25 mg/m^3 dose (Ma et al. 2006). In contrast to other reports, a study in marmosets dosed orally with 0, 100, 500, or 2500 mg/kg/day from weaning to sexual maturity showed that E_2 levels were elevated in the 500 mg/kg treatment group when compared to vehicle-treated controls (Tomonari et al. 2006).

Phthalate-induced impaired steroidogenesis has also been evaluated *in vitro* using granulosa, granulosa–lutein cell, and ovarian follicle culture systems. Specifically, rat granulosa cells treated with MEHP at 100 μM for 24 h had decreased P_4 production and decreased FSH-stimulated cAMP levels (Treinen et al. 1990), while MEHP (100 and 200 μM) significantly decreased E_2 production (Lovekamp and Davis 2001). In human granulosa–lutein cells, MEHP inhibited both basal (unstimulated) and FSH-, human chorionic gonadotropin-, and 8-bromoadenosine 3′5′-cyclic monophosphate-stimulated E_2 production. MEHP also inhibited both basal and stimulated P_4 production (Reinsberg et al. 2009). Interestingly, P_4 production was increased in porcine granulosa cells incubated for 72 h with dioctyl phthalate (DOP) and diisodecyl phthalate (DiDP) at 10^{-8} M, while an inhibitory effect was seen on E_2 production (Mlynarcíková et al. 2007). On the other hand, studies using ovarian follicle cultures systems have not only supported the observations from single-cell culture systems but have also revealed how different follicle types respond to increasing concentrations of phthalates. For example, MEHP (0.1 and 10 μg/mL; 96 h) was shown to significantly decrease E_2 production by cultured mouse antral follicles (Gupta et al. 2010); but when pre-antral mouse follicles were used at doses of MEHP (10–200 μM; 12 days), no significant deviations on E_2 production were observed (Lenie and Smitz 2009). Interestingly, estrone and testosterone levels were both significantly increased at the 100 μM dose, while P_4 production was increased in pre-antral follicles cultured with 200 μM MEHP (Lenie and Smitz 2009). Further, a recent study evaluated the effects of MEHP on steroidogenesis in secondary follicles and found that follicles treated with MEHP (30 and 100 μg/mL) had significantly increased P_4 in the culture media. Interestingly, levels of androstenedione, testosterone, and E_2 were increased in two lower-dose groups (10 and 30 μg/mL), but were significantly decreased at the 100 μg/mL dose. Further, the ratio of P_4 to androstenedione was significantly increased while no effects on the androstenedione to testosterone ratio and the testosterone to E_2 ratio were observed (Inada et al. 2012).

Finally, other studies have focused on developmental exposures but observed that phthalates could cause adverse pregnancy outcomes without altering the hormonal milieu of the offspring. For example, rats dosed daily throughout gestation and lactation with doses of DEHP ranging from 0.015 to 405 mg/kg had female offspring with normal E_2, P_4, FSH, and LH levels (Grande et al. 2007; Guerra et al. 2010). However, when Gray et al. exposed rats to DBP starting at weaning, through puberty, mating, and gestation, they found that DBP caused midpregnancy abortions, decreased serum P_4, and decreased *ex vivo* P_4 and increased E_2 production by the dam ovaries (Gray et al. 2006).

8.2.2 Effects on Ovarian Follicles, Oocytes, and Corpora Lutea

Increased numbers of atretic follicles present in the ovary have been reported in adult DEHP-treated rats (Ma et al. 2011) and the offspring of rats exposed to DEHP during gestation (Grande et al. 2007). However, most of what we know about the effects of phthalates on follicular development has been characterized using *in vitro* ovarian follicle culture systems. Specifically, pre-antral rat follicles cultured for 10 days with MEHP (40 and 80 μg/mL) have been shown to have a significantly lower survival rate and slower progression to the antral stage (Wan et al. 2010). Similarly, MEHP at 100 μg/mL also decreased *in vitro* growth and increased the number of apoptotic granulosa cells present in rat secondary follicles (Inada et al. 2012) and significantly decreased *in vitro* growth of mouse antral follicles (Gupta et al. 2010). Notably, *in vitro* exposure to DEHP (1, 10, or 100 μg/mL) or MEHP (0.1, 1, or 10 μg/mL) for 96 h significantly inhibited the expression of mRNAs for aromatase and the cell cycle regulators cyclin D2 and cyclin-dependent kinase 4. Interestingly, cotreatment with E_2 at 1 and 10 nM was able to prevent the effects of DEHP on mouse antral follicles (Gupta et al. 2010). In contrast, a similar study failed to detect any significant differences in growth and differentiation of mouse pre-antral follicles (Lenie and Smitz 2009).

MEHP has also been shown to negatively impact *in vitro* meiotic maturation in mouse (Dalman et al. 2008), bovine (Anas et al. 2003), and equine (Ambruosi et al. 2011) oocytes. Although one study using mouse pre-antral follicles as a model failed to observe significant differences in oocyte growth and maturation after MEHP treatment (Lenie and Smitz 2009), most recently, a study examined the effects of *in vitro* exposure to DEHP and MEHP (50 μM) on bovine cumulus–oocyte complexes and found that DEHP-treated oocytes produced a significantly smaller percentage of developing blastocysts than control-treated oocytes. Further, MEHP treatment (50 μM) resulted in a reduced number of oocytes advancing to metaphase II of meiosis (Grossman et al. 2012).

Finally, a recent study reported the ability of MEHP to enhance ovarian oxytocin production by bovine granulosa and luteal cells (Wang et al. 2010). Although it is most notably a pituitary gland hormone, oxytocin has been implicated in luteal function, specifically in the process of luteal regression in various species including the human (Fuchs 1988; LaFrance and Goff 1990). Therefore, taken together with findings in whole follicles and cumulus–oocyte complexes, phthalates have the potential to affect not only follicular development and oocyte maturation but also corpus luteum function.

8.3 MECHANISMS OF ACTION

One common observation following exposure to DEHP is decreased E_2 production. In fact, studies using rats (Davis et al. 1994a), rat granulosa cell cultures (Treinen et al. 1990), whole minced rat ovaries (Laskey and Berman 1993), and isolated mouse antral follicles (Gupta et al. 2010) have all observed decreased E_2 production. Because E_2 is mainly produced by the pre-ovulatory follicle and antral follicle, granulosa cells from DEHP-treated rats are smaller than those in control-treated animals, Davis et al. identified the granulosa cell as a target for DEHP ovarian toxicity (Davis et al. 1994a). *In vitro* studies using the rat granulosa cell as a model explored the mechanisms by which DEHP, via its metabolite MEHP, decreases E_2 production. Specifically, Treinen et al. showed that MEHP inhibits FSH-induced cAMP accumulation and progesterone production in cultured rat granulosa cells independently of protein kinase C signaling (PKC; Treinen et al. 1990). Further, Davis and coworkers showed that the mechanism by which MEHP suppresses E_2 production in rat granulosa cells is through altering the levels and/or availability of the aromatase enzyme (Davis et al. 1994b). DEHP- or MEHP-induced downregulation of aromatase has also been reported in whole rat ovaries (Xu et al. 2010), cultured rat granulosa cells (Lovekamp and Davis 2001), cultured mouse antral follicles (Gupta et al. 2010), and human granulosa–lutein cells (Reinsberg et al. 2009). However, at least one study has reported data in disagreement with these findings. Specifically, Ma et al. showed that prepubertal rats exposed to DEHP via inhalation (5 and 25 mg/m^3) had increased circulating E_2 and increased ovarian aromatase mRNA expression (Ma et al. 2006). Although the reason underlying this discrepancy is not clear, potential explanations include differences in experimental approaches such as *in vivo* vs. *in vitro* toxicokinetics, exposure routes, age of animals, exposure times, and doses used. Therefore, many mechanistic studies have been aimed at understanding the mechanisms by which DEHP, and possibly other phthalates, can downregulate aromatase expression and activity to decrease production of E_2 and alter granulosa cell function and/or survival. Two major areas have been identified and are discussed in the following: modulation of peroxisome proliferator-activated receptors (PPARs) and induction of oxidative stress. Figure 8.1 shows a schematic summarizing what we know of the effects of phthalates on the various cell types and compartments within the ovary.

8.3.1 Modulation of Peroxisome Proliferator-Activated Receptors

PPARs are bound and activated by a group of chemicals known as peroxisome proliferators. In the rat liver, peroxisome proliferators have been shown to act via PPARs to cause hepatic toxicity and carcinomas (Ward et al. 1986), and alter the expression of estrogen-metabolizing enzymes such as 17β-hydroxysteroid dehydrogenase IV (HSD17B4) (Corton et al. 1997). DEHP was initially proposed to activate PPARs because it causes hepatic toxicity and leads to hepatic lipidosis and carcinomas in mice via peroxisome proliferation (Ward et al. 1986). In fact, Maloney and Waxman showed that MEHP can activate both mouse and human PPARα and PPARγ in cell transactivation assays (Maloney and Waxman 1999). Studies using human and rat hepatoma cell lines showed that MEHP and DBP activated all three receptors, but that MEHP had a preference for PPARα (Lapinskas et al. 2005). In that same study, Lapinskas et al. used scintillation proximity assays to demonstrate that both MEHP and DBP directly interact with human PPARα and PPARγ. In MCF-7 breast cancer cells, MEHP activated both PPARα and PPARγ and had no effect on PPARβ/δ, while MBP antagonized both PPARγ and PPARβ/δ (Venkata et al. 2006). Hurst and Waxman reported that MEHP, MBzP, and mono-sec-butyl phthalate increased transcriptional activity of mouse PPARα in COS-1 cells, activated endogenous PPARα-activated genes in FAO rat liver cells, and stimulated PPARγ-dependent adipogenesis in the 3T3-L1 cell differentiation model (Hurst and Waxman 2003). Interestingly, MBzP also activated human PPARα and mouse and human PPARγ, while no significant activation was observed with monomethyl, mono-*n*-butyl, dimethyl or diethyl phthalates (Hurst and Waxman 2003). Kusu et al. (2008) used cell-free co-activator

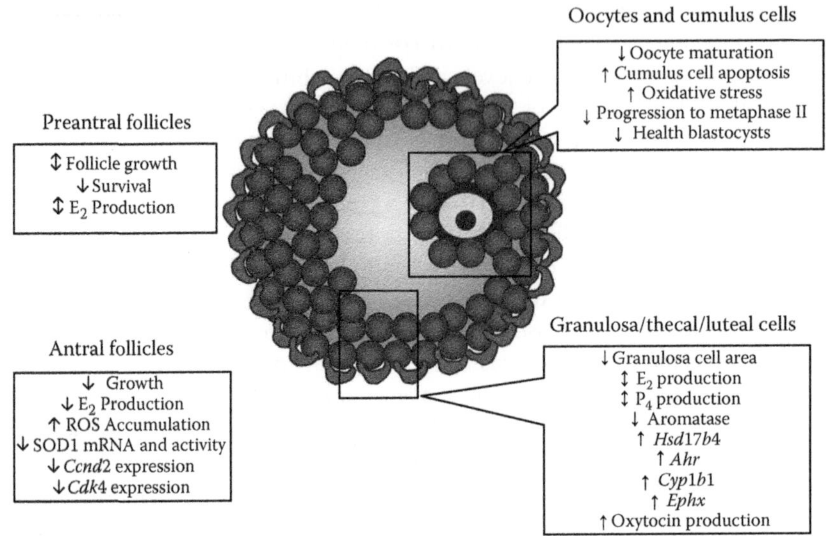

FIGURE 8.1 Ovarian processes affected by DEHP and MEHP exposure in animal models. The consequences of exposure to DEHP and its metabolite MEHP on ovarian processes are summarized according to the compartment targeted: oocytes and cumulus cells, granulosa/thecal/luteal cells, and whole preantral and antral follicles. Abbreviations and symbols: ↑ indicates an increase, ↓ indicates a decrease, ↕ indicates increased or decreased depending on study, E_2 indicates 17β-estradiol, P_4 indicates progesterone, *Hsd17b4* indicates 17β-hydroxysteroid dehydrogenase type 4 mRNA, *Ahr* indicates aryl hydrocarbon receptor mRNA, *Cyp1b1* indicates cytochrome P450 1b1 mRNA, *Ephx* indicates epoxide hydrolase mRNA, ROS indicates reactive oxygen species, SOD indicates superoxide dismutase 1, *Ccnd2* indicates cyclin D2 mRNA, and *Cdk4* indicates cyclin-dependent kinase 4 mRNA.

recruitment assays to show that some oxidative metabolites of DEHP also have the ability to influence PPAR activity (Kusu et al. 2008). Finally, the role of PPARα in DEHP toxicity was initially confirmed by the lack of hepatic toxicity in PPARα null mice (Ward et al. 1998). This was further supported by another study showing that *in vivo* exposure to DEHP or DBP failed to activate peroxisome proliferator-inducible gene products in livers of male mice lacking PPARα (Lapinskas et al. 2005). However, PPARα-independent mechanisms are also suspected in DEHP toxicity to other organs because PPARα null mice still developed DEHP-induced kidney and testis lesions (Ward et al. 1998).

Although, DEHP has been shown to act through PPARα in the liver (Ward et al. 1998), its actions on the ovary are thought to be also dependent on signaling via other PPARs. All PPAR subtypes have been shown to be expressed in the rat ovary (Braissant et al. 1996). Specifically, PPARα and β/δ are present in theca cells and stromal tissue, while PPARγ is present in granulosa cells (Komar et al. 2001). In fact, DEHP (150 and 500 mg/kg/day) increases the expression of PPARα protein in granulosa cells and corpora lutea in prepubertal rats (Ma et al. 2011). Lovekamp-Swan et al. hypothesized that MEHP suppresses aromatase expression in rat granulosa cells through PPAR pathways (Lovekamp-Swan et al. 2003). Specifically, they showed that PPARα and PPARγ agonists, similarly to MEHP, significantly decreased aromatase mRNA and E_2 production. Interestingly, a PPARγ-selective antagonist, GR 259662, partially blocked the suppression of aromatase by MEHP suggesting that PPARγ is involved. Further, they showed that MEHP and the PPARα-specific agonist, GW 327647, increased the expression of HSD17B4, a known PPARα-regulated gene in rat liver (Corton et al. 1997), as well as increased transcripts for proteins involved in xenobiotic metabolism such as the aryl hydrocarbon receptor (AHR), cytochrome P450 1B1 (CYP1B1; metabolizes E_2), and epoxide hydrolase (Lovekamp-Swan and Davis 2003). Thus, it has been proposed that MEHP decreases E_2 production in rat granulosa cells by transcriptionally downregulating aromatase via PPARγ, and upregulating HSD17B IV and CYP1B1 via PPARα (Lovekamp-Swan and Davis 2003; Lovekamp-Swan et al. 2003). Further, modulation of genes involved in xenobiotic metabolism has also been observed with other phthalates. For example, Chen et al. used the line of human immortalized granulosa cells, HO23, to investigate the effects of BBP on AHR signaling. In their study, BBP treatment (1 μM) resulted in increased *Ahr*, *Arnt*, and *Cyp1b1* mRNA and protein expression in HO23 cells. Further, specificity for the AHR signaling pathway was confirmed by the finding that treatment with the AHR antagonist, 3′,4′-dimethoxyflavone or *Ahr*-specific siRNAs blocked all BBP-induced gene and protein expression changes (Chen et al. 2012).

8.3.2 Induction of Oxidative Stress

The subjects of oxidative stress and its role in female reproduction and toxicity have been reviewed recently (Devine et al. 2012) and are further discussed in Chapter 4. Briefly, oxidative stress occurs when the production of reactive oxygen species (ROS) surpasses the ability of the cell's antioxidant system to quench the radicals produced. Under normal conditions, cells generate ROS from which it must protect itself through the action of several antioxidant enzymes and factors that include superoxide dismutase (SOD), glutathione peroxidase (GPX), glutathione *S*-transferase (GST), glutathione reductase (GSR), peroxiredoxin (PRDX), catalase (CAT), and glutathione itself (GSH). When the normal oxidative status of the cell is perturbed, damage to DNA, lipids, and proteins may occur. Several markers have been used in the evaluation of oxidative stress such as 8-hydroxyguanosine (8-OHdG; DNA damage), malondialdehyde (MDA; lipid peroxidation), thiobarbituric acid reactive substances (TBARS; lipid peroxidation), and the ratio of GSH to glutathione disulfide (GSH/GSSG; current oxidative status) among others. Further, oxidative stress can be ameliorated by supplementation with known antioxidant factors such as ascorbic acid, *N*-acetyl cysteine (NAC), resveratrol, selenium compounds, and vitamin E among others.

Several epidemiological studies have reported relationships between phthalate exposure and markers of oxidative stress in humans. Ferguson et al. studied the relationship between urinary phthalate metabolite concentrations and the serum marker for oxidative stress, gamma glutamyl transferase (GGT) in participants of NHANES from 1999 to 2006 and found that GGT was positively associated with MEHP levels (Ferguson et al. 2011). Another study investigated whether exposure to environmental chemicals, including phthalates, induces oxidative stress in adult dwelling in urban areas of Korea. Using simple regression analysis, Hong et al. observed that there was a significant dose–response relationship between urinary concentrations of all chemical exposure metabolites, including MEHP and MBP, and levels of oxidative stress markers (Hong et al. 2009). Also, long-term exposure to DEHP was shown to raise plasma MDA levels, in a study investigating the effects of long-term exposure to phthalates in infants and children undergoing cyclic long-term parenteral nutrition (Kambia et al. 2011). Taken together, these human studies support the idea that phthalate exposure may lead to increased oxidative stress.

While human studies showed relationships between phthalate exposure and markers of oxidative stress, animal studies have provided important clues regarding the potential mechanisms by which phthalates may cause oxidative stress. It is important to note that not much is known about the effect of phthalates on oxidative stress in the female reproductive system. In fact, most of what we know today about phthalates and oxidative stress has been elucidated in the male reproductive tract. Global gene expression analysis of fetal rat testis revealed that *in utero* exposure to a panel of phthalates resulted in downregulation of 11 genes involved in protection against oxidative stress including various GST and SOD isoforms (Liu et al. 2005). Exposure to DEHP in adult rats resulted in decreased testicular GSH/GSSG redox ratios, elevated TBARS levels (Erkekoglu et al. 2011a), increased ROS, and decreased levels of GSH and ascorbic acid (Kasahara et al. 2002). In the mouse Leydig cell line MA-10, MEHP (10 μM; IC_{50}=3 μM) was shown to cause cytotoxicity, increase ROS accumulation, decrease total GSH, and to decrease GPX, cytosolic thioredoxin reductase, and GST activities. At the IC_{50}, MEHP caused an increase in p53 protein, and led to DNA damage as shown by alkaline comet assays. Interestingly, all the effects of MEHP on MA-10 cells were prevented by cotreating with selenium (Erkekoglu et al. 2010b). Furthermore, similar observations were made in the LNCaP human prostate adenocarcinoma cell line in which DEHP and MEHP decreased cell viability, decreased GPX activity, and induced DNA damage. Like in MA-10 cells, selenium cotreatment was also protective in LNCaP cells (Erkekoglu et al. 2010a, 2011b, 2012). Botelho et al. assessed the influence of DEHP alone or associated with antioxidants on the reproductive system of newborn male rats and observed that DEHP exposure decreased GST activity (Botelho et al. 2009). However, and in contrast to other studies using other antioxidants, co-administration of DEHP and vitamin C and/or resveratrol did not ameliorate its toxicity. In fact, the authors observed that for some of the endpoints tested (e.g., catalase activity), cotreatment with an antioxidant resulted in greater disruptions. Unfortunately, it is not clear whether the contrasting observations of Botehlo et al. versus others are the result of differences in experimental design or antioxidant doses and relative potency (e.g., selenium vs. vitamin C or resveratrol). However, taken together, these findings provide strong evidence that DEHP causes oxidative stress in the male reproductive tract by downregulating antioxidant activity, but that this effect can be prevented with antioxidant supplementation.

Fewer studies have evaluated oxidative stress as a mechanism for phthalate toxicity in ovarian tissues. One study, using the horse as a model, evaluated the effects of *in vitro* exposure to DEHP on oocyte maturation, cumulus cell apoptosis, and oxidative status (Ambruosi et al. 2011). This study revealed that DEHP induced cumulus cell apoptosis and increased ROS production, and that these effects can be prevented by cotreating with the antioxidant NAC. Another study used an isolated mouse ovarian antral follicle culture system to evaluate the involvement of oxidative stress in DEHP-induced inhibition of *in vitro* antral follicle growth. Specifically, Wang et al. showed that DEHP exposure is associated with increased ROS accumulation, and decreased mRNA and activity of SOD1 in mouse antral follicles. Further, this study also demonstrated that all these DEHP-induced disruptions were prevented by cotreatment with NAC. Interestingly, DEHP exposure did not alter the mRNA expression or activity of GPX and CAT in mouse antral follicles (Wang et al. 2012a). In a similar study, MEHP, the active metabolite of DEHP, was shown to increase ROS accumulation and inhibit the expression of SOD1 and GPX1 in mouse antral follicles. Further, MEHP exposure resulted in decreased expression of important genes for progression through the cell cycle and favored pro-apoptotic gene expression. Like with DEHP, NAC treatment prevented all the detrimental effects of MEHP (Wang et al. 2012b). Although there are still many aspects to be studied, these studies have provided evidence that DEHP causes oxidative stress in ovarian tissues, and that these are likely mediated by accumulation of ROS and insufficiencies in the antioxidant system.

It is important to note that although DEHP and MEHP have been the most widely studied phthalates to date, there are a growing number of studies aimed at evaluating the toxicity of DBP and its effect on oxidative stress. Specifically, DBP and MBP were also recently shown to induce cytotoxicity and inhibit cell differentiation in cultured rat embryonic limb bud cells via an oxidative stress pathway (Kim et al. 2002). Interestingly, cotreatment with catalase and vitamin E acetate prevented DBP-induced cytotoxicity and inhibited differentiation, but these antioxidants afforded no protection against MBP treatment. Similar to the case of DEHP and MEHP, fewer studies have investigated the involvement of DBP and its metabolite MBP on induction of oxidative stress in reproductive tissues. Furthermore, all studies to date have evaluated DBP-induced oxidative stress in male reproductive tissues. For example, DBP (250 and/or 500 mg/kg/day; oral for 2 weeks) was shown to inhibit SOD and GPX activities, reduce GSH levels, and increase MDA levels in rat testes (Zhou et al. 2010). Similar findings were reported by others studying the rat testis (Wang et al. 2004), as well as the epididymis where DBP exposure results in decreased GPX and SOD activities, as well as increased MDA levels (Zhou et al. 2011). Further, rats treated with DBP showed altered hepatic α-tocopherol (a vitamin E) levels and SOD1 activity (O'Brien et al. 2001b), as well as decreased hepatic GSH levels and GST activity (O'Brien et al. 2001a).

Finally, a link between peroxisome proliferators, and thus PPAR ligands, and oxidative stress has been hypothesized because they increase the activities of enzymes involved in peroxisomal β-oxidation and omega-hydroxylation of fatty acids, which are thought to enhance the production of ROS in the cell (Lake et al. 1990; Lake 1995; Rao and Reddy 1991). In fact, clofibrate and Wy-14,643, two known peroxisome proliferators, have been shown to alter antioxidant enzyme levels and activity (clofibrate; Dobashi et al. 1999) and induce superoxide production (Wy-14,643; Rose et al. 1999). Therefore, the relationship between peroxisome proliferators and ROS generation suggests that PPAR modulation and oxidative stress may actually represent a continuum of events leading to toxicity rather than modulation of two strictly separate pathways.

8.4 SUMMARY

Phthalates are ubiquitous chemicals to which humans are exposed on a daily basis. Many years of research have identified phthalates as endocrine disruptors capable of disturbing normal development and reproduction in animal models. Phthalates are most widely known for disrupting steroidogenesis *in vivo* and *in vitro*, as well as disrupting ovarian follicle and oocyte development. Many studies have evaluated the mechanisms by which phthalates cause these effects. Thus, two major pathways have been explored: modulation of PPARs and induction of oxidative stress. Phthalates have been shown to bind and activate PPARs in the liver, breast, adipose tissue, and gonads. In the ovary, DEHP has been shown to act via both PPARα and PPARγ to decrease levels of E_2. Specifically, DEHP seems to downregulate E_2 synthesis by decreasing aromatase expression via PPARα, while it increases E_2 catabolism by upregulating E_2-metabolizing enzymes via PPARγ. DEHP and DBP, and their metabolites, have been shown to be associated with markers of oxidative stress in both humans and animals. Mechanistic studies have shown that these phthalates downregulate the expression and/or activity of important antioxidant defense factors and cause oxidative stress due to excessive ROS accumulation. Although the mechanism by which phthalates downregulate these antioxidant processes is not clear, we know that supplementing with selected antioxidants prevents phthalate-induced oxidative stress. Finally, future studies should be aimed at further elucidating the mechanisms by which DEHP and DBP compromise the oxidative balance of cells and understanding how PPAR signaling may cross-talk with oxidative stress pathways. Most importantly, further studies focusing on evaluating the effects of other nonwidely studied phthalates, including phthalate substitutes, are needed to gain a better understanding of the risks posed by this group of chemicals to women.

ACKNOWLEDGMENT

The authors thank Dr. Jodi A. Flaws (Comparative Biosciences, University of Illinois, Urbana, IL) for her kind mentoring and support.

REFERENCES

Ambruosi, B., Uranio, M., Sardanelli, A., Pocar, P., Martino, N., Paternoster, M., Amati, F., and Dell'Aquila, M. 2011. In vitro acute exposure to DEHP affects oocyte meiotic maturation, energy and oxidative stress parameters in a large animal model. *PLoS One* 6: e27452.

Anas, M., Suzuki, C., Yoshioka, K., and Iwamura, S. 2003. Effect of mono-(2-ethylhexyl) phthalate on bovine oocyte maturation in vitro. *Reprod Toxicol* 17: 305–310.

Blount, B., Silva, M., Caudill, S., Needham, L., Pirkle, J., Sampson, E., Lucier, G., Jackson, R., and Brock, J. 2000. Levels of seven urinary phthalate metabolites in a human reference population. *Environ Health Perspect* 108 (10): 979–982.

Botelho, G., Bufalo, A., Boareto, A., Muller, J., Morais, R., Martino-Andrade, A., Lemos, K., and Dalsenter, P. 2009. Vitamin C and resveratrol supplementation to rat dams treated with di(2-ethylhexyl)phthalate: Impact on reproductive and oxidative stress end points in male offspring. *Arch Environ Contam Toxicol* 57 (4): 785–793.

Braissant, O., Foufelle, F., Scotto, C., Dauça, M., and Wahli, W. 1996. Differential expression of peroxisome proliferator-activated receptors (PPARs): Tissue distribution of PPAR-alpha, -beta, and -gamma in the adult rat. *Endocrinology* 137 (1): 354–366.

Chen, H., Chiang, P., Wang, Y., Kao, M., Shieh, T., Tsai, C., and Tsai, E. 2012. Benzyl butyl phthalate induces necrosis by AhR mediation of CYP1B1 expression in human granulosa cells. *Reprod Toxicol* 33 (1): 67–75.

Corton, J., Bocos, C., Moreno, E., Merritt, A., Cattley, R., and Gustafsson, J. 1997. Peroxisome proliferators alter the expression of estrogen-metabolizing enzymes. *Biochimie* 79 (2–3): 151–162.

Dalman, A., Eimani, H., Sepehri, H., Ashtiani, S., Valojerdi, M., Eftekhari-Yazdi, P., and Shahverdi, A. 2008. Effect of mono-(2-ethylhexyl) phthalate (MEHP) on resumption of meiosis, in vitro maturation and embryo development of immature mouse oocytes. *Biofactors* 33 (2):149–155.

Davis, B. J., Maronpot, R. R., and Heindel, J. J. 1994a. Di-(2-ethylhexyl) phthalate suppresses estradiol and ovulation in cycling rats. *Toxicol Appl Pharmacol* 128: 216–223.

Davis, B. J., Weaver, R., Gaines, L. J., and Heindel, J. J. 1994b. Mono-(2-ethylhexyl) phthalate suppresses estradiol production independent of FSH-cAMP stimulation in rat granulosa cells. *Toxicol Appl Pharmacol* 128 (2): 224–228.

Devine, P., Perreault, S., and Luderer, U. 2012. Roles of reactive oxygen species and antioxidants in ovarian toxicity. *Biol Reprod* 86 (2): 27.

Dobashi, K., Asayama, K., Nakane, T., Hayashibe, H., Kodera, K., Uchida, N., and Nakazawa, S. 1999. Effect of peroxisome proliferator on extracellular glutathione peroxidase in rat. *Free Radic Res* 31 (3): 181–190.

Erkekoglu, P., Giray, B., Kizilgün, M., Rachidi, W., Hininger-Favier, I., Roussel, A., Favier, A., and Hincal, F. 2012. Di(2-ethylhexyl) phthalate-induced renal oxidative stress in rats and protective effect of selenium. *Toxicol Mech Methods* 22 (6): 415–423.

Erkekoglu, P., Giray, B., Rachidi, W., Hininger-Favier, I., Roussel, A.-M., Favier, A., and Hincal, F. 2011. Effects of di(2-ethylhexyl)phthalate on testicular oxidant/antioxidant status in selenium-deficient and selenium-supplemented rats. *Environ Toxicol.* doi: 10.1002/tox.20776.

Erkekoglu, P., Rachidi, W., De Rosa, V., Giray, B., Favier, A., and Hincal, F. 2010a. Protective effect of selenium supplementation on the genotoxicity of di(2-ethylhexyl) phthalate and mono(2-ethylhexyl) phthalate treatment in LNCaP cells. *Free Radic Biol Med* 49 (4): 559–566.

Erkekoglu, P., Rachidi, W., Yuzugullu, O., Favier, A., Ozturk, M., and Hincal, F. 2010b. Evaluation of cytotoxicity and oxidative DNA damaging effects of di(2-ethylhexyl)-phthalate (DEHP) and mono(2-ethylhexyl)-phthalate (MEHP) on MA-10 Leydig cells and protection by selenium. *Toxicol Appl Pharmacol* 248 (1): 52–62.

Erkekoglu, P., Rachidi, W., Yuzugullu, O., Giray, B., Ozturk, M., and Hincal, F. 2011b. Induction of ROS, p53, p21 in DEHP- and MEHP-exposed LNCaP cells-protection by selenium. *Food Chem Toxicol* 49 (7): 1565–1571.

Ferguson, K., Loch-Caruso, R., and Meeker, J. 2011. Urinary phthalate metabolites in relation to biomarkers of inflammation and oxidative stress: NHANES 1999–2006. *Environ Res* 111 (5): 718–726.

Fuchs, A. 1988. Oxytocin and ovarian function. *J Reprod Fertil Suppl* (36): 39–47.

Grande, S. W., Andrade, A. J. M., Talsness, C. E., Grote, K., Golombiewski, A., and Sterner-Kock, A. C. I. 2007. A dose–response study following in utero and lactational exposure to di-(2-ethylhexyl) phthalate (DEHP): Reproductive effects on adult female offspring rats. *Toxicology* 229 (1–2): 114–122.

Gray, L. E., Laskey, J., and Ostby, J. 2006. Chronic Di-n-butyl phthalate exposure in rats reduces fertility and alters ovarian function during pregnancy in female Long Evans Hooded Rats. *Toxicol Sci* 93 (1): 189–195.

Grossman, D., Kalo, D., Gendelman, M., Roth, Z. 2012. Effect of di-(2-ethylhexyl) phthalate and mono-(2-ethylhexyl) phthalate on in vitro developmental competence of bovine oocytes. *Cell Biol Toxicol* 28 (6): 383–396.

Guerra, M., Scarano, W., de Toledo, F., Franci, J., and Kempinas, W. G. 2010. Reproductive development and function of female rats exposed to di-eta-butyl-phthalate (DBP) in utero and during lactation. *Reprod Toxicol* 29 (1): 99–105.

Gupta, R. K., Singh, J. M., Leslie, T. C., Meachum, S., Flaws, J. A., and Yao, H. H. 2010. Di-(2-ethylhexyl) phthalate and mono-(2-ethylhexyl) phthalate inhibit growth and reduce estradiol levels of antral follicles in vitro. *Toxicol Appl Pharmacol* 242: 224–230.

Heudorf, U., Mersch-Sundermann, V., and Angerer, J. 2007. Phthalates: Toxicology and exposure. *Int J Hyg Environ Health* 210: 623–634.

Hines, E., Calafat, A., Silva, M., Mendola, P., and Fenton, S. 2009. Concentrations of phthalate metabolites in milk, urine, saliva, and serum of lactating North Carolina women. *Environ Health Perspect* 117 (1): 86–92.

Hirosawa, N., Yano, K., Suzuki, Y., and Sakamoto, Y. 2006. Endocrine disrupting effect of di-(2-ethylhexyl)phthalate on female rats and proteome analyses of their pituitaries. *Proteomics* 6 (3): 958–971.

Hong, Y., Park, E., Park, M., Ko, J., Oh, S., Kim, H., Lee, K., Leem, J., and Ha, E. 2009. Community level exposure to chemicals and oxidative stress in adult population. *Toxicol Lett*, 184 (2): 139–144.

Howdeshell, K. L., Rider, C. V., Wilson, V. S., and Gray, L. E. 2008. Mechanisms of action of phthalate esters, individually and in combination, to induce abnormal reproductive development in male laboratory rats. *Environ Res* 108: 168–176.

Hurst, C. and Waxman, D. 2003. Activation of PPARalpha and PPARgamma by environmental phthalate monoesters. *Toxicol Sci* 74 (2): 297–308.

Inada, H., Chihara, K., Yamashita, A., Miyawaki, I., Fukuda, C., Tateishi, Y., Kunimatsu, T., Kimura, J., Funabashi, H., and Miyano, T. 2012. Evaluation of ovarian toxicity of mono-(2-ethylhexyl) phthalate (MEHP) using cultured rat ovarian follicles. *J Toxicol Sci* 37 (3): 483–490.

Kambia, N., Dine, T., Gressier, B., Frimat, B., Cazin, J., Luyckx, M., Brunet, C., Michaud, L., and Gottrand, F. 2011. Correlation between exposure to phthalates and concentrations of malondialdehyde in infants and children undergoing cyclic parenteral nutrition. *JPEN* 35 (3): 395–401.

Kasahara, E., Sato, E., Miyoshi, M., Konaka, R., Hiramoto, K., Sasaki, J., Tokuda, M., Nakano, Y., and Inoue, M. 2002. Role of oxidative stress in germ cell apoptosis induced by di(2-ethylhexyl) phthalate. *Biochem J* 365 (Pt 3): 849–856.

Kim, S., Kim, S., Kwon, Q., Sohn, K., Kwack, S., Choi, Y., Han, S., Lee, M., and Park, K. 2002. Effects of dibutyl phthalate and monobutyl phthalate on cytotoxicity and differentiation in cultured rat embryonic limb bud cells; protection by antioxidants. *J Toxicol Environ Health A* 65 (5–6): 461–472.

Komar, C., Braissant, O., Wahli, W., and Curry, T. J. 2001. Expression and localization of PPARs in the rat ovary during follicular development and the periovulatory period. *Endocrinology* 142 (11): 4831–4838.

Krotz, S., Carson, S., Tomey, C., and Buster, J. 2012. Phthalates and bisphenol do not accumulate in human follicular fluid. *J Assist Reprod Genet* 29: 773–777.

Kusu, R., Oishi, A., Kakizawa, K., Kimura, T., Toda, C., Hashizume, K., Ueda, K., and Kojima, N. 2008. Effects of phthalate ester derivatives including oxidized metabolites on coactivator recruiting by PPARalpha and PPARgamma. *Toxicol In Vitro* 22 (6): 1534–1538.

LaFrance, M. and Goff, A. 1990. Control of bovine uterine prostaglandin F2 alpha release in vitro. *Biol Reprod* 42 (2): 288–293.

Lake, B. 1995. Mechanisms of hepatocarcinogenicity of peroxisome-proliferating drugs and chemicals. *Annu Rev Pharmacol Toxicol* 35: 483–507.

Lake, B., Gray, T., Smith, A., and Evans, J. 1990. Hepatic peroxisome proliferation and oxidative stress. *Biochem Soc Trans* 18 (1): 94–97.

Lapinskas, P., Brown, S., Leesnitzer, L., Blanchard, S., Swanson, C., Cattley, R., and Corton, J. 2005. Role of PPARalpha in mediating the effects of phthalates and metabolites in the liver. *Toxicology* 207 (1): 149–163.

Laskey, J. and Berman, E. 1993. Steroidogenic assessment using ovary culture in cycling rats: Effects of bis (2-diethylhexyl) phthalate on ovarian steroid production. *Reprod Toxicol* 7 (1): 25–33.

Latini, G., De Felice, C., Presta, G., Del Vecchio, A., Paris, I., Ruggieri, F., and Mazzeo, P. 2003. Exposure to Di(2-ethylhexyl) phthalate in humans during pregnancy. A preliminary report. *Biol Neonate* 83 (1): 22–24.

Lenie, S. and Smitz, J. 2009. Steroidogenesis-disrupting compounds can be effectively studied for major fertility-related endpoints using in vitro cultured mouse follicles. *Toxicol Lett* 185: 143–152.

Lin, L., Zheng, L., Gu, Y., Wang, J., Zhang, Y., and Song, W. 2008. Levels of environmental endocrine disruptors in umbilical cord blood and maternal blood of low-birth-weight infants. *Zhonghua Yu Fang Yi Xue Za Zhi* 42 (3): 177–180.

Liu, K., Lehman, K., Sar, M., Young, S., and Gaido, K. 2005. Gene expression profiling following in utero exposure to phthalate esters reveals new gene targets in the etiology of testicular dysgenesis. *Biol Reprod* 73 (1): 180–192.

Lovekamp, T. and Davis, B. 2001. Mono-(2-ethylhexyl) phthalate suppresses aromatase transcript levels and estradiol production in cultured rat granulosa cells. *Toxicol Appl Pharmacol* 172: 217–224.

Lovekamp-Swan, T. and Davis, B. J. 2003. Mechanisms of phthalate ester toxicity in the female reproductive system. *Environ Health Perspect* 111 (2): 139–145.

Lovekamp-Swan, T., Jetten, A., and Davis, B. 2003. Dual activation of PPARalpha and PPARgamma by mono-(2-ethylhexyl)phthalate in rat ovarian granulosa cells. *Mol Cell Endocrinol* 201 (1–2): 133–141.

Lyche, J. L., Gutleb, A. C., Bergman, A., Eriksen, G. S., Murk, A. J., Ropstad, E., Saunders, M., and Skaare, J. U. 2009. Reproductive and developmental toxicity of phthalates. *J Toxicol Environ Health B: Crit Rev* 12 (4): 225–249.

Ma, M., Kondo, T., Ban, S., Umemura, T., Kurahashi, N., Takeda, M., and Kishi, R. 2006. Exposure of prepubertal female rats to inhaled di(2-ethylhexyl)phthalate affects the onset of puberty and postpubertal reproductive functions. *Toxicol Sci* 93 (1): 164–171.

Ma, M., Zhang, Y., Pei, X., and Duan, Z. 2011. Effects of di-(2-ethylhexyl) phthalate exposure on reproductive development and PPARs in prepubertal female rats. *Wei Sheng Yan Jiu* 40 (6): 688–692.

Maloney, E. and Waxman, D. 1999. trans-Activation of PPARalpha and PPARgamma by structurally diverse environmental chemicals. *Toxicol Appl Pharmacol* 161 (2): 209–218.

Mlynarcíková, A., Ficková, M., and Scsuková, S. 2007. The effects of selected phenol and phthalate derivatives on steroid hormone production by cultured porcine granulosa cells. *Altern Lab Anim* 35 (1): 71–77.

National Center for Environmental Health. 2005. *Third National Report on Human Exposure to Environmental Chemicals*, Department of Health and Human Services, Centers for Disease Control and Prevention, NCEH Pub. No. 05-0570.

O'Brien, M., Cunningham, M., Spear, B., and Glauert, H. 2001a. Effects of peroxisome proliferators on glutathione and glutathione-related enzymes in rats and hamsters. *Toxicol Appl Pharmacol* 171 (1): 27–37.

O'Brien, M., Twaroski, T., Cunningham, M., Glauert, H., and Spear, B. 2001b. Effects of peroxisome proliferators on antioxidant enzymes and antioxidant vitamins in rats and hamsters. *Toxicol Sci* 60 (2): 271–278.

Rao, M. and Reddy, J. 1991. An overview of peroxisome proliferator-induced hepatocarcinogenesis. *Environ Health Perspect* 93: 205–209.

Reinsberg, J., Wegener-Toper, P., van der Ven, K., van der Ven, H., and Klingmueller, D. 2009. Effect of mono-(2-ethylhexyl) phthalate on steroid production of human granulosa cells. *Toxicol Appl Pharmacol* 239: 116–123.

Rose, M., Rivera, C., Bradford, B., Graves, L., Cattley, R., Schoonhoven, R., Swenberg, J., and Thurman, R. 1999. Kupffer cell oxidant production is central to the mechanism of peroxisome proliferators. *Carcinogenesis* 20 (1): 27–33.

Svechnikova, I., Svechnikov, K., and Söder, O. 2007. The influence of di-(2-ethylhexyl) phthalate on steroidogenesis by the ovarian granulosa cells of immature female rats. *J Endocrinol* 194: 603–609.

Tomonari, Y., Kurata, Y., David, R., Gans, G., Kawasuso, T., and Katoh, M. 2006. Effect of di(2-ethylhexyl) phthalate (DEHP) on genital organs from juvenile common marmosets: I. Morphological and biochemical investigation in 65-week toxicity study. *J Toxicol Environ Health A* 69 (17): 1651–1672.

Treinen, K. A., Dodson, W. C., and Heindel, J. J. 1990. Inhibition of FSH-stimulated cAMP accumulation and progesterone production by mono(2-ethylhexyl) phthalate in rat granulosa cell cultures. *Toxicol Appl Pharmacol* 106 (2): 334–340.

Venkata, N., Robinson, J., Cabot, P., Davis, B., Monteith, G., and Roberts-Thomson, S. 2006. Mono(2-ethylhexyl) phthalate and mono-n-butyl phthalate activation of peroxisome proliferator activated-receptor alpha and gamma in breast. *Toxicol Lett* 163 (3): 224–234.

Wan, X., Zhu, Y., Ma, X., Zhu, J., Zheng, Y., Hou, J., Wang, F., Liu, Z., and Zhang, T. 2010. Effect of DEHP and its metabolite MEHP on in vitro rat follicular development. *Wei Sheng Yan Jiu* 39 (3): 268–270.

Wang, W., Craig, Z., Basavarajappa, M., Gupta, R., and Flaws, J. 2012a. Di (2-ethylhexyl) phthalate inhibits growth of mouse antral follicles through an oxidative stress pathway. *Toxicol Appl Pharmacol* 258: 288–295.

Wang, W., Craig, Z., Basavarajappa, M., Hafner, K., and Flaws, J. 2012b. Mono (2-ethylhexyl) phthalate induces oxidative stress and inhibits growth of mouse ovarian antral follicles. *Biol Reprod*. In press, no. PMID 23077170.

Wang, X., Shang, L., Wang, J., Wu, N., and Wang, S. 2010. Effect of phthalate esters on the secretion of prostaglandins (F2alpha and E2) and oxytocin in cultured bovine ovarian and endometrial cells. *Domest Anim Endocrinol* 39 (2): 131–136.

Wang, Y., Song, L., Chen, J., He, J., Liu, R., Zhu, Z., and Wang, X. 2004. Effects of di-butyl phthalate on sperm motility and oxidative stress in rats. *Zhonghua Nan Ke Xue* 10 (4): 253–256.

Ward, J., Diwan, B., Ohshima, M., Hu, H., Schuller, H., and Rice, J. 1986. Tumor-initiating and promoting activities of di(2-ethylhexyl) phthalate in vivo and in vitro. *Environ Health Perspect* 65: 279–291.

Ward, J., Peters, J., Perella, C., and Gonzalez, F. 1998. Receptor and nonreceptor-mediated organ-specific toxicity of di(2-ethylhexyl)phthalate (DEHP) in peroxisome proliferator-activated receptor alpha-null mice. *Toxicol Pathol* 26: 240–246.

Xu, C., Chen, J.-A., Qiu, Z., Zhao, Q., Luo, J., Yang, L., Zeng, H., Huang, Y., Zhang, L., Cao, J., and Shu, W. 2010. Ovotoxicity and PPAR-mediated aromatase downregulation in female Sprague-Dawley rats following combined oral exposure to benzo[a]pyrene and di-(2-ethylhexyl) phthalate. *Toxicol Lett* 199: 323–332.

Zhou, D., Wang, H., and Zhang, J. 2011. Di-n-butyl phthalate (DBP) exposure induces oxidative stress in epididymis of adult rats. *Toxicol Ind Health* 27 (1): 65–71.

Zhou, D., Wang, H., Zhang, J., Gao, X., Zhao, W., and Zheng, Y. 2010. Di-n-butyl phthalate (DBP) exposure induces oxidative damage in testes of adult rats. *Syst Biol Reprod Med* 56 (6): 413–419.

9 Heavy Metals and the Ovary

Sakhila K. Banu

CONTENTS

Metals may be divided into four groups: (1) those with greatest toxicological significance that are widespread in the human environment [arsenic (As), cadmium (Cd), lead (Pb), mercury (Hg), chromium (Cr), and uranium (U)], (2) essential trace metals [cobalt (Co), copper (Cu), iron (Fe), manganese (Mn), selenium (Se), and zinc (Zn)], (3) other metals with evident biological interest (nickel and vanadium), and (4) metals of pharmacological interest (aluminum, gallium, and lithium) (Domingo 1994).

9.1 HISTORIC BACKGROUND OF HEAVY METAL USAGE

Heavy metals have been in anthropologic use from the ancient history to modern civilization. Use of heavy metals started long before the beginning of the industrial revolution. The earliest use of heavy metals by humans dates back to about 6000 BC (Adebowale 2004). *Stone age* is a large prehistoric period that lasted for about 3.4 million years, and ended between 4500 BC and 2000 BC with the advent of metal usage. The subsequent periods or ages of human history were named after the usage of metals such as the *copper age* (that started by 6000 BC and was widespread by 4500 BC), *bronze age* (around 3200 BC), and *iron age* (around 1200 BC) (Harper 1987). In fact, humans during the copper age used an iron/nickel alloy, naturally occurring in iron–nickel meteorites. The production and usage of heavy metals exponentially increased after the industrial revolution (1750–1850 AD) (Tylecote 1991).

9.2 HEAVY METAL ENDOCRINE DISRUPTORS

An endocrine-disrupting chemical (EDC) or endocrine disruptor is a man-made synthetic chemical or natural phytoestrogen (*naturally occurring plant or fungal metabolite-derived estrogen*) that acts on the endocrine systems of humans and animals by mimicking, blocking, and/or interfering in some manner with the natural cell signaling pathway of hormones in cells (Andrew et al. 2010). Heavy metals are the earliest EDCs in human history to disrupt endocrine functions. Even though heavy metal EDCs have their impact on almost all systems including those of the male and female reproductive tracts, the current chapter is focused as an update on the effects of widely used heavy metal EDCs on the ovary. General information about the anatomy, development, and functions of the ovary has been discussed in several earlier chapters of this volume. *Background* information for each metal in the following sections provides brief details about environmental exposure and occupational usage of these metals.

9.3 ARSENIC

9.3.1 Background

Arsenic (As), one of the major heavy metal water pollutants, exerts carcinogenic and toxic effects in mammals (Pott et al. 2001). Arsenic toxicity is a major global health concern due to its wide distribution and adverse health effects. AsIII is used in herbicides, insecticides, rodenticides, and food preservatives resulting in contamination of the environment and food (Cooksey 2012). Most recent reports from the Environmental Working Group (EWG) documented high levels of As present in rice due to the heavy usage of As-containing pesticides as well as the natural tendency of rice plants to retain As (EWG 2012). Therefore, long-term eating of rice might predispose consumers to the development of various cancers and infertility. Two new reports from the U.S. Food and Drug Administration and *Consumer Reports* magazine highlight the worrisome amounts of As in rice and popular rice-based processed foods (EWG 2012, Lunder and Undurraga 2012). Excluding occupational exposures from metal-smelting and glass-making industries, drinking water is the principal source of human exposure to As (Petrusevski et al. 2007). Therefore, ingestion of As-containing food, inhalation of arsine gas (AsH_3, one of the simplest As containing compounds in industrial settings), and exposure to arsenal herbicides and pesticides can also contribute to As intake (Akter et al. 2005). The shallow ground water of the western United States is more vulnerable than the eastern United States. Arizona, Utah, Nevada, and California in particular are hotspots for As contamination (Welch et al. 2000). The U.S. Environmental Protection Agency (USEPA) has recently revised the maximum contaminant level for As as 10 μg/L (USEPA 2001) based on recommendations from the National Academy of Sciences. The oxidized form of As (arsenate) is the principal inorganic As species found in drinking water. Glutathione (GSH) or arsenate reductase catalyzes the reduction of arsenate to arsenite *in vivo*. Arsenite is more toxic due to an increased reactivity of the trivalent form with biomacromolecules (Bode and Dong 2002). Toxicity of arsenal compounds results in the production of free radicals and reactive oxygen species (ROS) (Ercal et al. 2001) that can cause DNA single-strand breakage (Li et al. 2001). Exposure to As induces oxidative stress in several organs by a significant reduction in GSH (Li et al. 2002, Messarah et al. 2012, Mishra and Flora 2008).

9.3.2 Arsenic and the Ovary

Sodium arsenate treatment (0.4 ppm) of rats for 28 days through drinking water disrupted the estrous cycle causing a persistent diestrous phase, suppressed activities of 3β-HSD and 17β-HSD, and decreased LH, FSH, and estradiol (Chattopadhyay and

Ghosh 2010). Arsenate also decreased the number of healthy follicles and increased follicular atresia. Vitamin C mitigates As-induced ovarian toxicity and steroidogenic dysfunction. As binds to GSH and is exported by the multidrug resistance protein MRP-1 (Leslie 2012). Therefore, possible mechanisms of vitamin C intervention of As-toxicity may include its antioxidant property and facilitating the elimination of As from the body.

Gestational exposure to sodium arsenite (up to 84 ppm) induced epithelial ovarian tumors in F1 offspring of mice (Chen et al. 2004). As III induced oocyte meiotic abnormalities and compromised pre-implantation development in mice (Navarro et al. 2004). In female CD-1 mice injected with 0, 8, or 16 mg/kg sodium arsenite (i.p.) every 2 days for a period of 14 days, metaphase II oocytes exhibited increased meiotic aberrations, characterized by spindle disruption and chromosomal misalignment. Zygotes from As-treated mice had lower rates of cleavage, decreased morula formation, and decreased development to blastocysts with an increased number of apoptotic nuclei.

9.3.3 Clinical Use of Arsenic to Treat Ovarian Cancer

As promotes both oxidative stress and impairs DNA repair, and both of these effects tend to amplify mutation rates, thereby, increasing the likelihood of ovarian cancer. As persistently alters the production of inflammatory cytokines over time (Germolec et al. 1996). *In vitro* treatment with As (1–8 μM) increased cytotoxicity in the ovarian carcinoma cell line, MDAH 2774 (Terek et al. 2006). Clinically achievable concentrations (i.e., 2 μM) of As induced apoptosis in the platinum-resistant human ovarian cancer cell line CI80-13S, and the platinum-sensitive human ovarian cancer cell line OVCAR. As appeared to slow down the growth of cisplatin-sensitive human ovarian cancer cell lines, GG and JAM (Du and Ho 2001). Arsenic trioxide (As_2O_3) and cisplatin had additive effects on human ovarian carcinoma MDAH2774 cells (Uslu et al. 2000). As_2O_3 slowed the growth without apparent apoptotic cell death in human ovarian carcinoma cells, SKOV3 (Bornstein et al. 2005). As_2O_3 increased the Fas receptor, also known as apoptosis antigen 1 (APO-1 or APT), or cluster of differentiation 95 (CD95) in human ovarian cancer cells 3AO (Huang et al. 2002). As has been reported to induce apoptosis in a cisplatin-resistant derivative cell line 3AO/CDDP (Huang et al. 2002). An increased population of cells in S-phase associated with a decrease in percentage of cells in G2/M phase transition was observed at a dose <1 μM As_2O_3, whereas there was a decrease in the percentage of cells in G1 at >3 μM. As_2O_3 injection (i.p.) decreased peritoneal metastasis of human ovarian cancer cells (3AO, SW626, HO-8910PM) in nude mice (Zhang and Wang 2006). This was achieved through inhibition of matrix metalloproteinase (MMP)-2 and MMP-9 expression. MMPs promote ovarian cancer progression by enhancing cancer cell growth, migration and invasion, metastasis, and angiogenesis by degrading basement membranes allowing cancer cell invasion (Belotti et al. 2003). As_2O_3 is considered as useful in combination therapy because polyunsaturated fatty acids appear to sensitize As-resistant tumor cells, including SKOV3 cells, to As_2O_3-induced cytotoxicity and apoptosis.

9.4 CADMIUM

9.4.1 Background

Various modern industries use cadmium (Cd) including foundry, metallurgical, and electroplating industries (Kah et al. 2012). About 13,000 tons of Cd is produced yearly worldwide, mainly for manufacturing nickel–Cd batteries, pigments, chemical stabilizers, metal coatings, and alloys. Soluble Cd salts accumulate in mammals and result in toxicity to the kidney, liver, lungs, brain, testes, heart, and central nervous system. Cd is listed by the U.S. Environmental Protection Agency as one of 126 priority pollutants (Irwin et al. 1997). General population in the United States and developing countries are exposed to Cd either through the ingestion of contaminated foods (meat, fish, and fruit) or through contact with consumer products containing this metal (Jarup and Akesson 2009). Cd exposure is linked to numerous human health problems, including infertility, renal failure, osteoporosis, leukemia, hypertension, and lung cancer (Krivosheev et al. 2012). Unlike other heavy metals, Cd has a very long biological half-life (15–30 years), because it is excreted very slowly from the body even though it is mainly stored in the liver and kidney (Klimisch 1993).

9.4.2 Cadmium and the Ovary

Cd accumulates in the ovary, uterus, and pituitary of humans and alters the histopathology of these endocrine organs (Zhang et al. 2008). In the population, different groups and subjects have been identified as being more susceptible to Cd exposure (e.g., individuals with a low iron status, mainly women). Therefore, it is important to identify vulnerable groups, especially when setting recommendations for daily intake of Cd (Piasek and Laskey 1994). Experiments on laboratory animals have shown that Cd can alter ovarian morphogenesis (Piasek and Laskey 1999, Wan et al. 2010, Zhang and Jia 2007) and inhibit the normal growth and development of ovarian follicles. In mature cycling animals like hamsters, mice, and rats, ovarian hemorrhagic necrosis was seen within 24 h after administration of 1–3 mg Cd/kg of body weight (Kar et al. 1959, Rehm and Waalkes 1988). Cd administration to rats and hens alters ovarian steroidogenesis, associated with a reduction in progesterone secretion and release in a dose- and age-dependent manner (Piasek and Laskey 1994, Yang et al. 2012). Wistar rats exposed to Cd *in vivo* (at 2.5, 5, 7.5 mg/kg, as a single s.c. dose) had decreased progesterone levels. Ovarian granulosa cells treated with 0, 10, 20, or 40 μM $CdCl_2$ *in vitro* had dose-dependent decreases in progesterone levels as a result of decreased expression of StAR and P450scc (Zhang and Jia 2007). Cd suppressed FSH-induced expansion of cumulus–oocyte complexes, granulosa cell differentiation and decreased progesterone production (Mlynarcíkova et al. 2004). Cd also decreased progesterone production in primary cultures of rat and human ovarian granulosa cells (Paksy et al. 1997, Zhang and Jia 2007). Cd, at concentrations as low as 1 μM, significantly decreased the germ cell density in human fetal ovaries and increased germ cell apoptosis (Angenard et al. 2010). High concentrations of Cd exposure (1.2 mg/mL) inhibited germinal vesicle breakdown and oocyte maturation (Wan et al. 2010). In the porcine granulosa cell line JC-410, high concentrations (5 μM) of $CdCl_2$ inhibited P450scc gene promoter activity and caused a reduction in cell number. Low concentrations of Cd (0.6–3 μM) activated expression of the P450scc gene (Smida et al. 2004). Cd affects estrous cycles of rats by inhibiting ovulation and thus inducing infertility (Paksy et al. 1990). Ovarian hemorrhagic necrosis was reported in hamsters and rats injected with 20–45 μmol/kg of $CdCl_2$ (s.c) after 24–96 h (Rehm and Waalkes 1988). Small arteries of the developing follicles and stroma are selectively vulnerable to Cd toxicity. Electron microscopy of the ovary treated with Cd revealed undulation of the nuclear membrane in granulosa cells while theca cells exhibited dilated endoplasmic reticulum (ER), and cytoplasmic vacuolization was observed in the stromal cells. Ovarian endothelial cells exhibited dilated mitochondria with altered inner membranes missing cristae (Massányi et al. 2007a). Long-term treatment with Cd disintegrates chromatin and alters mitochondrial architecture (Massányi et al. 2007b). Pretreatment with zinc acetate and selenium markedly reduced Cd-induced ovarian lesions in hamsters (Khan et al. 1992). It is evident from various studies that a Cd-induced adverse effect on the ovary is through oxidative stress and depletion of antioxidants, such as superoxide dismutase (SOD) and glutathione peroxidase (GPx). Subcutaneous injection of $CdCl_2$ in pregnant rats on day 6 of gestation reduced the size of the ovary, inhibited folliculogenesis, and diminished numbers of primordial, growing, and antral follicles of F1 females on postnatal day 21. Cd also induced hypertrophy of follicular cells with cytoplasmic vacuolization (Bekheet 2011).

Cd-induced atresia of primary and growing follicles was reduced by co-administration of Zn and Se (Nad et al. 2007). Since Zn is a Cd antagonist, adequate Zn in the diet affords some protection from the adverse effects of Cd. Adult zebrafish exposed to 0.4 mg/L Cd in water and supplemented with Zn (5 mg/kg) in their diet for 21 days decreased the expression of Zn transporter 1 (ZnT1) and caused upregulation of Zrt-, Irt-related protein 10 (ZIP10), and metallothionein (MT) gene expression. These changes were accompanied by increased Cd and MT accumulation, decreased Zn content, as well as by histopathological damage in ovarian tissues. The co-exposure of zebrafish to Cd and Zn abolished ZnT1 downregulation and increased ZIP10 mRNA levels. Zn treatment also decreased Cd and MT accumulation, reversed Cd-induced Zn depletion, and partially restored Cd-induced histological changes in ovarian tissues. Thus, the protective effect of dietary Zn supplementation against Cd-induced ovarian toxicity is mediated by increased bioavailability of Zn, and through increased Zn transport (Chouchene et al. 2011). The concentrations of Ca, Cu, Zn, Fe, and Se in the diet can have a dramatic effect on Cd absorption and metabolism (He et al. 2005, Massanyi et al. 2005). Moderating the doses of these metals in the diet could serve as an intervention strategy to control the levels of Cd intake in the body.

9.5 CHROMIUM

9.5.1 Background

Hexavalent chromium (CrVI) is widely used in various industries such as chrome plating, welding, wood processing, and tanneries (Nriagu 1988). The extensive toxicokinetic and genotoxic literature associated with oral exposures to CrVI in animals and humans indicates that CrVI causes various health hazards including cancers, dermatitis, damage to the liver and kidneys, infertility in both males and females, defects in embryo/fetal development, and developmental problems in young children (Junaid et al. 1996, Kamath et al. 1997, Kanojia et al. 1998, Makarov and Shimtova 1978, Murthy et al. 1996, Zhitkovich 2005). Chromium (Cr) usage is increasing exponentially worldwide; and Cr pollution is a continuous, ongoing problem (Blacksmith Institute 2007, Sutton 2010, Zhitkovich 2005, Zhitkovich et al. 2005). CrVI gets into water supplies after being discharged from steel and pulp mills as well as metal plating and leather-tanning facilities (Sutton 2010). It can also pollute water through erosion of soil and rock (Sutton 2010). According to the Blacksmith Institute, various drinking water sources such as lakes, rivers, and wells in developing countries are highly polluted with CrVI, where its concentration far exceeds the USEPA approved safer limits in drinking water of 0.05 mg/L for total Cr (Blacksmith Institute 2007). A recent report from the Environmental Working Group (EWG) indicates increasing CrVI levels in 35 cities in the United States (Sutton 2010). At least 74 million people in nearly 7000 communities drink tap water polluted with total chromium; and 1.7 million people in 42 communities from New Jersey drink tap water polluted with total Cr which includes hexavalent and other forms of the metal in the United States (Sutton 2010).

Unlike most other divalent metal ions, CrVI is unique, specific, and behaves like an anion due to its structural similarity with anions (such as $CrO4^{2-}$, $HCrO^{4-}$ and $SO4^{2-}$) (Sahmoune and Mitiche 2009). Due to its anionic nature, CrVI is rapidly transported into cells through anion transporters and reduced to CrIII by various antioxidants such as ascorbate (vitamin C), GSH, cysteine, and antioxidant enzymes (Jomova and Valko 2011, Valko et al. 2005). CrIII has been considered to be less toxic than CrVI. However, *in utero* exposure of mice to CrIII (chromium chloride, 375 or 750 mg/kg body weight/day) or CrVI (potassium dichromate, 12.5 or 25 mg/kg body weight/day) resulted in significantly increased genotoxicity by CrIII rather than CrVI in postnatal day 20 offspring (Kirpnick-Sobol et al. 2006). Thus, it is evident that CrIII is more toxic than CrVI once inside the cells.

Once CrVI crosses a biological membrane, it is reduced to CrIII by various antioxidants, predominantly by vitamin C and GSH. Eventually, all the CrVI that enters a cell is reduced to CrIII. Vitamin C reduces CrVI in target tissues such as lung, liver, and kidney (Zhitkovich 2005, Zhitkovich et al. 2005). In general, the intracellular concentration of vitamin C is very high, and maximum levels of vitamin C (~1 to 5 mM) are present in the ovary, brain, and placenta. Vitamin C is concentrated in granulosa and theca cells of the ovarian follicle, luteal cells of the corpus luteum, and cytoplasm of the oocyte (Deane 1952, Hoch-Ligeti and Bourne 1948). Vitamin C uptake by granulosa cells in rats is hormonally regulated. Vitamin C plays a vital role in follicular development, implantation, and maintenance of healthy pregnancy. Conversely, vitamin C deficiency in guinea pigs results in anovulation with marked follicular degeneration (Kramer et al. 1933). Vitamin C has been considered to be one of the major fertility factors in primates as it prevents apoptosis in cultured ovarian follicles and inhibits follicular atresia (Millar 1992). Vitamin C acts as a potent water-soluble antioxidant in biological fluids by scavenging physiologically relevant reactive oxygen and nitrogen species (Carr and Frei 1999, Padayatty et al. 2003). These include free radicals including hydroxyl radicals, aqueous peroxyl radicals, superoxide anion, and nitrogen dioxide, as well as nonradical species such as hypochlorous acid, ozone, singlet oxygen, nitrosating species, nitroxide, and peroxynitrite. Vitamin C interacts with free radicals scavenging reactive oxygen and nitrogen species. It can also regenerate other antioxidants, such as α-tocopherol, GSH, and β-carotene, from their respective radical species (Berger et al. 1997, Padayatty et al. 2003, Padayatty and Levine 2001). Therefore, vitamin C is not only a reducing agent of CrVI but also an essential antioxidant for female reproductive functions.

9.5.2 Chromium and the Ovary

9.5.2.1 Exposure to Chromium Disrupts Follicle Development and Decreases Steroid Hormone Synthesis

Oral administration of mice with 5 or 10 mg/kg body weight potassium dichromate (CrVI) resulted in increased lipid peroxide (LPO) levels indicating increased oxidative stress, and decreased GSH, vitamin C, SOD, and catalase in the ovary. Vitamin E supplementation mitigated CrVI-induced oxidative stress, and prevented depletion of antioxidants (Rao et al. 2009). Cr disrupted ovarian function in women working in chromium industries who exhibited increased levels of Cr in their blood and urine. Those women experienced abnormal menses, infertility, or increased postpartum bleeding (Makarov and Shimtova 1978). Oral treatment of rabbits with sodium dichromate produces sclerotic and atrophic changes in the ovaries (Kucher 1966). Swiss albino female mice (90 days old) treated with either high doses (250, 500, and 750 ppm) or low doses (0.05, 0.5, and 5 ppm) of potassium dichromate for 20 days caused reduction in the number of small, medium, and large follicles, and reduced the number of oocytes collected after superovulation. The highest-dosed group (750 ppm Cr) revealed a large number of atretic follicles having degenerative cumulus cells showing dense pyknotic nuclei and karyorrhexis in follicular cells (Murthy et al. 1996). A few ovaries (30%) were completely hemolytic, showing erythrocytes throughout the stromal spaces. Most of the oocytes were surrounded by an incomplete layer of cumulus cells or were without the surrounding cumulus cells. Effective communication between cumulus cells and the oocyte is critical for the development of the oocyte and successful maturation and fertilization (Huang and Wells 2010). Thus, CrVI targets cumulus granulosa cells in mice.

Findings from our laboratory demonstrated toxic effects of Cr on the ovary and multiple mechanisms behind the adverse effects of exposure to CrVI (Banu et al. 2008, 2011, Stanley et al. 2011, 2013). When lactating mother rats were exposed to CrVI (50, 100, and 200 ppm) from postpartum day 1–21, CrVI is converted to CrIII in cells and body fluids (Barceloux 1999, Zhitkovich 2011) and transferred through the breast milk. This resulted in the accumulation of CrIII in the blood and the ovary of F1 pups. Lactational exposure to CrIII during postnatal age extended estrous cycle, delayed follicular development, arrested the growth or development of follicles at the secondary follicle stage, decreased the number of healthy follicles (primordial, primary, secondary, and antral), and increased follicular atresia in PND 21 rats (Figure 9.1). Cr also delayed pubertal onset, and decreased levels of testosterone, estradiol, and progesterone in F1 rats. Vitamin C protected ovaries from the deleterious effects of CrIII *in vivo*. When spontaneously immortalized rat granulosa

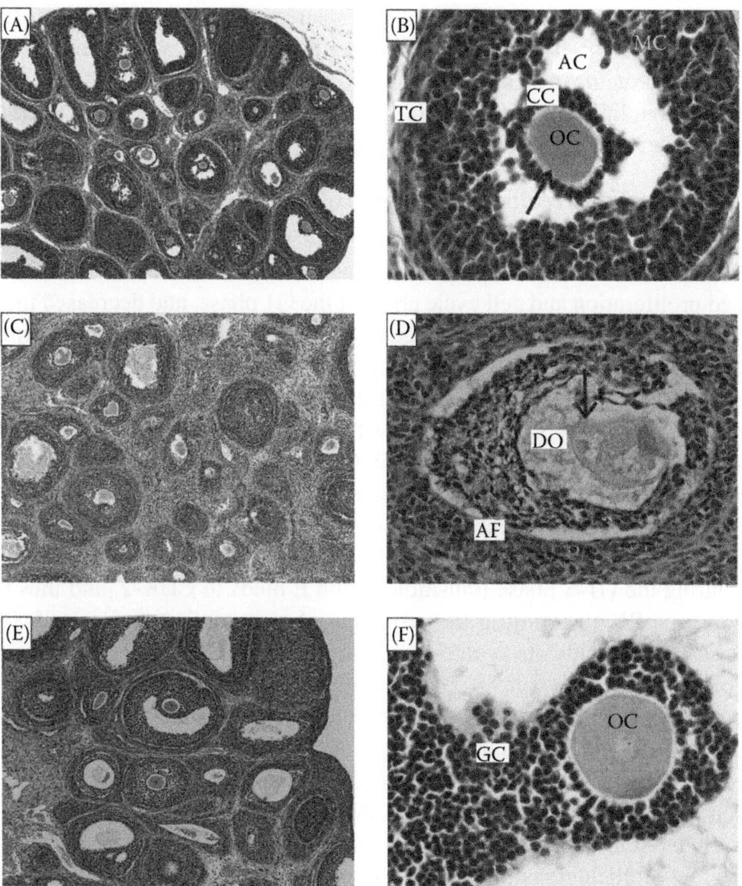

FIGURE 9.1 **(See color insert.)** Histology of the ovary in postnatal day (PND) 21 rats exposed to chromium through mother's milk from PND 1–21: Lactating mother rats were divided into three groups and given the following treatments from postpartum (PP) days 1–21: (A and B): Group 1 ($n=5$) received regular drinking water (control); (C and D): Group 2 ($n=5$) received drinking water with 'CrVI (50 ppm potassium dichromate); and (E and F): Group 3 ($n=5$) received drinking water with CrVI (50 ppm potassium dichromate) and were supplemented with vitamin C (500 mg/kg body weight) through gavage. During this period, the F1 female offsprings ($n=20$, i.e., five pups per mother) were exposed to Cr through mother's milk from PND 1–21. On PND 21, F1 female rats were euthanized and the ovaries were fixed in 4% buffered formalin for 24 h, transferred to cold 70% ethanol until paraffin embedding, sectioned at 5 μm, and stained with H and E. High-power magnification of a healthy follicle (B) shows a single oocyte (OC), several layers of mural granulosa cells (MC) and cumulus cells (CC), an intact basal lamina and theca cell layers (TC). High-power magnification of a follicle from a Cr-exposed rat (D) shows that the oocyte has degenerated (DO) and the somatic cells have undergone atresia. Vitamin C inhibited the adverse effects of Cr on the ovary. High-power magnification of a follicle from a Cr-exposed rat supplemented with vitamin C (F) shows a healthy follicle with an oocyte and several layers of granulosa cells. OC, oocyte; AC, antral cavity; CC, cumulus cells; MC, mural cells; AF, atretic follicle; DO, degenerated oocyte. (A,C,E) = 10× magnification; (B,D,F) = 40× magnification.

cells (SIGC) were treated with CrVI *in vitro*, decreased mRNA expression of StAR, SF-1, 17β-HSD-1, 17β-HSD-2, LHR, FSHR, ERα, and ERβ was observed, each of which are key proteins in steroid biosynthetic and signaling machinery that regulate ovarian function. Interestingly, vitamin C mitigated the adverse effect of CrIII on the ovary and protected the follicles from atresia.

9.5.2.2 Chromium Treatment Delayed Follicle Development by Altering Cell Cycle Regulatory Proteins

Granulosa cells isolated from prepubertal rats treated with 10 μM CrVI exhibited decreased proliferation and cell cycle arrest at the G1 phase, and decreased the number of cells in S and G2-M phases. In granulosa cells, CrVI decreased protein levels of G1-S phase regulators CDK-4, -6 and cyclins D2 and D3, and vitamin C mitigated CrVI effects on CDK-4, -6, and cyclin D2. These data suggest that accumulation of granulosa cells at the G1-phase is due to downregulation of CDK-4, -6/D-type cyclins. Pretreatment of cells with vitamin C (1 mM) mitigated or prevented CrVI-induced changes in G1-phase CDKs and cyclins (Stanley et al. 2011).

Treatment with CrVI decreased S-phase granulosa cell populations. The association of cyclin E with CDK2 is active at the G1/S transition and directs entry into S phase. During the G1-S phase transition, cyclin E binds to CDK-2, and thus hyperphosphorylates Rb, resulting in the activation of transcription factors and S-phase proteins such as thymidylate synthase and dihydrofolate reductase. S-phase progression is directed by the cyclin A/CDK2 complex (Malumbres 2011). CrVI treatment downregulated cyclin E2 and CDK-2 in granulosa cells, whereas vitamin C mitigated CrVI effects on cyclin E2 and its counterpart CDK-2 in granulosa cells.

Exposure to CrVI *in vitro* also altered CDK inhibitors p15, p16, and p27. p27 negatively regulates cyclin E/CDK2 and cyclin A/CDK2 complexes, and is a predominant CDK-inhibitor in the mammalian ovary, which tightly regulates primordial to primary follicle transition. p27-knockout mice have an accelerated primordial to primary follicle transition that exhausts follicle reserve prematurely leading to infertility (Edson et al. 2009). CrVI treatment upregulated p15, p16, and p27 in granulosa cells, while vitamin C mitigated CrVI effects. PCNA is required during DNA replication (Jaskulski et al. 1988), and is expressed in the nuclear matrix of cells during all phases of the cell cycle, reaching a maximum in S and G2-phase (Casasco et al. 1988). Expression of PCNA in granulosa cells begins with the formation of a primary follicle and its level of expression increases during the FSH-dependent stages of preovulatory follicular development (Oktay et al. 1995). CrVI treatment decreased PCNA in granulosa cells and vitamin C mitigated the CrVI-induced decrease in PCNA. This observation suggested that the CrVI-induced decrease in follicle number and delay/arrest in follicle development at the secondary follicular stage (Banu et al. 2011) might also be due to decreased PCNA levels, in addition to its effects on cell cycle machinery. In G2-M phase check point, cyclin A associates with CDK1 (also known as cdc2). CDK1/cyclin B assembly is active for mitosis to occur (Pomerening 2009). CrVI treatment decreased cell populations in the G2-M phase in granulosa cells, and vitamin C mitigated the effect of CrVI. CrVI treatment decreased cyclin B1/CDK-1 in granulosa cells, which was mitigated by vitamin C. Thus, *in vitro* exposure to CrVI delayed cells from entering into, and progressing through the G2-M phase by decreasing the levels of cyclins A and B1, and CDK-1, which could be prevented by vitamin C (Stanley et al. 2011).

9.5.2.3 Chromium Treatment Induced Granulosa Cell Apoptosis by Altering Subcellular Localization of Bcl-2 Family Members, p53 and ERK1/2

CrVI-induced apoptosis in Chinese hamster ovary (CHO) cells involves disruption of mitochondrial stability. Treatment with sodium chromate increased time-dependent release of mitochondrial cytochrome *c* (cyt *c*) in cytosolic extracts of CHO cells. Co-treatment of these cells with cyclosporine A (a cytochrome *c* inhibitor) inhibited the release of cyt *c* and abrogated CrVI-induced apoptosis and DNA fragmentation. In contrast, the general caspase inhibitor, Z-VAD-FMK, markedly inhibited most of the morphological and biochemical parameters of apoptosis, but did not prevent cyt *c* release. These results suggest that the mitochondrial permeability transition plays an important role in the regulation of ovarian cells (Pritchard et al. 2000). Lactational exposure of rat offspring (F1) to CrIII, accelerated granulosa cell apoptosis and follicular atresia (Stanley et al. 2013). Figure 9.1 shows representative images of the paraffin-embedded sections of the ovary, stained with hematoxylin and eosin. The underlying molecular and cellular mechanisms that regulate CrIII-induced follicular atresia/apoptosis are not known. Findings from our laboratory reveal that CrVI treatment induced apoptosis of granulosa cells *in vitro* through multiple mechanisms such as mitochondria-mediated intrinsic apoptosis, p53-mediated apoptosis, and ROS-mediated apoptosis (Banu et al. 2011, Stanley et al. 2011). Bcl-2 family members Bcl-2, Bcl-XL, Bax, and Bad proteins are the key mediators of the intrinsic apoptotic pathway. In addition, HSP70 protects cells against apoptosis by inhibiting translocation of BAX protein from the cytosol to the mitochondria, release of cytochrome *c* from the mitochondria into the cytosol, and activation of caspase-3 and PARP proteins (Bivik et al. 2007, Joly et al. 2010, Stankiewicz et al. 2005). Treatment with CrVI decreased expression of anti-apoptotic and cell survival proteins Bcl-2, Bcl-XL, HSP70, and HSP90; translocated BAX and BAD proteins from cytosol to the mitochondria; increased mitochondrial membrane permeability facilitating the release of cytochrome *c*; and activated caspase-3 and PARP proteins leading to apoptosis of granulosa cells (Banu et al. 2011). These results suggest that treatment with CrVI attenuates anti-apoptotic pathways in order to stabilize pro-apoptotic members to execute apoptosis of granulosa cells.

DNA damage promotes phosphorylation and subsequent stabilization of p53 and leads to apoptosis (Meek and Anderson 2009). Phosphorylation of p53 at multiple serine residues is required for apoptosis (Kurihara et al. 2007). Phosphorylation of p53 at ser-15 can be induced by oxidative stress (Long et al. 2007), H_2O_2 (Verschoor et al. 2010), ionization (Sluss et al. 2010), and UV irradiation (Milne et al. 1995). Treatment with CrVI induced selective translocation of active p53 protein into mitochondria in granulosa cells *in vitro*. p53-mediated cell death is primarily routed through mitochondrial pathways (Schuler and Green 2001), which require translocation of p53 protein into mitochondria (Zhao et al. 2005). Recent studies showed translocation of p53 from the cytosol to mitochondria and its association with antioxidants and apoptotic proteins (Galluzzi et al. 2011, Holley et al. 2010,

Pani et al. 2004, Siu et al. 2009). Mitochondrial translocation of p53 triggers a rapid pro-apoptotic response (Erster and Moll 2004). After translocation, p53 protein could interact with endogenous anti-apoptotic Bcl-XL and/or Bcl-2 protein, induce oligomerization of Bak protein, increase permeabilization of the outer mitochondrial membrane in order to facilitate cytochrome *c* release (Mihara et al. 2003), or interact with MnSOD and inhibit its ability to scavenge free radicals (Holley et al. 2010).

Lactational exposure to CrIII (50, 100, and 200 ppm) increased free radical generation, depleted antioxidant levels including vitamin C in plasma and the ovary of F1 female rats. Furthermore, CrVI (10 μM) decreased mRNA levels of cytosolic and mitochondrial antioxidant enzymes in primary cultures of granulosa and theca cells *in vitro* (Stanley et al. 2013). Moreover, recent findings have documented a role for delayed and sustained ERK activation in apoptosis (Gladys et al. 1999, Stanciu and DeFranco 2002). It is evident that CrVI induced increased activation and selective translocation of ERK1/2 into nuclei and mitochondria. ERK1/2 also is one of the upstream candidates for p53 phosphorylation in granulosa cells exposed to CrVI. Mono-ubiquitination has been found to be involved in the selective translocation of proteins (Li et al. 2003), while poly-ubiquitination plays key roles in proteasome-mediated degradation of proteins (Burger and Seth 2004, Glickman and Ciechanover 2002). At this point, it is not clear whether Cr is involved in these processes in the ovary. Clearly, multiple mechanisms are involved in Cr-induced apoptosis of granulosa cells and follicular atresia. Figure 9.2 shows schematic diagrams of chromium-mediated apoptosis of granulosa cells and atresia of ovarian follicles and cell cycle arrest and delayed development of ovarian follicles.

9.6 COPPER

9.6.1 Background

Based on the results of the U.S. Department of Agriculture 1989–1991 survey of food consumption, about 40% of dietary copper (Cu) comes from yeast breads, white potatoes, tomatoes, cereals, beef, and dried beans and lentils (Subar et al. 1998). Cu plumbing was hailed as a great advance in the 1940s, and today the majority of homes in the United States have Cu plumbing. In areas with acidic water, Cu can be leached from pipes, leaving in severe cases a greenish ring on bathroom fixtures. Water coolers and ice-makers in refrigerators also use Cu tubing. Water from these units can contain very high levels of Cu. Cu tea kettles and other Cu cookware can be a source of Cu toxicity if used frequently over a period of time (Eck and Wilson 1989). Some areas of the United States have high amounts of naturally occurring Cu in their water supply. Also, Cu sulfate is added to some municipal drinking water supplies to kill yeast and fungi. Cu sulfate is added to swimming pools and may be sprayed on fruits and vegetables to retard growth of algae and fungus. Plumbers, welders, machinists, and others who work with Cu are at risk for Cu toxicity. Cu is also used in dental alloys in fillings, crowns, and other appliances. The majority of plasma Cu is transported bound to ceruloplasmin (>75%), whereas the remainder is bound to albumin, transcuprein, and Cu–amino acid complexes (Blakley and Hamilton 1985). The concentration of free Cu ions in human plasma is 10^{-13} M.

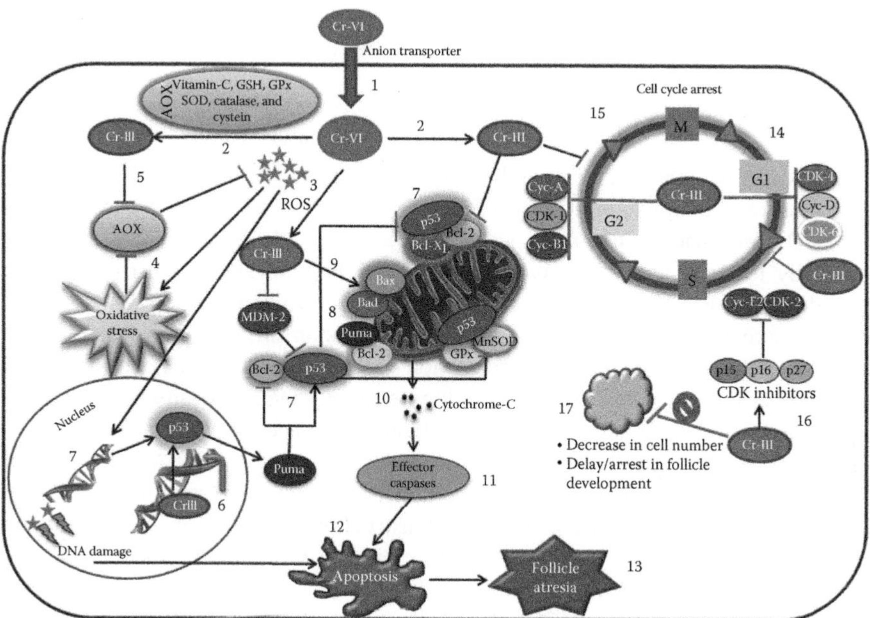

FIGURE 9.2 Schematic diagram of chromium-mediated apoptosis in granulosa cells, atresia of ovarian follicles (1–13), cell cycle arrest, and delayed development of ovarian follicles (14–17). (1) CrVI is taken up by cells via the anionic transport system; (2) CrVI is reduced to CrIII by antioxidants (AOX), predominantly vitamin C and GSH; (3) Large amounts of reactive oxygen species (ROS) are generated during the reduction of CrVI to CrIII; (4) AOX are consumed by cells to quench excess ROS resulting in decreased AOX levels; (5) CrIII downregulates mRNA expression of AOX genes, and decreases AOX; (6) CrIII binds to DNA, forms DNA-adducts, and induces mutation; (7) Free radicals can also directly induce DNA damage. DNA damage/mutation results in the upregulation of p53; (8) P53 increases p53 upregulated modulator of apoptosis (PUMA) and binds to Bcl2 localized on the mitochondrial membrane; (9) CrIII upregulates pro-apoptotic Bax and Bad proteins. All of these events change the mitochondrial membrane potential, and (10) are accompanied by the release of cytochrome *c* and (11) activation of effector caspases, resulting in (12) apoptosis of granulosa cells and (13) atresia of ovarian follicles. CrIII arrests the G1-S (14) and G2-M (15) phases of the cell cycle by decreasing cyclins and CDKs required for progression of cells through the cell cycle. (16) CrIII upregulates CDK inhibitors (p15, p16, and p27), resulting in cell cycle arrest and a (17) delay in follicle development. ⊣-indicates inhibition and arrow indicates stimulation.

Cu bound to these carriers has been reported to be the less tightly bound and is exchangeable (Gupte and Mumper 2009). The relationship between Cu and GSH has been investigated. Cu is a biological ligand forming binary complexes with GSH (Picco et al. 2012). A large store of GSH during oocyte maturation was shown to be important for cumulus expansion *in vitro* and embryo protection up to the blastocyst stage (Furnus et al. 1998, Takahashi et al. 1993). Cu is a component of a number of metalloenzymes, including cytochrome C oxidase, superoxide dismutase, glutathione peroxidase and transferase, tyrosine, dopamine β-hydroxylase, amino oxidase, lysyl oxidase, ceruloplasmin, and enzymes of fatty acid metabolism (Ferrer and Moreno 1992, Prohaska 1983, Sharma and Sharma 1997).

9.6.2 Copper and the Ovary

Cu is toxic in its unbound form, and causes redox imbalance due to its highly redox active nature (Cunningham et al. 1995, Evans et al. 2002). Cu intrauterine devices (Cu-IUDs) are one of the most cost-effective reversible birth control methods, especially for long-term use (Avecilla-Palau and Moreno 2003). Cu release from these devices is necessary for their contraceptive effect (Zipper et al. 1979). However, overexposure can produce a wide spectrum of effects on surrounding cells. The biological response depends on the concentration of ions released and the exposure time, among other factors. Since Cu-IUD is in long-term intimate proximity with local tissue, it may exert significant *in situ* adverse effects. Cu concentrations of uterine washings were 0.7 and 0.9 mg/L for IUD nonusers, while those with T-380A IUDs showed concentrations that varied according to their menstrual cycle (i.e., proliferative phase: 5.9 ± 1.8; secretory phase: 10.4 ± 4.9 and menstruation: 12.6 ± 5.4 mg/L) (Arancibia et al. 2003). Cu extracts (5.67–7.42 mg/L, clinically relevant Cu concentration of IUD users) cause potential cytotoxicity and genotoxicity in Chinese hamster ovary (CHO-K1) cells (Grillo et al. 2010). Cu ions reduced cell viability and increased DNA fragmentation in CHO cells (Jose et al. 2011). Six- to eight-week-old mice treated by gavage with 100 or 200 mg/kg CuSO4 for 5 weeks revealed an increased number of atretic follicles with degenerated oocytes and pyknotic granulosa cells (Fasano et al. 2011). Thus, Cu toxicity results in the death of ovarian follicles. In another study, estimates of Cu, Mn, and Fe in follicular fluid and granulosa cells of small, medium, and large atretic follicles as well as healthy follicles were obtained from ovaries collected from normal cycling goats. All three metals were higher in the atretic follicles compared to healthy follicles (Bhardwaj and Sharma 2011).

9.6.3 Copper and Cancer of the Ovary

The mean serum Cu level was significantly higher in ovarian carcinoma patients (316 μg/dL) compared to the control group (116 μg/dL). Rate of metastasis was also higher in ovarian cancer patients exhibiting increased Cu levels in serum (Zowczak et al. 2001a,b). Cu chelators are known to reduce angiogenesis in cancers and recommended as a potential anticancer strategy (Finney et al. 2009). Moreover, the serum Cu/Zn ratio also increased in patients with benign and malignant ovarian cancer compared to controls indicating that the Cu/Zn ratio may be used as a marker for malignancy and prognosis for ovarian cancers (Finney et al. 2009). Tumor cells contain relatively high concentrations of Cu compared to normal healthy tissues (Daniel et al. 2005). In cancer and inflammation, plasma Cu and ceruloplasmin concentrations rise and rates of synthesis and secretion of ceruloplasmin by the liver are also enhanced. Increases in ceruloplasmin and serum Cu levels in ovarian cancer patients have been reported (Nayak et al. 2004). The elevated ceruloplasmin concentrations increase Cu uptake by cells in both normal tissues and cancer cells. Ceruloplasmin also functions as an endogenous angiogenic stimulator (Brewer 2005) as Cu enhances angiogenesis in cancer (Zowczak et al. 2001b). Cu is exported from cells by one of two efflux pumps, ATP7A and ATP7B. ATP7A is expressed in most tissues other than liver, whereas ATP7B is expressed predominantly in the liver. Interestingly, increased expression of Cu efflux transporter ATP7A provides ovarian carcinoma cells with increased resistance to the chemotherapeutic drug cisplatin (Samimi et al. 2004). There is an association between high levels of mRNA for ATP7B in ovarian cancer and poor survival of ovarian cancer patients (Nakayama et al. 2002). These studies clearly indicate the importance of Cu in the pathogenesis of ovarian cancer. However, more studies are needed to understand the mechanism of Cu in promoting ovarian cancers.

9.7 IRON

9.7.1 Background

Iron (Fe) is an metallic element that makes up about 5% of the Earth's crust. Rainwater percolating through soil and rock dissolves minerals containing iron and holds them in solution. The water's hardness and acidity influence the amount of iron that will dissolve during the percolation process. These iron-rich waters recharge surface waters and aquifers that inevitably serve as drinking water sources. Often, corrosion also can be a source of iron in drinking water. Iron contamination as a result of corroded pipes is a common occurrence in many cities that have very old water systems (Colter and Mahler 2006).

9.7.2 Iron and the Ovary

Iron toxicity to the anterior pituitary results in decreased synthesis of lutenizing hormone (LH) and follicle-stimulating hormone (FSH) (Bergeron and Kovacs 1978). A recent study evaluated the effect of iron burden on hypogonadism and diminished ovarian reserve, and on infertility in thalassemia major (TM) women (Singer et al. 2011). Iron burden in the ovary of TM women has an inverse correlation with anti-mullerian hormone (AMH) levels and non-transferrin-bound iron (NTBI) (Cabantchik et al. 2005). An increase in ROS and lower enzymatic antioxidant defense mechanisms have been shown to accelerate follicle aging (Tarin 1996). High redox activity in the ovarian follicular fluid of a TM woman was reported, signifying that redox-active iron ions mediate free radical production, inducing oxidative injury in ovarian tissue (Reubinoff et al. 1996). A low antioxidant capacity is demonstrated in TM patients with low ascorbic acid levels. Overweight and obese women with PCOS have increased serum ferritin levels indicating increased iron stores. In PCOS patients, increased iron stores contribute to insulin resistance and hyperinsulinemia. Therefore, the reduction in body iron stores with the drug metformin may be favorable in overweight and obese women with PCOS (Escobar-Morreale 2012).

During follicular atresia and luteal regression, heme oxygenase-1 (HO-1), an enzyme-catalyzing heme degradation, was observed in apoptotic granulosa cells in atretic follicles (Harada et al. 2004), resulting in the release of iron ions from heme structures. Free iron ions, particularly ferrous iron ions, increase free radical generation through the Haber-Weiss reaction (Crichton et al. 2002, Gutteridge and Halliwell 1989, 2000), resulting in oxidative damage. Distribution of nonheme iron in ovarian tissue was studied in the ovaries of mice at 7 weeks of age (immature), at 13 weeks of age (adult), and at 46 and 63 weeks of age (aged, including late- and postreproductive age) (Asano 2012). The results demonstrated accumulation of nonheme iron in mouse ovarian stromal tissue during aging. In addition, the colocalization of nonheme ferric iron [NHF-III] and nonheme ferrous iron [NHF-II] in the mouse ovary strongly suggested the elevation of redox-active iron levels in aged ovaries. Elucidation of the molecular mechanisms of nonheme iron accumulation in the aging ovary may help us to understand the role of nonheme iron on the decline in ovarian function with aging.

Increased iron uptake associated with the iron storage disease hemochromatosis is also associated with a higher incidence of ovarian cancer. The frequency of two mutations (C282Y, H63D) in heterozygous carriers of the hemochromatosis gene was assessed in 677 women consisting of 80 controls, 124 benign, 96 with low metastatic potential, and 264 women with invasive ovarian tumors. The proportion of women with a single allele of the C282Y mutation was significantly elevated in women with benign tumors and ovarian cancers (8%–9%) compared with the control group (2.5%). This was reflected in a 4.9-fold increase in the risk of developing ovarian cancer. Survival rates for women with high-grade serous ovarian cancer with the heterozygous C282Y mutation were reduced from 39 to 19 months (Gannon et al. 2011, Robertson 2011). It is evident from the previous reports that increased iron burden is deleterious to the ovary, and could predispose to the development of ovarian cancers.

9.8 LEAD

9.8.1 Background

Lead (Pb) is an ubiquitous environmental and industrial pollutant (Schell et al. 2010). Pb concentrations have increased in the atmosphere as a consequence of extensive industrialization and environmental pollution (Bindler 2011). Major sources of Pb exposure include Pb in paint, gasoline, water distribution systems, food, and Pb used in hobby activities. Pb has been used to make petroleum products, glass panels, crafts, batteries, jewelry pencils, colored newsprints, etc. Between 1976 and 1990, Pb used in gasoline declined by 99.8% in the United States, but not in other countries where Pb is permitted in gasoline (Jooste and Anelich 2008). Pb poisoning is an environmental and public health hazard of global proportions. Children and adults in virtually every region of the world are being exposed to unsafe levels of lead in the environment. In fact, children are exposed to lead from different sources, such as paint, gasoline, and solder, and through different pathways such as air, food, water, dust, and soil. Although all U.S. children are exposed to some lead from food, air, dust, and soil, some children are exposed to high-dose sources of Pb. Pb-based paint is the most widespread source of Pb exposure for preschool children (Morrison et al. 2012). Throughout the 1940s and 1950s, lead-based paint was in widespread use. It continued to be used in lower concentrations until the mid-1970s. The manufacture of paint containing high concentrations of lead for interior and exterior residential surfaces, toys, and furniture was banned in 1978 by the Consumer Product Safety Commission. Although lead-containing paint was banned for residential use in the United States in 1978, residential paint in older buildings is the most frequent source of Pb exposure in young children (Mushak and Crocetti 1990). High Pb content is estimated to be in 74% of all housing built before 1980. Those housing units containing deteriorating Pb-based are a major concern. Of even greater concern are these homes that have young children as occupants (GAO 1993).

9.8.2 Lead and the Ovary

Pb disrupts follicle development and maturation and increases follicular atresia in the mouse ovary (Crystel et al. 2001, Junaid et al. 1995, Ouarda and Abdennour 2008). It decreases the cumulus cell population (Hilderbrand et al. 1973) and steroidogenesis (Thoreux-Manlay et al. 1995). Pb decreases binding affinity of LH and FSH to their respective receptors, which is mitigated by GSH (Priya et al. 2004). Intraperitoneal (i.p.) injection of $Pb(NO_3)$ to female mice (10 mg/kg/day) for 15 days or 15 weeks resulted in Pb accumulation in several soft tissues including the ovary. Pb increased antral follicle degeneration and decreased primordial follicle number and decreased the number of corporea lutea (Hilderbrand et al. 1973). The ovaries from Pb-exposed mice contained atretic antral follicles with detached granulosa cells, pyknotic nuclei in the granulosa cells, and a hypertrophy of theca cell layers (Taupeau et al. 2001). Pb also induced premature germinal vesicle breakdown and early resumption of meiosis in the oocytes (Shen et al. 2000). In addition, Pb induced ovulation failure with decreased number of healthy antral follicles (Pollack et al. 2011). Pb-intoxicated Rhesus monkeys (Vermande and Meigs 1960) and rats (Stowe and Moore 1971) had decreased healthy follicle numbers with increased follicle atresia.

When adult pregnant female rats were subcutaneously injected with Pb acetate (0.05 mg/kg of body weight per day) throughout the gestational and lactational periods and sacrificed on postnatal day 56, the activities of key steroidogenic enzymes (17β-hydroxysteroid dehydrogenase and 3β-hydroxysteroid dehydrogenase) were decreased in the ovary. Pb also decreased serum estradiol and progesterone levels, ovarian steroidogenic acute regulatory protein (StAR) and CYP11 mRNA levels, and ovarian cholesterol content. The Pb-induced decrease in ovarian steroidogenesis was mediated through increased oxidative stress and diminished antioxidant levels (superoxide dismutase, catalase, and glutathione peroxidase).

9.9 MANGANESE

9.9.1 Background

Manganese (Mn) is an essential trace element. Mn is used as a fungicide, an antiknock agent in gasoline, and a contrasting agent in nuclear magnetic resonance tomography. Millions of kilograms of Mn is released into the air and surface waters each year in the United States (Howe et al. 2004), but releases prior to the mid-twentieth century are unreported. Steel, iron, and ferroalloy manufacturing industries are the primary industrial emitters of Mn (80%), although coal burning, gasoline, and refuse incineration also emit Mn (Herndon and Brantley 2011). Mn generally precipitates as redox-sensitive, poorly crystalline oxides in soils, which can mobilize or strongly absorb metal contaminants such as Cr, Co, and Ni (Herndon and Brantley 2011, Pohl 2011, Suarez and Langmuir 1976). High Mn bioavailability in soils can lead to Mn toxicity in plants and has been implicated in the dieback (a plant disease caused by acid rain, heavy metal pollution, or pathogens) of sugar maples throughout the northeastern United States (Adriano 2001, Kogelmann and Sharpe 2006). According to the Toxics Release Inventory (TRI), in 2006, a total of 12,290 MT of Mn was released to the environment from 2,040 large processing facilities (TRI06 2008). An additional 90,630 MT of Mn compounds was released from 1,748 facilities in the United States (ATSDR 2008). Mn has been identified in at least 869 of the 1,699 hazardous waste sites that have been proposed for inclusion on the EPA National Priorities List (NPL) (HazDat 2008). Mn may also be released to the environment through the use of MMT (methylcyclopentadienyl manganese tricarbonyl) as a gasoline additive. Human exposure to Mn is therefore widespread (Crump 2000).

9.9.2 Manganese and the Ovary

High doses of Mn affect DNA replication and repair in bacteria and cause mutations. In mammalian cells, Mn causes DNA damage and chromosome aberrations (Gerber et al. 2002). Large amounts of Mn affect fertility in mammals and are toxic to the embryo and fetus (Colomina et al. 1996). Mn is a component of the mitochondrial enzymes, pyruvate carboxylase, superoxide dismutase (MnSOD), glutamine synthetase, alkaline phosphatase, and arginase. Mn also activates several enzymes. MnSOD, also known as SOD2, is a mitochondrial enzyme with potent antioxidant activity (St Clair 2004). Mn is an antagonist of iron and can replace Mg^{2+} in certain enzymes. Because of its similar ionic radius, Mn can also interfere with the metabolism of calcium (Marbaniang 2012). Prepubertal exposure to Mn caused precocious puberty in female rats by stimulating the prepubertal secretion of luteinizing hormone–releasing hormone (LHRH) from the hypothalamus (Dees et al. 2009, Lee et al. 2007, Pine et al. 2005). An increase in LHRH secretion causes enhanced pulsatile release of luteinizing hormone, and is responsible for initiating puberty in all mammals, including humans (Wetsel et al. 1992). However, induction of LHRH secretion can be detrimental if it occurs too early during development. Mn caused elevated serum levels of LH, FSH, and estradiol (Pine et al. 2005). Therefore, it is possible that Mn could induce early menarche in women. However, information is lacking on the direct toxic effects of Mn on the ovary; and future studies are required to address direct effects of Mn on follicular development and steroidogenesis in the ovary.

9.10 MERCURY

9.10.1 Background

Environmental contamination with mercury (Hg) is mainly from the alkali and metal processing industry, incineration of coal, medical and other waste. Mining of gold (Au) and Hg contributes greatly to Hg concentrations in some areas, but atmospheric deposition is the dominant source of Hg over most of the landscape. Once in the atmosphere, Hg is widely disseminated and can circulate for years, accounting for its widespread distribution. Natural sources of atmospheric Hg include volcanoes, geologic deposits of Hg, and volatilization from the ocean. Although all rocks, sediments, water, and soils naturally contain small but varying amounts of Hg, some local mineral occurrences and thermal springs are naturally high in Hg (Gustin 2003). Atmospheric deposition contains the three principal forms of Hg, although inorganic divalent Hg (HgII) is the dominant form. Once in surface water, Hg enters a complex cycle in which one form can be converted to another. Hg attached to particles can settle onto the sediments where it can diffuse into the water column, be resuspended and buried by other sediments, or be methylated. Methylmecury can enter the food chain, or it can be released onto the atmosphere by volatilization (Mukherjee 2011). Skin-lightening creams and dental amalgam are important contributors to Hg exposure (Al-Saleh and Shinwari 1997). Elemental (metallic) Hg is a highly hazardous chemical that can cause serious adverse health effects. Elemental Hg is used in thermometers, fluorescent light bulbs, blood pressure instruments, and in dental amalgams (Clarkson et al. 2003). Inhaled Hg vapor easily crosses the pulmonary capillary membranes and can accumulate in distal tissues (Magos 1967). Intracellular Hg is rapidly oxidized by cytosolic catalase to mercuric Hg (Hg^{2+}), the reactive species for most Hg compounds. Hg^{2+} can be formed by oxidation of Hg, reduction of mercuric salts, or demethylation of methylmercury (Rowland et al. 1984). Hg^{2+} is highly reactive and rapidly combines with intracellular ligands such as sulfhydryls, potentially disrupting enzymes and proteins (Davis et al. 2001).

9.10.2 Mercury and the Ovary

Epidemiological studies indicate that occupational exposure to Hg in women resulted in abnormal menstrual cycles, in terms of bleeding pattern and cycle length (De Rosis et al. 1985). Dental assistants exposed to Hg vapor experience decreased fertility (Rowland et al. 1994). Exposure to Hg0 vapor (2 mg/m^3) for 6–8 days resulted in prolonged estrous cycles, increased Hg burden in the ovary, increased progesterone (P4), and decreased estradiol (Davis et al. 2001). Hg accumulates in human follicular fluid (Capcarová and Kolesárová 2012). Progesterone release by granulosa cells of pregnant gilts was significantly stimulated after *in vitro* Hg culture at doses of 0.25 and 0.083 mg/mL (Kolesarova et al. 2010).

Cyclic female hamsters, given 1 mg of mercuric chloride per day on each day of the 4 day estrous cycle, demonstrated alterations in histology of the reproductive tract, progesterone levels, and cyclicity. The ovaries of Hg-treated animals showed retarded follicular development and morphologically retained corpora lutea (Lamperti and Printz 1973). Hg inhibited protein synthesis, maturation of the ovary by inhibiting the response of the ovaries to gonad stimulating hormone in swamp crawfish, *Procambarus clarkia*. This served as a bioindicator for the toxic effects of various pollutants (Suárez-Serrano et al. 2010). Histochemical localization showed deposits of Hg in the ovaries of rats, particularly in macrophages of atretic ovarian follicles, corpora lutea, follicular fluid, and in the granulosa cells of atretic follicles of young rats fed with mercuric chloride (Stadnicka 1980).

9.11 NICKEL

9.11.1 Background

Nickel (Ni) and its compounds are naturally present in the Earth's crust, and released into the environment through windblown dust and volcanic eruptions, as well as from anthropogenic activities. It is estimated that 8.5 million kg of nickel is emitted into the atmosphere from natural sources such as windblown dust, volcanoes, and vegetation each year (Bennett 1984). Five times that quantity is estimated to come from anthropogenic sources (Cempel and Nikel 2006). The burning of residual waste and fuel oil is responsible for 62% of anthropogenic emissions, followed by Ni metal refining, municipal incineration, steel production, other Ni alloy production, and coal combustion (IARC 1990, Sutherland and Costa 2002). Occupational exposure to Ni may occur by dermal contact or by inhalation of aerosols, dusts, fumes, or mists containing Ni. Dermal contact may also occur with Ni solutions, such as those used in electroplating, Ni salts, and Ni metal or alloys. Ni-containing dust may be ingested where poor work practices exist or where poor personal hygiene is practiced. A National Occupational Exposure Survey (NOES) conducted by NIOSH from 1981 to 1983 estimates that 727,240 workers were potentially exposed to some form of Ni metal, alloys, salts, or inorganic nickel compounds in the United States (ATSDR 2005). The most probable route of Ni exposure from hazardous waste sites would be from consumption of contaminated drinking water, inhalation of dust, dermal contact with bath/shower water, soil, or dust, and ingestion of Ni-contaminated soil. Groundwater contamination may occur where the soil has a coarse texture and where acid waste, such as waste from plating industries, is discarded (De Brouwere et al. 2012).

9.11.2 Nickel and Ovary

Nickel (II) may induce genotoxic effects such as DNA–protein crosslinking, DNA strand breaks, sister chromatid exchange, and oxidative DNA base damage, including the mutagenic 8-oxo-29-deoxyguanosine and other lesions in CHO cells (Kasprzak 1995). Ni (16 mg/kg b.wt) increased free radical levels and decreased ascorbic acid, GSH, SOD, and catalase in the mouse ovary. Vitamin E protected the ovary against Ni toxicity (Rao et al. 2009). Ni (II) caused cell cycle arrest at G2/M stage and induced apoptosis through upregulation of p53 in CHO cells (Shiao et al. 1998). Ni can cause DNA strand breaks in CHO cells (Robison and Costa 1982). Ni compounds can increase lipid peroxidation and hydrogen peroxide, thus increasing oxidative stress in CHO cells (Huang et al. 1994). Oxidative stress induced by Ni compounds could be attenuated by catalase (Chen et al. 2003). In fish, $NiCl_2$ induced aberrant development and death of oocytes with yolk granules scattered in the ovarian cavity (Sioson and Herrera 1993). Ni^{2+} was found to be cytotoxic at 62.5 μM in primary cultures of granulosa cells from women (23–37 years of age) who undergo *in vitro* fertilization. Ni^{2+} decreased human chorionic gonadotropin (0.1 IU/mL hCG) or dibutyryl cyclic adenosine monophosphate (1 mM db-cAMP)-induced progesterone production (Révész et al. 2004). More studies are needed to address the effects of Ni on the development and function of the ovary and ovarian cancers.

9.12 TITANIUM

9.12.1 Background

Titanium tetrachloride ($TiCl_4$) is frequently used as a white pigment for a wide range of paints, paper, inks, and plastics. By virtue of its physical, chemical, and mechanical properties, Ti exhibits excellent resistance to corrosion and good biocompatibility, and is currently the best and most widely used material in the manufacture of orthopedic and dental implants (Thompson 2000, Williams 2001). Occupational exposure to Ti occurs through mining of ores, in the preparation of titanium dioxide (TiO_2) and in any of the industries in which the powder is stored and used. $TiCl_4$ enters the environment primarily in the air from factories that make it or use it in various chemical processes, or as a result of spills. $TiCl_4$ reacts rapidly with moisture in the air to form hydrochloric acid and other titanium compounds, such as titanium hydroxide and titanium oxychlorides. Some of the titanium compounds may settle out in soil or water. In water, they sink into the bottom sediments. The titanium compounds may remain for a long time in the soil or sediments (Freese et al. 2001).

TiO_2 nanoparticles are used for protection against UV ray exposure due to their high refractive index. Many sunscreens contain TiO_2 as well as surface coating products, which are colorless and reflect and scatter UV rays morc efficiently than larger particles (Oberdoerster et al. 2005, Rittner 2002). Some types of TiO_2 nanoparticles have been reported to cause toxicity both *in vitro* and *in vivo*, attributed to the generation of ROS resulting in apoptosis (Liu et al. 2010, Sun et al. 2012), micronuclei formation (Gurr et al. 2005, Rahman et al. 2002), mitochondrial abnormalities (Hussain et al. 2005), and other forms of cell toxicity.

9.12.2 Titanium and the Ovary

CHO cells treated with nano-TiO_2 rapidly formed extracellular aggregates with dimensions that were generally >100 nm. Aggregates were readily internalized by the CHO cells and appeared in vacuoles taken up by a phagocytotic or endocytotic process. Internalized aggregates were restricted to the cytoplasm and were not localized to any specific organelles or intracellular sites. Exposure to TiO_2 (5 and 200 nm size) aggregates with >3 mg/L dose increased the production of ROS in both short- and long-term exposures (Thomas et al. 2011). Superoxide dismutase quenched the ROS signal produced by nano-TiO_2 of human hepatocytes (Du et al. 2012). There are no studies indicating deleterious effects of Ti on the ovary. More studies are needed in the future to address the effects of Ti, particularly nanoparticles of Ti on ovarian development and function.

9.13 HEAVY METAL TOXICITY: MECHANISM OF ACTION

Commonly used metals such as Fe, Cu, Cd, Cr, Hg, Ni, Pb, and As possess the ability to generate free radicals, resulting in depletion of enzyme activities, damage to lipid bilayer and DNA (Stohs and Bagchi 1995). A schematic diagram of various heavy metal-induced apoptosis through oxidative stress is given in Figure 9.3. There are a

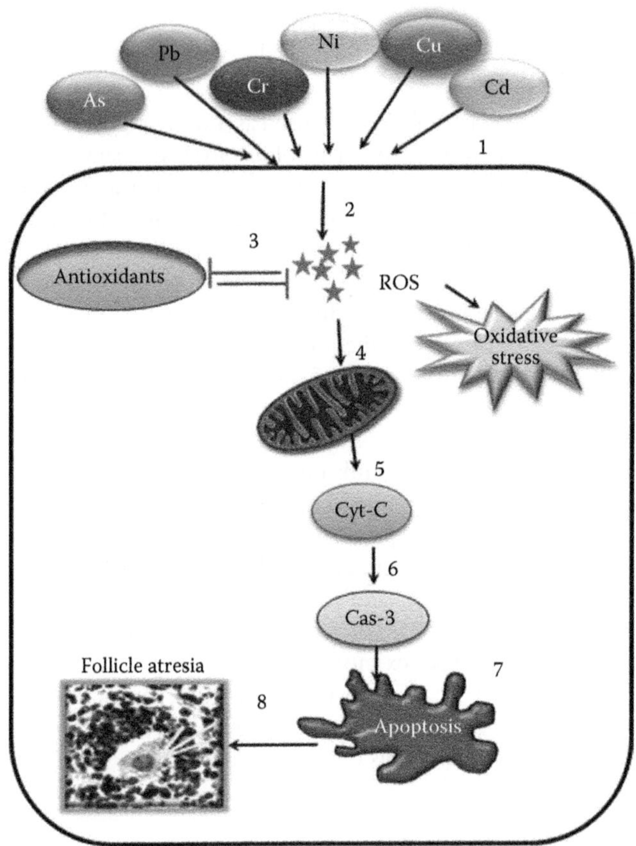

FIGURE 9.3 A schematic diagram of heavy metal–induced apoptosis through oxidative stress: (1) Heavy metals enter cells by active transport or passive diffusion, which results in the (2) generation of large amounts of reactive oxygen species (ROS). (3) ROS deplete antioxidants (AOX) and AOX quench ROS. (4) Increased oxidative stress generated by ROS changes mitochondrial membrane permeabilization. (5) Release of cytochrome *c* from the mitochondria and (6) activation of caspase-3 lead to (7) apoptosis of cells in the ovary, and (8) atresia of follicles. Arrow indicates a degenerated oocyte of an atretic follicle.

wide variety of oxygen-, carbon-, sulfur-, and nitrogen- radicals, originating not only from superoxides, hydrogen peroxide, and lipid peroxides but also from chelates of amino acids, peptides, and proteins complexed with the toxic metals (Dröge 2002). The resulting oxidative stress may affect the levels and functions of redox-sensitive signaling molecules, such as AP-1, NF-κB, and p53; derange the cell signaling and gene expression systems; and/or induce apoptosis (Genestra 2007, Trachootham et al. 2008). Both AP-1 and NF-κB are considered stress-response transcription factors that govern the expression of a variety of pro-inflammatory and cytotoxic genes (Hu et al. 2002). The heavy metals have electron-sharing affinities that can result in the formation of covalent attachments mainly between heavy metal and sulfhydryl groups of proteins. Several enzymes in antioxidant defense systems may protect the proper balance between pro-oxidant and antioxidant species but unfortunately, enzymes contain sulfhydryl groups which can bind metal ions at their active sites and, hence, become inactive due to direct binding of metal ions to sulfhydryl groups (Quig 1998). GSH is found in mammalian tissues at millimolar concentrations (Pastore et al. 2003). The oocyte has a GSH concentration of 10 mM which accounts for more than 90% of total nonprotein sulfur (Yoshida et al. 1993). Pb is also known to deplete GSH levels (Ghibelli et al. 1995).

Zn serves as a cofactor for most of the enzymes, and can be replaced by Pb, which inactivates the function of several Zn-dependent enzymes. The antioxidant enzymes SOD, catalase, and GPx are potential targets of Pb. Selenium is essential for GPx activity, and Pb forms a complex with Se and decreases GPx activity (Whanger 1992). Pb inhibits heme synthesis. Because catalase is a heme-containing enzyme, Pb decreases its activity (Mylroie et al. 1984). SOD requires Cu and Zn for its activity. Whereas, Cu ions play a functional role in the reaction by undergoing alternate oxidation, Zn ions seem to stabilize the SOD enzyme (Halliwell and Gutteridge 1989). Pb also replaces Cu and Zn, thus, decreasing the activity of Cu/Zn SOD. Therefore, inhibitory effects of metal ions such as Pb and Cu on various enzymes impair antioxidant defense mechanisms by cells and render them more vulnerable to oxidative stress.

Selenium (Se) is an essential trace element with antioxidative, antimutagenic, antiviral, and anticarcinogenic properties (Rahmanto and Davies 2012). An important property of Se is its interaction with other elements that may be present in foods, water, workplace, and the environment including As, Cu, Ni, Co, Cr, Mn, Zn, Cd, Sn, Pb, Hg, Bi, Mo, Ag, Au (Schrauzer 2009). The sequestration of elements by Se not only represents an efficient natural detoxification mechanism for some of these elements but also results in the physiological inactivation of Se. Se is essential for cellular antioxidant defense systems to scavenge free radicals (Machlin and Bendich 1987, Watson et al. 2012). Selenocysteine has a structure similar to that of cysteine, but with an atom of Se taking the place of the usual sulfur, forming a selenol group, which is deprotonated at physiological pH. Proteins that contain one or more selenocysteine residues are called selenoproteins (Low and Berry 1996). Se, which is found at the active site of glutathione peroxidase (GPx), can help to detoxify organic peroxides and inhibit lipid peroxidation, mainly as selenocysteine (Liu et al. 2008). Another important and essential metal with antioxidant properties is Zn, which is associated with several enzymes such as oxidoreductases, transferases, hydrolases, isomerases, lyases, ligases, and 3β-HSD. Any impairment in the bioavailability or transport of Zn will affect the performance of these enzymes by impairing their homeostatic mechanisms (Taneja and Mahajan 1999). For an example, one of the mechanisms of Cd toxicity on the reproductive processes is depletion of Zn (Gunn et al. 1963). Transport of Zn away from the cytosol, either into organelles or out of the cell, is mediated by members of the Zn transporter family (ZnT). Intracellular Zn is strictly regulated by binding to metallothionein (MTs) and GSH and by compartmentalization through the Zn transporters (Chimienti et al. 2003). MTs have high binding affinity for Zn and play a central role in maintaining stable intracellular Zn through sequestration or release of Zn (Tapiero and Tew 2003). Cd also induced downregulation of ZnT1 as well as the upregulation of ZIP10 in response to Zn depletion in the ovary (Chouchene et al. 2011). Supplementation of Se or Zn mitigated or inhibited the deleterious effects of Cd in causing follicular atresia in Japanese quail (Nad et al. 2007). Therefore, supplementation of an additional dose of Se and/or Zn (other than the dietary level) could help mitigate Cd toxicity, or other metal toxicities that respond to Se or Zn supplementation. As is one of the most extensively studied metals that induces ROS generation resulting in oxidative stress (Shi et al. 2004). As produces superoxide ($O2^{\bullet-}$), singlet oxygen, the peroxyl radical (ROO•), nitric oxide (NO•) (Pi et al. 2003), hydrogen peroxide (H_2O_2), dimethylarsinic peroxyl radicals (CH3)2AsOO•, and also the dimethylarsinic radical (CH3)2As• (Rin et al. 1995). Free radicals generated by As lead to the activation of oxidative signaling pathways that result in cell apoptosis. As decreased GSH levels and glutathione reductase (GR). Reduced GR levels lead to an increase in GSSG levels, which enhance As toxicity in guinea pigs (Wang et al. 1996).

Supplementation of vitamin C and E alters the extent of DNA damage by reducing TNF-α levels and inhibiting activation of the caspase cascade in As-intoxicated animals (Ramanathan et al. 2005). A combination of vitamin C and thiamine was effective in reducing Pb levels in blood, liver, and kidney. α-Lipoic acid (LA) is an endogenous thiol antioxidant, which possesses the potential to quench ROS, regenerate GSH, and chelate metals such as iron, Cu, Hg, and Cd. LA is also known to mediate free-radical damage in biological systems (Young and Woodside 2001). LA is readily available in the diet, absorbed through the gut, and easily passes through the blood–brain barrier. Exogenous supplementation with LA has been reported to increase unbound LA levels, which can act as a potent antioxidant and reduce oxidative stress both *in vitro* and *in vivo* (Bustamante et al. 1998). LA serves as a protective tool against Cd-induced membrane damage and cell dysfunction in hepatocytes (Müller 1989). Another hormone with antioxidant properties is melatonin. Melatonin stimulates several antioxidative enzymes, including glutathione reductase, GPx, and SOD; promotes quick disposal of H_2O_2 (Kotler et al. 1998); enhances the production of enzymes that are involved in the synthesis of GSH (Reiter et al. 1999); and prevents the reduction of membrane fluidity caused by lipid peroxidation. In this way, melatonin helps in scavenging free radicals (Garcia et al. 1997). Thus, it could be a possible intervention against metal toxicity.

As long as industries exist, heavy metal contamination in the environment is inevitable. Therefore, it is important to understand the molecular mechanisms of heavy metal toxicity and to identify potential intervention strategies to mitigate or inhibit metal-induced adverse effects on the ovary to protect/preserve fertility and reduce infertility in women. Even though heavy metals have been in anthropologic use from the prehistoric ages, very little information is available on their effects in the ovary. Hence, it is very important to uncover the mechanism of action of heavy metals within the ovary, as well as on other aspects of female reproduction. It is more common that the industrial effluents, fumes released into the air from industries, hazardous waste disposal in the water and soil, and cigarette smoke contain a mixture of several metals along with other chemicals. Therefore, it is also imperative to understand the effects of complex mixtures on female reproduction. More studies are needed in the future to understand the metal-induced adverse effects on the ovary, to preserve fertility in the present and future generations.

ACKNOWLEDGMENTS

The author acknowledges Dr. Robert C. Burghardt, Professor, Department of Veterinary Integrative Biosciences, Texas A&M University, for the critical review of the chapter. Most of the data on chromium and the ovary from the author's laboratory were generated and published with the funding support from the National Institute of Health (NIH)/National Institute of Environmental Health Sciences (NIEHS) grants ES016605-A2 and ES020561-01.

REFERENCES

Adebowale, A. 2004. *Bioremediation of Arsenic, Chromium, Lead, and Mercury*, ed. USEPA Office of Solid Waste and Emergency Response, pp. 1–43. Washington, DC: U.S. Environmental Protection Agency.

Adriano, D. C. 2001. *Trace Elements in Terrestrial Environments: Biogeochemistry, Bioavailability, and Risks of Metals*, pp. 91–132. New York: Springer-Verlag.

Akter, K. F., G. Owens, D. E. Davey, and R. Naidu. 2005. Arsenic speciation and toxicity in biological systems. *Rev Environ Contam Toxicol* 184: 97–149.

Al-Saleh, I. and N. Shinwari. 1997. Urinary mercury levels in females: Influence of skin-lightening creams and dental amalgam fillings. *Biometals* 10: 315–323.

Andrew, D. A. C., A. R. Edward, and F. O. J. Guillette Jr. 2010. Endocrine disrupting contaminants and hormone dynamics: Lessons from wild life. In *Environmental Endocrine Disruptors: An Evolutionary Perspective*, eds. L. J. Guillette Jr. and A. Crain, pp. 1–21. New York: Taylor & Francis Group.

Angenard, G., V. Muczynski, H. Coffigny et al. 2010. Cadmium increases human fetal germ cell apoptosis. *Environ Health Perspect* 118: 331–37.

Arancibia, V., C. Peña, H. E. Allen, and G. Lagos. 2003 Characterization of copper in uterine fluids of patients who use the copper T-380A intrauterine device. *Clin Chim Acta* 332: 69–78.

Asano, Y. 2012. Age-related accumulation of non-heme ferric and ferrous iron in mouse ovarian stroma visualized by sensitive non-heme iron histochemistry. *J Histochem Cytochem* 60: 229–242.

ATSDR. 2005. Toxicological profile for nickel, pp. 167–178. Atlanta, GA: Agency for Toxic Substances and Disease Registry.

ATSDR. 2008. Toxicological profile for manganese, pp. 341–350. Atlanta, GA: U.S. Department of Health and Human Services.

Avecilla-Palau, A. and V. Moreno. 2003. Uterine factors and risk of pregnancy in IUD users: A nested case-control study. *Contraception* 67: 235–239.

Banu, S. K., J. B. Samuel, J. A. Arosh, R. C. Burghardt, and M. M. Aruldhas. 2008. Lactational exposure to hexavalent chromium delays puberty by impairing ovarian development, steroidogenesis and pituitary hormone synthesis in developing Wistar rats. *Toxicol Appl Pharmacol* 232: 180–189.

Banu, S. K., J. A. Stanley, J. Lee et al. 2011. Hexavalent chromium-induced apoptosis of granulosa cells involves selective sub-cellular translocation of Bcl-2 members, ERK1/2 and p53. *Toxicol Appl Pharmacol* 251: 253–266.

Barceloux, D. G. 1999. Chromium. *J Toxicol Clin Toxicol* 37: 173–194.

Bekheet, S. H. 2011. Comparative effects of repeated administration of cadmium chloride during pregnancy and lactation and selenium protection against cadmium toxicity on some organs in immature rats' offsprings. *Biol Trace Elem Res* 144: 1008–1023.

Belotti, D., P. Paganoni, L. Manenti et al. 2003. Matrix metalloproteinases (MMP9 and MMP2) induce the release of vascular endothelial growth factor (VEGF) by ovarian carcinoma cells: Implications for ascites formation. *Cancer Res* 63: 5224–5229.

Bennett, B. G. 1984. Environmental nickel pathways to man. *IARC Sci Publ* 1984(53): 487–495.

Berger, T. M., M. C. Polidori, A. Dabbagh et al. 1997. Antioxidant activity of vitamin C in iron-overloaded human plasma. *J Biol Chem* 272: 15656–15660.

Bergeron, C. and K. Kovacs. 1978. Pituitary siderosis: A histologic, immunocytologic, and ultrastructural study. *Am J Pathol* 93: 295–309.

Bhardwaj, J. K. and R. K. Sharma. 2011. Changes in trace elements during follicular atresia in goat (Capra hircus) ovary. *Biol Trace Elem Res* 140: 291–298.

Bindler, R. 2011. Contaminated lead environments of man: Reviewing the lead isotopic evidence in sediments, peat, and soils for the temporal and spatial patterns of atmospheric lead pollution in Sweden. *Environ Geochem Health* 33: 311–329.

Bivik, C., I. Rosdahl, and K. Ollinger. 2007. Hsp70 protects against UVB induced apoptosis by preventing release of cathepsins and cytochrome c in human melanocytes. *Carcinogenesis* 28: 537–544.

Blacksmith Institute. 2007. The world's worst polluted places: The top ten, pp. 1–57. New York: The Blacksmith Institute.

Blakley, B. R. and D. L. Hamilton. 1985. Ceruloplasmin as an indicator of copper status in cattle and sheep. *Can J Camp Med* 49: 405–408.

Bode, A. M. and Z. Dong. 2002. The paradox of arsenic: Molecular mechanisms of cell transformation and chemotherapeutic effects. *Crit Rev Oncol Hematol* 42: 5–24.

Bornstein, J., S. Sagi, A. Haj, J. Harroch, and F. Fares. 2005. Arsenic Trioxide inhibits the growth of human ovarian carcinoma cell line. *Gynecol Oncol* 99: 726–729.

Brewer, G. 2005. Anticopper therapy against cancer and diseases of inflammation and fibrosis. *Drug Dis Today* 10: 1103–1109.

Burger, A. M. and A. K. Seth. 2004. The ubiquitin-mediated protein degradation pathway in cancer: Therapeutic implications. *Eur J Cancer* 40: 2217–2229.

Bustamante, J., J. K. Lodge, L. Marcocci et al. 1998. Lipoic acid in liver metabolism and disease. *Free Rad Biol Med* 24: 1023–1039.

Cabantchik, Z. I., W. Breuer, G. Zanninelli, and P. Cianciulli. 2005. LPI-labile plasma iron in iron overload. *Best Pract Res Clin Haematol* 18: 277–287.

Capcarová, M. and A. Kolesárová. 2012. Trace elements in follicular fluid and their effects on reproductive functions. *J Microbiol Biotechnol Food Sci* 1: 1039–1044.

Carr, A. and B. Frei. 1999. Does vitamin C act as a pro-oxidant under physiological conditions? *FASEB J* 13: 1007–1024.

Casasco, A., A. Calligaro, E. Casasco et al. 1988. An immunocytochemical method for studying embryo cytokinetics. *Basic Appl Histochem* 32: 293–296.

Cempel, M. and G. Nikel. 2006. Nickel: A review of its sources and environmental toxicology. *Polish J Environ Stud* 15: 375–382.

Chattopadhyay, S. and D. Ghosh. 2010. Role of dietary GSH in the amelioration of sodium arsenite-induced ovarian and uterine disorders. *Reprod Toxicol* 30: 481–488.

Chen, H., S. Li, J. Liu et al. 2004. Chronic inorganic arsenic exposure induces hepatic global and individual gene hypomethylation: implications for arsenic hepatocarcinogenesis. *Carcinogenesis* 25: 1779–1786.

Chen, C. Y., Y. F. Wang, Y. H. Lin, and S. F. Yen. 2003. Nickel-induced oxidative stress and effect of antioxidants in human lymphocytes. *Arch Toxicol* 77: 123–130.

Chimienti, F., M. Aouffen, A. Favier, and M. Seve. 2003. Zinc homeostasis-regulating proteins: New drug targets for triggering cell fate. *Curr Drug Targets* 4: 323–338.

Chouchene, L., M. Banni, A. Kerkeni, K. Saïd, and I. Messaoudi. 2011. Cadmium-induced ovarian pathophysiology is mediated by change in gene expression pattern of zinc transporters in zebrafish (Danio rerio). *Chem Biol Interact* 193: 172–179.

Clarkson, T. W., L. Magos, and G. J. Myers. 2003. The toxicology of mercury—Current exposures and clinical manifestations. *N Engl J Med* 249: 1731–1737.

Colomina, M. T., J. L. Domingo, J. M. Llobet, and J. Corbella. 1996. Effect of day of exposure on the developmental toxicity of manganese in mice. *Vet Hum Toxicol* 38: 7–9.

Colter, A. and R. L. Mahler. 2006. Iron in drinking water, pp. 1–4. Moscow, ID: University of Idaho.

Cooksey, C. 2012. Health concerns of heavy metals and metalloids. *Sci Prog* 95: 73–88.

Crichton, R. R., S. Wilmet, R. Legssyer, and R. J. Ward. 2002. Molecular and cellular mechanisms of iron homeostasis and toxicity in mammalian cells. *J Inorg Biochem* 91: 9–18.

Crump, K. S. 2000. Manganese exposures in Toronto during use of the gasoline additive, methylcyclopentadienyl manganese tricarbonyl. *J Expo Anal Environ Epidemiol* 10: 227–239.

Crystel, T., P. Joël, N. Françoise, and L. Brigitte. 2001. Lead accumulation in the mouse ovary after treatment-induced follicular atresia. *Reprod Toxicol* 15: 385–391.

Cunningham, J., M. Leffell, P. Mearkle, and P. Harmatz. 1995. Elevated plasma ceruloplasmin in insulin-dependent diabetes mellitus: Evidence for increased oxidative stress as a variable complication. *Metabolism* 44: 996–999.

Daniel, K., D. Chen, S. Orlu et al. 2005. Clioquinol and pyrrolidine dithiocarbamate complex with copper to form proteasome inhibitors and apoptosis inducers in human breast cancer cells. *Breast Cancer Res* 7: R897–R908.

Davis, B. J., H. C. Price, R. W. O'Connor et al. 2001. Mercury vapor and female reproductive toxicity. *Toxicol Sci* 59: 291–296.

De Brouwere, K., J. Buekers, C. Cornelis, C. E. Schlekat, and A. R. Oller. 2012. Assessment of indirect human exposure to environmental sources of nickel: Oral exposure and risk characterization for systemic effects. *Sci Total Environ Sci Total Environ* 419.

De Rosis, F., S. P. Anastasio, L. Selvaggi, A. Beltrame, and G. Moriani. 1985. Female reproductive health in two lamp factories: Effects of exposure to inorganic mercury vapour and stress factors. *Br J Ind Med* 42: 488–494.

Deane, H. W. 1952. Histochemical observations on the ovary and oviduct of the albino rat during the estrous cycle. *Am J Anat* 91: 363–393.

Dees, W., J. K. Hiney, and V. K. Srivastava. 2009. Influences of manganese on female puberty. *Curr Trend Neurol* 3: 85–92.

Domingo, J. L. 1994. Metal-induced developmental toxicity in mammals: A review. *J Toxicol Environ Health* 42: 123–141.

Dröge, W. 2002. Free radicals in the physiological control of cell function. *Physiological Reviews* 82: 47–95.

Du, H., X. Zhu, C. Fan et al. 2012. Oxidative damage and OGG1 expression induced by a combined effect of titanium dioxide nanoparticles and lead acetate in human hepatocytes. *Environ Toxicol* 27: 590–597.

Du, Y. H. and P. C. Ho. 2001. Arsenic compounds induce cytotoxicity and apoptosis in cisplatin-sensitive and -resistant gynecological cancer cell lines. *Cancer Chemother Pharmacol* 47: 481–490.

Eck, P. C. and L. Wilson. 1989. *Copper Toxicity*. Phoenix, AZ: The Eck Institute of Applied Nutrition and Bioenergetics, Ltd.

Edson, M. A., A. K. Nagaraja, and M. M. Matzuk. 2009. The mammalian ovary from genesis to revelation. *Endocr Rev* 30: 624–712.

Ercal, N., H. Gurer-Orhan, and N. Aykin-Burns. 2001. Toxic metals and oxidative stress part I: Mechanisms involved in metal-induced oxidative damage. *Curr Top Med Chem* 1: 529–539.

Erster, S. and U. M. Moll. 2004. Stress-induced p53 runs a direct mitochondrial death program: Its role in physiologic and pathophysiologic stress responses in vivo. *Cell Cycle* 3: 1492–1495.

Escobar-Morreale, H. F. 2012. Iron metabolism and the polycystic ovary syndrome. *Trends Endocrinol Metab* 23: 509–515.

Evans, J. L., I. D. Goldfine, B. A. Maddux, and G. M. Grodsky. 2002. Oxidative stressand stress-activated signaling pathways: A unifying hypothesis of type 2 diabetes. *Endocrin Rev* 23: 599–622.

EWG. 2012. Environmental Working Group's tips on reducing your exposure to arsenic. *Reducing Arsenic in Your Diet*, ed. E. W. Group, p.1. Washington, DC: Environmental Working Group.

Fasano, G., F. Moffa, J. Dechène, Y. Englert, and I. Demeestere. 2011. Vitrification of in vitro matured oocytes collected from antral follicles at the time of ovarian tissue cryopreservation. *Reprod Biol Endocrinol* 9: 150.

Ferrer, X. and J. J. Moreno. 1992. Effects of copper, iron and zinc on oedema formation induced by phospholipase A2. *Comp Biochem Physiol C* 102: 325–327.

Finney, L., S. Vogt, T. Fukai, and D. Glesne. 2009. Copper and angiogenesis: Unravelling a relationship key to cancer progression. *Clin Exp Pharmacol Physiol* 36: 88–94.

Freese, H. L., M. G. Volas, and J. R. Wood. 2001. Metallurgy and technological properties of titanium and titanium alloys. In *Titanium in Medicine: Material Science, Surface Science, Engineering, Biological Responses, and Medical Applications*, eds. D. M. Brunnette, P. Tengvall, M. Textor, and P. Thompsen, pp. 25–53. New York: Springer-Verlag.

Furnus, C. C., D. G. de Matos, and D. F. Moses. 1998. Cumulus expansion during in vitro maturation of bovine oocytes: Relationship with intracellular glutathione level and its role on subsequent embryo development. *Mol Reprod Dev* 51: 76–83.

Galluzzi, L., E. Morselli, O. Kepp et al. 2011. Mitochondrial liaisons of p53. *Antioxid Redox Signal* 15: 1691–1714.

Gannon, P. O., S. Medelci, C. Le Page et al. 2011. Impact of hemochromatosis gene (HFE) mutations on epithelial ovarian cancer risk and prognosis. *Int J Cancer* 128: 2326–2334.

GAO. 1993. Lead-based paint poisoning: Children not fully protected when federal agencies sell homes to public, pp. 1–15. Washington, DC: Central Accounting Office.

Garcia, J. J., R. J. Reiter, J. M. Guerrero et al. 1997. Melatonin prevents changes in microsomal membrane fluidity during induced lipid peroxidation. *FEBS Lett* 408: 297–300.

Genestra, M. 2007. Oxyl radicals, redox-sensitive signalling cascades and antioxidants. *Cell Signal* 19: 1807–1819.

Gerber, G. B., A. Léonard, and P. Hantson. 2002. Carcinogenicity, mutagenicity and teratogenicity of manganese compounds. *Crit Rev Oncol Hematol* 42: 25–34.

Germolec, D. R., T. Yoshida, K. Gaido et al. 1996. Arsenic induces overexpression of growth factors in human keratinocytes. *Toxicol Appl Pharmacol* 141: 308–311.

Ghibelli, L., S. Coppola, G. Rotilio et al. 1995. Non-oxidative loss of glutathione in apoptosis via GSH extrusion. *Biochem Biophys Res Commun* 216: 313–320.

Gladys, S., B. Van Meerbeek, P. Lambrechts, and G. Vanherle. 1999. Evaluation of esthetic parameters of resin-modified glass-ionomer materials and a polyacid-modified resin composite in Class V cervical lesions. *Quintessence Int* 30: 607–614.

Glickman, M. H. and A. Ciechanover. 2002. The ubiquitin-proteasome proteolytic pathway: Destruction for the sake of construction. *Physiol Rev* 82: 373–428.

Grillo, C. A., M. A. Reigosa, and M. A. de Mele. 2010. Does over-exposure to copper ions released from metallic copper induce cytotoxic and genotoxic effects on mammalian cells? *Contraception* 81: 343–349.

Gunn, S. A., T. C. Gould, and W. A. Anderson. 1963. The selective injurious response of testicular and epididymal blood vessels to cadmium and its prevention by zinc. *Am J Pathol* 42: 685–702.

Gupte, A. and R. J. Mumper. 2009. Elevated copper and oxidative stress in cancer cells as a target for cancer treatment. *Cancer Treat Rev* 35: 32–46.

Gurr, J. R., A. S. Wang, C. H. Chen, and K. Y. Jan. 2005. Ultrafine titanium dioxide particles in the absence of photoactivation can induce oxidative damage to human bronchial epithelial cells. *Toxicology* 213: 66–73.

Gustin, M. S. 2003. Are mercury emissions from geologic sources significant? A status report. *Sci Total Environ* 304: 153–167.

Gutteridge, J. M. and B. Halliwell. 1989. Iron toxicity and oxygen radicals. *Baillieres Clin Haematol* 2: 195–256.

Gutteridge, J. M. and B. Halliwell. 2000. Free radicals and antioxidants in the year 2000. A historical look to the future. *Ann NY Acad Sci* 899: 136–147.

Halliwell, B. and J. M. C. Gutteridge. 1989. *Free Radicals in Biology and Medicine*. Oxford, U.K.: Clarendon Press.

Harada, T., H. Koi, T. Kubota, and T. Aso. 2004. Haem oxygenase augments porcine granulosa cell apoptosis in vitro. *J Endocrinol Invest* 181: 191–205.

Harper, M. 1987. Possible toxic metal exposure of prehistoric bronze workers. *Br J Ind Med* 44: 652–656.

HazDat. 2008. Manganese. HazDat database: ATSDR's hazardous substance release and health effects database. Atlanta, GA: Agency for Toxic Substances and Disease Registry.

He, Z. L. L., X. E. Yang, and P. J. Stoffella. 2005. Trace elements in agroecosystems and impacts on the environment. *J Trace Elem Med Biol* 19: 125–140.

Herndon, E. M. and S. L. Brantley. 2011. Movement of manganese contamination through the Critical Zone. *Appl Geochem* 26: 40–43.

Hilderbrand, D. C., R. Der, W. T. Griffin, and M. S. Fahim. 1973. Effect of lead acetate on reproduction. *Am J Obstet Gynecol* 115: 1058–1065.

Hoch-Ligeti, C. and G. H. Bourne. 1948. Changes in the concentration and histological distribution of ascorbic acid in ovaries, adrenals and livers of rats during oestrus cycles. *Br J Pathol* 29: 400–407.

Holley, A. K., S. K. Dhar, and D. K. St Clair. 2010. Manganese superoxide dismutase versus p53: The mitochondrial center. *Ann NY Acad Sci* 1201: 72–78.

Howe, P., H. Malcolm, and S. Dobson. 2004. Manganese and its compounds: Environmental aspects. In *Concise International Chemical Assessment Documents*, pp. 1–61. Geneva, Switzerland: World Health Organization.

Hu, Y., X. Jin, and E. T. Snow. 2002. Effect of arsenic on transcription factor AP-1 and NF-κB DNA binding activity and related gene expression. *Toxicol Lett* 133: 33–45.

Huang, S., B. Kong, Y. Ma, and S. Jiang. 2002. Apoptosis of drug-resistant human ovarian carcinoma cell line 3AO/cDDP induced by arsenic trioxide and its mechanism. *Zhonghua Yi Xue Za Zhi* 82: 911–914.

Huang, Z. and D. Wells. 2010. The human oocyte and cumulus cells relationship: New insights from the cumulus cell transcriptome. *Mol Hum Reprod* 16: 715–725.

Huang, X., Z. Zhuang, K. Frenkel, C. B. Klein, and M. Costa. 1994. The role of nickel and nickel-mediated reactive oxygen species in the mechanism of nickel carcinogenesis. *Environ Health Perspect* 102: 281–284.

Hussain, S. M., K. L. Hess, J. M. Gearhart, K. T. Geiss, and J. J. Schlager. 2005. In vitro toxicity of nanoparticles in BRL 3A rat liver cells. *Toxicol in vitro* 19: 975–983.

IARC. 1990. Nickel and nickel compounds, pp. 257–445. Lyon, France: IARC Monographs on the Evaluation of Carcinogenic Risks to Humans.

Irwin, R. J., M. VanMouwerik, L. Stevens, M. D. Seese, and W. Basham. 1997. *Environmental Contaminants Encyclopedia: Cadmium*, pp. 1–88. Fruita, CO: National Park Service.

Jarup, L. and A. Akesson. 2009. Current status of cadmium as an environmental health problem. *Toxicol Appl Pharmacol* 238: 201–208.

Jaskulski, D., J. K. deRiel, W. E. Mercer, B. Calabretta, and R. Baserga. 1988. Inhibition of cellular proliferation by antisense oligodeoxynucleotides to PCNA cyclin. *Science* 240: 1544–1546.

Joly, A. L., G. Wettstein, G. Mignot, F. Ghiringhelli, and C. Garrido. 2010. Dual role of heat shock proteins as regulators of apoptosis and innate immunity. *J Innate Immun* 2: 238–247.

Jomova, K. and M. Valko. 2011. Advances in metal-induced oxidative stress and human disease. *Toxicology* 283: 65–87.

Jooste, P. J. and E. C. M. Anelich. 2008. Safety and quality of dairy products. In *Advanced Dairy Science and Technology*, eds. T. Britz and R. K. Robinson, pp. 153–78. Oxford, U.K.: Blackwell Publishing Ltd.

Jose, G. P., S. Santra, S. K. Mandal, and T. K. Sengupta. 2011. Singlet oxygen mediated DNA degradation by copper nanoparticles: Potential towards cytotoxic effect on cancer cells. *J Nanobiotechnol* 9: 1–9.

Junaid, M., D. K. Chowdhuri, R. Narayan, R. Shanker, and D. K. Saxena. 1995. Lead-induced changes in ovarian follicular development and maturation in mice. *J Toxicol Environ Health* 50: 31–40.

Junaid, M., R. C. Murthy, and D. K. Saxena. 1996. Embryotoxicity of orally administered chromium in mice: Exposure during the period of organogenesis. *Toxicol Lett* 84: 143–148.

Kah, M., L. Levy, and C. Brown. 2012. Potential for effects of land contamination on human health. 1.The case of cadmium. *J Toxicol Environ Health B Crit Rev* 15: 348–363.

Kamath, S. M., B. J. Stoecker, M. L. Davis-Whitenack et al. 1997. Absorption, retention and urinary excretion of chromium-51 in rats pretreated with indomethacin and dosed with dimethylprostaglandin E2, misoprostol or prostacyclin. *J Nutr* 127: 478–482.

Kanojia, R. K., M. Junaid, and R. C. Murthy. 1998. Embryo and fetotoxicity of hexavalent chromium: A long-term study. *Toxicol Lett* 95: 165–172.

Kar, A. B., R. P. Das, and J. N. Karkun. 1959. Ovarian changes in prepuberal rats after treatment with cadmium chloride. *Acta Biol Med Gerontol* 3: 372–399.

Kasprzak, K. S. 1995. Possible role of oxidative damage in metal-induced carcinogenesis. *Cancer Invest* 13: 411–430.

Khan, E. A., M. P. Sinha, N. Saxena, and P. N. Mehrotra. 1992. Biochemical effect of cadmium toxicity on a hill stream teleost Gara mullya (Sykes) during egg maturation II cholesterol and glycogen. *Poll Res* 11: 163–167.

Kirpnick-Sobol, Z., R. Reliene, and R. H. Schiestl. 2006. Carcinogenic Cr(VI) and the nutritional supplement Cr(III) induce DNA deletions in yeast and mice. *Cancer Res* 66: 3480–3484.

Klimisch, H. J. 1993. Lung deposition, lung clearance and renal accumulation of inhaled cadmium chloride and cadmium sulphide in rats. *Toxicology* 84: 103–124.

Kogelmann, W. J. and W. E. Sharpe. 2006. Soil acidity and manganese in declining and nondeclining sugar maple stands in Pennsylvania. *J Environ Qual* 35: 433–441.

Kolesarova, A., S. Roychoudhury, J. Slivkova et al. 2010. In vitro study on the effects of lead and mercury on porcine ovarian granulosa cells. *J Environ Sci Health A Tox Hazard Subst Environ Eng* 45: 320–331.

Kotler, M., C. Rodriguez, R. M. Sainz, I. Antolin, and A. Menendez-Peláe. 1998. Melatonin increases gene expression for antioxidant enzymes in rat brain cortex. *J Pineal Res* 24: 83–89.

Kramer, M. M., M. T. Harman, and A. K. Brill. 1933. Disturbances of reproduction and ovarian changes in the guinea-pig in relation to vitamin C deficiency. *Am J Physiol* 106: 611–622.

Krivosheev, A. B., E. L. Poteriaeva, B. N. Krivosheev, L. Kupriianova, and E. L. Smirnova 2012. Toxic effects of cadmium on the human body. *Med Tr Prom Ekol* 6: 35–42.

Kucher, I. M. 1966. A single dose of 10–45 mg sodium dichromate administered to rabbits resulted in 80% mortality. *Proceedings of the 5th Scientific Session of the Aktiubinsk Medical Institute*, pp. 24–26. Alma-Ata, Kazakhstan.

Kurihara, A., H. Nagoshi, M. Yabuki et al. 2007. Ser46 phosphorylation of p53 is not always sufficient to induce apoptosis: Multiple mechanisms of regulation of p53-dependent apoptosis. *Genes Cells* 12: 853–861.

Lamperti, A. A. and R. H. Printz. 1973. Effects of mercuric chloride on the reproductive cycle of the female hamster. *Biol Reprod* 8: 378–387.

Lee, B., J. K. Hiney, M. D. Pine, V. K. Srivastava, and W. L. Dees. 2007. Manganese stimulates luteinizing hormone releasing hormone secretion in prepubertal female rats: Hypothalamic site and mechanism of action. *J Physiol (Paris)* 578: 765–772.

Leslie, E. M. 2012. Arsenic-glutathione conjugate transport by the human multidrug resistance proteins (MRPs/ABCCs). *J Inorg Biochem* 108: 141–149.

Li, M., C. L. Brooks, F. Wu-Baer et al. 2003. Mono- versus polyubiquitination: Differential control of p53 fate by Mdm2. *Science* 302: 1972–1975.

Li, M., J. F. Cai, and J. F. Chiu. 2002. Arsenic induces oxidative stress and activates stress gene expressions in cultured lung epithelial cells. *J Cell Biochem* 87: 29–38.

Liu, L., S. Z. Mao, X. M. Liu et al. 2008. Functional mimicry of the active site of glutathione peroxidase by glutathione imprinted selenium-containing protein. *Biomacromolecules* 9: 363–368.

Li, D., K. Morimoto, T. Takeshita, and Y. Lu. 2001. Arsenic induces DNA damage via reactive oxygen species in human cells. *Environ Health Prev Med* 6: 27–32.

Liu, S., L. Xu, T. Zhang, G. Ren, and Z. Yang. 2010. Oxidative stress and apoptosis induced by nanosized titanium dioxide in PC12 cells. *Toxicology* 267: 172–177.

Long, X., M. J. Goldenthal, and J. Marin-Garcia. 2007. Oxidative stress enhances phosphorylation of p53 in neonatal rat cardiomyocytes. *Mol Cell Biochem* 303: 167–174.

Low, S. C. and M. J. Berry. 1996. Knowing when not to stop: Selenocysteine incorporation in eukaryotes. *Trends Biochem Sci* 21: 203–208.

Lunder, S. and D. Undurraga. 2012. *Getting Arsenic out of Your (and Your Kids') Diet*. Washington, DC: Environmental Working Group.

Machlin, L. J. and A. Bendich. 1987. Free radical tissue damage: Protective role of antioxidant nutrients. *FASEB J* 1: 441–445.

Magos, L. 1967. Mercury—Blood interaction and mercury uptake by the brain after vapor exposure. *Environ Res* 4: 323–337.

Makarov, Y. and L. A. Shimtova. 1978. Occupational conditions and gynecological illness in workers engaged in the production of chromium compounds. *Environ Health Perspect* 24: 1–128.

Malumbres, M. 2011. Physiological relevance of cell cycle kinases. *Physiol Rev* 91: 973–1007.

Marbaniang, D. G. 2012. Spectrophotometric determination of manganese in ground water in Shillong city using Bismuthate oxidation method. *Int J Environ Protect* 21: 22–26.

Massányi, P., N. Lukác, V. Uhrín et al. 2007a. Female reproductive toxicology of cadmium. *Acta Biol Hung* 58: 287–299.

Massányi, P., R. Stawarz, N. Lukac et al. 2007b. Cadmium associated microscopic and ultrastructural alterations in female reproductive organs of rabbits. *Acta Microscopica* 16: 114–115.

Massanyi, P., J. Trandzik, P. Nad et al. 2005. Concentration of copper, zinc, iron, cadmium, lead and nickel in bull, ram, boar, stallion and fox semen. *J Environ Sci Health* 40: 1097–1105.

Meek, D. W. and C. W. Anderson. 2009. Posttranslational modification of p53: Cooperative integrators of function. *Cold Spring Harb Perspect Biol* 1: a000950.

Messarah, M., F. Klibet, A. Boumendjel et al. 2012. Hepatoprotective role and antioxidant capacity of selenium on arsenic-induced liver injury in rats. *Exp Toxicol Pathol* 64: 167–174.

Mihara, M., S. Erster, A. Zaika et al. 2003. p53 has a direct apoptogenic role at the mitochondria. *Mol Cell* 11: 577–590.

Millar, J. 1992. Vitamin C—The primate fertility factor? *Med Hypotheses* 38: 292–295.

Milne, D. M., L. E. Campbell, D. G. Campbell, and D. W. Meek. 1995. p53 is phosphorylated in vitro and in vivo by an ultraviolet radiation-induced protein kinase characteristic of the c-Jun kinase, JNK1. *J Biol Chem* 270: 5511–5518.

Mishra, D. and S. J. Flora. 2008. Differential oxidative stress and DNA damage in rat brain regions and blood following chronic arsenic exposure. *Toxicol Ind Health* 24: 247–256.

Mlynarcíkova, A., S. Scsukova, S. Vrsanska et al. 2004. Inhibitory effect of cadmium and tobacco alkaloids on expansion of porcine oocyte-cumulus complexes. *Cent Eur J Public Health* 12(Suppl): S62–S64.

Morrison, D., Q. Lin, S. Wiehe et al. 2012. Spatial relationships between lead sources and children's blood lead levels in the urban center of Indianapolis (USA). *Environ Geochem Health* 35(2): 171.

Mukherjee, S. 2011. Essentials of mineralogy. In *Applied Mineralogy: Applications in Industry and Environment*, pp. 1–19. New Delhi, India: Springer-Capital Publishing Company.

Müller, L. 1989. Protective effects of DL-alpha-lipoic acid on cadmium-induced deterioration of rat hepatocytes. *Toxicology* 58: 175–185.

Murthy, R. C., M. Junaid, and D. K. Saxena. 1996. Ovarian dysfunction in mice following chromium (VI) exposure. *Toxicol Lett* 89: 147–154.

Mushak, P. and A. F. Crocetti. 1990. Methods for reducing lead exposure in young children and other risk groups: An integrated summary of a report to the U.S. Congress on childhood lead poisoning. *Environ Health Perspect* 89: 125–135.

Mylroie, A. A., C. Umbles, and J. Kyle. 1984. Effects of dietary copper supplementation on erythrocyte superoxide dismutase activity, ceruloplasmin and related parameters in rats ingesting lead acetate. *Trace Substances in Environ Health* 18: 497–504.

Nad, P., P. Massanyi, M. Skalicka et al. 2007. The effect of cadmium in combination with zinc and selenium on ovarian structure in Japanese quails. *J Environ Sci Health A Tox Hazard Subst Environ Eng* 42: 2017–2022.

Nakayama, K., A. Kanzaki, K. Ogawa et al. 2002. Copper-transporting P-type adenosine triphosphatase (ATP7B) as a cisplatin based chemoresistance marker in ovarian carcinoma: Comparative analysis with expression of MDR1, MRP1, MRP2, LRP and BCRP. *Int J Cancer* 101: 488–495.

Navarro, P. A., L. Liu, and D. L. Keefe. 2004. In vivo effects of arsenite on meiosis, preimplantation development, and apoptosis in the mouse. *Biol Reprod* 70: 980–985.

Nayak, S. B., V. R. Bhat, and S. S. Mayya. 2004. Serum copper, ceruloplasmin and thiobarbituric acid reactive substance status in patients with ovarian cancer. *Indian J Physiol Pharmacol* 48: 486–488.

Nriagu, J. O. 1988. Historical perspectives. In *Chromium in the Natural and Human Environments*, eds. J. O. Nriagu and E. Nieboer, pp. 1–19. New York: John Wiley & Sons.

Oberdoerster, G., E. Oberdoerster, and J. Oberdoerster. 2005. Nanotoxicology: An emerging discipline evolving from studies of ultrafine particles. *Environ Health Perspect* 113: 823–839.

Oktay, K., R. S. Schenken, and J. F. Nelson. 1995. Proliferating cell nuclear antigen marks the initiation of follicular growth in the rat. *Biol Reprod* 53: 295–301.

Ouarda, M. and C. Abdennour. 2008. Influence of sudden cystine supplementation and suppression on adrenal and ovary of lead exposed rat. *Eur J Sci Res* 23: 548–558.

Padayatty, S. J., A. Katz, Y. Wang et al. 2003. Vitamin C as an antioxidant: Evaluation of its role in disease prevention. *J Am Coll Nutr* 22: 18–35.

Padayatty, S. J. and M. Levine. 2001. New insights into the physiology and pharmacology of vitamin C. *CMAJ* 164: 353–355.

Paksy, K., K. Rajczy, Z. Forgács et al. 1997. Effect of cadmium on morphology and steroidogenesis of cultured human ovarian granulosa cells. *J Appl Toxicol* 17: 321–327.

Paksy, K., B. Varga, and G. Folly. 1990. Long-term effects of a single cadmium chloride injection on the ovulation, ovarian progesterone and estradiol-17 beta secretion in rats. *Acta Physiol Hung* 76: 245–252.

Pani, G., R. Colavitti, B. Bedogni et al. 2004. Mitochondrial superoxide dismutase: A promising target for new anticancer therapies. *Curr Med Chem* 11: 1299–1308.

Pastore, A., G. Federici, E. Bertini, and F. Piemonte. 2003. Analysis of glutathione: Implication in redox and detoxification. *Clin Chim Acta* 333: 19–39.

Petrusevski, B., S. K. Sharma, J. C. Schippers, and K. Shordt. 2007. Arsenic in drinking water, pp. 1–11. Hague, the Netherlands: IRC International Water and Sanitation Centre.

Pi, J., S. Horiguchi, Y. Sun et al. 2003. A potential mechanism for the impairment of nitric oxide formation caused by prolonged oral exposure to arsenate in rabbits. *Free Rad Biol Med* 35: 102–113.

Piasek, M. and J. Laskey. 1994. Acute cadmium exposure and ovarian steroidogenesis in cycling and pregnant rats. *Reprod Toxicol* 8: 495–507.

Piasek, M. and J. W. Laskey. 1999. Effects of in vitro cadmium exposure on ovarian steroidogenesis in rats. *J Appl Toxicol* 19: 211–217.

Picco, S. J., D. E. Rosa, J. P. Anchordoquy et al. 2012. Effects of copper sulphate concentrations during in vitro maturation of bovine oocytes. *Theriogenology* 77: 373–381.

Pine, M., B. Lee, R. Dearth, J. K. Hiney, and W. L. Dees. 2005. Manganese acts centrally to stimulate luteinizing hormone secretion: A potential influence on female pubertal development. *Toxicol Sci* 85: 880–885.

Pohl, W. L. 2011. *Economic Geology: Principles and Practice*, pp. 159–163. Oxford, U.K.: Wiley-Blackwell Publishers.

Pollack, A. Z., E. F. Schisterman, L. R. Goldman et al. 2011. Cadmium, lead, and mercury in relation to reproductive hormones and anovulation in premenopausal women. *Environ Health Perspect* 119: 1156–1161.

Pomerening, J. R. 2009. Positive-feedback loops in cell cycle progression. *FEBS Lett* 583: 3388–3396.

Pott, W. A., S. A. Benjamin, and R. S. Yang. 2001. Pharmacokinetics, metabolism, and carcinogenicity of arsenic. *Rev Environ Contam Toxicol* 169: 165–214.

Pritchard, D. E., J. Singh, D. L. Carlisle, and S. R. Patierno. 2000. Cyclosporin A inhibits chromium(VI)-induced apoptosis and mitochondrial cytochrome c release and restores clonogenic survival in CHO cells. *Carcinogenesis* 21: 2027–2033.

Priya, P. N., A. Pillai, and S. Gupta. 2004. Effect of simultaneous exposure to lead and cadmium on gonadotropin binding and steroidogenesis on granulosa cells: An in vitro study. *Indian J Exp Biol* 42: 143–148.

Prohaska, J. R. 1983. Comparison of copper metabolism between brindled mice and dietary copper deficient mice using 67Cu. *J Nutr* 113: 1212–1220.

Quig, D. 1998. Cysteine metabolism and metal toxicity. *Altern Med Rev* 3: 262–270.

Rahman, Q., M. Lohani, E. Dopp et al. 2002. Evidence that ultrafine titanium dioxide induces micronuclei and apoptosis in Syrian hamster embryo fibroblasts. *Environ Health Perspect* 110: 797–800.

Rahmanto, A. S. and M. J. Davies. 2012. Selenium-containing amino acids as direct and indirect antioxidants. *IUBMB Life* 64: 863–871.

Ramanathan, K., M. Anusuyadevi, S. Shila, and C. Panneerselvam. 2005. Ascorbic acid and tocopherol as potent modulators of apoptosis on arsenic induced toxicity in rats. *Toxicol Lett* 156: 297–306.

Rao, M. V., S. L. Chawla, and S. R. Sharma. 2009. Protective role of vitamin E on nickel and/or chromium induced oxidative stress in the mouse ovary. *Food Chem Toxicol* 47: 1368–1371.

Rehm, S. and M. P. Waalkes. 1988. Cadmium-induced ovarian toxicity in hamsters, mice, and rats. *Fundam Appl Toxicol* 10: 635–647.

Reiter, R. J., D. X. Tan, J. Cabrera et al. 1999. The oxidant/antioxidant network: Role of melatonin. *Biol Signal Recept* 8: 56–63.

Reubinoff, B. E., R. Har-El, N. Kitrossky et al. 1996. Increased levels of redox-active iron in follicular fluid: A possible cause of free radical-mediated infertility in beta-thalassemia major. *Am J Obstet Gynecol* 174: 914–918.

Révész, C., Z. Forgács, P. Lázár et al. 2004. Effect of nickel (ni(2+)) on primary human ovarian granulosa cells in vitro. *Toxicol Mech Method* 14: 287–292.

Rin, K., K. Kawaguchi, K. Yamanaka et al. 1995. DNA-strand breaks induced by dimethylarsinic acid, a metabolite of inorganic arsenics, are strongly enhanced by superoxide anion radicals. *Biol Pharm Bull* 18: 45–48.

Rittner, M. N. 2002. Market analysis of nanostructured materials. *Am Ceram Soc Bull* 81: 33–36.

Robertson, D. M. 2011. Hemochromatosis and ovarian cancer. *Womens Health (Lond Engl)* 7: 525–527.

Robison, S. H. and M. Costa. 1982. The induction of DNA strand breakage by nickel compounds in cultured Chinese hamster ovary cells. *Cancer Lett* 15: 35–40.

Rowland, A. S., D. D. Baird, C. R. Weinberg et al. 1994. The effect of occupational exposure to mercury vapour on the fertility of female dental assistants. *Occup Environ Med* 51: 28–34.

Rowland, I. R., R. D. Robinson, and R. A. Doherty. 1984. Effects of diet on mercury metabolism and excretion in mice given methylmercury: Role of gut flora. *Arch Environ Health* 39: 401–408.

Sahmoune, A. and L. Mitiche. 2009. Extraction and transport of chromium (VI) through a bulk liquid membrane containing triphenylphosphine. *Ann Chim* 94: 1–10.

Samimi, G., R. Safaei, K. Katano et al. 2004. Increased expression of the copper efflux transporter ATP7A mediates resistance to cisplatin, carboplatin, and oxaliplatin in ovarian cancer cells. *Clin Cancer Res* 10: 4661–4669.

Schell, L. M., K. K. Burnitz, and P. W. Lathrop. 2010. Pollution and human biology. *Ann Hum Biol* 37: 347–366.

Schrauzer, G. N. 2009. Selenium and selenium-antagonistic elements in nutritional cancer prevention. *Crit Rev Biotechnol* 29: 10–17.

Schuler, M. and D. R. Green. 2001. Mechanisms of p53-dependent apoptosis. *Biochem Soc Trans* 29: 684–688.

Sharma, R. K. and M. Sharma. 1997. Physiological perspectives of copper. *Indian J Exp Biol* 35: 696–713.

Shen, W., Y. Chen, C. Li, and L. Li. 2000. Effects of 6 kinds of metal elements on meiotic maturation and in vitro fertilization on mouse oocyte. *Wei Sheng Yan Jiu* 29: 202–204.

Shi, H., X. Shi, and K. J. Liu. 2004. Xidative mechanism of arsenic toxicity and carcinogenesis. *Mol Cell Biochem* 255: 67–78.

Shiao, Y. H., S. H. Lee, and K. S. Kasprzak. 1998. Cell cycle arrest, apoptosis and p53 expression in nickel(II) acetate-treated Chinese hamster ovary cells. *Carcinogenesis* 19: 1203–1207.

Singer, S. T., E. P. Vichinsky, G. Gildengorin et al. 2011. Reproductive capacity in iron overloaded women with thalassemia major. *Blood* 118: 2878–2881.

Sioson, C. and A. Herrera. 1993. Impact of nickel poisoning on the histology of the ovaries of Oreochromis mossambicus, eds. C. L. Marte, G. F. Quinitio, and A. C. Emata, p. 109. Tigbauan, Iloilo, Philippines: SEAFDEC Aquaculture Department.

Siu, P. M., Y. Wang, and S. E. Alway. 2009. Apoptotic signaling induced by H2O2-mediated oxidative stress in differentiated C2C12 myotubes. *Life Sci* 84: 468–481.

Sluss, H. K., H. Gannon, A. H. Coles et al. 2010. Phosphorylation of p53 serine 18 upregulates apoptosis to suppress Myc-induced tumorigenesis. *Mol Cancer Res* 8: 216–222.

Smida, A. D., X. P. Valderrama, M. C. Agostini, M. A. Furlan, and J. Chedrese. 2004. Cadmium stimulates transcription of the cytochrome p450 side chain cleavage gene in genetically modified stable porcine granulosa cells. *Biol Reprod* 70: 25–31.

St Clair, D. 2004. Manganese superoxide dismutase: Genetic variation and regulation. *J Nutr* 134: 3190S–3191S.

Stadnicka, A. 1980. Localization of mercury in the rat ovary after oral administration of mercuric chloride. *Acta Histochem* 67: 227–233.

Stanciu, M. and D. B. DeFranco. 2002. Prolonged nuclear retention of activated extracellular signal-regulated protein kinase promotes cell death generated by oxidative toxicity or proteasome inhibition in a neuronal cell line. *J Biol Chem* 277: 4010–4017.

Stankiewicz, A. R., G. Lachapelle, C. P. Foo, S. M. Radicioni, and D. D. Mosser. 2005. Hsp70 inhibits heat-induced apoptosis upstream of mitochondria by preventing Bax translocation. *J Biol Chem* 280: 38729–3839.

Stanley, J. A., J. Lee, T. K. Nithy et al. 2011. Chromium-VI arrests cell cycle and decreases granulosa cell proliferation by down-regulating cyclin-dependent kinases (CDK) and cyclins and up-regulating CDK-inhibitors. *Reprod Toxicol* 32: 112–123.

Stanley, J. A., K. K. Sivakumar, T. K. Nithy et al. 2013. Postnatal exposure to hexavalent chromium through mother's milk accelerates follicular atresia in F1 offspring through increased oxidative stress and depletion of antioxidant enzymes. *Free Rad Biol Med* 61C: 179–196.

Stohs, S. J. and D. Bagchi. 1995. Oxidative mechanisms in the toxicity of metal-ions. *Free Rad Biol Med* 18: 321–336.

Stowe, H. D. and R. A. Moore. 1971. The reproductive ability and progeny of F1 Pb-toxic rats. *Fertil Steril* 22: 755–760.

Suárez-Serrano, A., C. Alcaraz, C. Lbáñez, R. Trobajo, and C. Barata. 2010. Procambarus clarkii as a bioindicator of heavy metal pollution sources in the lower Ebro River and Delta. *Ecotoxicol Environ Saf* 73: 280–286.

Suarez, D. L. and D. Langmuir. 1976. Heavy metal relationships in a Pennsylvania soil. *Geochim Cosmochim Acta* 40: 589–598.

Subar, A. F., S. M. Krebs-Smith, A. Cook, and L. L. Kahle. 1998. Dietary sources of nutrients among US adults, 1989 to 1991. *J Am Diet Assoc* 98: 537–547.

Sun, Q., D. Tan, Q. Zhou et al. 2012. Oxidative damage of lung and its protective mechanism in mice caused by long-term exposure to titanium dioxide nanoparticles. *J Biomed Mater Res A* 100: 2554–2562.

Sutherland, E. and M. Costa. 2002. Nickel. In *Heavy Metals in the Environment*, ed. B. Sarkar, pp. 401–440. New York: CRC Press.

Sutton, R. 2010. Chromium-6 in U.S. tap water, pp. 1–22. Oakland, CA: Environmental Working Group.

Takahashi, M., T. Nagai, S. Hamano et al. 1993. Effect of thiol compounds on in vitro development and intracellular glutathione content of bovine embryo. *Biol Reprod Fertil Dev* 49: 228–232.

Taneja, S. K. and M. Mahajan. 1999. Zinc in obesity-a critical review. *JPAS* 1: 211–216.

Tapiero, H. and K. D. Tew. 2003. Trace elements in human physiology and pathology: Zinc and metallothioneins. *Biomed Pharmacother* 57: 399–411.

Tarin, J. J. 1996. Potential effects of age-associated oxidative stress on mammalian oocytes/embryos. *Mol Hum Reprod* 2: 717–724.

Taupeau, C., J. Poupon, F. Nomé, and B. Lefèvre. 2001. Lead accumulation in the mouse ovary after treatment-induced follicular atresia. *Reprod Toxicol* 15: 385–391.

Terek, M. C., B. Karabulut, N. Selvi et al. 2006. Arsenic trioxide-loaded, microemulsion-enhanced cytotoxicity on MDAH 2774 ovarian carcinoma cell line. *Int J Gynecol Cancer* 16: 532–537.

Thomas, K. V., J. Farkas, E. Farmen et al. 2011. Effects of dispersed aggregates of carbon and titanium dioxide engineered nanoparticles on rainbow trout hepatocytes. *J Toxicol Environ Health A* 74: 466–477.

Thompson, S. A. 2000. An overview of nickel–titanium alloys used in dentistry. *Int Endodontic J* 33: 297–310.

Thoreux-Manlay, A., C. Le Goascogne, D. Segretain, B. Jégou, and G. Pinon-Lataillade. 1995. Lead affects steroidogenesis in rat Leydig cells in vivo and in vitro. *Toxicology* 103: 53–62.

Trachootham, D., D. Lu, M. A. Ogasawara, R. Valle, and P. Huang. 2008. Redox regulation of cell survival. *Antioxid Redox Signal* 10: 1343–1374.

TRI06. 2008. TRI explorer: Providing access to EPA's toxics release inventory data. Washington, DC: U.S. Environmental Protection Agency.

Tylecote, R. F. 1991. *The Industrial Revolution in Metals*. London, U.K.: The Institute of Metals.

USEPA. 2001. National primary drinking water regulations: Arsenic and clarifications to compliance and new source contaminants monitoring, ed. E. P. Agency, pp. 6975–7066. Washington, DC: U.S. Environmental Protection Agency.

Uslu, R., U. A. Sanli, C. Sezgin et al. 2000. Arsenic trioxide-mediated cytotoxicity and apoptosis in prostate and ovarian carcinoma cell lines. *Clin Cancer Res* 6: 4957–4964.

Valko, M., H. Morris, and M. T. Cronin. 2005. Metals, toxicity and oxidative stress. *Curr Med Chem* 12: 1161–1208.

Vermande, G. J. and J. W. Meigs. 1960. Changes in the ovary of Rhesus monkey after chronic Pb intoxication. *Fertil Steril* 11: 223–234.

Verschoor, M. L., L. A. Wilson, and G. Singh. 2010. Mechanisms associated with mitochondrial-generated reactive oxygen species in cancer. *Can J Physiol Pharmacol* 88: 204–219.

Wan, X., J. Zhu, Y. Zhu et al. 2010. Rat ovarian follicle bioassay reveals adverse effects of cadmium chloride (CdCl2) exposure on follicle development and oocyte maturation. *Toxicol Ind Health* 26: 609–618.

Wang, T. S., C. F. Kuo, K. Y. Jan, and H. Huang. 1996. Arsenite induces apoptosis in Chinese hamster ovary cells by generation of reactive oxygen species. *J Cell Physiol* 169: 256–268.

Watson, M., L. van Leer, J. J. Vanderlelie, and A. V. Perkins. 2012. Selenium supplementation protects trophoblast cells from oxidative stress. *Placenta* 33: 1012–1019.

Welch, A. H., D. B. Westjohn, D. R. Helsel, and R. B. Wanty. 2000. Arsenic in ground water of the United States: Occurrence and geochemistry. *Ground Water* 38: 589–604.

Wetsel, W. C., M. M. Valença, I. Merchenthaler et al. 1992. Intrinsic pulsatile secretory activity of immortalized luteinizing hormone-releasing hormone-secreting neurons. *Proc Natl Acad Sci USA* 89: 4149–4153.

Whanger, P. D. 1992. Selenium in the treatment of heavy metals poisoning and chemical carcinogenesis. *J Trace Elem Elect* 6: 209–221.

Williams, D. F. 2001. Titanium for medical applications. In *Titanium in Medicine: Material Science, Surface Science, Engineering, Biological Responses, and Medical Applications*, eds. D. M. Brunnette, P. Tengvall, M. Textor, and P. Thompsen, pp. 13–25. New York: Springer-Verlag.

Yang, S., Z. Zhang, J. He et al. 2012. Ovarian toxicity induced by dietary cadmium in hen. *Biol Trace Elem Res* 148: 53–60.

Yoshida, M., K. Ishigaki, T. Nagai, M. Chikyu, and V. G. Pursel. 1993. Glutathione concentration during maturation and after fertilization in pig oocytes: Relevance to the ability of oocytes to form male pronucleus. *Biol Reprod* 49: 89–94.

Young, I. S. and I. S. Woodside. 2001. Antioxidants in health and disease. *J Clin Pathol* 54: 176–186.

Zhang, W. and H. Jia. 2007. Effect and mechanism of cadmium on the progesterone synthesis of ovaries. *Toxicology* 239: 204–212.

Zhang, W., F. Pang, Y. Huang, P. Yan, and W. Lin. 2008. Cadmium exerts toxic effects on ovarian steroid hormone release in rats. *Toxicol Lett* 182: 18–23.

Zhang, J. and B. Wang. 2006. Arsenic trioxide (As(2)O(3)) inhibits peritoneal invasion of ovarian carcinoma cells in vitro and in vivo. *Gynecol Oncol* 103: 199–206.

Zhao, Y., L. Chaiswing, J. M. Velez et al. 2005. p53 translocation to mitochondria precedes its nuclear translocation and targets mitochondrial oxidative defense protein-manganese superoxide dismutase. *Cancer Res* 65: 3745–3750.

Zhitkovich, A. 2005. Importance of chromium-DNA adducts in mutagenicity and toxicity of chromium(VI). *Chem Res Toxicol* 18: 3–11.

Zhitkovich, A. 2011. Chromium in drinking water: Sources, metabolism, and cancer risks. *Chem Res Toxicol* 24: 1617–1629.

Zhitkovich, A., E. Peterson-Roth, and M. Reynolds. 2005. Killing of chromium-damaged cells by mismatch repair and its relevance to carcinogenesis. *Cell Cycle* 4: 1050–1052.

Zipper, J. A., H. J. Tatum, M. Medel, L. Pastene, and M. Rivera. 1979. Contraception through the use of intrauterine metals. I. Copper as an adjunct to the T device. *Am J Obstet Gynecol* 109: 771–774.

Zowczak, M., M. Iskra, J. Paszkowski et al. 2001a. Oxidase activity of ceruloplasmin and concentrations of copper and zinc in serum of cancer patients. *J Trace Elem Med Biol* 15: 193–196.

Zowczak, M., M. Iskra, L. Torliñski, and S. Cofta. 2001b. Analysis of serum copper and zinc concentrations in cancer patients. *Biol Trace Elem Res* 82: 1–8.

10 Cigarette Smoking and Ovarian Function

Anne M. Gannon, J.C. Sadeu, S.K. Agarwal, Claude L. Hughes, and Warren G. Foster

CONTENTS

10.1 INTRODUCTION

The global prevalence of infertility is estimated to be 9% [1] and between 50 and 80 million people worldwide are infertile [2]. Advanced age, diet, prescription medication use, preexisting health status, and infections are among the known risk factors for infertility; however, for many women, the cause of their infertility is unknown. Environmental toxicants and lifestyle factors are thought to adversely affect human fertility in part via impaired ovarian function [3–5]. Of the many environmental chemicals to which women are exposed, we have focused on cigarette smoking because it is the one activity that a woman chooses to engage in that is known to kill eggs, decreases fertility, and brings forward the age of menopause. The health-care costs in 2008, in the United States, associated with cigarette smoking were 96 billion dollars [6] with secondhand cigarette smoke exposure adding another 10 billion dollars [7]. A well-documented general health hazard, cigarette smoke also has serious consequences for reproductive health in women. Indeed, compared to women who have never smoked or been exposed to cigarette smoke, cigarette smoking has been linked to longer time to pregnancy, earlier age at menopause, decreased follicle counts, and diminished response to ovulation induction [8–15]. Despite the documented adverse health effects of cigarette smoking on women's reproductive health, the number of young women commencing smoking is increasing [16], suggesting that current smoking prevention strategies are ineffective in this population. Hence, women represent a growing population who are exposed to the single most preventable toxic exposure and documented health risk.

The increase in the number of young women who smoke coupled with the trend toward delayed childbearing [17] plus the well-documented decrease in fertility with advancing age [18–20] highlights cigarette smoking as a serious reproductive health issue. In the United States, the proportion of first births to women aged 30 years or greater has increased from 5% in 1975 to 24% in 2006 [21]. A mathematical model of follicular growth dynamic suggests that the number of primordial follicles initiating growth daily in the ovary of a 25-year-old woman is approximately 37. With increasing age, the population of these specific follicles progressively decreases to reach an ovarian reserve that is less than 1000 follicles by the median menopausal age of 51 [22,23]. The decline in fertility begins generally in the fourth decade of life where a significant change in the dynamic of follicle growth occurs with the rate of primordial follicle depletion increasing by 2–3-fold from around age 37 onward. Hence, we predict that the young women who are smoking today will place even greater demands on fertility clinics in the future. The decreased number of ova retrieved in women who smoke [24] and the decreased success of assisted reproductive techniques in smokers [25,26] underscore the health concern. The problem is compounded by the fact that most women are unaware of the risks to reproductive health attributable to cigarette smoking [27]. Furthermore, nicotine addiction is very powerful; even successful "quitters" typically require multiple attempts over several years to successfully stop smoking [28–31]. Thus, merely counseling women to stop smoking is likely to have only modest benefits for ovarian function and reproductive health. Moreover, it is not known if smoking cessation can reverse the ovarian toxic effects of cigarette smoking. It is therefore imperative that we develop a better understanding of the mechanisms underlying the adverse effect of cigarette smoke on ovarian function and follicle loss to enable novel therapeutic options and targeted advice for women.

10.2 CIGARETTE SMOKE AND A MODE OF ACTION

Compared to nonsmokers, cigarette smoke exposure has been associated with longer time to pregnancy, altered ovarian steroidogenesis, depleted ovarian reserves, impaired oocyte function and viability, reduced IVF success rates, and earlier mean age of menopause [8,10,12,24–26,32–45]; however, the underlying mechanism(s) remains ill defined. Cigarette smoke is a complex mixture of toxic chemicals known to contain more than 4000 compounds including polycyclic aromatic hydrocarbons (PAHs), metals, cyanide, and nicotine [46–49]. Of the toxicants present in cigarette smoke, we are chiefly interested in the PAHs for several reasons. First, PAHs are chemicals produced from the incomplete combustion of fossil fuels and are found ubiquitously in air pollution, tobacco smoke (mainstream cigarette smoke and secondhand smoke), diet (barbecued foods and cereal grains), soot, and coal tar [50–58]. Hence, human exposure to these chemicals is unavoidable. Second, PAHs are known to act as ovarian toxicants [59–64]; and benzo[a]pyrene (B[*a*]P), an aryl hydrocarbon receptor (AhR)-ligand, has been quantified in serum and follicular fluid [65], and B[*a*]P-induced DNA adducts have been demonstrated in granulosa cells of women who smoke [66]. We have shown that concentrations of B[*a*]P representative of human exposure attenuate follicle development and steroidogenesis and decrease follicle survival [67–69]. Thus, we believe that PAHs are central to the ovarian toxic effects of cigarette smoke. The adverse effects on ovarian function found in women who smoke may also be present in nonsmokers who are unwittingly and chronically exposed to PAHs through other environmental sources such as secondhand smoke, air pollution, and diesel exhaust [70].

Extensive evidence demonstrates that most of the toxic actions of PAHs are mediated through the AhR [71]. Specifically, the adverse effects of PAHs on the ovary require the presence of a functional AhR, a ligand-activated transcription factor [72] ubiquitously expressed in many human tissues and cell lines [73,74], including oocytes and granulosa cells of ovarian follicles at all stages of development [72]. In the absence of a ligand, the AhR exists in an inactive form in the cytoplasm (Figure 10.1). Upon ligand binding, the AhR undergoes a conformational change resulting in exposure of the nuclear localization signal (NLS) leading to translocation of the AhR-ligand complex to the nucleus where it binds to the AhR nuclear translocator (ARNT) and subsequently recognizes and binds to specific DNA sequences in the 5′-flanking region of AhR-regulated genes (dioxin response element) (DRE) thereby altering gene expression. Commonly recognized AhR-regulated genes include but are not limited to the following: cytochrome P450 isoenzymes CYP1A1, 1A2, 1B1, 2S1, NAD(P)H:quinone acceptor oxidoreductase, and UDP glucouronyltransferase [75–81]. Furthermore, the AhR has been inculpated in the regulation of ovarian

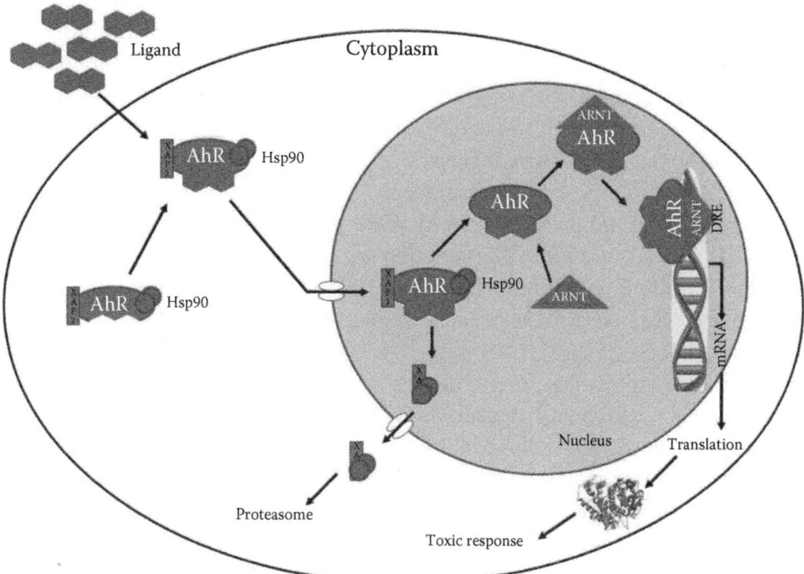

FIGURE 10.1 (See color insert.) The AhR is present in the cytoplasm coupled to heat shock protein (hsp90). Upon binding of the ligand with the AhR, the complex is transported to the nucleus of the cell where the receptor–ligand complex binds with the ARNT and hsp90 exits the nucleus to be degraded in the proteasome. The ligand–receptor–ARNT complex then binds with the dioxin response element (DRE) in AhR-regulated genes, resulting in their expression.

follicle numbers [72,82,83]. Therefore, we propose that the AhR has a central and incompletely understood role in follicle development and demise. Several distinct lines of evidence lend support to this hypothesis. First, there were more follicles at birth in $AhR^{-/-}$ mice compared to wild-type mice [72]. Second, activation of the AhR and its downstream target CYP1A1 has been demonstrated in smokers suggesting that toxic chemical constituents of cigarette smoke reach concentrations in the circulation sufficient to induce signaling through this receptor [84–86].

10.3 OVARY

The ovary is composed of a medulla surrounded by a cortex containing follicles at different stages of development. Follicles are composed of two theca layers, the externa and interna (androgen production), a basement membrane, granulosa cells (sites of estradiol [E_2] and antimüllerian hormone [AMH] synthesis), and an oocyte. In mammals, females are born with a finite population of primordial follicles that represent the resting pool of follicles. In adult humans, a cohort of primordial follicles constitutes one of the several waves of growing follicles with each menstrual cycle [87,88]. Typically, one follicle from the pool of growing follicles is selected to ovulate while the remainder become atretic. Of the estimated 500,000 follicles present in the human ovary at the start of reproductive life, only about 400 reach the preovulatory stage and ovulate. Therefore, follicle atresia is the fate for the vast majority of female germ cells [89]. Although the possibility of an ovarian or bone marrow stem cell population that could lead to repopulation of the ovary [90–95] has been suggested, this issue remains controversial [96] and does not obviate the role of primordial follicle depletion in triggering ovarian failure and menopause [97]. Thus, stem cell recruitment, were it to occur, is unlikely to counter the adverse effects of environmental toxicant exposure including cigarette smoke exposure.

Folliculogenesis (follicle recruitment and growth to ovulation) is regulated in a stage-dependent manner by oocyte-derived factors (e.g., bone morphogenetic protein-15 [BMP-15], growth differentiation factor-9 [GDF-9], kit, and kit ligand), gonadotropins (follicle-stimulating hormone [FSH] and luteinizing hormone [LH] in early antral and Graafian follicles), and several growth regulators (e.g., transforming growth factor-β [TGF-β], AMH, inhibin-B, activin, vascular endothelial growth factor, FOXL2, and insulin-like growth factors and binding proteins), reviewed in [98]. The mechanisms regulating primordial follicle recruitment are unknown; however, recent studies demonstrate that AMH, a member of the TGF-β family, is produced exclusively by healthy growing follicles, is positively correlated with antral follicle count, and is a negative regulator of primordial follicle recruitment [99–101]. AMH is therefore thought to have clinical value as a marker of ovarian aging [99–114]. Of note, circulating levels of AMH decline with age [115] and are lower in women who smoke compared to nonsmokers [26,116,117] although others have not found a similar relationship [13,105], potentially owing to differences in methods and age of study subjects. Circulating concentrations of AMH were lower in mice exposed to cigarette smoke compared to controls [63] as well as in rat [68] and mouse [69] follicles cultured in the presence of B[*a*]P, a key chemical constituent of cigarette smoke. Thus, measurement of AMH concentrations could provide a clinical marker of follicle reserve in women who smoke and provide clinicians with an objective marker for decision-making purposes in this population.

10.4 CIGARETTE SMOKE–INDUCED FOLLICLE LOSS

The ovary is a dynamic organ that, with each cycle, undergoes extensive cell proliferation, inflammation, tissue remodeling, angiogenesis, and removal of damaged cells or cells whose function is no longer needed. Cells generally die through one of at least three distinct processes including necrosis, terminal differentiation leading to cell death [118], and apoptosis. Although all three mechanisms are important, apoptosis (programmed cell death) is thought to be the main route of follicle atresia in the mammalian ovary [119–125]. Therefore, apoptosis is the most common target pathway assessed to explain environmental toxicant and cigarette smoke–induced ovarian follicle loss. Apoptosis is characterized by nuclear condensation, cell membrane blebbing, and degradation of the DNA into nucleosome fragments. Resulting nucleosomes can be detected by gel electrophoresis as a classical laddering pattern of 180 base pair fragments or by terminal deoxynucleotidyl transferase dUTP nick-end labeling (TUNEL). Contrary to our expectations, follicle loss in cigarette smoke–exposed mice was not associated with activation of either the intrinsic or extrinsic apoptosis pathways as shown by absence of an effect on TUNEL staining, DNA laddering, and activated caspase-3, or caspase-8 and 9 expression compared to controls [63]. While apoptosis is thought to be the primary mechanism of follicle atresia [119–125], emerging data challenges this notion [63,64], and we suggest that an alternative/accessory AhR-dependent cell death pathway is important in regulating cigarette smoke exposure–induced follicle loss.

Previous studies have shown that Bax is an important factor in the regulation of follicular endowment in mice [126]. Mice deficient in Bax have an increased number of follicles compared to wild-type mice. Destruction of developing fetal ovarian germ cells and induction of premature ovarian failure has been achieved in mice treated with AhR-ligands that activated the intrinsic pathway leading to enhanced Bax expression [82,83,127]. In mice, maternal exposure to high concentrations of the PAHs, B[*a*]P, and 7,12 dimethylbenz[a]anthracene (DMBA) (1 mg/kg each/week for 6 weeks) significantly depleted primordial follicle numbers via increased expression of Bax that, in a subsequent experiment, was shown to involve induction of *harakiri*, a gene that codes for a Bcl-2 interacting protein [128]. However, we note that AhR ligand–induced apoptosis may be both tissue and concentration dependent. Unlike the results earlier, treatment of pregnant mice with high concentrations of B[*a*]P and DMBA (1 mg/kg each/week for 6 weeks) inhibited apoptosis in the murine placenta [129]. In this study, treatments increased expression of FasL and Xiap (a prosurvival protein) but decreased Bax and apoptosis in the placenta, suggesting tissue specificity. Moreover, developmental exposure to the AhR-ligand tetrachlorodibenzo-*p*-dioxin (TCDD) is associated with vaginal dysmorphogenesis in mice through attenuated apoptosis [130]. We therefore postulate that AhR-mediated effects on apoptosis are target tissue dependent. The effects of AhR-ligands may also be concentration dependent.

In our studies, we consistently find that cigarette smoke exposure produces a significant decrease in ovarian weight (absolute and relative) and loss of follicles

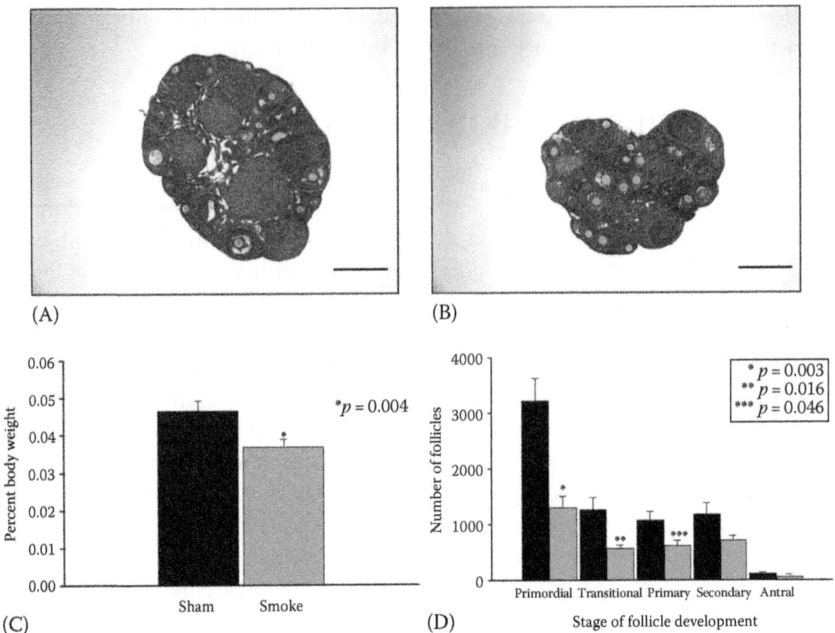

FIGURE 10.2 Mice were exposed to cigarette smoke (12 cigarettes twice a day/5 days/week) or to room air (sham exposure) for 8 weeks in a whole-body inhalation chamber. Cigarette smoke exposure did not prevent follicle development. Follicles in all stages of development are visible in both (A) sham- and (B) smoke-exposed ovaries. Cigarette smoke exposure significantly reduced body weight at necropsy and (C) relative ovarian weight compared to sham controls. The total number of follicles and the number of primordial, transitional, and primary follicles (D) were also decreased by cigarette smoke exposure compared to the control animals; however, although decreased in number, there were no differences in the number of secondary or antral follicles between the two groups. Data were analyzed by *t*-test. A $p < 0.05$ was considered significant.

at all stages of development in mice exposed to cigarette smoke (Figure 10.2). However, cigarette smoke exposure does not induce apoptosis as shown by absence of an effect on TUNEL staining, DNA laddering, and activated caspase-3, or caspase-8 and 9 expression versus controls [63]. Our results diverge from those of prior studies [82,128] using profoundly higher concentrations of B[*a*]P than are found in cigarette smoke. In addition, B[*a*]P treatment of 4-day-old mouse ovaries *in vitro* decreased Bcl-2 protein expression, while Bax remained unchanged, suggesting a concentration-dependent effect of cigarette smoke and B[*a*]P exposure on ovarian follicle loss [63]. Thus, in addition to being target tissue dependent, the AhR-mediated effects on apoptosis in the ovary are also concentration dependent. We suggest that prior studies showing evidence of PAH-induced follicle destruction via Bax activation are phenomenological and not relevant to human health because of the high concentrations of B[*a*]P and DMBA used. Moreover, we suggest that alternate mechanisms of ovarian follicle loss may be more relevant at lower concentrations, especially concentrations that are representative of human exposure. The existence of an alternative or accessory pathway for follicle loss is also suggested from studies in which mice lacking both the proapoptosis members Bax and Bak are completely resistant to apoptosis, yet cell death proceeded normally with the appearance of autophagosomes and autolysosomes [131]. Nonapoptotic cell death in these mice was dependent on the autophagic proteins Atg5 and Beclin-I, the disassociation of which from Bcl-2/Bcl-X_L in the endoplasmic reticulum (ER) but not the mitochondria is a key driver of autophagy (Atg) [132]. Thus, Atg is potentially an alternative/accessory cell death pathway important in ovarian function and response to environmental insults. We suggest that Atg may be more sensitive to toxic insult than apoptosis and thus may be more relevant than apoptosis at lower exposure concentrations.

10.5 AUTOPHAGY

Atg is a fundamental cellular process that removes long-lived proteins and damaged organelles (mitochondria and ER) through lysosomal degradation. In Atg, damaged proteins and cell organelles are engulfed in a double membrane-bound vesicle called an autophagosome, which subsequently fuses with a lysosome to become an autophagolysosome. Approximately 35 Atg genes have been identified and established as important regulators of Atg in yeast, many of which have human homologues [133,134]. Atg serves an adaptive response to various stresses including oxidative stress, nutrient starvation, and genotoxic agents [135,136] that lead to activation of Beclin-I and membrane nucleation. Beclin-I is part of the class III PI3 kinase complex and is crucial for Atg but is inhibited by Bcl-2 [137–139]. LC3 is another key mediator of Atg [140–142]. During the autophagic process, LC3-I is processed to LC3-II and sequestered in the membranes of the autophagosome. Mechanisms regulating cross talk between the apoptosis and Atg pathways are unclear; however, we note that Bcl-2 is at the interface between both pathways. We and others [64,136,143,144] have identified Atg as an important alternative/accessory cell death pathway in human and rodent granulosa cells. In human granulosa cells, unchecked oxidative stress led to increased expression of lectin-like oxidized low-density receptor (LOX-I), a scavenger receptor and membrane glycoprotein that is activated by oxidized low-density lipoprotein [136]. Indeed, reparative Atg was higher in young normal weight women versus older and obese women. However, the mechanistic steps leading to Atg and follicle loss are unknown.

We have shown that cigarette smoke exposure decreases the number of primordial and growing follicles in the absence of increased apoptosis [63,64]. Results of our recent study demonstrated that cigarette smoke exposure induced increased oxidative stress and Atg as shown by increased SOD-II, Beclin-I, and LC3 expression together with an increase in the number of autophagolysosomes/cell ($p<0.001$; Figure 10.3) [64]. Therefore, we think that Atg is an important alternative/accessory cell death pathway in ovarian follicle physiology and loss. A central role of Atg in cell loss is supported by studies in which cigarette smoke exposure increases Atg-mediated cell death in lung cells from patients with chronic obstructive pulmonary disease [145]. Cigarette smoke extract (CSE) increased processing of LC3-I to LC3-II and increased Atg in cultures of human bronchial epithelial cells [146]. Similarly, CSE treatment induced Atg in lung epithelial cells, macrophages, and fibroblasts [147].

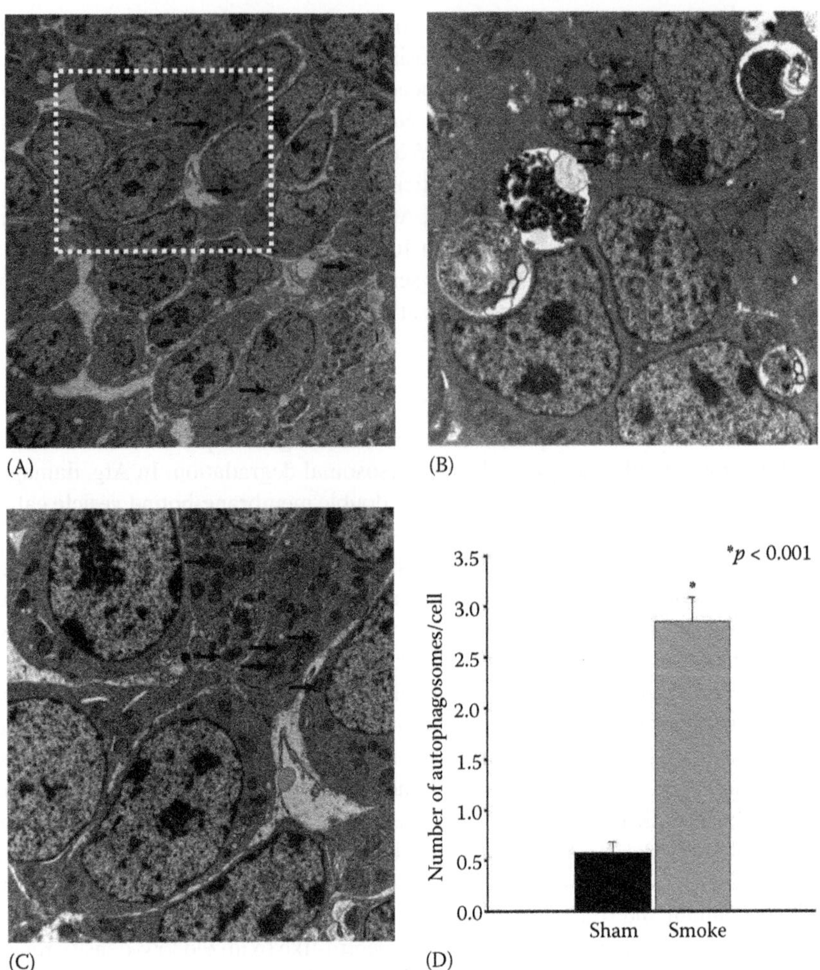

FIGURE 10.3 Autophagolysosomes (arrows) were present as membrane-bound structures containing degenerating cellular organelles including mitochondria and potentially endoplasmic reticulum in (A) room air (sham control; $n=5$) versus cigarette smoke (B; $n=5$)–exposed mice. (C) High-power magnification of dashed box in (A) showing mitochondria in granulosa cells of sham controls. Mitochondria appear normal and are abundant. (D) The number of autophagolysosomes/cell was markedly greater in cigarette smoke–exposed ovarian granulosa cells versus room air exposure mice. Images were evaluated by two independent investigators blinded to treatment group. (A) and (B): original magnification 7,500×. (C): original magnification 10,000×.

Hence, we postulate that cigarette smoke exposure can induce mitochondrial oxidative stress leading to Atg in granulosa cells as previously demonstrated [63,64]. Furthermore, it is noteworthy that the adverse effects of cigarette smoke on follicle development include retarded follicle growth and suboptimal function as shown by decreased E_2 and AMH output and decreased follicle survival [148]. We believe that cigarette smoke exposure acts via AhR-dependent mitochondrial oxidative stress to activate the autophagic pathway and cause follicle loss (Figure 10.3). TCDD, a well-established AhR-ligand, has been shown to induce dose- and time-dependent oxidative stress, lipid peroxidation, and DNA damage in multiple rodent tissues [149–157]. TCDD treatment produced an AhR-dependent increase in liver superoxide and H_2O_2 concentration in hepatic mitochondria [153,155]. Furthermore, DRE have been documented in the promoter region of several different electron transport chain genes including NADH dehydrogenase, cytochrome *c* reductase, cytochrome *c* oxidase, and adenosine triphosphate (ATP) synthase [158]. Thus, TCDD and potentially other PAHs such as B[*a*]P can affect the proton gradient, ATP synthesis, and chaperone protein activities, all leading to mitochondrial oxidative stress.

10.5.1 Dysregulation of Mitochondrial Dynamics and Mitophagy

Mitochondria are essential organelles that generate ATP to power the cell. The mitochondria exist in a dynamic interconnected network or reticulum that is constantly reshaped by a balance between fission and fusion [159]. The balance between fission and fusion is precisely regulated in order to maintain appropriate mitochondrial content in daughter cells and allow repair of damaged mitochondria. During fission, protein kinase A activates PTEN-induced kinase-1 (PINK-1), a mitochondrial kinase, which causes translocation of Parkin from the cytosol to damaged mitochondria where it promotes ubiquitination and degradation of the central fusion proteins MFN1 and MFN2 [160–162]. Furthermore, dynamin-related protein-1 (Drp-1) translocates from the cytosol to mitochondria where it is thought to bind with fission receptors such as hFis on the outer membrane [163]. Oligomerization of Drp-1 provides the mechanical force to constrict and fragment the mitochondrion [164]. During apoptosis, mitochondrial cristae are remodeled opening their tubular junctions leading to release of proapoptotic factors such as cytochrome c and activation of the apoptosis cascade [165,166], a process that we have consistently shown to be unaffected by cigarette smoke exposure [63,64]. In contrast to fission, optic atrophy-1 (OPA1), MFN1, and MFN2, key regulatory proteins in mitochondrial fusion, drive mitochondrial elongation, increased cristae density, and maintenance of ATP output [167,168] to sustain cell viability. OPA1 encodes a 96 amino acid mitochondrial dynamin–related guanosine triphosphatase (GTPase) that is associated with sequestration of cytochrome c in the mitochondria and regulation of mitochondrial fusion. MFN1 and MFN2 are outer membrane proteins that act as antiapoptotic GTPases to protect the cell from apoptotic stimuli [169,170]. Dysregulation of mitochondrial dynamics and inhibition of mitochondrial fusion has been documented in neurodegenerative diseases [171–175]; however, changes in mitochondrial dynamics have not been explored in granulosa cells previously. Several distinct lines of evidence lead us to propose that cigarette smoke–induced suboptimal growth and decreased follicle survival is mediated via inhibition of mitochondrial fusion and activation of Atg including mitochondrial Atg (mitophagy). Specifically, cigarette smoke condensate and B[*a*]P exposure both delayed follicle development and decreased E_2 and AMH output of follicles in isolated ovarian follicle cultures [69,148]. Furthermore, cigarette smoke exposure induced oxidative stress as shown by increased hsp-25/27 and decreased SOD-II expression but did not induce apoptosis in mice [63,64]. Moreover, we have shown [176] that MFN1 and MFN2 gene and protein expression were profoundly decreased, while Parkin gene and protein expression was significantly increased in the ovaries of mice exposed to cigarette smoke versus controls (Figure 10.4). Taken together, we suggest that cigarette smoke exposure induces

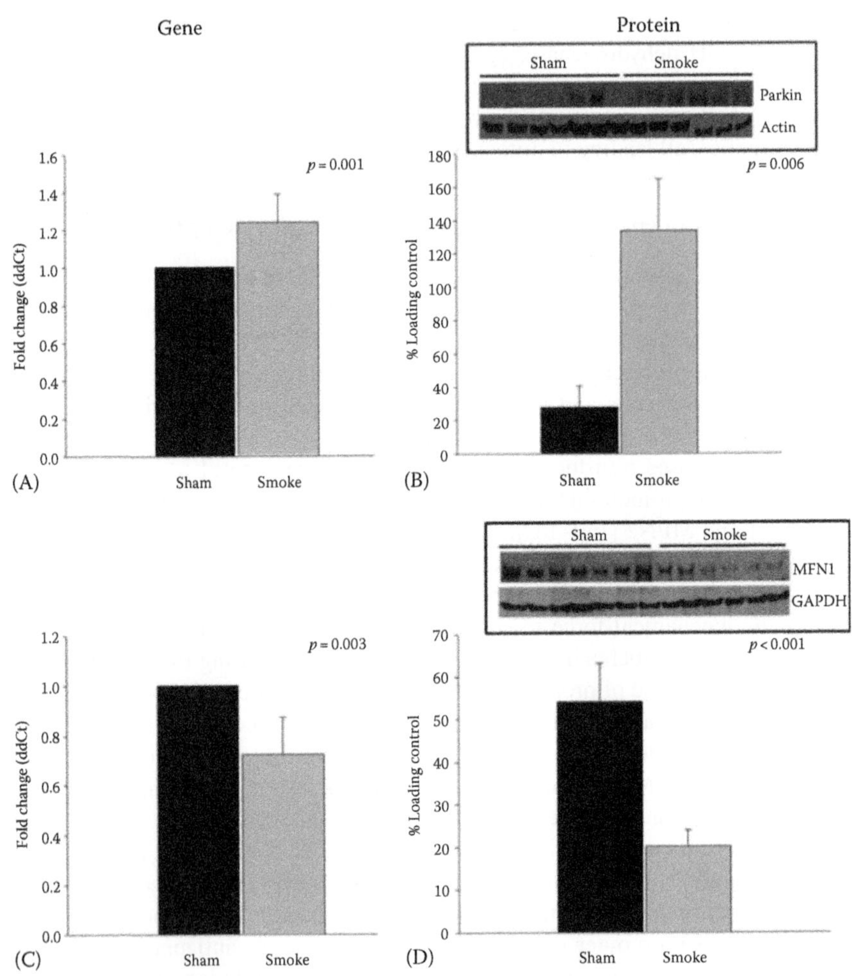

FIGURE 10.4 Cigarette smoke exposure resulted in an increase in both the gene and protein expression of PARK2 (A, B) and a significant decrease in the gene and protein expression of MFN1 (C, D) and MFN2 (E, F). Mice were exposed to cigarette smoke (12 cigarettes twice a day/5 days/week) or to room air (sham exposure) for 8 weeks in a whole-body inhalation chamber. We have shown that this exposure produces serum cotinine concentrations (metabolite of nicotine and marker of cigarette smoke exposure) that is equivalent to an average smoker (a pack/day smoker). Data were checked for normality and equal variance and treatment effects were tested using *t*-test. Values are expressed as mean (±SEM). A $p<0.05$ was considered significant ($n=6$–7/group). (From Gannon, A.M. et al., *Biol. Reprod.*, 88(3), 63, 2013. With permission.)

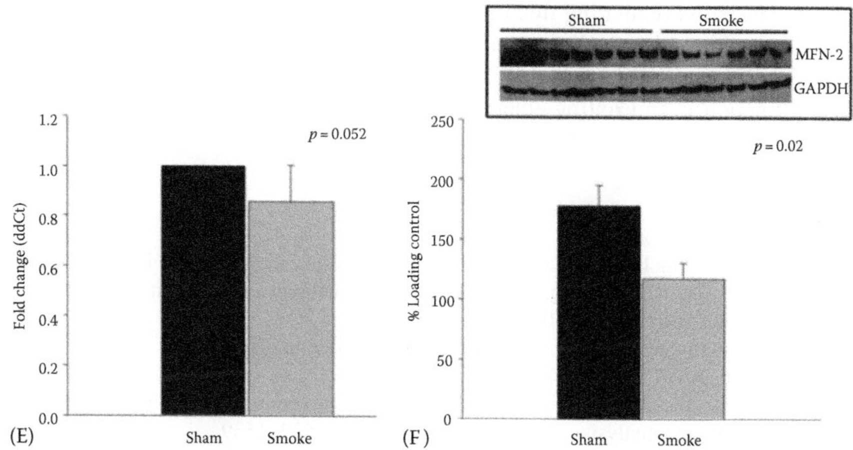

FIGURE 10.4 (continued) Cigarette smoke exposure resulted in an increase in both the gene and protein expression of PARK2 and a significant decrease in the gene and protein expression of MFN1 and MFN2. Mice were exposed to cigarette smoke (12 cigarettes twice a day/5 days/week) or to room air (sham exposure) for 8 weeks in a whole-body inhalation chamber. We have shown that this exposure produces serum cotinine concentrations (metabolite of nicotine and marker of cigarette smoke exposure) that is equivalent to an average smoker (a pack/day smoker). Data were checked for normality and equal variance and treatment effects were tested using *t*-test. Values are expressed as mean (±SEM). A $p<0.05$ was considered significant ($n=6$–7/group). (From Gannon, A.M. et al., *Biol. Reprod.*, 88(3), 63, 2013. With permission.)

mitochondrial oxidative stress via an AhR-dependent process that leads to dysfunction of mitochondrial dynamics, impaired follicle development, and dysregulation of the Atg machinery ultimately culminating in follicle loss. The potential for other environmental toxicants to exploit this pathway is unexplored.

10.6 SUMMARY AND CONCLUSIONS

Exposure to cigarette smoke is a reproductive and development hazard that is potentially avoidable. At concentrations representative of human exposure, we have shown that cigarette smoke disrupts mitochondrial homeostasis and activates Atg in granulosa cells rather than inducing widespread apoptosis as previously suggested from studies using high concentrations of PAHs. Insights into the cellular and molecular mechanisms underlying cigarette smoke–induced ovarian follicle loss are important as they imply the existence of a specific toxicopathologic pathway that mediates ovarian injury by the broad class of PAH compounds. Further study of this pathway might reveal points of entry by which other classes of compounds could exacerbate or mitigate toxic insult to the ovary. As young women around the globe are taking up cigarette smoking, knowledge about these mechanisms will be important for development of wise and effective regulatory, health policy, and therapeutic interventions to protect this vulnerable population. Furthermore, we suggest that reparative Atg is a fundamental process essential to follicle development, and a better understanding of the mechanisms regulating this important cellular process could have important implications for understanding subfertility and fertility preservation. Hence, we propose that the role of Atg and mitochondrial physiology in folliculogenesis and ovarian function is an exciting emerging area of study in reproductive biology and toxicology.

REFERENCES

1. Boivin J, Bunting L, Collins JA, Nygren KG. International estimates of infertility prevalence and treatment-seeking: potential need and demand for infertility medical care. *Hum Reprod* 2007; 22(6):1506–1512.
2. World Health Organization. Infections, pregnancies, and infertility: Perspectives on prevention. *Fertil Steril* 1987; 47(6):964–968.
3. Augood C, Duckitt K, Templeton AA. Smoking and female infertility: a systematic review and meta-analysis. *Hum Reprod* 1998; 13(6):1532–1539.
4. Foster WG. Do environmental contaminants adversely affect human reproductive physiology? *J Obstet Gynaecol Can* 2003; 25(1):33–44.
5. Pocar P, Brevini TA, Fischer B, Gandolfi F. The impact of endocrine disruptors on oocyte competence. *Reproduction* 2003; 125(3):313–325.
6. Centers for Disease Control and Prevention. Smoking-attributable mortality, years of potential life lost, and productivity losses—United States 2000–2004. *Morb Mortal Week Rep* 2008; 57(45):1226–1228.
7. Behan DF, Eriksen MP, Lin Y. Economic effects of environmental tobacco smoke report, 2005. www.soa.org/files/research/projects/etsreportfinaldraft(final-3.pdf)
8. Baird DD, Wilcox AJ. Cigarette smoking associated with delayed conception. *JAMA* 1985; 253(20):2979–2983.
9. Pattinson HA, Taylor PJ, Pattinson MH. The effect of cigarette smoking on ovarian function and early pregnancy outcome of in vitro fertilization treatment. *Fertil Steril* 1991; 55(4):780–783.
10. Sharara FI, Beatse SN, Leonardi MR, Navot D, Scott RT, Jr. Cigarette smoking accelerates the development of diminished ovarian reserve as evidenced by the clomiphene citrate challenge test. *Fertil Steril* 1994; 62(2):257–262.
11. Soares SR, Simon C, Remohi J, Pellicer A. Cigarette smoking affects uterine receptiveness. *Hum Reprod* 2007; 22(2):543–547.
12. Waylen AL, Metwally M, Jones GL, Wilkinson AJ, Ledger WL. Effects of cigarette smoking upon clinical outcomes of assisted reproduction: a meta-analysis. *Hum Reprod Update* 2009; 15(1):31–44.
13. Waylen AL, Jones GL, Ledger WL. Effect of cigarette smoking upon reproductive hormones in women of reproductive age: a retrospective analysis. *Reprod Biomed Online* 2010; 20(6):861–865.
14. Windham GC, Elkin EP, Swan SH, Waller KO, Fenster L. Cigarette smoking and effects on menstrual function. *Obstet Gynecol* 1999; 93(1):59–65.
15. Windham GC, Mitchell P, Anderson M, Lasley BL. Cigarette smoking and effects on hormone function in premenopausal women. *Environ Health Perspect* 2005; 113(10):1285–1290.
16. Cohen B, Evers S, Manske S, Bercovitz K, Edward HG. Smoking, physical activity and breakfast consumption among secondary school students in a southwestern Ontario community. *Can J Public Health* 2003; 94(1):41–44.
17. Ventura SJ, Mosher WD, Curtin SC, Abma JC, Henshaw S. Trends in pregnancies and pregnancy rates by outcome: estimates for the United States, 1976–96. *Vital Health Stat 21* 2000;(56):1–47.

18. Dunson DB, Baird DD, Colombo B. Increased infertility with age in men and women. *Obstet Gynecol* 2004; 103(1):51–56.
19. Menken J, Trussell J, Larsen U. Age and infertility. *Science* 1986; 233(4771):1389–1394.
20. van Noord-Zaadstra BM, Looman CW, Alsbach H, Habbema JD, te Velde ER, Karbaat J. Delaying childbearing: effect of age on fecundity and outcome of pregnancy. *BMJ* 1991; 302(6789):1361–1365.
21. Macaluso M, Wright-Schnapp TJ, Chandra A et al. A public health focus on infertility prevention, detection, and management. *Fertil Steril* 2010; 93(1):16–20.
22. Faddy MJ, Gosden RG. A model conforming the decline in follicle numbers to the age of menopause in women. *Hum Reprod* 1996; 11(7):1484–1486.
23. Faddy MJ, Gosden RG. A mathematical model of follicle dynamics in the human ovary. *Hum Reprod* 1995; 10(4):770–775.
24. Fuentes A, Munoz A, Barnhart K, Midwife BA, Diaz M, Pommer R. Recent cigarette smoking and assisted reproductive technologies outcome. *Fertil Steril* 2010; 93(1):89–95.
25. Neal MS, Hughes EG, Holloway AC, Foster WG. Sidestream smoking is equally as damaging as mainstream smoking on IVF outcomes. *Hum Reprod* 2005; 20(9):2531–2535.
26. Freour T, Masson D, Mirallie S et al. Active smoking compromises IVF outcome and affects ovarian reserve. *Reprod Biomed Online* 2008; 16(1):96–102.
27. Roth LK, Taylor HS. Risks of smoking to reproductive health: assessment of women's knowledge. *Am J Obstet Gynecol* 2001; 184(5):934–939.
28. Westmaas JL, Brandon TH, Lokitis J. Altering risk in patients who smoke. *Respir Care Clin N Am* 2003; 9(2):259–268, viii–ix.
29. Borland R, Yong HH, Balmford J et al. Motivational factors predict quit attempts but not maintenance of smoking cessation: findings from the International Tobacco Control Four country project. *Nicotine Tob Res* 2010; 12 Suppl:S4–S11.
30. West R. The multiple facets of cigarette addiction and what they mean for encouraging and helping smokers to stop. *COPD* 2009; 6(4):277–283.
31. Coleman T, Agboola S, Leonardi-Bee J, Taylor M, McEwen A, McNeill A. Relapse prevention in UK Stop Smoking Services: current practice, systematic reviews of effectiveness and cost-effectiveness analysis. *Health Technol Assess* 2010; 14(49):1–152, iii–iv.
32. Curtis KM, Savitz DA, Arbuckle TE. Effects of cigarette smoking, caffeine consumption, and alcohol intake on fecundability. *Am J Epidemiol* 1997; 146(1):32–41.
33. El Nemr A, Al Shawaf T, Sabatini L, Wilson C, Lower AM, Grudzinskas JG. Effect of smoking on ovarian reserve and ovarian stimulation in in-vitro fertilization and embryo transfer. *Hum Reprod* 1998; 13(8):2192–2198.
34. Hughes EG, Yeo J, Claman P et al. Cigarette smoking and the outcomes of in vitro fertilization: measurement of effect size and levels of action. *Fertil Steril* 1994; 62(4):807–814.
35. Hughes EG, Brennan BG. Does cigarette smoking impair natural or assisted fecundity? *Fertil Steril* 1996; 66(5):679–689.
36. Jick H, Porter J. Relation between smoking and age of natural menopause. Report from the Boston Collaborative Drug Surveillance Program, Boston University Medical Center. *Lancet* 1977; 1(8026):1354–1355.
37. Rosevear SK, Holt DW, Lee TD, Ford WC, Wardle PG, Hull MG. Smoking and decreased fertilisation rates in vitro. *Lancet* 1992; 340(8829):1195–1196.
38. Rowlands DJ, McDermott A, Hull MG. Smoking and decreased fertilisation rates in vitro. *Lancet* 1992; 340(8832):1409–1410.
39. Van Voorhis BJ, Dawson JD, Stovall DW, Sparks AE, Syrop CH. The effects of smoking on ovarian function and fertility during assisted reproduction cycles. *Obstet Gynecol* 1996; 88(5):785–791.

40. Zenzes MT, Reed TE, Casper RF. Effects of cigarette smoking and age on the maturation of human oocytes. *Hum Reprod* 1997; 12(8):1736–1741.
41. Zenzes MT, Wang P, Casper RF. Cigarette smoking may affect meiotic maturation of human oocytes. *Hum Reprod* 1995; 10(12):3213–3217.
42. Zenzes MT. Smoking and reproduction: gene damage to human gametes and embryos. *Hum Reprod Update* 2000; 6(2):122–131.
43. Sterzik K, Strehler E, De SM et al. Influence of smoking on fertility in women attending an in vitro fertilization program. *Fertil Steril* 1996; 65(4):810–814.
44. Crha I, Hruba D, Fiala J, Ventruba P, Zakova J, Petrenko M. The outcome of infertility treatment by in-vitro fertilisation in smoking and non-smoking women. *Cent Eur J Public Health* 2001; 9(2):64–68.
45. Weigert M, Hofstetter G, Kaipl D et al. The effect of smoking on oocyte quality and hormonal parameters of patients undergoing in vitro fertilization-embryo transfer. *J Assist Reprod Genet* 1999; 16(6):287–293.
46. Swauger JE, Steichen TJ, Murphy PA, Kinsler S. An analysis of the mainstream smoke chemistry of samples of the U.S. cigarette market acquired between 1995 and 2000. *Regul Toxicol Pharmacol* 2002; 35(2 Pt 1):142–156.
47. Kaiserman MJ, Rickert WS. Carcinogens in tobacco smoke: benzo[a]pyrene from Canadian cigarettes and cigarette tobacco. *Am J Public Health* 1992; 82(7):1023–1026.
48. Roemer E, Stabbert R, Rustemeier K et al. Chemical composition, cytotoxicity and mutagenicity of smoke from US commercial and reference cigarettes smoked under two sets of machine smoking conditions. *Toxicology* 2004; 195(1):31–52.
49. Rustemeier K, Stabbert R, Haussmann HJ, Roemer E, Carmines EL. Evaluation of the potential effects of ingredients added to cigarettes. Part 2: chemical composition of mainstream smoke. *Food Chem Toxicol* 2002; 40(1):93–104.
50. Buckley TJ, Lioy PJ. An examination of the time course from human dietary exposure to polycyclic aromatic hydrocarbons to urinary elimination of 1-hydroxypyrene. *Br J Ind Med* 1992; 49(2):113–124.
51. Sinha R, Kulldorff M, Gunter MJ, Strickland P, Rothman N. Dietary benzo[a]pyrene intake and risk of colorectal adenoma. *Cancer Epidemiol Biomarkers Prev* 2005; 14(8):2030–2034.
52. Sinha R, Peters U, Cross AJ et al. Meat, meat cooking methods and preservation, and risk for colorectal adenoma. *Cancer Res* 2005; 65(17):8034–8041.
53. Ibanez R, Agudo A, Berenguer A et al. Dietary intake of polycyclic aromatic hydrocarbons in a Spanish population. *J Food Prot* 2005; 68(10):2190–2195.
54. Viau C, Diakite A, Ruzgyte A et al. Is 1-hydroxypyrene a reliable bioindicator of measured dietary polycyclic aromatic hydrocarbon under normal conditions? *J Chromatogr B Analyt Technol Biomed Life Sci* 2002; 778(1–2):165–177.
55. Phillips DH. Polycyclic aromatic hydrocarbons in the diet. *Mutat Res* 1999; 443(1–2):139–147.
56. Ovrebo S, Hewer A, Phillips DH, Haugen A. Polycyclic aromatic hydrocarbon-DNA adducts in coke-oven workers. *IARC Sci Publ* 1990;(104):193–198.
57. Pan CH, Chan CC, Huang YL, Wu KY. Urinary 1-hydroxypyrene and malondialdehyde in male workers in Chinese restaurants. *Occup Environ Med* 2008; 65(11):732–735.
58. Lodovici M, Akpan V, Evangelisti C, Dolara P. Sidestream tobacco smoke as the main predictor of exposure to polycyclic aromatic hydrocarbons. *J Appl Toxicol* 2004; 24(4):277–281.
59. Borman SM, Christian PJ, Sipes IG, Hoyer PB. Ovotoxicity in female Fischer rats and B6 mice induced by low-dose exposure to three polycyclic aromatic hydrocarbons: comparison through calculation of an ovotoxic index. *Toxicol Appl Pharmacol* 2000; 167(3):191–198.

60. Mattison DR, Shiromizu K, Nightingale MS. Oocyte destruction by polycyclic aromatic hydrocarbons. *Am J Ind Med* 1983; 4(1–2):191–202.
61. Mattison DR, Nightingale MS. Oocyte destruction by polycyclic aromatic hydrocarbons is not linked to the inducibility of ovarian aryl hydrocarbon (benzo(a)pyrene) hydroxylase activity in (DBA/2N X C57BL/6N) F1 X DBA/2N backcross mice. *Pediatr Pharmacol (New York)* 1982; 2(1):11–21.
62. Miller MM, Plowchalk DR, Weitzman GA, London SN, Mattison DR. The effect of benzo(a)pyrene on murine ovarian and corpora lutea volumes. *Am J Obstet Gynecol* 1992; 166:1535–1541.
63. Tuttle AM, Stampfli M, Foster WG. Cigarette smoke causes follicle loss in mice ovaries at concentrations representative of human exposure. *Hum Reprod* 2009; 24(6):1452–1459.
64. Gannon AM, Stampfli MR, Foster WG. Cigarette smoke exposure results in significant follicle loss via an alternative ovarian cell death pathway in mice. *Toxicol Sci* 2012; 125(1):274–284.
65. Neal MS, Zhu J, Foster WG. Quantification of benzo[a]pyrene and other PAHs in the serum and follicular fluid of smokers versus non-smokers. *Reprod Toxicol* 2008; 25(1):100–106.
66. Zenzes MT, Puy LA, Bielecki R. Immunodetection of benzo[a]pyrene adducts in ovarian cells of women exposed to cigarette smoke. *Mol Hum Reprod* 1998; 4(2):159–165.
67. Neal MS, Zhu J, Holloway AC, Foster WG. Follicle growth is inhibited by benzo-[a]-pyrene, at concentrations representative of human exposure, in an isolated rat follicle culture assay. *Hum Reprod* 2007; 22(4):961–967.
68. Neal MS, Mulligan Tuttle AM, Casper RF, Lagunov A, Foster WG. Aryl hydrocarbon receptor antagonists attenuate the deleterious effects of benzo[a]pyrene on isolated rat follicle development. *Reprod Biomed Online* 2010; 21(1):100–108.
69. Sadeu JC, Foster WG. Effect of in vitro exposure to Benzo[a]pyrene, a component of cigarette smoke, on folliculogenesis, steroidogenesis, and oocyte maturation. *Reprod Toxicol* 2011; 31(4):402–408.
70. Legro RS, Sauer MV, Mottla GL et al. Effect of air quality on assisted human reproduction. *Hum Reprod* 2010; 25(5):1317–1324.
71. Safe S. Polychlorinated biphenyls (PCBs), dibenzo-p-dioxins (PCDDs), dibenzofurans (PCDFs), and related compounds: environmental and mechanistic considerations which support the development of toxic equivalency factors (TEFs). *Crit Rev Toxicol* 1990; 21(1):51–88.
72. Robles R, Morita Y, Mann KK et al. The aryl hydrocarbon receptor, a basic helix-loop-helix transcription factor of the PAS gene family, is required for normal ovarian germ cell dynamics in the mouse. *Endocrinology* 2000; 141(1):450–453.
73. Harper PA, Prokipcak RD, Bush LE, Golas CL, Okey AB. Detection and characterization of the Ah receptor for 2,3,7,8-tetrachlorodibenzo-p-dioxin in the human colon adenocarcinoma cell line LS180. *Arch Biochem Biophys* 1991; 290(1):27–36.
74. Li W, Harper PA, Tang BK, Okey AB. Regulation of cytochrome P450 enzymes by aryl hydrocarbon receptor in human cells: CYP1A2 expression in the LS180 colon carcinoma cell line after treatment with 2,3,7,8-tetrachlorodibenzo-p-dioxin or 3-methylcholanthrene. *Biochem Pharmacol* 1998; 56(5):599–612.
75. Ciolino HP, Yeh GC. Inhibition of aryl hydrocarbon-induced cytochrome P-450 1A1 enzyme activity and CYP1A1 expression by resveratrol. *Mol Pharmacol* 1999; 56(4):760–767.
76. Nebert DW, Petersen DD, Fornace AJ, Jr. Cellular responses to oxidative stress: the [Ah] gene battery as a paradigm. *Environ Health Perspect* 1990; 88:13–25.
77. Nebert DW, Roe AL, Vandale SE, Bingham E, Oakley GG. NAD(P)H:quinone oxidoreductase (NQO1) polymorphism, exposure to benzene, and predisposition to disease: a huge review. *Genet Med* 2002; 4(2):62–70.

78. Schmidt JV, Bradfield CA. Ah receptor signaling pathways. *Annu Rev Cell Dev Biol* 1996; 12:55–89.
79. Hankinson O. The aryl hydrocarbon receptor complex. *Annu Rev Pharmacol Toxicol* 1995; 35:307–340.
80. Hankinson O. The role of the aryl hydrocarbon receptor nuclear translocator protein in aryl hydrocarbon receptor action. *Trends Endocrinol Metab* 1994; 5(6):240–244.
81. Ciolino HP, Daschner PJ, Yeh GC. Resveratrol inhibits transcription of CYP1A1 in vitro by preventing activation of the aryl hydrocarbon receptor. *Cancer Res* 1998; 58(24):5707–5712.
82. Matikainen T, Perez GI, Jurisicova A et al. Aromatic hydrocarbon receptor-driven Bax gene expression is required for premature ovarian failure caused by biohazardous environmental chemicals. *Nat Genet* 2001; 28(4):355–360.
83. Matikainen TM, Moriyama T, Morita Y et al. Ligand activation of the aromatic hydrocarbon receptor transcription factor drives Bax-dependent apoptosis in developing fetal ovarian germ cells. *Endocrinology* 2002; 143(2):615–620.
84. Hincal F. Effects of exposure to air pollution and smoking on the placental aryl hydrocarbon hydroxylase (AHH) activity. *Arch Environ Health* 1986; 41(6):377–383.
85. Huel G, Godin J, Moreau T et al. Aryl hydrocarbon hydroxylase activity in human placenta of passive smokers. *Environ Res* 1989; 50(1):173–183.
86. Manchester DK, Parker NB, Bowman CM. Maternal smoking increases xenobiotic metabolism in placenta but not umbilical vein endothelium. *Pediatr Res* 1984; 18(11):1071–1075.
87. Baerwald AR, Adams GP, Pierson RA. A new model for ovarian follicular development during the human menstrual cycle. *Fertil Steril* 2003; 80(1):116–122.
88. Baerwald AR, Adams GP, Pierson RA. Characterization of ovarian follicular wave dynamics in women. *Biol Reprod* 2003; 69(3):1023–1031.
89. Byskov AGS. Follicle atresia. In: RE Jones., ed. *The Vertebrate Ovary*. New York: Plenum Press, 1978, pp. 533–562.
90. Johnson J, Canning J, Kaneko T, Pru JK, Tilly JL. Germline stem cells and follicular renewal in the postnatal mammalian ovary. *Nature* 2004; 428(6979):145–150.
91. Gong SP, Lee ST, Lee EJ et al. Embryonic stem cell-like cells established by culture of adult ovarian cells in mice. *Fertil Steril* 2010; 93(8):2594–2601.
92. Johnson J, Bagley J, Skaznik-Wikiel M et al. Oocyte generation in adult mammalian ovaries by putative germ cells in bone marrow and peripheral blood. *Cell* 2005; 122(2):303–315.
93. Niikura Y, Niikura T, Tilly JL. Aged mouse ovaries possess rare premeiotic germ cells that can generate oocytes following transplantation into a young host environment. *Aging* 2009; 1(12):971–978.
94. Selesniemi K, Lee HJ, Niikura T, Tilly JL. Young adult donor bone marrow infusions into female mice postpone age-related reproductive failure and improve offspring survival. *Aging* 2009; 1(1):49–57.
95. Tilly JL, Telfer EE. Purification of germline stem cells from adult mammalian ovaries: a step closer towards control of the female biological clock? *Mol Hum Reprod* 2009; 15(7):393–398.
96. Byskov AG, Faddy MJ, Lemmen JG, Andersen CY. Eggs forever? *Differentiation* 2005; 73(9–10):438–446.
97. Skaznik-Wikiel M, Tilly JC, Lee HJ et al. Serious doubts over "Eggs forever?" *Differentiation* 2007; 75(2):93–99.
98. Oktem O, Oktay K. The ovary: anatomy and function throughout human life. *Ann N Y Acad Sci* 2008; 1127:1–9.
99. Durlinger AL, Gruijters MJ, Kramer P et al. Anti-Mullerian hormone inhibits initiation of primordial follicle growth in the mouse ovary. *Endocrinology* 2002; 143(3):1076–1084.

100. Durlinger AL, Kramer P, Karels B et al. Control of primordial follicle recruitment by anti-Mullerian hormone in the mouse ovary. *Endocrinology* 1999; 140(12):5789–5796.
101. Themmen AP. Anti-Mullerian hormone: its role in follicular growth initiation and survival and as an ovarian reserve marker. *J Natl Cancer Inst Monogr* 2005;(34):18–21.
102. Gnoth C, Schuring AN, Friol K, Tigges J, Mallmann P, Godehardt E. Relevance of anti-Mullerian hormone measurement in a routine IVF program. *Hum Reprod* 2008; 23(6):1359–1365.
103. Kwee J, Schats R, McDonnell J, Themmen A, de JF, Lambalk C. Evaluation of anti-Mullerian hormone as a test for the prediction of ovarian reserve. *Fertil Steril* 2008; 90(3):737–743.
104. Massin N, Meduri G, Bachelot A, Misrahi M, Kuttenn F, Touraine P. Evaluation of different markers of the ovarian reserve in patients presenting with premature ovarian failure. *Mol Cell Endocrinol* 2008; 282(1–2):95–100.
105. Nardo LG, Christodoulou D, Gould D, Roberts SA, Fitzgerald CT, Laing I. Anti-Mullerian hormone levels and antral follicle count in women enrolled in in vitro fertilization cycles: relationship to lifestyle factors, chronological age and reproductive history. *Gynecol Endocrinol* 2007; 23(8):486–493.
106. Nilsson E, Rogers N, Skinner MK. Actions of anti-Mullerian hormone on the ovarian transcriptome to inhibit primordial to primary follicle transition. *Reproduction* 2007; 134(2):209–221.
107. Salmon NA, Handyside AH, Joyce IM. Oocyte regulation of anti-Mullerian hormone expression in granulosa cells during ovarian follicle development in mice. *Dev Biol* 2004; 266(1):201–208.
108. Shin SY, Lee JR, Noh GW et al. Analysis of serum levels of anti-Mullerian hormone, inhibin B, insulin-like growth factor-I, insulin-like growth factor binding protein-3, and follicle-stimulating hormone with respect to age and menopausal status. *J Korean Med Sci* 2008; 23(1):104–110.
109. Visser JA, De Jong FH, Laven JS, Themmen AP. Anti-Mullerian hormone: a new marker for ovarian function. *Reproduction* 2006; 131(1):1–9.
110. Visser JA, Themmen AP. Anti-Mullerian hormone and folliculogenesis. *Mol Cell Endocrinol* 2005; 234(1–2):81–86.
111. Andersen CY, Schmidt KT, Kristensen SG, Rosendahl M, Byskov AG, Ernst E. Concentrations of AMH and inhibin-B in relation to follicular diameter in normal human small antral follicles. *Hum Reprod* 2010; 25(5):1282–1287.
112. La Marca A, Giulini S, Tirelli A et al. Anti-Mullerian hormone measurement on any day of the menstrual cycle strongly predicts ovarian response in assisted reproductive technology. *Hum Reprod* 2007; 22(3):766–771.
113. La Marca A, Volpe A. Anti-Mullerian hormone (AMH) in female reproduction: is measurement of circulating AMH a useful tool? *Clin Endocrinol (Oxf)* 2006; 64(6):603–610.
114. La Marca A., Sighinolfi G, Radi D et al. Anti-Mullerian hormone (AMH) as a predictive marker in assisted reproductive technology (ART). *Hum Reprod Update* 2010; 16(2):113–130.
115. Yeh J, Kim B, Peresie J, Liang YJ, Arroyo A. Serum and ovarian Mullerian inhibiting substance, and their decline in reproductive aging. *Fertil Steril* 2007; 87(5):1227–1230.
116. Plante BJ, Cooper GS, Baird DD, Steiner AZ. The impact of smoking on anti-Mullerian hormone levels in women aged 38 to 50 years. *Menopause* 2010; 17(3):571–576.
117. Freour T, Dessolle L, Jean M, Masson D, Barriere P. Predictive value of ovarian reserve markers in smoking and non-smoking women undergoing IVF. *Reprod Biomed Online* 2010; 20(6):857–860.
118. Van Wezel I, Dharmarajan AM, Lavranos TC, Rodgers RJ. Evidence for alternative pathways of granulosa cell death in healthy and slightly atretic bovine antral follicles. *Endocrinology* 1999; 140(6):2602–2612.

119. Boone DL, Carnegie JA, Rippstein PU, Tsang BK. Induction of apoptosis in equine chorionic gonadotropin (eCG)-primed rats ovaries by anti-eCG antibody. *Biol Reprod* 1997; 57:420–427.
120. Boone DL, Tsang BK. Identification and localization of deoxyribonuclease I in the rat ovary. *Biol Reprod* 1997; 57:813–821.
121. Boone DL, Tsang BK. Caspase-3 in the rat ovary: Localization and possible role in follicular atresia and luteal regression. *Biol Reprod* 1998; 58:1533–1539.
122. Dharma SJ, Kelkar RL, Nandedkar TD. Fas and Fas ligand protein and mRNA in normal and atretic mouse ovarian follicles. *Reproduction* 2003; 126(6):783–789.
123. Flaws JA, Hirshfield AN, Hewitt JA, Babus JK, Furth PA. Effect of Bcl-2 on primordial follicle endowment in the mouse ovary. *Biol Reprod* 2001; 64:1153–1159.
124. Kim J-M, Boone DL, Auyeung A, Tsang BK. Granulosa cell apoptosis induced at the penultimate stage of follicular development is associated with increased levels of Fas and Fas ligand in the rat ovary. *Biol Reprod* 1998; 58:1170–1176.
125. Tilly JL. Molecular and genetic basis of normal and toxicant-induced apoptosis in female germ cells. *Toxicol Lett* 1998; 102–103:497–501.
126. Greenfeld CR, Pepling ME, Babus JK, Furth PA, Flaws JA. BAX regulates follicular endowment in mice. *Reproduction* 2007; 133(5):865–876.
127. Kee K, Flores M, Cedars MI, Reijo Pera RA. Human primordial germ cell formation is diminished by exposure to environmental toxicants acting through the AHR signaling pathway. *Toxicol Sci* 2010; 117(1):218–224.
128. Jurisicova A, Taniuchi A, Li H et al. Maternal exposure to polycyclic aromatic hydrocarbons diminishes murine ovarian reserve via induction of Harakiri. *J Clin Invest* 2007; 117(12):3971–3978.
129. Detmar J, Rennie MY, Whiteley KJ et al. Fetal growth restriction triggered by polycyclic aromatic hydrocarbons is associated with altered placental vasculature and AhR-dependent changes in cell death. *Am J Physiol Endocrinol Metab* 2008; 295(2):E519–E530.
130. Gray LE, Jr., Ostby JS. In utero 2,3,7,8-tetrachlorodibenzo-p-dioxin (TCDD) alters reproductive morphology and function in female rat offspring. *Toxicol Appl Pharmacol* 1995; 133(2):285–294.
131. Shimizu S, Kanaseki T, Mizushima N et al. Role of Bcl-2 family proteins in a non-apoptotic programmed cell death dependent on autophagy genes. *Nat Cell Biol* 2004; 6(12):1221–1228.
132. Maiuri MC, Criollo A, Kroemer G. Crosstalk between apoptosis and autophagy within the Beclin 1 interactome. *EMBO J* 2010; 29(3):515–516.
133. Reggiori F, Klionsky DJ. Autophagosomes: biogenesis from scratch? *Curr Opin Cell Biol* 2005; 17(4):415–422.
134. Reggiori F, Klionsky DJ. Autophagy in the eukaryotic cell. *Eukaryot Cell* 2002; 1(1):11–21.
135. Bursch W. The autophagosomal-lysosomal compartment in programmed cell death. *Cell Death Differ* 2001; 8(6):569–581.
136. Vilser C, Hueller H, Nowicki M, Hmeidan FA, Blumenauer V, Spanel-Borowski K. The variable expression of lectin-like oxidized low-density lipoprotein receptor (LOX-1) and signs of autophagy and apoptosis in freshly harvested human granulosa cells depend on gonadotropin dose, age, and body weight. *Fertil Steril* 2010; 93(8):2706–2715.
137. Liang XH, Yu J, Brown K, Levine B. Beclin 1 contains a leucine-rich nuclear export signal that is required for its autophagy and tumor suppressor function. *Cancer Res* 2001; 61(8):3443–3449.
138. Liang XH, Jackson S, Seaman M et al. Induction of autophagy and inhibition of tumorigenesis by beclin 1. *Nature* 1999; 402(6762):672–676.

139. Pattingre S, Tassa A, Qu X et al. Bcl-2 antiapoptotic proteins inhibit Beclin 1-dependent autophagy. *Cell* 2005; 122(6):927–939.
140. Levine B, Klionsky DJ. Development by self-digestion: molecular mechanisms and biological functions of autophagy. *Dev Cell* 2004; 6(4):463–477.
141. Levine B, Yuan J. Autophagy in cell death: An innocent convict? *J Clin Invest* 2005; 115(10):2679–2688.
142. Klionsky DJ, Codogno P, Cuervo AM et al. A comprehensive glossary of autophagy-related molecules and processes. *Autophagy* 2010; 6(4):438–448.
143. Choi JY, Jo MW, Lee EY, Yoon BK, Choi DS. The role of autophagy in follicular development and atresia in rat granulosa cells. *Fertil Steril* 2010; 93(8):2532–2537.
144. Gawriluk TR, Hale AN, Flaws JA, Dillon CP, Green DR, Rucker EB, III. Autophagy is a cell survival program for female germ cells in the murine ovary. *Reproduction* 2011; 141(6):759–765.
145. Chen ZH, Kim HP, Sciurba FC et al. Egr-1 regulates autophagy in cigarette smoke-induced chronic obstructive pulmonary disease. *PLoS ONE* 2008; 3(10):e3316.
146. Kim HP, Wang X, Chen ZH et al. Autophagic proteins regulate cigarette smoke-induced apoptosis: protective role of heme oxygenase-1. *Autophagy* 2008; 4(7):887–895.
147. Hwang J, Chung S, Sundar IK et al. Cigarette smoke-induced autophagy is regulated by SIRT1-PARP-1-dependent mechanism: Implication in pathogenesis of COPD. *Arch Biochem Biophys* 2010; 500:203–209.
148. Sadeu JC, Foster WG. Cigarette smoke condensate exposure delays follicular development and function in a stage-dependent manner. *Fertil Steril* 2011; 95(7):2410–2417.
149. Hassoun EA, Wang H, Abushaban A, Stohs SJ. Induction of oxidative stress in the tissues of rats after chronic exposure to TCDD, 2,3,4,7,8-pentachlorodibenzofuran, and 3,3′,4,4′,5-pentachlorobiphenyl. *J Toxicol Environ Health A* 2002; 65(12):825–842.
150. Hassoun EA, Li F, Abushaban A, Stohs SJ. Production of superoxide anion, lipid peroxidation and DNA damage in the hepatic and brain tissues of rats after subchronic exposure to mixtures of TCDD and its congeners. *J Appl Toxicol* 2001; 21(3):211–219.
151. Hassoun EA, Li F, Abushaban A, Stohs SJ. The relative abilities of TCDD and its congeners to induce oxidative stress in the hepatic and brain tissues of rats after subchronic exposure. *Toxicology* 2000; 145(2–3):103–113.
152. Hassoun EA, Wilt SC, DeVito MJ et al. Induction of oxidative stress in brain tissues of mice after subchronic exposure to 2,3,7,8-tetrachlorodibenzo-p-dioxin. *Toxicol Sci* 1998; 42(1):23–27.
153. Senft AP, Dalton TP, Nebert DW et al. Mitochondrial reactive oxygen production is dependent on the aromatic hydrocarbon receptor. *Free Radic Biol Med* 2002; 33(9):1268–1278.
154. Senft AP, Dalton TP, Nebert DW, Genter MB, Hutchinson RJ, Shertzer HG. Dioxin increases reactive oxygen production in mouse liver mitochondria. *Toxicol Appl Pharmacol* 2002; 178(1):15–21.
155. Shen D, Dalton TP, Nebert DW, Shertzer HG. Glutathione redox state regulates mitochondrial reactive oxygen production. *J Biol Chem* 2005; 280(27):25305–25312.
156. Shertzer HG, Genter MB, Shen D, Nebert DW, Chen Y, Dalton TP. TCDD decreases ATP levels and increases reactive oxygen production through changes in mitochondrial F(0) F(1)-ATP synthase and ubiquinone. *Toxicol Appl Pharmacol* 2006; 217(3):363–374.
157. Slezak BP, Hamm JT, Reyna J, Hurst CH, Birnbaum LS. TCDD-mediated oxidative stress in male rat pups following perinatal exposure. *J Biochem Mol Toxicol* 2002; 16(2):49–52.
158. Forgacs AL, Burgoon LD, Lynn SG, LaPres JJ, Zacharewski T. Effects of TCDD on the expression of nuclear encoded mitochondrial genes. *Toxicol Appl Pharmacol* 2010; 246(1–2):58–65.

159. Detmer SA, Chan DC. Functions and dysfunctions of mitochondrial dynamics. *Nat Rev Mol Cell Biol* 2007; 8(11):870–879.
160. Glauser L, Sonnay S, Stafa K, Moore DJ. Parkin promotes the ubiquitination and degradation of the mitochondrial fusion factor mitofusin 1. *J Neurochem* 2011; 118(4):636–645.
161. Tanaka A, Cleland MM, Xu S et al. Proteasome and p97 mediate mitophagy and degradation of mitofusins induced by Parkin. *J Cell Biol* 2010; 191(7):1367–1380.
162. Gegg ME, Cooper JM, Chau KY, Rojo M, Schapira AH, Taanman JW. Mitofusin 1 and mitofusin 2 are ubiquitinated in a PINK1/parkin-dependent manner upon induction of mitophagy. *Hum Mol Genet* 2010; 19(24):4861–4870.
163. Cereghetti GM, Stangherlin A, Martins de BO et al. Dephosphorylation by calcineurin regulates translocation of Drp1 to mitochondria. *Proc Natl Acad Sci U S A* 2008; 105(41):15803–15808.
164. Meeusen SL, Nunnari J. How mitochondria fuse. *Curr Opin Cell Biol* 2005; 17(4):389–394.
165. Cipolat S, Rudka T, Hartmann D et al. Mitochondrial rhomboid PARL regulates cytochrome c release during apoptosis via OPA1-dependent cristae remodeling. *Cell* 2006; 126(1):163–175.
166. Pellegrini L, Scorrano L. A cut short to death: Parl and Opa1 in the regulation of mitochondrial morphology and apoptosis. *Cell Death Differ* 2007; 14(7):1275–1284.
167. Gomes LC, Di BG, Scorrano L. During autophagy mitochondria elongate, are spared from degradation and sustain cell viability. *Nat Cell Biol* 2011; 13(5):589–598.
168. Gomes LC, Scorrano L. Mitochondrial elongation during autophagy: A stereotypical response to survive in difficult times. *Autophagy* 2011; 7(10):1251–1253.
169. Chen H, Chan DC. Emerging functions of mammalian mitochondrial fusion and fission. *Hum Mol Genet* 2005; 14 Spec No. 2:R283–R289.
170. Chen H, Chomyn A, Chan DC. Disruption of fusion results in mitochondrial heterogeneity and dysfunction. *J Biol Chem* 2005; 280(28):26185–26192.
171. Alexander C, Votruba M, Pesch UE et al. OPA1, encoding a dynamin-related GTPase, is mutated in autosomal dominant optic atrophy linked to chromosome 3q28. *Nat Genet* 2000; 26(2):211–215.
172. Thiselton DL, Alexander C, Morris A et al. A frameshift mutation in exon 28 of the OPA1 gene explains the high prevalence of dominant optic atrophy in the Danish population: evidence for a founder effect. *Hum Genet* 2001; 109(5):498–502.
173. Delettre C, Lenaers G, Griffoin JM et al. Nuclear gene OPA1, encoding a mitochondrial dynamin-related protein, is mutated in dominant optic atrophy. *Nat Genet* 2000; 26(2):207–210.
174. Zuchner S, Mersiyanova IV, Muglia M et al. Mutations in the mitochondrial GTPase mitofusin 2 cause Charcot-Marie-Tooth neuropathy type 2A. *Nat Genet* 2004; 36(5):449–451.
175. Nicholson GA, Magdelaine C, Zhu D et al. Severe early-onset axonal neuropathy with homozygous and compound heterozygous MFN2 mutations. *Neurology* 2008; 70(19):1678–1681.
176. Gannon AM, Stampfli MR, Foster WG. Cigarette smoke exposure elicits increased autophagy and dysregulation of mitochondrial dynamics in murine granulosa cells. *Biol Reprod* 2013; 88(3):63, 1–11.

11 Bisphenol A and the Ovary

Ronit Machtinger and Catherine Racowsky

CONTENTS

11.1 INTRODUCTION

Bisphenol A (BPA) is a synthetic chemical, which is one of the highest volume industrial chemicals produced worldwide. There is substantial evidence that this substance alters the normal function of the endocrine system (Schug et al., 2011) and, therefore, is called an endocrine-disrupting chemical (EDC). Potential sources of BPA include the lining of cans used for food and beverages, polycarbonate bottles, thermal receipts, and dental sealants (Vandenberg et al. 2007; Caserta et al., 2008; Talsness et al., 2009). Public health concerns regarding exposure to BPA are reflected by its detection in the urine of more than 90% of participants in the U.S. National Health and Nutrition Examination Survey (Calafat et al., 2008).

There is accumulating evidence that human fertility is decreasing (Guzick and Swan, 2006; Hamilton and Ventura, 2006). One of the suggested explanations for this decline has been the increasing chronic exposure to EDCs (Mendola et al., 2008). According to prevailing dogma, there is a finite pool of oogonial stem cells, which undergoes a progressive decline during the fetal period from the second trimester until menopause (Baker, 1963). Of specific relevance to this chapter is the fact that BPA has been detected in the human ovary *in vivo*, in the follicular fluid that surrounds the oocyte (Ikezuki, 2002).

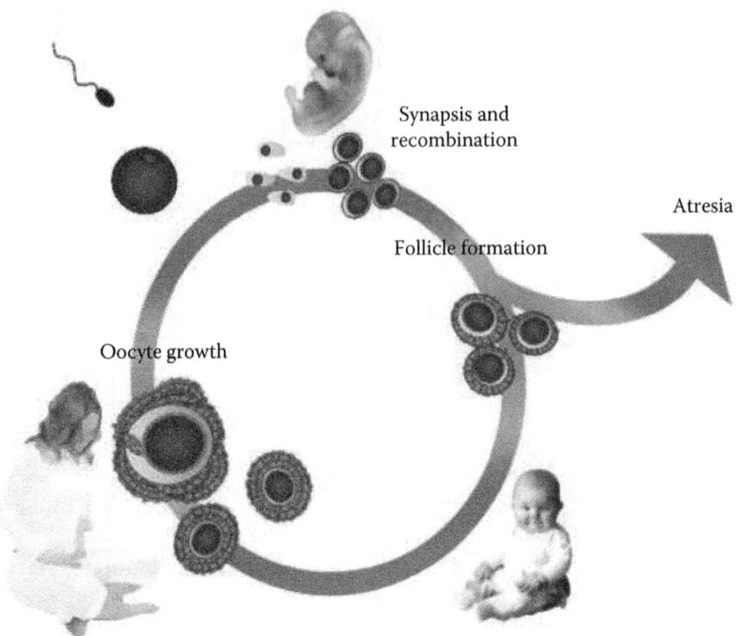

FIGURE 11.1 **(See color insert.)** The three vulnerable stages of oogenesis: (i) the meiotic prophase events of synapsis and recombination, which occur in the fetal ovary; (ii) follicle formation, which occurs during the second trimester of fetal development and is associated with a dramatic loss of oocytes caused by atresia, and (iii) oocyte growth, which occurs in the adult ovary and culminates in the resumption and completion of meiosis I and ovulation of a metaphase II–arrested egg. Figure by Crystal Lawson. (From Hunt, P.A. and Hassold, T.J., *Trends Genet.*, 24(2), 86, 2008. With permission, Figure 1, p. 87).

Exposure to environmental toxicants at several life stages may adversely affect oocyte quality. As discussed by Hunt and Hassold (2008), particularly vulnerable stages to endocrine disruptors include (1) entry of oocytes into prophase I in the fetal ovary, which is the stage of synapsis and recombination; (2) follicular formation, which occurs in the fetal ovary during the second trimester of pregnancy; and (3) the final stages of oocyte maturation, in the adult ovary (Figure 11.1).

The scope of this chapter is to consider the effect of BPA on the ovary. We will specifically consider current knowledge regarding BPA effects on meiosis in both animal models and the human, as well as review the literature regarding BPA levels and outcome following *in vitro* fertilization (IVF).

11.2 BPA EXPOSURE AND EARLY OOGENESIS (PROPHASE I)

Prophase of meiosis I occurs in the fetal ovary; this is the stage in which pairing, synapsis, and recombination between homologous chromosomes take place. The effect of BPA on this first stage of meiosis was evaluated by treating pregnant mice with low doses of BPA (implanted pellets that released 400 ng [1.7 μM] of BPA daily) during midgestation (Susiarjo et al., 2007). Oocytes from female fetuses that were exposed to BPA demonstrated abnormalities in prophase I, including synaptic defects and increased levels of recombination as well as an increase in chromosomal abnormalities.

In order to determine whether these effects in rodents were reproducible in primates, Rhesus monkeys were exposed to BPA during the second trimester of pregnancy, the stage of germ cell differentiation and entry into meiosis (Hunt et al., 2012). Similar to the findings in mice, chronic exposure to BPA adversely affected prophase events in Rhesus monkeys with a significant increase in recombination rates per cell in oocytes as compared with controls.

Similar results, albeit with a higher concentration of BPA, were reported in the human. Brieño-Enríquez et al. (2011) investigated the effect of BPA on the early stages of meiosis in the human. Oocytes from fetal ovaries were cultured for 7, 14, or 21 days with/without BPA. Oocytes cultured with at least 1 μM of BPA showed higher degeneration rates. Exposure of oocytes to BPA concentrations of ≥10 μM was associated with an increase in the incidence of crossing over, i.e., interference with pairing synapsis and recombination processes. The same researchers then investigated changes in gene expression in human oocytes in correlation with BPA exposure (Brieño-Enríquez et al., 2012). Ovarian fetal tissue was cultured with/without 30 μM BPA and analyzed before culture and after 7, 14, and 21 days. Gene expression associated with pairing-synapsis, double-strand break, and estrogen receptors was compared between tissue that was incubated with/without BPA using real-time PCR (RT-PCR). BPA exposure was associated with upregulation of genes involved in double-strand break generation, signaling, and repair.

The data mentioned earlier indicate that exposure to BPA during entry into meiosis I is associated with abnormalities in meiotic prophase I including synaptic defects, increased levels of recombination and chromosomal abnormalities.

11.3 BPA AND FOLLICULOGENESIS

Precisely, orchestrated follicular growth is critical for formation of a meiotically mature and developmentally competent oocyte. Any perturbations in follicle growth are likely to interfere with abnormalities in follicular steroidogenesis and may lead to follicular atresia (Eppig et al., 1996; Peretz et al., 2012). Peretz et al. (2012) conducted an *in vitro* study to determine whether exposure to BPA inhibits antral follicle growth and induces follicular atresia. These investigators cultured antral follicles in a medium containing vehicle control (DMSO) or BPA (1–100 μg/mL) (4.4–440 μM). Follicles were measured for growth every 24 h for 96–120 h. They showed that exposure to BPA at a concentration of 100 μg/mL (440 μM) significantly decreased follicle growth and increased atresia rates compared to controls.

Hunt et al. (2012) compared the rates of growing follicles in Rhesus monkeys exposed to BPA as compared with controls. Among females that were treated with a single daily dose of BPA (400 μg/kg body weight), there was a significantly higher number of secondary and antral follicles containing 2–3 oocytes, 4–5 oocytes, or >5 oocytes compared with controls ($p < 0.001$). Among the animals that were exposed to a continuous BPA regimen of unconjugated deuterated BPA administered as silastic tubing implants producing serum levels ranging from 2.2 to 3.3 ng/mL

(10–15 nM), the proportion of follicles with more than five oocytes was significantly increased compared with controls. Growing follicles from animals chronically exposed to BPA also contained oocytes of different sizes and the medullary region of ovaries from monkeys in this group showed many small, unenclosed oocytes.

The previously mentioned findings indicate that exposure to BPA during folliculogenesis is associated with impairment to follicular growth and an increased incidence of atresia.

11.4 BPA AND OOCYTE MEIOTIC MATURATION

11.4.1 Oocyte Meiotic Maturation

After a prolonged period of quiescence in which the oocytes remain arrested at prophase I, selected follicles are recruited into growing cohorts. Around days 3–5 of the menstrual cycle, one growing follicle is selected to become the dominant follicle, which ultimately responds to the midcycle surge of luteinizing hormone (LH), resulting in release of the oocyte from prophase I (i.e., the germinal vesicle [GV] stage) and its progression through meiotic maturation, ultimately to become a mature oocyte which is ovulated (Hodgen, 1982; Sowers et al., 2008). Progression of meiosis from prophase I through telophase I, and then on through prophase II to metaphase II is referred to as oocyte meiotic maturation. The process of oocyte meiotic maturation therefore occurs in the adult ovary.

11.4.2 In Vivo Studies on BPA and Oocyte Meiotic Maturation

The first observation that BPA may interfere with meiotic maturation in mammals was made serendipitously (Hodges et al., 2002). A sudden increase in meiotic disturbances and aneuploidy were observed in oocytes collected from female mice that were housed in damaged polycarbonate cages that were leaching BPA (Hodges et al., 2002; Hunt et al., 2003).

An additional study by Hunt et al. (2003) demonstrated that exposure of mouse oocytes to BPA induced alterations in the meiotic spindle, abnormalities in chromosome alignment, and an increase in the incidence of meiotic arrest and even aneuploidy. In this experiment, juvenile mice were injected with daily doses of 0, 20, 40, and 100 ng/g BPA per body weight for 6–8 days. GV-stage oocytes were collected from these animals, cultured overnight and then fixed, labeled, and analyzed. The authors showed that BPA exposure during the final stages of oocyte maturation was associated with meiotic abnormalities and increased rates of chromosome congression failure.

Eichenlaub-Ritter et al. (2008) exposed mice to low oral doses of BPA for a week. Denuded GV oocytes were matured *in vitro*, and BPA exposure was found to be associated with aberrant spindle morphology and decreased Metaphase II oocytes. However, this study did not reveal a BPA-related increase in aneuploidy.

Pacchierotti et al. (2008) also investigated the effects of *in vivo* exposure on meiotic maturation of mouse oocytes. Exposure was in three forms: acute, 0.2 mg/kg, once;

subchronic, 0.04 mg/kg for 7 days; and chronic, 0.5 mg/L in drinking water for 7 weeks. They found a significant increase in the incidence of MII oocytes with prematurely segregated chromatids after the treatment involving chronic exposure.

To our knowledge, no *in vivo* studies have been published reporting a direct relationship between follicular BPA concentrations and oocyte meiotic status in the human. However, BPA at a concentration of 1–2 ng/mL has been detected in follicular fluid aspirated during oocyte retrieval in a small series of IVF patients (Ikezuki, 2002).

11.4.3 In Vitro Studies on BPA and Oocyte Meiotic Maturation

11.4.3.1 Animal Studies

Lenie et al. (2008) analyzed the effects of chronic exposure of mice to BPA for 12 days on follicle-enclosed growth, and on *in vitro* meiotic maturation and cytoskeletal structure of the oocytes. Follicles were cultured in various concentrations of BPA (3 nM–30 μM). Exposure to 30 μM BPA resulted in a reduction in granulosa cell proliferation and estrogen production, although the follicles were still able to grow. Follicles that were exposed to this concentration showed a significant increase in Metaphase I-arrested oocytes with spindle aberrations and unaligned chromosomes, and an increase in abnormal Telophase I. There was a nonlinear, dose-dependent effect of BPA on the meiotic spindle with abnormal chromosome alignment in MII oocytes exposed for prolonged periods to low concentrations of BPA (3 nM–3 μM).

Can et al. (2005) tested the potential effect of BPA on meiotic maturation in mouse follicle-free cumulus–oocyte complexes (COCs). *In vitro* exposure of oocytes to BPA (10 and 30 μM) during the first meiotic division caused a significant reversible dose-dependent meiotic delay as well as spindle abnormalities. Depending on the BPA dose, oocytes showed loosening and elongation of meiotic spindles and compaction/dispersion of pericentriolar material.

Eichenlaub-Ritter et al. (2008) exposed mouse oocytes *in vitro* to a wide range of concentrations of BPA (50 ng/mL–10 μg/mL) (0.2–44 μM). Oocytes cultured in a medium containing 10 μg/mL BPA exhibited a significantly higher incidence of meiotic arrest, spindle abnormalities, and chromosome alignment compared with controls.

11.4.3.2 Human Studies

To our knowledge, there are no published studies investigating the effect of BPA on meiotic progression in human oocytes. However, based on the results in mice, we have recently conducted a series of experiments to evaluate whether *in vitro* exposure of GV-stage human oocytes to BPA interferes with meiotic maturation *in vitro*. Using otherwise discarded GV-stage oocytes from consenting patients undergoing IVF procedures, we have cultured oocytes in BPA concentrations ranging from 20 ng/mL (0.09 μM) to 20,000 ng/mL (88 μM). We observed that as BPA dose increased, there was a significant decrease in the likelihood of an oocyte reaching MII and a significant increase in the likelihood of an oocyte becoming degenerate or undergoing activation when a polar body was present (Machtinger et al., *unpublished observations*).

11.5 CLINICAL STUDIES: BPA AND IVF OUTCOME

A few studies have investigated the association between BPA and IVF outcome. Mok-Lin et al. (2009) investigated the association between urinary BPA levels among 84 women undergoing 112 IVF cycles, peak estradiol levels, and the number of oocytes retrieved. The authors showed an inverse correlation between urinary BPA levels, the number of oocytes retrieved, and peak estradiol levels. Bloom et al. (2011) evaluated serum BPA concentrations and follicular response to exogenous ovarian stimulation. Forty four women undergoing IVF were included in this preliminary study. BPA levels were inversely correlated with estrogen levels although no association was found between BPA levels and the number of oocytes retrieved.

Ehrlich et al. (2012a) evaluated the association between urinary BPA levels and implantation failure among women undergoing IVF. One hundred and thirty seven women undergoing 180 IVF cycles were included. The authors observed increased odds of implantation failure with higher quartiles of urinary BPA concentrations compared with the lowest quartile, and showed a positive, linear dose–response association between urinary levels of BPA and implantation failure.

In a subsequent study, this same group of researchers investigated the association between urinary levels of BPA, oocyte maturation, fertilization, embryo morphology on day 3, and blastocyst formation among IVF patients. They showed an inverse correlation between BPA levels, the number of mature (MII) oocytes, and the number of blastocysts formed (Ehrlich et al. 2012b).

11.6 SUMMARY

This chapter reviews current literature regarding the effect of BPA on the mammalian ovary, specifically with regard to perturbation of folliculogenesis, oogenesis, and oocyte maturation. Available data indicate that exposure to BPA is associated with impairment to folliclar growth and an increased incidence of atresia. When exposed to BPA at various stages of oogenesis, meiosis is impaired in murine oocytes, both *in vitro* and *in vivo*, and in human oocytes *in vitro*. Clinical data have also shown an inverse correlation between urinary BPA levels and peak estrogen levels, the number of oocytes retrieved, and implantation rates among IVF patients. However, further studies are needed to investigate the effect of prolonged exposure of oocytes to BPA and oocyte quality *in vivo*.

REFERENCES

Baker TG. A quantitative and cytological study of germ cells in human ovaries. 1963. *Proc R Soc Lond B Biol Sci*. 22;158:417–433.

Bloom MS, Kim D, Vom Saal FS et al. 2011. Bisphenol A exposure reduces the estradiol response to gonadotropin stimulation during in vitro fertilization. *Fertil Steril*. 96(3):672–677.

Brieño-Enríquez MA, Robles P, Camats-Tarruella N et al. 2011. Human meiotic progression and recombination are affected by Bisphenol A exposure during in vitro human oocyte development. *Hum Reprod*. 26(10):2807–2818.

Brieño-Enríquez MA, Reig-Viader R, Cabero L. 2012. Gene expression is altered after bisphenol A exposure in human fetal oocytes in vitro. *Mol Hum Reprod.* 18(4):171–183.

Calafat AM, Ye X, Wong LY et al. 2008. Exposure of the U.S. population to bisphenol A and 4-tertiary-octylphenol: 2003–2004. *Environ Health Perspect.* 116(1):39–44.

Can A, Semiz O, Cinar O. 2005. BSA induces cell cycle delay and alters centrosome and spindle in oocytes during meiosis. *Molec Hum Reprod.* 11:389–396.

Caserta D, Maranghi L, Mantovani A et al. 2008. Impact of endocrine disruptor chemicals in gynecology. *Hum Reprod Update.* 14(1):59–72.

Ehrlich S, Williams PL, Missmer SA et al. 2012a. Urinary bisphenol A concentrations and implantation failure among women undergoing in vitro fertilization. *Environ Health Perspect.* 120(7):978–983.

Ehrlich S, Williams PL, Missmer SA et al. 2012b. Urinary bisphenol A concentrations and early reproductive health outcomes among women undergoing IVF. Ehrlich S, Williams PL, Missmer SA, Flaws JA, Ye X, Calafat AM, Petrozza JC, Wright D, Hauser R. *Hum Reprod.* September 26. 27(12):3583–3592.

Eichenlaub-Ritter U, Vogt E, Cukurcam S. 2008. Exposure of mouse oocytes to bisphenol A causes meiotic arrest but not aneuploidy. *Mutat Res.* 12;651(1–2):82–92.

Eppig JJ, O'Brien M, Wigglesworth K. 1996. Mammalian oocyte growth and development in vitro. *Mol Reprod Dev.* 44:260–273.

Guzick DS, Swan S. 2006. The decline of infertility: apparent or real? *Fertil Steril.* 86:524–526.

Hamilton BE, Ventura SJ. 2006. Fertility and abortion rates in the United States, 1960–2002. *Int J Androl.* 29:34–45.

Hodgen GD. 1982. The dominant ovarian follicle. *Fertil Steril.* 38(3):281–300.

Hodges CA, Ilagan A, Jennings D et al. 2002. Experimental evidence that changes in oocyte growth influence meiotic chromosome segregation. *Hum Reprod.* 17:1171–1180.

Hunt PA, Hassold TJ. 2008. Human female meiosis: what makes a good egg go bad? Human female meiosis: what makes a good egg go bad? *Trends Genet.* 24(2):86–93.

Hunt PA, Koehler KE, Susiarjo M et al. 2003. Bisphenol A exposure causes meiotic aneuploidy in the female mouse. *Curr Biol.* 1:13(7):546–553.

Hunt PA, Lawson C, Gieske M et al. 2012. Bisphenol A alters early oogenesis and follicle formation in the fetal ovary of the rhesus monkey. *Proc Natl Acad Sci USA.* 23;109(43):17525–17530.

Ikezuki Y. 2002. Determination of bisphenol A concentrations in human biological fluids reveals significant early prenatal exposure. *Hum Reprod.* 17(11):2839–2841.

Lenie S, Cortvrindt R, Eichenlaub-Ritter U et al. 2008. Continuous exposure to bisphenol A during in vitro follicular development induces meiotic abnormalities. *Mutat Res.* 12:651(1–2):71–81.

Mendola P, Messer LC, Rappazzo K. 2008. Science linking environmental contaminant exposures with fertility and reproductive health impacts in the adult female. *Fertil Steril.* 89:e81–e94.

Mok-Lin E, Ehrlich S, Williams PL et al. 2009. Urinary bisphenol A concentrations and ovarian response among women undergoing IVF. *Int J Androl.* 32:1–9.

Pacchierotti F, Ranaldi R, Eichenlaub-Ritter U et al. 2008. Evaluation of aneugenic effects of bisphenol A in somatic and germ cells of the mouse. *Mutat Res.* 12;651(1–2):64–70.

Peretz J, Craig ZR, Flaws JA. 2012. Bisphenol A inhibits follicle growth and induces atresia in cultured mouse antral follicles independently of the genomic estrogenic pathway. *Biol Reprod.* 21;87(3):63.

Schug TT, Janesick A, Blumberg B et al. 2011. Endocrine disrupting chemicals and disease susceptibility. *J Steroid Biochem Mol Biol.* 127(3–5):204–215.

Sowers MR, Zheng H, McConnell D et al. 2008. Follicle stimulating hormone and its rate of change in defining menopause transition stages. *J Clin Endocrinol Metab.* 93(10):3958–3964.

Susiarjo M, Hassold TJ, Freeman E et al. 2007. Bisphenol A exposure in utero disrupts early oogenesis in the mouse. *PLoS Genet.* 12;3(1):e5.

Talsness CE, Andrade AG, Kuriyama SN et al. 2009. Components of plastic: experimental studies in animals and relevance for human health. *Philos Trans R Soc Lond B Biol Sci.* 27:2079–2096.

Vandenberg LN, Hauser R, Marcus M et al. 2007. Human exposure to bisphenol A (BPA). *Reprod Toxicol.* 24(2):139–177.

Part III

Ovarian Cancer

12 Endocrine Effects on Ovarian Cancer
Insight from Animal Models

Kendra Hodgkinson and Barbara C. Vanderhyden

CONTENTS

12.1 INTRODUCTION

Ovarian cancer is the fifth most frequently occurring cancer in North American women, and is the leading cause of gynecological cancer death in this population. Although the etiology of ovarian cancer remains unclear, certain risk factors have been implicated for this disease. These include hereditary factors such as mutations in the tumor suppressor proteins BRCA1 or BRCA2, reproductive factors such as nulliparity, and hormonal factors such as menopausal hormone therapy (Cramer 2012, Hunn and Rodriguez 2012). Infertility or later onset of menopause contributes to greater risk of developing ovarian cancer, while pregnancy, tubal ligation, and hysterectomy reduce risk (Hunn and Rodriguez 2012, Cramer 2012). Oral contraceptive use is strongly protective against ovarian cancer, whereas large epidemiological studies found menopausal hormone therapy to be a risk factor for ovarian cancer (Cramer 2012, Hunn and Rodriguez 2012). The marked influence of hormones and reproductive factors on ovarian cancer risk suggests that environmental toxins with endocrine-disrupting activity may impact risk; however, there is a notable lack of research in this area (Salehi et al. 2008).

During the past decade, a variety of animal models of ovarian cancer with clinically relevant genetic and phenotypic characteristics have been developed. This chapter summarizes the literature on animal models of ovarian cancer, with emphasis on their ability to reveal the origins of ovarian cancer, the genes that contribute to tumor susceptibility, and the endocrine factors that alter ovarian cancer incidence or progression. The relevance of these models to human disease is dependent upon their ability to replicate a number of features that contribute to mortality, including age of onset, pattern of tumor dissemination, ascites accumulation, and rate of disease progression. It is anticipated that as animal models become more clinically relevant, they will become valuable resources for future toxicology testing and for the study of risk factors that may contribute to the initiation and/or progression of ovarian cancer.

12.2 BIOLOGY OF OVARIAN CANCER

Ovarian cancer is the most lethal gynecological malignancy in developed countries. Approximately 90% of ovarian cancers are epithelial ovarian cancers, which are divided into five histological subtypes: serous, mucinous, endometrioid, clear cell, and undifferentiated (Romero and Bast 2012). Epithelial ovarian cancers can also be divided into two groups based on molecular phenotype, clinical progression, and histological grade. Type I cancers are typically slow-growing tumors with mucinous, clear-cell, low-grade serous, or low-grade endometrioid histologies (Kurman and Shih 2010). Mutations in *K-RAS*, *BRAF*, *PTEN*, or the β-catenin pathway are frequently seen in type I cancers, whereas *TP53* and *BRCA1/2* mutations are rare in this group (Kurman and Shih 2010, Romero and Bast 2012). By contrast, type II cancers are aggressive and are usually diagnosed at advanced stages, with high-grade serous, high-grade endometrioid, or undifferentiated histology (Kurman and Shih 2010, Romero and Bast 2012). Genomic instability is very high and mutations of *TP53* and *BRCA1/2* are common, whereas mutations in *K-RAS*, *BRAF*, *PTEN*, and the β-catenin pathway are rare. Type II cancers, which are mainly serous, represent 75% of ovarian cancers and 90% of ovarian cancer deaths (Kurman and Shih 2010). This predominance of high-grade serous cancers can mask the heterogeneity of ovarian cancer, and many research findings apply only to serous tumors and not to other histological subtypes. Due to the molecular and clinical differences between histological subtypes, animal models that recapitulate one subtype of ovarian cancer are unlikely to accurately model other subtypes.

12.2.1 Origins of Ovarian Cancer

A challenge in the generation of animal models of ovarian cancer is that the tissue of origin for ovarian cancer remains controversial. The ovarian surface epithelium (OSE) has historically been considered the initiation site of epithelial ovarian cancer (Fathalla 1971). Invaginations of the OSE form ovarian inclusion cysts, which are believed to be a precursor to ovarian cancer (Scully 1977, Fleming et al. 2006). Unlike OSE, inclusion cysts and ovarian cancers have a Müllerian morphology and molecular signature (Li et al. 2012). The cause of this Müllerian phenotype is still unclear. Local factors such as ovulation-associated inflammation and steroid hormones may induce a metaplastic change in the OSE (Auersperg 2011). An alternative explanation for the Müllerian morphology of inclusion cysts is that they may derive from nonovarian cells, which have transplanted to the ovary (Kurman and Shih 2010, Li et al. 2011).

Considerable evidence has recently accumulated implicating the distal fallopian tube as a site of origin for type II ovarian cancers, based on the discovery of dysplasias and adenocarcinomas in the fallopian tubes of women at high risk for ovarian cancer (Piek et al. 2001, Medeiros et al. 2006, Levanon et al. 2008). It has been suggested that the fallopian tube fimbria and OSE, which share an embryological origin, form a single transitional epithelium rather than two independent epithelia (Auersperg 2011). The OSE and fimbria are anatomically contiguous and molecular markers such as calretinin and cadherins do not show a defined boundary, suggesting that the OSE and fimbrial cells are incompletely differentiated and may be susceptible to neoplastic transformation (Auersperg 2011). Recent evidence suggests that carcinogenesis may occur in a similar transitional zone, the fallopian tube–peritoneal junction (Seidman et al. 2011).

The current evidence suggests that many or all type II ovarian tumors derive from the fimbria of the fallopian tube, and that type I tumors can develop from ovarian inclusion cysts but may also originate in nonovarian tissues (Kurman and Shih 2010, Vaughan et al. 2011). Molecular and histological comparisons have suggested that low-grade endometrioid and clear-cell carcinomas may originate in endometriotic lesions, whereas some mucinous tumors may develop from gastrointestinal tissue (Vaughan et al. 2011). Further research is needed to elucidate the origin of cells which eventually form type I ovarian tumors.

12.2.2 Modeling Human Ovarian Cancer in Rodents: Xenografted and Syngeneic Transplants

The earliest models of ovarian cancer, developed in the 1970s, used carcinogens to induce ovarian tumors in rodents; however, these tumors did not have a consistent origin or histology, limiting their ability to model human ovarian cancer (reviewed in Shan and Liu 2009). Adams and Auersperg (1981) developed a xenograft mouse model, which grew ovarian tumors after injection of rat OSE that had been transformed *in vitro* by Kirsten sarcoma virus; however, the tumors were sarcomas, which did not accurately model epithelial ovarian cancer. Godwin et al. (1992) improved on this model by using spontaneously transformed rat OSE, which formed epithelial tumors when injected into immunocompromised mice. Additional xenograft models have been developed using transformed human OSE, resected tumors, or ovarian cancer cell lines injected into immunocompromised mice (Davy et al. 1977, Fogh et al. 1977, Liu et al. 2004). Xenograft models are useful for studying tumor progression *in vivo*, but have at least three major drawbacks. First, the requirement for a suppressed immune system means that the normal immune response to tumors is impaired or eliminated, reducing the relevance of the model system. Second, because fully transformed cells are injected, it is impossible to study tumorigenesis or early stages of disease progression. Third, it is unclear how well the cell lines used in those studies resemble the original tumors; cell behavior and genotype may be altered by culture, and a recent study suggested that several commonly used ovarian cancer cell lines may be misidentified (Korch et al. 2012).

Despite these limitations, xenograft models are still commonly used for rapid testing of new therapies and for the examination of molecular events in cancer progression. To enable the use of immunocompetent mice, syngeneic models were developed using transformed mouse OSE (Roby et al. 2000, Orsulic et al. 2002, Roberts et al. 2005) or, more recently, serial allografts of a spontaneous rat ovarian tumor (Sharrow et al. 2010). Although these syngeneic models allow a normal immune response to tumor progression, they still have little value in the study of early disease.

12.2.3 Modeling Human Ovarian Cancer in Transgenic Mice

In the past decade, research has focused on the development of transgenic mouse models of ovarian cancer in order to study the cellular and molecular events associated with tumor initiation and progression in an immunocompetent animal. Because the fallopian tube was only recently given considerable attention as a site of cancer origin, most animal models of ovarian cancer were designed to target OSE (reviewed in Mullany and Richards 2012, Vanderhyden et al. 2003, Garson et al. 2005). Genetic manipulations based on both well-known and novel genetic pathways have led to a diverse collection of transgenic mouse models representing various subtypes of ovarian tumors, including benign tumors. Ovarian cystadenomas (benign epithelial tumors) form in mice with *Disabled-2* haplodeficiency (Yang et al. 2006), *Brca1* deletion in granulosa cells (Chodankar et al. 2005), or knockout of receptors for follicle stimulating hormone (FSH; Chen et al. 2007).

Recapitulating the histology and molecular characteristics of the various histological subtypes of epithelial ovarian cancer has been a challenge with limited success. Activation of the β-catenin pathway and deletion of *Pten* in the OSE leads to low-grade endometrioid ovarian cancer in two different mouse models (Wu et al. 2007, Tanwar et al. 2011). In another model, deletion of *Pten* alone leads to endometriotic lesions, which develop into aggressive endometrioid ovarian cancer when mutant *K-ras* is activated (Dinulescu et al. 2005). *PTEN* deletion is a frequent event in endometrioid ovarian cancer, but *K-RAS* mutation is rarely seen in this subtype, although it is common in mucinous and low-grade serous cancers (Dinulescu et al. 2005, Rosen et al. 2009). Knockout of *p53* and *Rb* in the OSE leads to serous or undifferentiated epithelial ovarian cancer in another mouse model (Flesken-Nikitin et al. 2003). Similar tumors with mixed histology (serous/poorly differentiated) were seen after induction of SV40 T antigen (TAg) under the control of the promoter region of anti-Müllerian hormone receptor-2 (Amhr2; also known as Müllerian-inhibiting substance receptor type II, MISIIR; Connolly et al. 2003). Cell lines established from ascites of these mice form tumors with high-grade serous or poorly differentiated histology when injected into syngeneic mice (Quinn et al. 2010). In a mouse model with inducible activation of TAg selectively in the OSE, mice developed epithelial ovarian tumors with poorly differentiated/sex cord stromal histology (Laviolette et al. 2010).

Recently, the first mouse model with high-grade serous ovarian cancer originating in the fallopian tube was developed (Kim et al. 2012). This model inactivates *Dicer* and *Pten* in the female reproductive tract by crossing floxed *Dicer*/*Pten* mice with Amhr2-Cre mice. Offspring form high-grade serous cancers arising in the fallopian tube and spreading to the ovaries before metastasizing further and developing ascites (Kim et al. 2012). Microarray analysis of the tumors showed molecular similarities to human high-grade serous cancers, suggesting that this mouse model accurately reflects molecular as well as clinical progression of this subtype of ovarian cancer (Kim et al. 2012). While very promising, this model has several drawbacks, including the fact that in this model tumors arise from the stroma rather than the epithelium, the cell type where early lesions and carcinomas have been found in humans (Kurman and Shih 2010). Furthermore, *PTEN* mutations are common in low-grade endometrioid and clear-cell cancers, but are rarely found in high-grade serous cancers (Rosen et al. 2009). Despite these limitations, this mouse has the potential to be a very useful model to study high-grade cancer arising from the fallopian tube.

12.2.4 Nonmammalian Models of Ovarian Cancer

An alternative to transgenic mouse models is the hen, which has a high rate of spontaneous ovarian cancer due to its extremely high ovulation rate (Barnes et al. 2002). After several years of daily ovulation, birds develop ascites and metastasizing tumors with histologies similar to all the histological subtypes seen in human ovarian cancer. The varied histologies and spontaneous development of these tumors are significant advantages of this model. However, there are key molecular differences between birds and mammals, which may limit the ability to translate some findings from this model. Another drawback of this model is the requirement for long-term maintenance of large numbers of birds in order to achieve sufficient numbers of spontaneous ovarian cancers.

The development of accurate animal models of ovarian cancer, particularly those in which tumors develop *in situ*, enables the study of how various endogenous and exogenous factors affect ovarian cancer initiation and progression. Endogenous factors that may be relevant include circulating hormones and inflammatory cytokines present in follicular fluid. Relevant exogenous factors include pharmaceutical hormones such as menopausal hormone therapy and oral contraceptives, which both alter the risk of developing ovarian cancer. There is substantial evidence indicating that estrogen tends to promote ovarian cancer development, and there is also support for the involvement of other hormones including progesterone, testosterone, and gonadotropins. Environmental toxins with estrogenic or endocrine-disrupting activity may affect the risk of ovarian cancer, although further research is needed to draw any conclusions in this area. The remainder of this chapter addresses what has been learned from animal models about the hormonal risk factors associated with ovarian cancer.

12.3 EFFECTS OF ESTROGENS ON OVARIAN CANCER

12.3.1 Effects of Estrogens on Tumor Susceptibility and Initiation

Estrogens in menopausal hormone therapy increase the risk of developing ovarian cancer, as shown by two recent meta-analyses; Pearce et al. (2009) analyzed 14 population-based studies, and Greiser et al. (2007) analyzed 42 studies that were either population-based or drawn from cancer registry data. The mechanism explaining the increased risk has not been determined, although experimental evidence suggests that increased proliferation may be a factor. The surface of the ovary and the fimbriae of the fallopian tube are exposed to high endogenous levels of estrogens after ovulation (Wu et al. 1977). At this time, OSE cells proliferate rapidly in order to close the postovulatory wound. This wound-healing process is thought to increase the risk of ovarian cancer (Fathalla 1971), which may be explained by DNA damage caused by oxidative stress (King et al. 2011) or increased proliferation. In rabbit ovaries, OSE proliferation following ovulation leads to papillary structures forming over the corpora lutea (Osterholzer et al. 1985a). Similarly, treatment with exogenous estradiol (E2) caused a 20-fold increase in OSE DNA synthesis and a 16-fold increase in papillary structures compared to control injections, and long-term E2 treatment induced papillomas (Bai et al. 2000). In this rabbit model, OSE cells isolated as tissue fragments remained responsive to E2 *in vitro*, whereas OSE isolated by trypsin digestion lost the proliferative response (Bai et al. 2000). Interestingly, OSE cultured with stromal cells had an increased proliferative response to E2, suggesting that paracrine interactions may be important in the regulation of OSE proliferation (Bai et al. 2000). E2 treatment increased proliferation of primary cultures of human OSE, although in primate OSE, E2 induced growth arrest (Syed et al. 2001, Wright et al. 2002). These differences may indicate species-specific responses or differences in methodology. In rodent ovaries, E2 treatment increases OSE proliferation and drives putative preneoplastic changes such as stratification, hyperplasia, and dysplasia (Stewart et al. 2004a, Gotfredson and Murdoch 2007, Perniconi et al. 2008, Laviolette et al. 2010). Interestingly, surgical injury to the ovary increased the mitogenic actions of E2 (Stewart et al. 2004a). In rhesus macaques, changes in OSE morphology and physiology were observed throughout the menstrual cycle (Wright et al. 2011). In guinea pigs, E2 treatment resulted in ovarian serous cystadenomas whereas diethylstilbestrol, a synthetic estrogen, induced papillary structures on the ovarian surface (Silva et al. 1998). A transgenic mouse with *Brca1* deleted in the granulosa cells, causing increased circulating E2 levels, also developed serous cystadenomas (Chodankar et al. 2005, Hong et al. 2010).

Fallopian tube epithelium is increasingly accepted as the initiation site of some epithelial ovarian cancers, particularly those of the high-grade serous histological subtype (Kurman and Shih 2010). The potential role of E2 in the formation of preneoplastic lesions of the fallopian tube has not been investigated, although the fallopian tube contains receptors for E2 and progesterone and is sensitive to both endogenous and exogenous steroid hormones (reviewed in Jansen 1984). In the mammalian oviduct, endogenous or exogenous E2 stimulation induces differentiation of ciliated and secretory cells, and progesterone opposes this E2-induced differentiation (Jansen 1984). E2 may also play a role in proliferation, although the adult oviduct has a very low mitotic index (Jansen 1984). Exogenous E2 stimulated proliferation of epithelial cells in chick and mammalian oviducts (Oka and Schimke 1969, Laugier et al. 1983, Kamwanja and Hansen 1993, Wollenhaupt et al. 2002, Okada et al. 2004), but not in mouse oviducts (King et al. 2011). In ovariectomized cats, E2 treatment increased oviductal epithelial cell hypertrophy and mitotic index (Bareither and Verhage 1981). Similar effects were seen in ovariectomized primates (Verhage et al. 1990). However, primary cultures of human fallopian tube epithelium did not proliferate in response to E2 treatment (Takeuchi et al. 1991). Further studies are required to determine whether E2-induced changes in proliferation and differentiation contribute to risk of malignant transformation.

Although E2 exposure causes preneoplastic changes and benign tumors in the mammalian OSE and induces proliferation in both OSE and oviductal epithelial cells, it does not appear to be sufficient to induce malignant epithelial ovarian tumors in these animal models. Because these short-lived animals rarely or never develop spontaneous epithelial ovarian cancer, it remains unclear whether E2 is sufficient to induce tumors in humans or whether additional factors such as mutations or environmental toxins are required for tumor initiation. One mechanism by which E2 might promote tumor initiation is through the induction of DNA mutations; CYP1B1, an enzyme catalyzing E2 to genotoxic 4-OHE2, is increased in hen ovarian cancer relative to normal ovaries (Zhuge et al. 2009). Similarly, it has been shown in breast epithelial cells that estrogens can be converted to metabolites that form DNA adducts, leading to mutations and increased risk of tumorigenesis (Cavalieri et al. 2006).

12.3.2 Effects of Estrogens on Tumor Growth and Progression

The contribution of E2 to human ovarian cancer progression has been modeled with xenografts of human ovarian cancer cell lines injected into immunocompromised mice. Early experiments with BG-1 cells showed that ovariectomy caused an increase in tumor growth, and that an injection of E2 in ovariectomized mice strongly inhibited tumor growth relative to either ovariectomized or intact mice (Zimniski et al. 1989). However, more recent studies have shown that E2 increases tumor growth of BG-1 cells injected subcutaneously into ovariectomized mice (Salvo et al. 2006). These contradictory results may be explained by differences in methodology, particularly E2 administration and dose; Zimniski et al. gave a single 0.2 mg intramuscular E2 injection whereas Salvo et al. used a slow-release subcutaneous implant (0.72 mg/60 days). Notably, some BG-1 cells have recently been identified by short-tandem repeat analysis to be MCF-7 breast cancer cells, and the identity of cells used in past publications is unclear (Korch et al. 2012). Acceleration of tumor growth by E2 has been shown in xenografted SKOV-3, SKOV3ip1, HEYA8, PE04, OVA-5, and OVCAR3 human ovarian cancer cells (Sawada et al. 1990, Armaiz-Pena et al. 2009, Spillman et al. 2010, Laviolette et al. 2011), and anti-estrogens have been shown to slow the growth of xenografted PE04 cells (Langdon et al. 1994) and BG-1 cells (Zimniski et al. 1989). Similarly, Armaiz-Pena et al. (2009) showed that when SKOV3ip1 and HEYA8 cells were injected during proestrus, when mice have high endogenous estrogen levels, the resulting tumors grew faster than those injected during the estrus phase. Vascular endothelial growth factor (VEGF) levels and microvessel density were increased in tumors from mice injected during proestrus, suggesting that enhanced angiogenesis may be partially responsible for the increased growth (Armaiz-Pena et al. 2009). It is likely that growth is mainly stimulated through ERα, as ovarian cancer xenografts lacking this receptor failed to respond to E2 (Spillman et al. 2010).

Although xenograft models recapitulate tumor growth more accurately than cell culture methods, they have several significant disadvantages. Because the mice are immunocompromised, the ability to evaluate how the immune system responds to the treatment is limited. Interactions between mouse and human cells may alter the dynamics of the extracellular matrix of the tumor, potentially changing tumor growth and response to treatment. Furthermore, because the cells that are injected are already fully transformed, it is not clear how well the progression of tumors formed by transplanted cells resembles the progression of tumors developing *in situ*.

Transgenic and carcinogenesis animal models allow monitoring of both tumor initiation and progression in an immunocompetent animal, enabling the identification of factors that promote risk and/or disease progression. An additional benefit of transgenic models is the ability to recapitulate genetic mutations frequently occurring in human cancer, whereas carcinogenesis models present with variable mutations. Laviolette et al. (2010) investigated the effects of E2 on the initiation and progression of ovarian cancer in the tgCAG-LS-TAg mouse model, which uses the Cre/Lox system to selectively induce TAg. TAg is a potent oncogene due to its ability to bind and deactivate p53 and Rb (reviewed in Pipas 2009). When adenovirus expressing Cre recombinase (AdCre) is injected into the ovarian bursal membrane, TAg is expressed in the OSE and the epithelial cells lining the oviduct, leading to bilateral ovarian tumors initiating within 80–90 days (Laviolette et al. 2010). This long latency period allows the evaluation of factors affecting tumor initiation as well as progression. Disease characteristics parallel those seen in humans, including extensive peritoneal metastases and ascites. In this model, E2 promoted a more papillary histology and also accelerated tumor onset, decreasing median survival to 50 days in E2-treated mice, whereas control mice had a median survival of 113 days with no microscopic ovarian lesions visible until 80 days after induction of TAg expression (Laviolette et al. 2010). A syngeneic rat model using 7,12-dimethylbenz(a)anthracene (DMBA)-derived tumor transplants found that E2 treatment increased tumor growth (Lee et al. 1992), supporting the role of E2 in promoting tumor progression. The mechanism(s) by which E2 accelerates the onset and progression of disease remain unknown.

In a study of aged hens, which spontaneously develop ovarian cancer at a high incidence, E2 (25 mg slow-release implant) did not alter incidence but showed a trend for higher stage and a larger proportion of serous tumors, indicating a potential role for E2 in tumor progression and histology (Trevino et al. 2012). E2 did not alter proliferation or apoptosis of the hen OSE, suggesting that avian OSE may not be as responsive to E2 as mammalian OSE (Trevino et al. 2012).

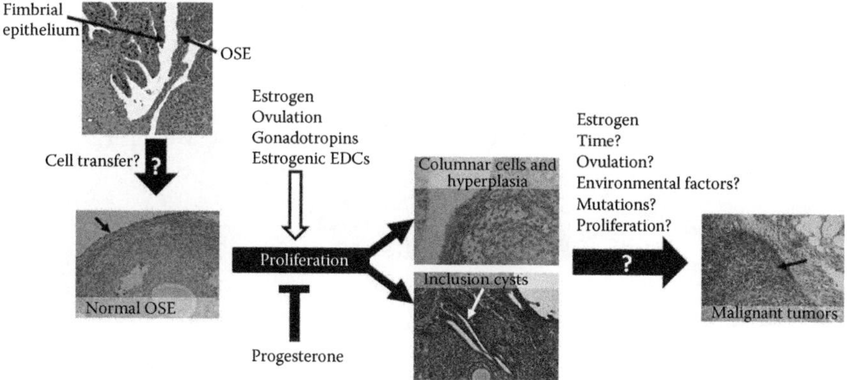

FIGURE 12.1 Hormones alter OSE morphology and proliferation, leading to putative preneoplastic lesions in mouse models. Cells lining inclusion cysts resemble oviductal (fallopian tube) epithelial cells and may derive from oviductal cells transplanted to the OSE and/or in growth of OSE cells. The origin of ovarian cancer is further complicated by the fact that, in mice and humans, the fimbrial epithelium is contiguous with the OSE, forming a transitional zone. Ovulations or exposure to exogenous estrogen, gonadotropins, or endocrine-disrupting chemicals (EDCs) increases areas of epithelial hyperplasia, columnar cells, and inclusion cysts. Evidence from mouse models indicate that estrogen can decrease the latency period of tumor initiation (Laviolette et al. 2010), but it is likely that other triggers are involved, such as time, ovulations, environmental factors, mutations, proliferation, or other undefined factors. In animal models, progestins generally suppress or block the tumor-initiating actions of estrogen.

Animal models have revealed that E2 stimulates both the initiation (Figure 12.1) and progression (Figure 12.2) of epithelial ovarian cancer, and may alter tumor histology. Epidemiological evidence suggests that the role of E2 in human cancer is similar to that seen in animal models, but further research is needed to evaluate the role of E2 in different subtypes of ovarian cancer, to identify the mechanism of action for E2-stimulated tumor growth, and to identify other factors that may influence the actions of E2.

12.4 EFFECTS OF PROGESTINS ON OVARIAN CANCER

12.4.1 Effects of Progestins on Tumor Susceptibility and Initiation

The role of progesterone (P4) in the development of ovarian cancer has not been studied as extensively as that of E2. In most contexts, P4 appears to oppose the actions of estrogen. P4 has been reported to stimulate apoptosis, which may be a mechanism to eliminate cells damaged by rapid proliferation or genotoxic effects induced by E2. The layer of OSE in mouse ovaries normally contains some areas of columnar or stratified cells. It has been suggested that these may be early events in the initiation of epithelial ovarian cancer, notably because these areas are increased by E2 treatment (Gotfredson and Murdoch 2007, Laviolette et al. 2010). Tok et al. (2006) found that incidence of ovarian surface papillomatosis was associated with a longer duration of menopausal hormone therapy. In contrast to E2, P4 treatment

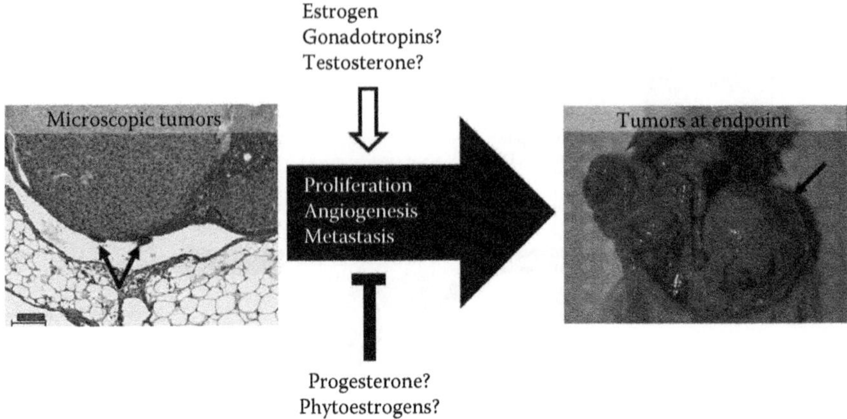

FIGURE 12.2 Estrogen alters tumor progression in mouse models, leading to changes in histology, rate of tumor growth, and survival. Estrogen decreases the time between tumor initiation and the development of tumors that are sufficient to shorten survival in the tgCAG-LS-TAg mouse model (Laviolette et al. 2010). In most animal models, estrogen promotes tumor growth and metastasis, whereas progesterone has little to no effect on estrogen-stimulated tumor progression in established tumors. However, progesterone treatment prior to injection with cancer cells slowed tumor progression in a xenograft model (McDonnel et al. 2005), and Armaiz-Pena et al. (2009) showed that adding progesterone eliminated the tumor-promoting actions of estrogen in another xenograft model, suggesting that progesterone can inhibit ovarian cancer in some situations. Phytoestrogens were able to inhibit tumor growth in a xenograft model (Salvo et al. 2006), but more studies are needed to determine if and how phytoestrogens act on ovarian cancer. The impact of other hormones on tumor progression has not been studied sufficiently to make firm conclusions.

completely eliminated columnar and stratified OSE, suggesting that apoptosis was induced in these putative preneoplastic cells (Gotfredson and Murdoch 2007). This is supported by a study in rhesus macaques in which the progestin levonorgestrel increased the percentage of OSE cells undergoing apoptosis (Rodriguez et al. 1998). Combination oral contraceptives containing levonorgestrel and ethinyl estradiol also increased the proportion of apoptotic OSE, although not as much as levonorgestrel alone (Rodriguez et al. 1998). The lack of spontaneous epithelial ovarian cancer in these models prevents direct assessment of any preventative actions of P4 on tumor initiation.

P4 opposes the E2-stimulated differentiation of secretory and ciliated cells in the oviductal epithelium; regardless of E2 level, high P4 levels will induce dedifferentiation (reviewed in Jansen 1984). P4 may similarly oppose the proliferation induced by E2. P4 has been reported to inhibit proliferation in quail oviductal epithelium (Perche et al. 1989). In pigs, P4 had no effect on the proliferation of the oviductal cells and decreased transcriptional activity, whereas E2 increased both proliferation and transcription (Wollenhaupt et al. 2002). In cats and primates, P4 reduced cell height and induced apoptosis in E2-stimulated oviductal epithelial cells, opposing the effects of E2 (Bareither and Verhage 1981, Verhage et al. 1990). It appears consistent across mammalian species that P4 inhibits proliferation and/or induces apoptosis in a manner that could counteract the mitogenic actions of E2 in both the ovarian and the oviductal epithelium, and may thereby inhibit tumorigenesis.

In aged hens, the progestin medroxyprogesterone acetate (MPA) profoundly reduced the incidence of spontaneous epithelial ovarian cancer (Barnes et al. 2002, Trevino et al. 2012), perhaps by suppressing ovulation, a key factor in the development of spontaneous ovarian cancer in this model (Giles et al. 2010, Carver et al. 2011). MPA did not alter apoptosis or proliferation in the OSE, and exposure to exogenous E2 did not alter the protective actions of MPA, suggesting that the decreased cancer incidence was caused by the reduction of ovulation rather than by direct hormone action on the OSE (Trevino et al. 2012).

12.4.2 Effects of Progestins on Tumor Growth and Progression

P4 has been reported to have variable effects on the growth of ovarian cancer xenografts. Early experiments showed that injections of P4 had no effect on growth or histology of OVA-5 xenografts (Sawada et al. 1990). P4 similarly had no effect on growth of SKOV3ip1 or HeyA8 xenografts, but interestingly, P4 treatment abrogated E2-stimulated tumor growth of both cell lines (Armaiz-Pena et al. 2009). McDonnel et al. (2005) found that P4 treatment one day before injection with SKOV-3 cells reduced peritoneal dissemination and invasiveness and increased survival in athymic mice. However, in that study, P4 treatment 3 weeks after SKOV-3 cell injection had no effect on tumor progression or survival, suggesting that P4 has no relevant actions on established tumors. P4 was reported to increase cisplatin sensitivity in established tumors by increasing platinum concentrations in tumors, leading to reduced numbers and diameters of intestinal tumors in the cisplatin-resistant SKOV-3 and OVCAR-3 xenografts (Murdoch et al. 2008). The authors proposed that P4 alters membrane fluidity, inhibiting cisplatin excretion from the cells. P4 did not affect apoptosis in the tumors, suggesting that P4 may act on different pathways in normal OSE versus ovarian cancer cells (Murdoch et al. 2008). Interestingly, the anti-progestin mifepristone has been reported to significantly decrease tumor growth of SKOV-3 xenografts (Goyeneche et al. 2007), although the mechanism of this growth suppression is not yet clear.

In a syngeneic rat model, P4 did not alter growth of transplanted DMBA-induced tumors, but changed tumor histology to a less differentiated form (Lee et al. 1992). Progestin action has been examined in two transgenic mouse models of ovarian cancer. After treatment with AdCre, the LSL-K-ras^{G12D}/Pten$^{loxP/loxP}$ mouse expresses mutant *K-ras* and loses *Pten* expression; AdCre injected into the bursal membrane induces epithelial ovarian tumors arising from the OSE, with endometrioid histology (Dinulescu et al. 2005). *PTEN* is frequently mutated in endometrioid ovarian cancer, whereas *K-RAS* is mutated in other subtypes of ovarian cancer but very rarely in the endometrioid subtype (Rosen et al. 2009). In this model, the progestin norethindrone reduced tumor growth by 42%, but due to high variation in response among the tumors, the difference was not statistically significant (Romero et al. 2009). Similar results were seen for norethindrone in combination with ethinyl estradiol (Romero et al. 2009). By contrast, in the tgCAG-LS-TAg transgenic mouse model of ovarian cancer, P4 had no effect on survival or tumor characteristics (Laviolette et al. 2010), which may be a reflection of the different histological subtypes observed in this model.

The contribution of P4 to the initiation and progression of ovarian cancer remains unclear (Figures 12.1 and 12.2). Collectively, the data suggest that although P4 can suppress the initial growth of ovarian cancer xenografts, it has limited or no effects on the growth of established epithelial ovarian tumors in animal models. However, P4 may synergize with cisplatin; it would be interesting to evaluate the effect of P4 on cisplatin plus taxol treatment, a standard first-line therapy for epithelial ovarian cancer. Epidemiological studies suggest that the increased risk of ovarian cancer caused by estrogenic menopausal hormone therapy is reduced or eliminated by the addition of a progestin (Pearce et al. 2009). P4 may counteract some of the mitogenic or genotoxic actions of E2, but the evidence is not yet conclusive. Further research is needed to elucidate the potential interactions between E2 and P4 in the development of ovarian cancer.

12.5 EFFECTS OF GONADOTROPINS ON OVARIAN CANCER

12.5.1 Risk Factors of Ovarian Cancer Associated with Ovulation and Gonadotropins

Ovulation and gonadotropins are strongly implicated in the initiation of epithelial ovarian cancer. Epidemiological evidence has shown that the number of ovulations is a risk factor for ovarian cancer. Factors that decrease lifetime ovulation such as pregnancy, breastfeeding, late menarche, and use of oral contraceptives decrease the risk of ovarian cancer (reviewed in Cramer 2012, Hunn and Rodriguez 2012). It has been proposed that each ovulation increases the risk of developing ovarian cancer due to the OSE rapidly proliferating to close the postovulatory wound, in the presence of estrogen-rich follicular fluid (Fathalla 1971). Because most factors that alter ovulation also alter hormone levels, the impact of ovulation on the risk of developing ovarian cancer is difficult to distinguish from the effects of hormones. However, hormones have been shown to affect ovarian cancer incidence in cases where ovulation is not altered, such as menopausal hormone therapy. Menopause, which is associated with high serum levels of FSH and luteinizing hormone (LH), may be a risk factor for ovarian cancer (reviewed in Vanderhyden et al. 2005). Both human OSE and fallopian tube epithelium express receptors for both LH and FSH (Lei et al. 1993, Zheng et al. 1996, Kuroda et al. 2001), implying that gonadotropins can act directly on these tissues. Gonadotropins have been reported to stimulate proliferation of OSE, which may promote ovarian tumorigenesis (Cramer and Welch 1983).

Ovulation causes changes in the ovarian surface, which are associated with an increased risk of developing ovarian cancer, including increased proliferation and altered morphology (Figure 12.1). OSE proliferation after hCG-induced ovulation in rabbit ovaries leads to papillary structures forming over the corpora lutea (Osterholzer et al. 1985a). Superovulation induced in rodents by sequential treatment with pregnant mare's serum gonadotropin (PMSG) and human chorionic gonadotropin (hCG) increased OSE proliferation and stratification (Davies et al. 1999, Stewart et al. 2004a, Burdette et al. 2006, Gotfredson and Murdoch 2007). Davies et al. (1999)

found that recombinant LH or FSH alone also increased OSE proliferation, suggesting that gonadotropins can act on OSE through mechanisms that do not involve ovulation. This conclusion is supported by reports of gonadotropins stimulating proliferation of primary cultures of rabbit OSE (Osterholzer et al. 1985b). Primary cultures of human OSE also proliferate in response to gonadotropins, although primate OSE did not (Syed et al. 2001, Kuroda et al. 2001, Wright et al. 2002). It is unclear whether these differing responses are due to physiological differences between species or changes in methodology. In guinea pigs, gonadotropins induced the formation of benign epithelial ovarian cysts in two of three treated animals (Silva et al. 1997). Ovulation induced by PMSG and hCG did not alter oviductal epithelial cell proliferation in mice (King et al. 2011).

12.5.2 Effects of Gonadotropins on Ovarian Cancer Growth and Progression

It has been suggested that gonadotropins promote ovarian cancer because postmenopausal women, who are at higher risk of developing ovarian cancer, have higher levels of gonadotropins (Cramer and Welch 1983). However, the role of gonadotropins in ovarian cancer progression is poorly understood. Some studies have examined the effects of ovariectomy, which causes low E2 and P4 and high FSH and LH (due to the lack of negative feedback by E2). The results are difficult to interpret because it is unclear whether high levels of gonadotropins and/or low levels of steroid hormones are responsible for the observed results. Ovariectomy increased tumor growth of xenografted MLS ovarian cancer spheroids, which may have been caused by the increased angiogenesis observed in these tumors (Schiffenbauer et al. 1997). Administration of FSH and LH also increased tumor growth of xenografted OC109 spheroids (Schiffenbauer et al. 1997). Similar results were seen when minced BG-1 tumors were injected into nude mice; ovariectomy increased tumor growth and a single injection of E2 prevented this increase (Zimniski et al. 1989).

Gonadotropin releasing hormone (GnRH) agonists and antagonists have yielded mixed results. BG-1 xenograft growth was inhibited by the GnRH agonist leuprolide whereas a different agonist, Depot-Leupron, increased tumor growth in the transgenic LSL-K-ras^{G12D}/Pten$^{loxP/loxP}$ mouse by 71%, although large variation in tumor response prevented statistical significance (Zimniski et al. 1989, Romero et al. 2009). A GnRH antagonist inhibited growth of OV-1063 cells both *in vitro* and in xenografts (Yano et al. 1994a,b). In a DMBA-induced carcinogenesis rat model, the GnRH agonist buserelin suppressed LH, FSH, and P4 levels, leading to tumors with increased necrosis and decreased the number of tumor cells relative to tumors in control mice; however, buserelin did not alter tumor growth rate (Maruuchi et al. 1998). Stewart et al. (2004b) used a slightly different model to evaluate the effects of hormones on ovarian cancer initiation; DMBA-coated sutures embedded within the bursal membrane led to preneoplastic or neoplastic lesions in 43% of the rats within 12 months of surgery. Six cycles of superovulation with PMSG and hCG did not increase lesion incidence, but lesions appeared more advanced histologically (Stewart et al. 2004b). In a different rat carcinogenesis model using N-nitrosobis(2-oxopropyl) amine (BOP), the GnRH agonist D-Trp-LH-RH decreased tumor incidence and size, and eliminated metastasis (Pour et al. 1988). Chemically induced follicular loss, which resulted in high serum FSH and LH levels, altered tumor histology and modestly prolonged survival in the tgCAG-LS-TAg transgenic mouse model of ovarian cancer (Laviolette et al. 2011).

Several studies indicate that gonadotropins stimulate ovarian cancer progression, but the evidence remains mixed. It is still unclear what factors modulate the effects of gonadotropins on ovarian cancer, and whether gonadotropins act mainly through direct stimulation of OSE proliferation or indirectly by inducing ovulation and altering circulating hormone levels. There has been some suggestions that gonadotropins used to treat infertility may increase the risk of developing ovarian cancer, but the evidence so far has been inconsistent (reviewed in Vlahos et al. 2010). Because ovarian cancer has a relatively low incidence, few studies have sufficient power to evaluate whether fertility drugs are linked to ovarian cancer.

12.6 EFFECTS OF ANDROGENS ON OVARIAN CANCER

The hypothesis that androgens may play a role in developing cancer arises from studies showing that women who have taken testosterone supplements have an increased incidence of ovarian cancer (Olsen et al. 2008). However, conditions associated with high androgen levels such as polycystic ovarian syndrome (PCOS), acne, and hirsutism do not correlate with increased ovarian cancer risk, although women with PCOS have an increased risk of serous borderline tumors (Olsen et al. 1998). Isolated human OSE cells express androgen receptor, and a synthetic androgen increased proliferation in five out of nine of the isolated cultures (Edmondson et al. 2002).

In guinea pigs, exogenous testosterone induced epithelial ovarian cysts in all three animals treated (Silva et al. 1997), but there are otherwise few studies that have examined the potential effects of androgens on ovarian cancer *in vivo*. Xenograft studies have yielded conflicting results. Neither testosterone nor two anti-androgens altered tumor growth of BG-1 xenografts (Zimniski et al. 1989), whereas OVA-5 xenografts grew more rapidly with 5α-dihydrotestosterone treatment (Sawada et al. 1990). In syngeneic transplants of DMBA-induced tumors in rats, exogenous testosterone treatment slowed tumor growth and altered tumor histology (Lee et al. 1992). The explanation for these inconsistent results remains elusive; responses may vary depending on individual cell line characteristics and hormone dose. No studies have yet evaluated the effects of androgens on ovarian cancer arising in transgenic mouse models.

12.7 ENVIRONMENTAL RISK FACTORS FOR OVARIAN CANCER

There have been very few studies examining potential environmental risk factors for ovarian cancer (reviewed in Salehi et al. 2008). None of the animal models described previously have examined the effect of endocrine-disrupting chemicals on ovarian cancer initiation or progression. However, several animal studies have shown that environmental pollutants can induce putative preneoplastic lesions in the OSE, including hyperplasia and a shift from squamous to columnar cell morphology (Iatropoulos et al. 1976, Babineau et al. 1991, Sims et al. 1991, Borgeest et al. 2002).

Recently, there has been the suggestion that phytoestrogens may be protective against ovarian cancer, although the evidence is not yet conclusive. A meta-analysis in 2009 examining seven studies concluded that high soy intake was protective against ovarian cancer (Myung et al. 2009). In contrast, two recent studies found that dietary phytoestrogens did not impact ovarian cancer risk, although one study showed a near-significant decrease in risk with an odds ratio of 0.62 (Bandera et al. 2011, Hedelin et al. 2011). Glyceollin is a particularly interesting anti-estrogenic soy compound, which was able to suppress E2-stimulated growth of tumors developing from BG-1 cells in athymic mice (Salvo et al. 2006).

Exogenous hormones strongly influence the initiation and progression of ovarian cancer, and therefore endocrine-disrupting chemicals may also alter disease characteristics. Further research evaluating the actions of common pollutants in animal models of ovarian cancer is necessary in order to determine how they may influence human disease.

12.8 SUMMARY

Animal models have greatly improved our understanding of ovarian cancer biology. Processes that are difficult to evaluate in humans, such as hormone actions, can be modeled in other organisms. Because millions of women are exposed to hormones from various sources (e.g., menopausal hormone therapy; contraceptives; fertility treatments; endocrine-disrupting chemicals), it is critical to understand the effects of these hormones on the initiation and early progression of ovarian cancer. Menopausal hormone therapy increases the risk of developing ovarian cancer, but it is unclear how the hormones are promoting ovarian cancer. Oral contraceptives substantially decrease the risk of developing ovarian cancer, but the mechanisms of prevention are only partially understood (reviewed in Fraser and Kovacs 2003). Prevention of ovulation is likely to be a primary factor in decreasing the incidence of ovarian cancer, but it is still unclear whether other mechanisms are involved. The impact of fertility drugs on ovarian cancer incidence is still unclear; several studies have shown conflicting results (Vlahos et al. 2010).

Many of the most clinically relevant animal models have been developed in the past decade, and very few have been used to test the actions of hormones. It would be particularly interesting to test the effect of hormones on the model of high-grade serous cancer arising from the fallopian tube, as this may be the most accurate model for a large proportion of ovarian cancers (Kim et al. 2012). Because the majority of ovarian cancers are high-grade serous, and because ovarian cancer is relatively rare, it is difficult to perform epidemiological studies with sufficient power to examine the role of hormones on other histological subtypes. Due to the large molecular differences between the histological subtypes of ovarian cancer, the development of additional animal models accurately recapitulating all the histological subtypes of ovarian cancer is crucial. No animal models currently exist for mucinous cancers, and models of clear-cell carcinomas are limited to xenografts of certain cell lines (Shaw et al. 2004). Most of the transgenic mouse models of endometrioid and serous ovarian cancers have been generated with genetic alterations that do not accurately reflect the changes most commonly seen in the human disease. Despite these limitations, the current models can still be used to evaluate potential prevention strategies, biomarkers, risk factors, and treatments.

By increasing our understanding of the early events in epithelial ovarian cancer, it may be possible to reduce its incidence, accelerate diagnosis, and improve treatments, leading to an increase in survival for women diagnosed with this disease. The ovary is highly responsive to hormones, and it is frequently targeted either intentionally by pharmaceutical agents or unintentionally by exposure to endocrine-disrupting chemicals that are increasingly found in the environment. By using animal models to examine how hormones alter the initiation and progression of ovarian cancer, we may be able to develop strategies to mitigate the risk factors for this disease.

ACKNOWLEDGMENTS

The authors thank Dr. Laura Laviolette, Dr. Katherine Clark-Knowles, and Lisa Gamwell for the photographs used in the figures, and Dr. Ken Garson for his critical review of this manuscript. KH is supported by a scholarship from the Canadian Institutes of Health Research (CIHR) Strategic Training Program in Reproduction, Embryonic Development and its Impact on Health, and an Ovarian Cancer Canada Teal Heart Scholarship. The study of estrogen effects on ovarian cancer is supported by a CIHR grant to BCV.

REFERENCES

Adams, A.T. and Auersperg, N. 1981, Transformation of cultured rat ovarian surface epithelial cells by Kirsten murine sarcoma virus, *Cancer Research*, 41 (6), 2063–2072.

Armaiz-Pena, G.N., Mangala, L.S., Spannuth, W.A., Lin, Y.G., Jennings, N.B., Nick, A.M., Langley, R.R. et al. 2009, Estrous cycle modulates ovarian carcinoma growth, *Clinical Cancer Research: An Official Journal of the American Association for Cancer Research*, 15 (9), 2971–2978.

Auersperg, N. 2011, The origin of ovarian carcinomas: A unifying hypothesis, *International Journal of Gynecological Pathology: Official Journal of the International Society of Gynecological Pathologists*, 30 (1), 12–21.

Babineau, K.A., Singh, A., Jarrell, J.F., and Villeneuve, D.C. 1991, Surface epithelium of the ovary following oral administration of hexachlorobenzene to the monkey, *Journal of Submicroscopic Cytology and Pathology*, 23 (3), 457–464.

Bai, W., Oliveros-Saunders, B., Wang, Q., Acevedo-Duncan, M.E., and Nicosia, S.V. 2000, Estrogen stimulation of ovarian surface epithelial cell proliferation, *In Vitro Cellular & Developmental Biology. Animal*, 36 (10), 657–666.

Bandera, E.V., King, M., Chandran, U., Paddock, L.E., Rodriguez-Rodriguez, L., and Olson, S.H. 2011, Phytoestrogen consumption from foods and supplements and epithelial ovarian cancer risk: A population-based case control study, *BMC Women's Health*, 11, 40.

Bareither, M.L. and Verhage, H.G. 1981, Control of the secretory cell cycle in cat oviduct by estradiol and progesterone, *The American Journal of Anatomy*, 162 (2), 107–118.

Barnes, M.N., Berry, W.D., Straughn, J.M., Kirby, T.O., Leath, C.A., Huh, W.K., Grizzle, W.E., and Partridge, E.E. 2002, A pilot study of ovarian cancer chemoprevention using medroxyprogesterone acetate in an avian model of spontaneous ovarian carcinogenesis, *Gynecologic Oncology*, 87 (1), 57–63.

Borgeest, C., Symonds, D., Mayer, L.P., Hoyer, P.B., and Flaws, J.A. 2002, Methoxychlor may cause ovarian follicular atresia and proliferation of the ovarian epithelium in the mouse, *Toxicological Sciences: An Official Journal of the Society of Toxicology*, 68 (2), 473–478.

Burdette, J.E., Kurley, S.J., Kilen, S.M., Mayo, K.E., and Woodruff, T.K. 2006, Gonadotropin-induced superovulation drives ovarian surface epithelia proliferation in CD1 mice, *Endocrinology*, 147 (5), 2338–2345.

Carver, D.K., Barnes, H.J., Anderson, K.E., Petitte, J.N., Whitaker, R., Berchuck, A., and Rodriguez, G.C. 2011, Reduction of ovarian and oviductal cancers in calorie-restricted laying chickens, *Cancer Prevention Research (Philadelphia, Pa.)*, 4 (4), 562–567.

Cavalieri, E., Chakravarti, D., Guttenplan, J., Hart, E., Ingle, J., Jankowiak, R., Muti, P. et al. 2006, Catechol estrogen quinones as initiators of breast and other human cancers: Implications for biomarkers of susceptibility and cancer prevention, *Biochimica et Biophysica Acta*, 1766 (1), 63–78.

Chen, X., Aravindakshan, J., Yang, Y., and Sairam, M.R. 2007, Early alterations in ovarian surface epithelial cells and induction of ovarian epithelial tumors triggered by loss of FSH receptor, *Neoplasia (New York, N.Y.)*, 9 (6), 521–531.

Chodankar, R., Kwang, S., Sangiorgi, F., Hong, H., Yen, H.Y., Deng, C., Pike, M.C., Shuler, C.F., Maxson, R., and Dubeau, L. 2005, Cell-nonautonomous induction of ovarian and uterine serous cystadenomas in mice lacking a functional Brca1 in ovarian granulosa cells, *Current Biology: CB*, 15 (6), 561–565.

Connolly, D.C., Bao, R., Nikitin, A.Y., Stephens, K.C., Poole, T.W., Hua, X., Harris, S.S., Vanderhyden, B.C., and Hamilton, T.C. 2003, Female mice chimeric for expression of the simian virus 40 TAg under control of the MISIIR promoter develop epithelial ovarian cancer, *Cancer Research*, 63 (6), 1389–1397.

Cramer, D.W. 2012, The epidemiology of endometrial and ovarian cancer, *Hematology/Oncology Clinics of North America*, 26 (1), 1–12.

Cramer, D.W. and Welch, W.R. 1983, Determinants of ovarian cancer risk. II. Inferences regarding pathogenesis, *Journal of the National Cancer Institute*, 71 (4), 717–721.

Davies, B.R., Finnigan, D.S., Smith, S.K., and Ponder, B.A. 1999, Administration of gonadotropins stimulates proliferation of normal mouse ovarian surface epithelium, *Gynecological Endocrinology: The Official Journal of the International Society of Gynecological Endocrinology*, 13 (2), 75–81.

Davy, M., Mossige, J., and Johannessen, J. 1977, Heterologous growth of human ovarian cancer: A new in vivo testing system, *Acta Obstetricia et Gynecologica Scandinavica*, 56 (1), 55–59.

Dinulescu, D.M., Ince, T.A., Quade, B.J., Shafer, S.A., Crowley, D., and Jacks, T. 2005, Role of K-ras and Pten in the development of mouse models of endometriosis and endometrioid ovarian cancer, *Nature Medicine*, 11 (1), 63–70.

Edmondson, R.J., Monaghan, J.M., and Davies, B.R. 2002, The human ovarian surface epithelium is an androgen responsive tissue, *British Journal of Cancer*, 86 (6), 879–885.

Fathalla, M.F. 1971, Incessant ovulation—A factor in ovarian neoplasia? *Lancet*, 2 (7716), 163.

Fleming, J.S., Beaugie, C.R., Haviv, I., Chenevix-Trench, G., and Tan, O.L. 2006, Incessant ovulation, inflammation and epithelial ovarian carcinogenesis: Revisiting old hypotheses, *Molecular and Cellular Endocrinology*, 247 (1–2), 4–21.

Flesken-Nikitin, A., Choi, K.C., Eng, J.P., Shmidt, E.N., and Nikitin, A.Y. 2003, Induction of carcinogenesis by concurrent inactivation of p53 and Rb1 in the mouse ovarian surface epithelium, *Cancer Research*, 63 (13), 3459–3463.

Fogh, J., Fogh, J.M., and Orfeo, T. 1977, One hundred and twenty-seven cultured human tumor cell lines producing tumors in nude mice, *Journal of the National Cancer Institute*, 59 (1), 221–226.

Fraser, I.S. and Kovacs, G.T. 2003, The efficacy of non-contraceptive uses for hormonal contraceptives, *The Medical Journal of Australia*, 178 (12), 621–623.

Garson, K., Shaw, T.J., Clark, K.V., Yao, D.S., and Vanderhyden, B.C. 2005, Models of ovarian cancer—Are we there yet? *Molecular and Cellular Endocrinology*, 239 (1–2), 15–26.

Giles, J.R., Elkin, R.G., Trevino, L.S., Urick, M.E., Ramachandran, R., and Johnson, P.A. 2010, The restricted ovulator chicken: A unique animal model for investigating the etiology of ovarian cancer, *International Journal of Gynecological Cancer: Official Journal of the International Gynecological Cancer Society*, 20 (5), 738–744.

Godwin, A., Testa, J., Handel, L., Liu, Z., Vanderveer, L., Tracey, P., and Hamilton, T. 1992, Spontaneous transformation of rat ovarian surface epithelial cells: Association with cytogenetic changes and implications of repeated ovulation in the etiology of ovarian cancer, *Journal of the National Cancer Institute*, 84 (8), 592–601.

Gotfredson, G.S. and Murdoch, W.J. 2007, Morphologic responses of the mouse ovarian surface epithelium to ovulation and steroid hormonal milieu, *Experimental Biology and Medicine (Maywood, N.J.)*, 232 (2), 277–280.

Goyeneche, A.A., Caron, R.W., and Telleria, C.M. 2007, Mifepristone inhibits ovarian cancer cell growth in vitro and in vivo, *Clinical Cancer Research: An Official Journal of the American Association for Cancer Research*, 13 (11), 3370–3379.

Greiser, C.M., Greiser, E.M., and Doren, M. 2007, Menopausal hormone therapy and risk of ovarian cancer: Systematic review and meta-analysis, *Human Reproduction Update*, 13 (5), 453–463.

Hedelin, M., Lof, M., Andersson, T.M., Adlercreutz, H., and Weiderpass, E. 2011, Dietary phytoestrogens and the risk of ovarian cancer in the women's lifestyle and health cohort study, *Cancer Epidemiology, Biomarkers & Prevention: A Publication of the American Association for Cancer Research, Cosponsored by the American Society of Preventive Oncology*, 20 (2), 308–317.

Hong, H., Yen, H.Y., Brockmeyer, A., Liu, Y., Chodankar, R., Pike, M.C., Stanczyk, F.Z., Maxson, R., and Dubeau, L. 2010, Changes in the mouse estrus cycle in response to BRCA1 inactivation suggest a potential link between risk factors for familial and sporadic ovarian cancer, *Cancer Research*, 70 (1), 221–228.

Hunn, J. and Rodriguez, G.C. 2012, Ovarian cancer: Etiology, risk factors, and epidemiology, *Clinical Obstetrics and Gynecology*, 55 (1), 3–23.

Iatropoulos, M.J., Hobson, W., Knauf, V., and Adams, H.P. 1976, Morphological effects of hexachlorobenzene toxicity in female rhesus monkeys, *Toxicology and Applied Pharmacology*, 37 (3), 433–444.

Jansen, R.P. 1984, Endocrine response in the fallopian tube, *Endocrine Reviews*, 5 (4), 525–551.

Kamwanja, L.A. and Hansen, P.J. 1993, Regulation of proliferation of bovine oviductal epithelial cells by estradiol. Interactions with progesterone, interferon-tau and interferon-alpha, *Hormone and Metabolic Research = Hormon- und Stoffwechselforschung = Hor mones et metabolisme*, 25 (9), 500–502.

Kim, J., Coffey, D.M., Creighton, C.J., Yu, Z., Hawkins, S.M., and Matzuk, M.M. 2012, High-grade serous ovarian cancer arises from fallopian tube in a mouse model, *Proceedings of the National Academy of Sciences of the United States of America*, 109 (10), 3921–3926.

King, S.M., Hilliard, T.S., Wu, L.Y., Jaffe, R.C., Fazleabas, A.T., and Burdette, J.E. 2011, The impact of ovulation on fallopian tube epithelial cells: Evaluating three hypotheses connecting ovulation and serous ovarian cancer, *Endocrine-Related Cancer*, 18 (5), 627–642.

Korch, C., Spillman, M., Jackson, T., Jacobsen, B., Murphy, S., Lessey, B., Jordan, V., and Bradford, A. 2012, DNA profiling analysis of endometrial and ovarian cell lines reveals misidentification, redundancy and contamination, *Gynecologic Oncology*, 127 (1), 241–248.

Kurman, R.J. and Shih, I. 2010, The origin and pathogenesis of epithelial ovarian cancer: A proposed unifying theory, *The American Journal of Surgical Pathology*, 34 (3), 433–443.

Kuroda, H., Mandai, M., Konishi, I., Tsuruta, Y., Kusakari, T., Kariya, M., and Fujii, S. 2001, Human ovarian surface epithelial (OSE) cells express LH/hCG receptors, and hCG inhibits apoptosis of OSE cells via up-regulation of insulin-like growth factor-1, *International Journal of Cancer. Journal International du Cancer*, 91 (3), 309–315.

Langdon, S.P., Crew, A.J., Ritchie, A.A., Muir, M., Wakeling, A., Smyth, J.F., and Miller, W.R. 1994, Growth inhibition of oestrogen receptor-positive human ovarian carcinoma by anti-oestrogens in vitro and in a xenograft model, *European Journal of Cancer (Oxford, England: 1990)*, 30A (5), 682–686.

Laugier, C., Pageaux, J.F., Soto, A.M., and Sonnenschein, C. 1983, Mechanism of estrogen action: Indirect effect of estradiol-17 beta on proliferation of quail oviduct cells, *Proceedings of the National Academy of Sciences of the United States of America*, 80 (6), 1621–1625.

Laviolette, L.A., Ethier, J.F., Senterman, M.K., Devine, P.J., and Vanderhyden, B.C. 2011, Induction of a menopausal state alters the growth and histology of ovarian tumors in a mouse model of ovarian cancer, *Menopause (New York, N.Y.)*, 18 (5), 549–557.

Laviolette, L.A., Garson, K., Macdonald, E.A., Senterman, M.K., Courville, K., Crane, C.A., and Vanderhyden, B.C. 2010, 17beta-Estradiol accelerates tumor onset and decreases survival in a transgenic mouse model of ovarian cancer, *Endocrinology*, 151 (3), 929–938.

Lee, K.S., Sugiyama, T., Kataoka, A., Hirakawa, N., Maruuchi, T., Nishida, T., and Yakushiji, M. 1992, A study of the role of sex hormones in rat ovarian cancer, *The Kurume Medical Journal*, 39 (4), 285–290.

Lei, Z.M., Toth, P., Rao, C.V., and Pridham, D. 1993, Novel coexpression of human chorionic gonadotropin (hCG)/human luteinizing hormone receptors and their ligand hCG in human fallopian tubes, *The Journal of Clinical Endocrinology and Metabolism*, 77 (3), 863–872.

Levanon, K., Crum, C., and Drapkin, R. 2008, New insights into the pathogenesis of serous ovarian cancer and its clinical impact, *Journal of Clinical Oncology: Official Journal of the American Society of Clinical Oncology*, 26 (32), 5284–5293.

Li, J., Abushahin, N., Pang, S., Xiang, L., Chambers, S.K., Fadare, O., Kong, B., and Zheng, W. 2011, Tubal origin of 'ovarian' low-grade serous carcinoma, *Modern Pathology: An Official Journal of the United States and Canadian Academy of Pathology, Inc*, 24 (11), 1488–1499.

Li, J., Fadare, O., Xiang, L., Kong, B., and Zheng, W. 2012, Ovarian serous carcinoma: Recent concepts on its origin and carcinogenesis, *Journal of Hematology & Oncology*, 5, 8.

Liu, J., Yang, G., Thompson-Lanza, J.A., Glassman, A., Hayes, K., Patterson, A., Marquez, R.T. et al. 2004, A genetically defined model for human ovarian cancer, *Cancer Research*, 64 (5), 1655–1663.

Maruuchi, T., Sugiyama, T., Kataoka, A., Nishida, T., and Yakushiji, M. 1998, Effects of a gonadotropin-releasing hormone agonist on rat ovarian adenocarcinoma cell lines in vitro and in vivo, *Japanese Journal of Cancer Research: Gann*, 89 (9), 977–983.

McDonnel, A.C., Van Kirk, E.A., Isaak, D.D., and Murdoch, W.J. 2005, Effects of progesterone on ovarian tumorigenesis in xenografted mice, *Cancer Letters*, 221 (1), 49–53.

Medeiros, F., Muto, M.G., Lee, Y., Elvin, J.A., Callahan, M.J., Feltmate, C., Garber, J.E., Cramer, D.W., and Crum, C.P. 2006, The tubal fimbria is a preferred site for early adenocarcinoma in women with familial ovarian cancer syndrome, *The American Journal of Surgical Pathology*, 30 (2), 230–236.

Mullany, L.K. and Richards, J.S. 2012, Minireview: Animal models and mechanisms of ovarian cancer development, *Endocrinology*, 153 (4), 1585–1592.

Murdoch, W.J., Van Kirk, E.A., Isaak, D.D., and Shen, Y. 2008, Progesterone facilitates cisplatin toxicity in epithelial ovarian cancer cells and xenografts, *Gynecologic Oncology*, 110 (2), 251–255.

Myung, S.K., Ju, W., Choi, H.J., Kim, S.C., and Korean Meta-Analysis (KORMA) Study Group 2009, Soy intake and risk of endocrine-related gynaecological cancer: A meta-analysis, *BJOG: An International Journal of Obstetrics and Gynaecology*, 116 (13), 1697–1705.

Oka, T. and Schimke, R.T. 1969, Interaction of estrogen and progesterone in chick oviduct development. I. Antagonistic effect of progesterone on estrogen-induced proliferation and differentiation of tubular gland cells, *The Journal of Cell Biology*, 41 (3), 816–831.

Okada, A., Ohta, Y., Brody, S.L., Watanabe, H., Krust, A., Chambon, P., and Iguchi, T. 2004, Role of foxj1 and estrogen receptor alpha in ciliated epithelial cell differentiation of the neonatal oviduct, *Journal of Molecular Endocrinology*, 32 (3), 615–625.

Olsen, C.M., Green, A.C., Nagle, C.M., Jordan, S.J., Whiteman, D.C., Bain, C.J., Webb, P.M., and Australian Cancer Study Group (Ovarian Cancer) and the Australian Ovarian Cancer Study Group 2008, Epithelial ovarian cancer: Testing the 'androgens hypothesis', *Endocrine-Related Cancer*, 15 (4), 1061–1068.

Orsulic, S., Li, Y., Soslow, R.A., Vitale-Cross, L.A., Gutkind, J.S., and Varmus, H.E. 2002, Induction of ovarian cancer by defined multiple genetic changes in a mouse model system, *Cancer Cell*, 1 (1), 53–62.

Osterholzer, H.O., Johnson, J.H., and Nicosia, S.V. 1985a, An autoradiographic study of rabbit ovarian surface epithelium before and after ovulation, *Biology of Reproduction*, 33 (3), 729–738.

Osterholzer, H.O., Streibel, E.J., and Nicosia, S.V. 1985b, Growth effects of protein hormones on cultured rabbit ovarian surface epithelial cells, *Biology of Reproduction*, 33 (1), 247–258.

Pearce, C.L., Chung, K., Pike, M.C., and Wu, A.H. 2009, Increased ovarian cancer risk associated with menopausal estrogen therapy is reduced by adding a progestin, *Cancer*, 115 (3), 531–539.

Perche, O., Laine, M.C., Pageaux, J.F., Laugier, C., and Sandoz, D. 1989, Modification of cell evagination and cell differentiation in quail oviduct hyperstimulated by progesterone, *Biology of the Cell/Under the Auspices of the European Cell Biology Organization*, 67 (2), 123–134.

Perniconi, S.E., Simoes Mde, J., Simoes Rdos, S., Haidar, M.A., Baracat, E.C., and Soares, J.M. Jr. 2008, Proliferation of the superficial epithelium of ovaries in senile female rats following oral administration of conjugated equine estrogens, *Clinics (Sao Paulo, Brazil)*, 63 (3), 381–388.

Piek, J., van Diest, P., Zweemer, R., Jansen, J., Poort-Keesom, R., Menko, F., Gille, J. et al. 2001, Dysplastic changes in prophylactically removed Fallopian tubes of women predisposed to developing ovarian cancer, *The Journal of Pathology*, 195 (4), 451–456.

Pipas, J.M. 2009, SV40: Cell transformation and tumorigenesis, *Virology*, 384 (2), 294–303.

Pour, P.M., Redding, T.W., Paz-Bouza, J.I., and Schally, A.V. 1988, Treatment of experimental ovarian carcinoma with monthly injection of the agonist D-Trp-6-LH-RH: A preliminary report, *Cancer Letters*, 41 (1), 105–110.

Quinn, B.A., Xiao, F., Bickel, L., Martin, L., Hua, X., Klein-Szanto, A., and Connolly, D.C. 2010, Development of a syngeneic mouse model of epithelial ovarian cancer, *Journal of Ovarian Research*, 3, 24.

Roberts, P.C., Mottillo, E.P., Baxa, A.C., Heng, H.H., Doyon-Reale, N., Gregoire, L., Lancaster, W.D., Rabah, R., and Schmelz, E.M. 2005, Sequential molecular and cellular events during neoplastic progression: A mouse syngeneic ovarian cancer model, *Neoplasia (New York, N.Y.)*, 7 (10), 944–956.

Roby, K.F., Taylor, C.C., Sweetwood, J.P., Cheng, Y., Pace, J.L., Tawfik, O., Persons, D.L., Smith, P.G., and Terranova, P.F. 2000, Development of a syngeneic mouse model for events related to ovarian cancer, *Carcinogenesis*, 21 (4), 585–591.

Rodriguez, G.C., Walmer, D.K., Cline, M., Krigman, H., Lessey, B.A., Whitaker, R.S., Dodge, R., and Hughes, C.L. 1998, Effect of progestin on the ovarian epithelium of macaques: Cancer prevention through apoptosis? *Journal of the Society for Gynecologic Investigation*, 5 (5), 271–276.

Romero, I. and Bast, R.C. Jr. 2012, Minireview: Human ovarian cancer: Biology, current management, and paths to personalizing therapy, *Endocrinology*, 153 (4), 1593–1602.

Romero, I.L., Gordon, I.O., Jagadeeswaran, S., Mui, K.L., Lee, W.S., Dinulescu, D.M., Krausz, T.N., Kim, H.H., Gilliam, M.L., and Lengyel, E. 2009, Effects of oral contraceptives or a gonadotropin-releasing hormone agonist on ovarian carcinogenesis in genetically engineered mice, *Cancer Prevention Research (Philadelphia, Pa.)*, 2 (9), 792–799.

Rosen, D.G., Yang, G., Liu, G., Mercado-Uribe, I., Chang, B., Xiao, X.S., Zheng, J., Xue, F.X., and Liu, J. 2009, Ovarian cancer: Pathology, biology, and disease models, *Frontiers in Bioscience: A Journal and Virtual Library*, 14, 2089–2102.

Salehi, F., Dunfield, L., Phillips, K.P., Krewski, D., and Vanderhyden, B.C. 2008, Risk factors for ovarian cancer: An overview with emphasis on hormonal factors, *Journal of Toxicology and Environmental Health. Part B, Critical Reviews*, 11 (3–4), 301–321.

Salvo, V.A., Boue, S.M., Fonseca, J.P., Elliott, S., Corbitt, C., Collins-Burow, B.M., Curiel, T.J. et al. 2006, Antiestrogenic glyceollins suppress human breast and ovarian carcinoma tumorigenesis, *Clinical Cancer Research: An Official Journal of the American Association for Cancer Research*, 12 (23), 7159–7164.

Sawada, M., Terada, N., Wada, A., Mori, Y., Yamasaki, M., Saga, T., and Endo, K. 1990, Estrogen- and androgen-responsive growth of human ovarian adenocarcinoma heterotransplanted into nude mice, *International Journal of Cancer. Journal International du Cancer*, 45 (2), 359–363.

Schiffenbauer, Y.S., Abramovitch, R., Meir, G., Nevo, N., Holzinger, M., Itin, A., Keshet, E., and Neeman, M. 1997, Loss of ovarian function promotes angiogenesis in human ovarian carcinoma, *Proceedings of the National Academy of Sciences of the United States of America*, 94 (24), 13203–13208.

Scully, R.E. 1977, Ovarian tumors. A review, *The American Journal of Pathology*, 87 (3), 686–720.

Seidman, J., Yemelyanova, A., Zaino, R., and Kurman, R. 2011, The fallopian tube-peritoneal junction: A potential site of carcinogenesis, *International Journal of Gynecological Pathology*, 30 (1), 4–11.

Shan, W. and Liu, J. 2009, Epithelial ovarian cancer: Focus on genetics and animal models, *Cell Cycle (Georgetown, Tex.)*, 8 (5), 731–735.

Sharrow, A.C., Ronnett, B.M., Thoburn, C.J., Barber, J.P., Giuntoli, R.L. II, Armstrong, D.K., Jones, R.J., and Hess, A.D. 2010, Identification and characterization of a spontaneous ovarian carcinoma in Lewis rats, *Journal of Ovarian Research*, 3, 9.

Shaw, T.J., Senterman, M.K., Dawson, K., Crane, C.A., and Vanderhyden, B.C. 2004, Characterization of intraperitoneal, orthotopic, and metastatic xenograft models of human ovarian cancer, *Molecular Therapy: The Journal of the American Society of Gene Therapy*, 10 (6), 1032–1042.

Silva, E.G., Tornos, C., Deavers, M., Kaisman, K., Gray, K., and Gershenson, D. 1998, Induction of epithelial neoplasms in the ovaries of guinea pigs by estrogenic stimulation, *Gynecologic Oncology*, 71 (2), 240–246.

Silva, E.G., Tornos, C., Fritsche, H.A. Jr., el-Naggar, A., Gray, K., Ordonez, N.G., Luna, M., and Gershenson, D. 1997, The induction of benign epithelial neoplasms of the ovaries of guinea pigs by testosterone stimulation: A potential animal model, *Modern Pathology: An Official Journal of the United States and Canadian Academy of Pathology, Inc*, 10 (9), 879–883.

Sims, D.E., Singh, A., Donald, A., Jarrell, J., and Villeneuve, D.C. 1991, Alteration of primate ovary surface epithelium by exposure to hexachlorobenzene: A quantitative study, *Histology and Histopathology*, 6 (4), 525–529.

Spillman, M.A., Manning, N.G., Dye, W.W., Sartorius, C.A., Post, M.D., Harrell, J.C., Jacobsen, B.M., and Horwitz, K.B. 2010, Tissue-specific pathways for estrogen regulation of ovarian cancer growth and metastasis, *Cancer Research*, 70 (21), 8927–8936.

Stewart, S.L., Querec, T.D., Gruver, B.N., O'Hare, B., Babb, J.S., and Patriotis, C. 2004a, Gonadotropin and steroid hormones stimulate proliferation of the rat ovarian surface epithelium, *Journal of Cellular Physiology*, 198 (1), 119–124.

Stewart, S.L., Querec, T.D., Ochman, A.R., Gruver, B.N., Bao, R., Babb, J.S., Wong, T.S. et al. 2004b, Characterization of a carcinogenesis rat model of ovarian preneoplasia and neoplasia, *Cancer Research*, 64 (22), 8177–8183.

Syed, V., Ulinski, G., Mok, S.C., Yiu, G.K., and Ho, S.M. 2001, Expression of gonadotropin receptor and growth responses to key reproductive hormones in normal and malignant human ovarian surface epithelial cells, *Cancer Research*, 61 (18), 6768–6776.

Takeuchi, K., Maruyama, I., Yamamoto, S., Oki, T., and Nagata, Y. 1991, Isolation and monolayer culture of human fallopian tube epithelial cells, *In Vitro Cellular & Developmental Biology: Journal of the Tissue Culture Association*, 27A (9), 720–724.

Tanwar, P.S., Zhang, L., Kaneko-Tarui, T., Curley, M.D., Taketo, M.M., Rani, P., Roberts, D.J., and Teixeira, J.M. 2011, Mammalian target of rapamycin is a therapeutic target for murine ovarian endometrioid adenocarcinomas with dysregulated Wnt/beta-catenin and PTEN, *PloS One*, 6 (6), e20715.

Tok, E.C., Ertunc, D., Tataroglu, C., Yazici, G., Kanat, H., and Dilek, S. 2006, Clinicopathologic study of the putative precursor lesions of epithelial ovarian cancer in low-risk women, *International Journal of Gynecological Cancer: Official Journal of the International Gynecological Cancer Society*, 16 (2), 501–506.

Trevino, L.S., Buckles, E.L., and Johnson, P.A. 2012, Oral contraceptives decrease the prevalence of ovarian cancer in the hen, *Cancer Prevention Research (Philadelphia, Pa.)*, 5 (2), 343–349.

Vanderhyden, B.C., Shaw, T.J., and Ethier, J.F. 2003, Animal models of ovarian cancer, *Reproductive Biology and Endocrinology: RB&E*, 1, 67.

Vanderhyden, B.C. 2005, Loss of ovarian function and the risk of ovarian cancer. *Cell and Tissue Research,* 322(1), 117–124.

Vaughan, S., Coward, J.I., Bast, R.C. Jr., Berchuck, A., Berek, J.S., Brenton, J.D., Coukos, G. et al. 2011, Rethinking ovarian cancer: Recommendations for improving outcomes, *Nature Reviews. Cancer*, 11 (10), 719–725.

Verhage, H.G., Mavrogianis, P.A., Boice, M.L., Li, W., and Fazleabas, A.T. 1990, Oviductal epithelium of the baboon: Hormonal control and the immuno-gold localization of oviduct-specific glycoproteins, *The American Journal of Anatomy*, 187 (1), 81–90.

Vlahos, N.F., Economopoulos, K.P., and Creatsas, G. 2010, Fertility drugs and ovarian cancer risk: A critical review of the literature, *Annals of the New York Academy of Sciences*, 1205, 214–219.

Wollenhaupt, K., Tomek, W., Brussow, K.P., Tiemann, U., Viergutz, T., Schneider, F., and Nurnberg, G. 2002, Effects of ovarian steroids and epidermal growth factor (EGF) on expression and bioactivation of specific regulators of transcription and translation in oviductal tissue in pigs, *Reproduction (Cambridge, England)*, 123 (1), 87–96.

Wright, J.W., Jurevic, L., and Stouffer, R.L. 2011, Dynamics of the primate ovarian surface epithelium during the ovulatory menstrual cycle, *Human Reproduction (Oxford, England)*, 26 (6), 1408–1421.

Wright, J.W., Toth-Fejel, S., Stouffer, R.L., and Rodland, K.D. 2002, Proliferation of rhesus ovarian surface epithelial cells in culture: Lack of mitogenic response to steroid or gonadotropic hormones, *Endocrinology*, 143 (6), 2198–2207.

Wu, R., Hendrix-Lucas, N., Kuick, R., Zhai, Y., Schwartz, D.R., Akyol, A., Hanash, S. et al. 2007, Mouse model of human ovarian endometrioid adenocarcinoma based on somatic defects in the Wnt/beta-catenin and PI3K/Pten signaling pathways, *Cancer Cell*, 11 (4), 321–333.

Wu, C.H., Mastroianni, L. Jr., and Mikhail, G. 1977, Steroid hormones in monkey oviductal fluid, *Fertility and Sterility*, 28 (11), 1250–1256.

Yang, D.H., Fazili, Z., Smith, E.R., Cai, K.Q., Klein-Szanto, A., Cohen, C., Horowitz, I.R., and Xu, X.X. 2006, Disabled-2 heterozygous mice are predisposed to endometrial and ovarian tumorigenesis and exhibit sex-biased embryonic lethality in a p53-null background, *The American Journal of Pathology*, 169 (1), 258–267.

Yano, T., Pinski, J., Halmos, G., Szepeshazi, K., Groot, K., and Schally, A.V. 1994a, Inhibition of growth of OV-1063 human epithelial ovarian cancer xenografts in nude mice by treatment with luteinizing hormone-releasing hormone antagonist SB-75, *Proceedings of the National Academy of Sciences of the United States of America*, 91 (15), 7090–7094.

Yano, T., Pinski, J., Radulovic, S., and Schally, A.V. 1994b, Inhibition of human epithelial ovarian cancer cell growth in vitro by agonistic and antagonistic analogues of luteinizing hormone-releasing hormone, *Proceedings of the National Academy of Sciences of the United States of America*, 91 (5), 1701–1705.

Zheng, W., Magid, M.S., Kramer, E.E., and Chen, Y.T. 1996, Follicle-stimulating hormone receptor is expressed in human ovarian surface epithelium and fallopian tube, *The American Journal of Pathology*, 148 (1), 47–53.

Zhuge, Y., Lagman, J.A., Ansenberger, K., Mahon, C.J., Daikoku, T., Dey, S.K., Bahr, J.M., and Hales, D.B. 2009, CYP1B1 expression in ovarian cancer in the laying hen Gallusdomesticus, *Gynecologic Oncology*, 112 (1), 171–178.

Zimniski, S.J., Garola, R.E., Fendl, K., and Peterson, C.M. 1989, Endocrine characterization of a human ovarian carcinoma (BG-1) established in nude mice, *Steroids*, 54 (6), 593–606.

13 New Perspectives in Chemoresistant Ovarian Cancer

*Ahmed Y. Ali, Lee Farrand,
Ji Young Kim, Akechai Im-Aram,
Sanguine Byun, Elaine Lai-Han Leung,
Hyong Joo Lee, and Benjamin K. Tsang*

CONTENTS

13.1 INTRODUCTION

Ovarian cancer (OVCA) is the most lethal of all gynecological malignancies and the fifth most frequent cause of cancer-related death in women. It ranks second among all gynecological cancers in the number of new cases and the first in the number of deaths each year.[1] One of the major obstacles in OVCA treatment has been the failure to detect the disease at early stages due to lack of presentable symptoms until the tumors are too advanced to be contained by available therapeutic options. Even in the absence of metastasis, late detection presents two complications: a need for more complex surgical debulking with higher probability of residual tumor cells, which exhibit greater heterogeneity. Due to the existence of cancer stem cells and higher mutational frequencies in heterogeneous subpopulations, late-stage cancers often contain tumor cells that do not respond to chemotherapeutic challenge.[2]

Systemic administration of current chemotherapeutics for OVCA and the high dosages required to penetrate the tumor tissue often results in nonspecific toxicity. The side effects range from moderate (alopecia, nausea, and erythema) to severe (neuropathy, nephrotoxicity, ototoxicity, myelotoxicity, hemolytic anemia, and compromised immunity leading to higher rates of infections). Despite the use of combination chemotherapy (e.g., cisplatin, taxol, and their derivatives) at low dosages, adverse side effects remain a concern. These therapeutic issues are further complicated by the fact that higher dosages of chemotherapeutic agents are often used to overcome chemoresistance.

For the past 30 years, despite considerable resources that have been invested to combat cancer, significant reductions in the incidence and deaths have not been evident. The discovery of molecular pathways involved in the control of tumorigenesis and chemoresistance has offered potential targets for the identification of biomarkers and therapeutic intervention with minimal adverse side effects. An emerging concept in the treatment of cancer is the use of natural compounds found in food products. Recent evidence indicates that functional food compounds (molecules extracted from food products) have been shown to have cancer chemopreventive capabilities as well as anticarcinogenic effects. Due to the toxic nature of available chemotherapeutics, the use of functional food compounds may prevent tumor development in high-risk individuals and sensitization of tumors to conventional chemotherapy.

In the current chapter, we have focused our discussion on the recent advances in the understanding of the molecular signaling pathways frequently dysregulated

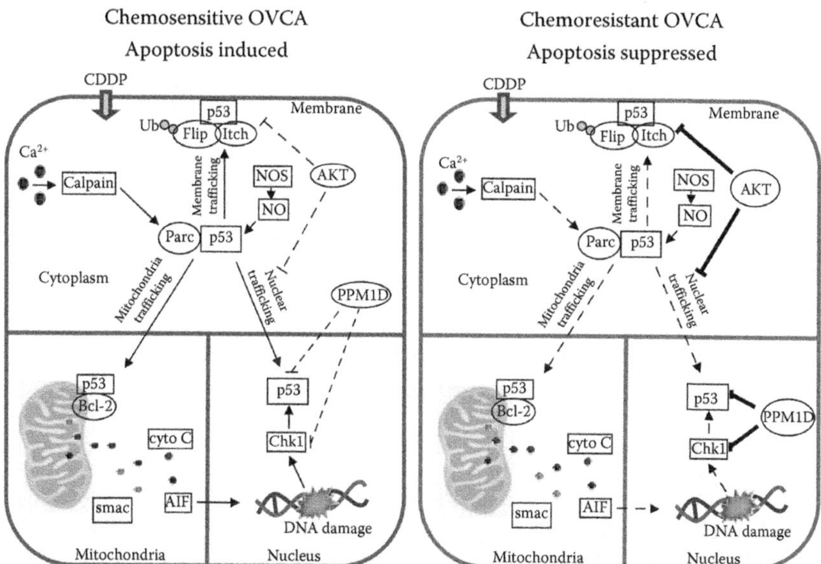

FIGURE 13.1 A hypothetical model illustrating the differences in subcellular interactions and functions of p53, PPM1D, FLIP, Akt, and NO in the regulation of apoptosis in chemosensitive and chemoresistant OVCA cells in response to CDDP treatment. p53 is pro-apoptotic following CDDP treatment, whereas Akt, PARC, FLIP, and PPM1D are anti-apoptotic and regulate chemosensitivity of OVCA through interactions at the plasma membrane, cytoplasm, mitochondria, and nucleus. In chemosensitive cells and in response to CDDP, p53 induces apoptosis by facilitating (i) gene transcription at the nucleus; (ii) FLIP ubiquitination and degradation at the plasma membrane; and (iii) mitochondrial cytochrome c and AIF release; p53 availability and activation results from calpain-mediated PARC degradation and PPM1D downregulation and cytoplasmic retention. The expression and stability of p53 are regulated by nitric oxide (NO), produced by nitric oxide synthases (NOSs) in response to CDDP. Low level of Akt has minimal influence on these processes in chemosensitive cells. In contrast, in chemoresistant cells where Akt activity and/or content are high, Akt suppresses p53 activation and the above processes.

in chemoresistant OVCA, particularly in relation to the p53 tumor suppressor, the nitric oxide/cyclic GMP, and the PI3K/Akt/mTOR pathway as potential molecular determinants of chemosensitivity. In addition, we have reviewed the latest discoveries in the field of functional food compounds for possible use in chemoprevention and adjuvant chemotherapy (Figure 13.1).

13.1.1 Ovarian Cancer and Chemoresistance

Cisplatin (CDDP) and its derivatives are the first-line chemotherapeutic agents in the treatment of OVCA. CDDP induces apoptosis through irreversible intercalation of DNA strands by creating inter- and intrastrand DNA adducts, thereby activating the DNA damage response and the subsequent induction of apoptosis. Most patients are initially responsive to chemotherapy; however, the development of drug resistance is a major obstacle to successful treatment. Recurrence of ovarian tumors is quite common and is characterized by highly aggressive tumors, which disseminate to secondary target tissues (omentum, liver, bladder, spleen, gastrointestinal tract, etc.) and acquire resistance to conventional chemotherapeutics. CDDP resistance is a multifactorial event in OVCA cells and may result from enhanced DNA damage repair, increased drug clearance, detoxification, altered drug metabolism, and finally loss of apoptotic capacity due to acquired genetic mutations.[3] However, the mechanisms of CDDP resistance in human OVCA remain obscure and warrant extensive investigation.

13.2 INVOLVEMENT OF P53 FAMILY MEMBERS IN CHEMORESISTANCE IN OVARIAN CANCER

13.2.1 p53 Pathway

The tumor suppressor p53 is a transcription factor, which plays an important role within the cell as a guardian of genomic integrity. We have shown that CDDP induces p53 activation through specific phosphorylation of serine residues 15 and 20,[4] which stabilizes it by suppressing its binding to the E3 ubiquitin ligase minute double murine 2 (MDM2) and its subsequent ubiquitination and degradation through a proteasomal-dependent mechanism.[5] We have also demonstrated through site-directed mutagenesis studies that p53 phosphorylation on those two serine residues effectively enhances the pro-apoptotic properties of p53.[4,6] Moreover, p53 phosphorylation results in its activation as a transcription factor, leading to the transcription of several genes whose protein products such as p21, are anti-proliferative, and ultimately cause cell cycle arrest.[6]

p53 is involved in the regulation of cellular proliferation and apoptosis by controlling numerous molecular pathways. p53 elicits its actions through both transcription-dependent and -independent mechanisms.[7,8] We have previously shown that a functional p53 signaling pathway is necessary in the chemosensitization of OVCA cells to DNA-damaging agents, such as CDDP.[7–10] In response to genomic insults, p53 is activated by the DNA damage sensors ataxia talengiectasia mutated (ATM) protein and its related family member ataxia talengiectasia and Rad3-related (ATR) protein and their respective effectors, checkpoint kinases 1 and 2 (Chk1 and Chk2). In turn, p53 sustains cell cycle arrest at the G_1 and the G_2/M phases by enhancing the expression of the cyclin-dependent kinase inhibitor p21 and 14-3-3σ, which sequesters CDC25C phosphatase in the cytoplasm.[6,11,12] Moreover, p53 induces the release of mitochondrial death proteins through the expression of several pro-apoptotic proteins, which act on the mitochondria. These include Bcl-2 family members Bax and Bid,[13,14] p53 upregulated modulator of apoptosis (PUMA),[15,16] apoptotic peptidase activating factor 1 (Apaf-1),[17] and NADPH oxidase activator (NOXA).[16] p53 also upregulates the expression of the death receptors Fas, DR4, and DR5.[18–20] We have demonstrated that p53 facilitates the ubiquitination and proteasomal degradation of the anti-apoptotic Fas-associated death domain-like interleukin-1b-converting enzyme (FLICE)-like inhibitory protein (FLIP) by promoting its interaction with the E3 ubiquitin ligase Itch.[21] These few examples of p53-regulated genes belong to a growing list that emphasizes the multifunctional role of the p53 network in tumor suppression. Mutations and/or functional inactivation of p53 are frequent events in many human malignancies, including OVCA.

13.2.2 Role of p73

Another member of the p53 family, p73, has been implicated in the transduction of drug-induced DNA damage signals to the cell fate machinery. p73 shares similar structure to p53 in containing a transactivation domain (TAD) located in the amino terminal, a DNA-binding domain (DBD), and an oligomerization domain (OD) located in the carboxy terminal. The p73 gene (*TP73*) contains two distinct promoters located in noncoding regions (promoter 1 in exon 1 and promoter 2 in intron 3). Transcription of *TP73* from promoter 1 produces several full-length functional isoforms with different carboxy terminals, which contain all three domains necessary for p73 function and are aptly termed TA isoforms (α–η). On the other hand, the use of promoter 2 produces shorter, nonfunctional isoforms lacking the important amino terminal TAD that are largely considered to function in a dominant-negative manner through competitive promoter binding of TAp73-regulated genes and/or inhibition of hetero-oligomerization and activation of TAp73 isoforms. These isoforms are termed ΔNp73α–η.[22,23] *TP73* gene is located in a region (1q36) frequently altered in human malignancies.[24] and the general trend of *TP73* alterations is either methylation of promoter 1 to inhibit the expression of functional p73 isoforms or the overexpression of the dominant-negative ΔN isoforms.[25]

TAp73 has been shown to control the expression of target genes similar to p53 such as p21, PUMA, NOXA, Bax, and BAD, suggesting its involvement in the apoptotic response. However, TAp73 also regulates different genes and shows distinct p53-independent functions.[22] We have recently shown that the overexpression of TAp73α enhanced the sensitivity of chemosensitive OVCA cell lines and sensitized several chemoresistant cell lines to drug-induced apoptosis. Moreover, siRNA-mediated downregulation of p73α significantly decreased CDDP sensitivity in a chemosensitive OVCA cell line.[26] While TAp73 possesses pro-apoptotic properties, the ΔN variants antagonize its action and inhibit its activity. ΔNp73 variants have been shown to be overexpressed in 95 of 100 specimens in a panel of ovarian tumors.[25] ΔNp73 also has the ability to inhibit p53 activity in a dominant-negative manner.

p73 can be partially processed through ubiquitin-mediated proteasomal degradation. The E3 ubiquitin ligase Itch has been established as a regulator of p73 stability.[24] Furthermore, we have demonstrated that p73 stability can be affected by drug-induced changes in intracellular calcium concentration. Calpains, a family of calcium-dependent proteases, were shown to target p73 for proteolytic cleavage *in vitro*. Moreover, p73 contains several consensus calpain cleavage sites at both the amino and the carboxy terminals.[26] We have demonstrated that CDDP treatment in chemosensitive OVCA cells caused a significant increase in intracellular calcium concentration. This response is due to calcium release from intracellular stores, which lead to calpain activation, and subsequent p73α proteolytic cleavage and downregulation. However, those responses were not observed in chemoresistant cells treated with CDDP.[26]

13.3 SUBCELLULAR ACTIONS OF P53

13.3.1 Regulation of Nuclear p53 Activity: Inactivation by PPM1D

Protein phosphatase magnesium/manganese-dependent 1D (PPM1D), also known as protein phosphatase type 2C delta (PP2Cδ) and wild-type p53 inducible phosphatase 1 (Wip1), was first identified as a transcriptional target of p53 in response to ionizing and ultraviolet irradiation. It is a type 2C serine/threonine phosphatase belonging to the magnesium/manganese-dependent subfamily of PPM1 phosphatases. It has been recently identified as a p53-induced phosphatase, preferentially targeting phosphoserine and phosphothreonine residues in the SQ/TQ motifs and phosphothreonine residues in the TXY motifs.[27–32] It dephosphorylates both phospho-p53 (Ser^{15})[33] and phospho-Chk1 (Ser^{345}), significantly reducing their activities.[34–36] It has been demonstrated that p38 mitogen-activated protein kinase (p38 MAPK), which activates p53 during genotoxic stress, is dephosphorylated by PPM1D, thereby, negatively regulating the activation of p53.[37,38] Recent studies have shown that PPM1D also interacts with several proteins involved in numerous cellular processes: MDM2 and MDMX in the DNA damage response[39,40]; UNG2 in base excision repair[28]; and NF-κB in the inflammatory response.[41] PPM1D is also regulated by several transcription factors, including E2F1,[42] cyclic AMP response element binding protein (CREB),[43] estrogen receptor α (ERα),[44] c-Jun,[45] and NF-κB.[41]

PPM1D has two functional isoforms. While full-length PPM1D (PPM1D605) is ubiquitously expressed, the shorter PPM1D isoform (PPM1D430) is exclusively expressed in testes where it is involved in spermatogenesis, and leukocytes where it plays an important role in lymphocyte maturation.[46] The two isoforms share a common target profile of proteins destined for dephosphorylation as they both retain phosphatase activity. PPM1D605 contains two putative nuclear localization signal (NLS) domains and is believed to be a strictly nuclear phosphatase, while PPM1D430 contains only one NLS and shows both nuclear and cytoplasmic localizations. However, we have found that PPM1D605 localization is differentially regulated between CDDP-sensitive and resistant OVCA cells, with PPM1D605 displaying cytoplasmic localization and nuclear exclusion in sensitive cells, and significant nuclear localization in resistant cells in response to CDDP (unpublished data).

Following a genomic insult, PPM1D functions in restoring homeostasis to the cells by inducing cell cycle arrest at the G_2/M phase in collaboration with p53, thus allowing a sufficient amount of time for the repair of the DNA damage.[47–50] However, high PPM1D activity due to either amplification and/or enhanced stability sustains the inhibition of proteins involved in the DNA damage response. Numerous human malignancies, including OVCA, exhibit PPM1D overexpression, and its level is directly related to reduced responsiveness to therapy and poor overall prognosis.[37,38,51–59] The primary oncogenic function of PPM1D is the modulation of apoptotic and DNA damage responses following a genomic insult. This is achieved by the regulation of the p53 and ATM/ATR pathways. PPM1D expression is induced by p53 in response to DNA damage and it negatively regulates the pro-apoptotic activity of p53 by dephosphorylating it at Ser^{15}, an essential residue for p53 stabilization and subsequent activation. We have observed that PPMID is important in the regulation of p53 activation and chemosensitivity in OVCA cells (Figure 13.2). Furthermore, we have demonstrated that PPM1D silencing enhances p53 activation through increasing Ser[15] phosphorylation (Figure 13.2a through c), leading to the sensitization of resistant OVCA cells to CDDP-induced apoptosis, while the overexpression of PPM1D in sensitive OVCA cells decreased phospho-Ser[15]-p53 content and significantly reduced CDDP sensitivity (Figure 13.2d).[10] However, the role of PPM1D in the modulation of p53 activity goes beyond direct regulation. PPM1D can also regulate p53 activation and stability indirectly by modulation of the function of known regulators of p53 activation and stabilization such as ATM,[60,61] Chk1,[10,36,62] and Chk2,[63–66] as well as MDM2[33] and MDMX.[40,67] Furthermore, PPM1D inhibits p38 MAPK and attenuates the expression of its downstream effectors p16[Ink4a] and p19[ARF], which are important tumor suppressors and regulators of p53 activity.[29,68,69] It attenuates both base excision repair by dephosphorylating uracil DNA glycosylase (UNG2),[28,32] and nucleoside excision repair by dephosphorylating excision repair proteins xeroderma pigmentosum complementation group A (XPA) and complementation group C (XPC).[70,71] Thus, PPM1D attenuates apoptosis, cell cycle checkpoints, and ultimately DNA repair. By these means, PPM1D enhances oncogenic transformation and tumor growth.

13.3.2 p53 Function at the Plasma Membrane: Interaction with FLIP and Itch

Although p53 and FLIP are major determinants of CDDP sensitivity in OVCA,[3,72] the complex mechanism of interplay between p53 and FLIP in the control of apoptosis is poorly understood. The importance of the p53-Itch-FLIP interaction at the plasma membrane has been clearly demonstrated to regulate CDDP sensitivity in OVCA cells, resulting in FLIP ubiquitination and degradation prior to the induction of apoptosis.[9,21] FLIP inhibits the activation of caspase-8 by binding to Fas-associated death domain (FADD), thereby suppressing apoptosis.[73,74] CDDP downregulates both splice variants, $FLIP_L$ (long isoform, 55 kDa) and $FLIP_S$ (short isoform, 28 kDa), allowing for the activation of caspase-8, caspase-3, and the induction of apoptosis in chemosensitive OVCA cells but not their resistant counterparts. siRNA-mediated FLIP downregulation *in vitro* sensitized chemoresistant OVCA cells to CDDP-induced apoptosis,[72] while CDDP induced FLIP proteasomal degradation via the E3 ubiquitin ligase, Itch (Figure 13.3a and b).[21] This response was accomplished by p53 activation and the interaction of FLIP-p53-Itch, forming a complex at the plasma membrane (Figure 13.3a). The overexpression of activated Akt attenuated CDDP-induced FLIP-p53-Itch interaction and colocalization in chemosensitive cells, and this response was abolished by the downregulation of Akt activity via dominant-negative Akt overexpression, which facilitated FLIP degradation, caspase activation, and apoptosis in chemoresistant OVCA cells.[9] Together, these findings point to a novel action of p53 in the modulation of FLIP content, which may contribute to a therapeutic strategy for OVCA.

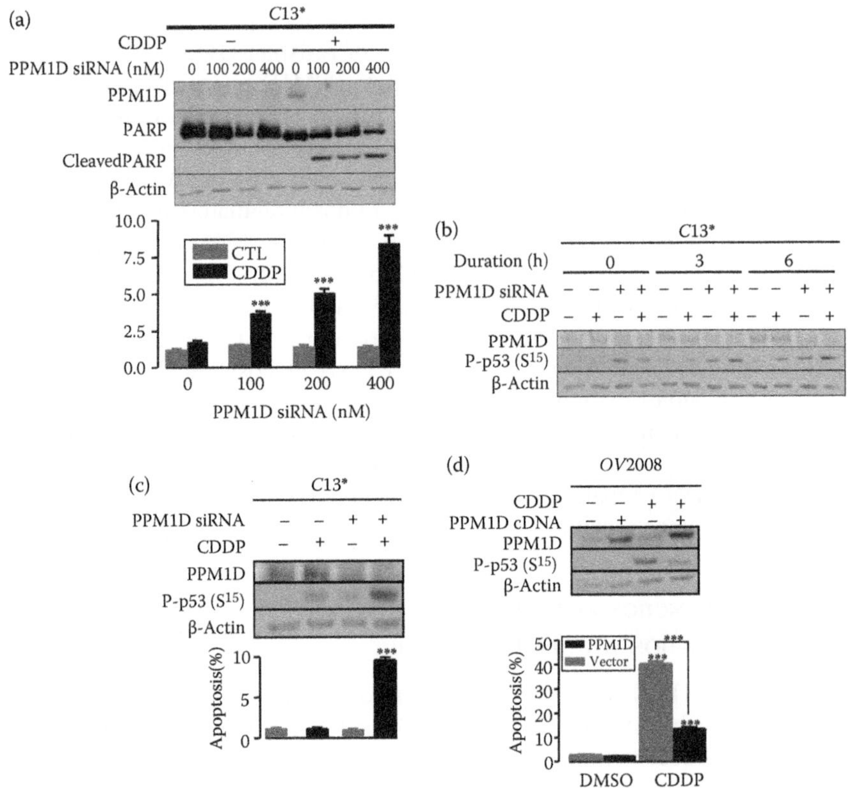

FIGURE 13.2 PPM1D suppresses CDDP-induced p53 activation and apoptosis in OVCA cells, thus decreasing CDDP sensitivity. (a) siRNA-mediated PPM1D downregulation sensitized chemoresistant cells (C13*) to CDDP-induced apoptosis (increased apoptotic cell count and PARP cleavage), suggesting that PPM1D has an inhibitory role in CDDP-induced apoptosis in chemoresistant cells. C13* cells were incubated with PPM1D siRNA or control siRNA (0–400, 24 h), treated with CDDP (0–10 μM, 24 h; $n = 3$). (b) PPM1D knockdown in C13* cells significantly upregulated phospho-S^{15}-p53 content, suggesting PPM1D significantly suppresses p53 activation in chemoresistant cells. C13* cells were incubated with PPM1D siRNA or control siRNA (0–400 nM, 24 h), treated with CDDP (0–10 μM, 0–6 h; $n = 3$, $P < 0.001$). (c) Upregulation of phospho-S^{15}-p53 content following PPM1D knockdown in C13* cells sensitized them to CDDP-induced apoptosis. C13* cells were treated with PPM1D siRNA (0–400 nM, 24 h), treated with CDDP (0–10 μM, 24 h; $n = 3$, $P < 0.001$). (d) Overexpression of PPM1D in chemosensitive cells (OV2008) significantly decreased CDDP-induced apoptosis, which was associated with decreased phospho-S^{15}-p53 contents. OV2008 cells were transfected (1 μg, 24 h) with PPM1D cDNA or empty vector, treated with CDDP (0–10 μM, 24 h; $n = 3$, $P < 0.001$). (Adapted from Ali, A.Y. et al., *Oncogene*, 31(17), 2175, 2012.)

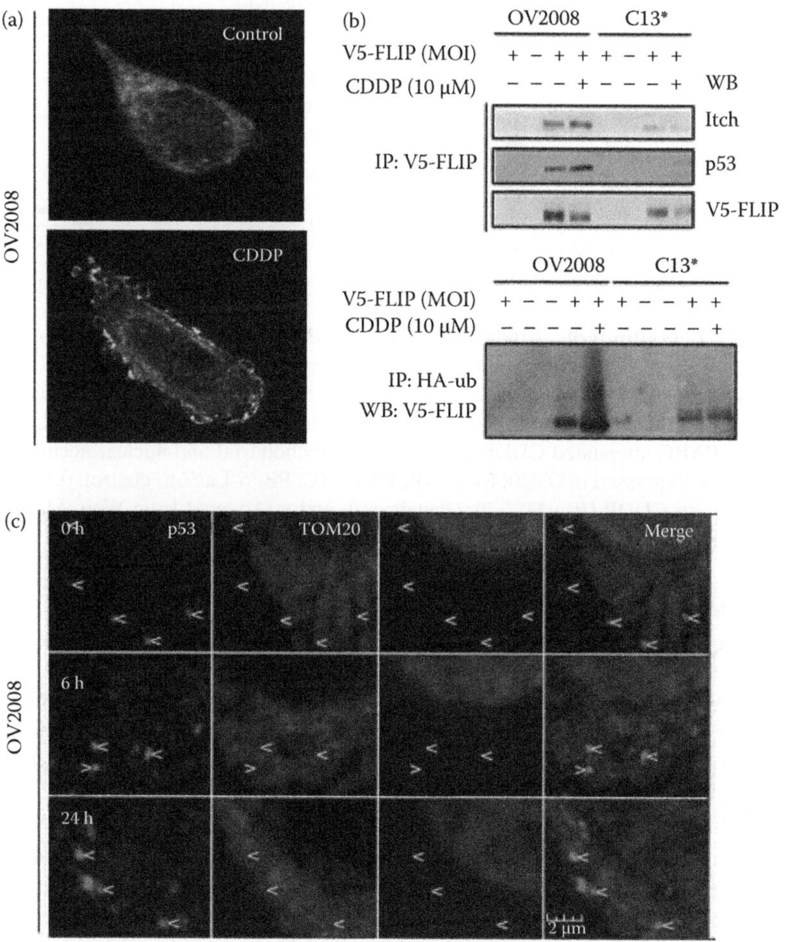

FIGURE 13.3 Effect of CDDP on p53, FLIP, and Itch interactions at the plasma membrane and p53 mitochondrial and nuclear accumulation in chemosensitive OVCA cells. (a) CDDP induces p53-FLIP-Itch colocalization at the cell membrane in chemosensitive cells (OV2008; Adapted from Abedini, M.R. et al., *Cancer Res.*, 68(12), 4511, 2008. With permission.) (b) CDDP induces p53-FLIP-Itch interaction (Co-IP) and FLIP ubiquitination in OV2008 cells, but not in C13* cells. (Adapted from Abedini, M.R. et al., *Oncogene*, 29(1), 11, 2010. With permission.) (c) CDDP induces p53 mitochondrial and nuclear accumulation in chemosensitive OV2008 cells. Arrows indicate exact locations across fields and serve to highlight the presence or absence of p53 colocalization with a translocase of the outer mitochondrial membrane (TOM20) and DAPI, by immunofluorescence/confocal microscopy. PARC was overexpressed in OV2008 cells (PEF6-PARC; PEF6-LacZ as control; 0.5 μg, 24 h) and treated with CDDP (10 μM, 6 h). (Panels c, d, and e: Adapted from Woo, M.G. et al., *J. Biol. Chem.*, 287(6), 3963, 2012. With permission.)

(*continued*)

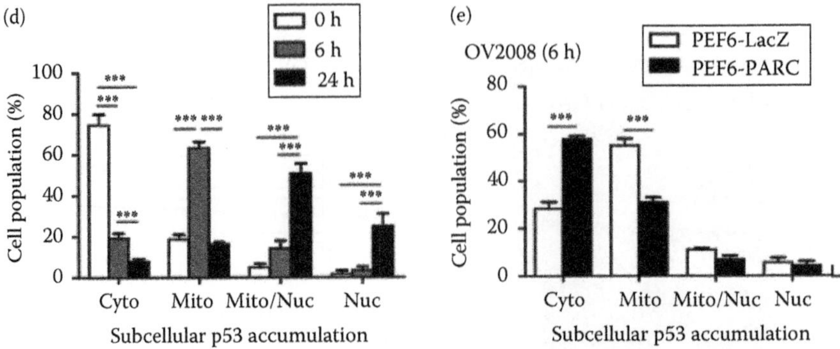

FIGURE 13.3 (continued) Effect of CDDP on p53, FLIP, and Itch interactions at the plasma membrane and p53 mitochondrial and nuclear accumulation in chemosensitive OVCA cells. (d) Quantification of the confocal images shows the population of cells exhibiting p53 accumulation in the cytoplasm, mitochondria, both mitochondria and nucleus, and only the nucleus. (e) PARC attenuated CDDP-induced p53 mitochondrial and nuclear accumulation. PARC was overexpressed in OV2008 cells (PEF6-PARC; PEF6-LacZ as control; 0.5 μg, 24 h) and treated with CDDP (10 μM, 6 h). (Panels c, d, and e: Adapted from Woo, M.G. et al., *J. Biol. Chem.*, 287(6), 3963, 2012. With permission.)

13.3.3 Modulation of Cytosolic p53 Activity: Regulation by MDM2 and Parc

Under a variety of cellular stress conditions, cytosolic p53 can directly translocate to the mitochondria and nucleus to induce apoptosis.[75,76] The action, expression, and subcellular localization of p53 are tightly regulated by posttranslational modifications including phosphorylation, ubiquitination, and acetylation.[77] MDM2 is an E3 ubiquitin ligase that plays an important role in the regulation of p53 content and activity via proteasomal degradation.[5] In the presence of excess MDM2, a herpesvirus-associated ubiquitin-specific protease (HAUSP) can stabilize p53 through de-ubiquitination, allowing for apoptosis to proceed.[78] However, HAUSP mainly localizes to the nucleus and may not be able to inhibit cytosolic p53 degradation.[79] Recently, Yuan and colleagues have observed that USP10, a cytoplasmic HAUSP, deubiquitinates p53 directly and reverses MDM2-mediated p53 degradation. Following DNA damage, USP10 was upregulated and translocated to the nucleus.[80] The role of USP10 in the regulation of p53-mediated apoptosis and CDDP sensitivity in OVCA warrants further investigation in the near future.

Parc (p53-associated, parkin-like cytoplasmic protein, Cul9) exists as a multiprotein complex in the cytoplasm where it acts as a molecular anchor for p53. The amino terminal of Parc strongly interacts with the carboxy terminal of p53, regulating its localization and subsequent function.[81] Parc, a large 270 kDa protein, contains Ring-IBR-Ring and carboxy terminal Cullen homology domain (CCH) signature motifs, commonly present in proteins exhibiting ubiquitin ligase activities.[81,82] However, Parc alone seems unable to degrade p53. siRNA-mediated Parc downregulation promotes nuclear p53 accumulation, transcriptional activation, and apoptosis in neuroblastoma cells and peyronie's disease fibroblasts.[81,83] Recently, the role of Parc in the regulation of mitochondrial p53 import and p53-mediated apoptosis in overcoming chemoresistance has been elucidated in our laboratory.[7] CDDP downregulates Parc content in a calpain-dependent manner, allowing for p53 mitochondrial and nuclear translocation to induce apoptosis in chemosensitive but not chemoresistant OVCA cells (Figure 13.3c and d). Forced expression of Parc attenuated CDDP-induced p53 translocation and apoptosis (Figure 13.3e). Moreover, the inhibition of Akt function was required to sensitize chemoresistant OVCA cells to CDDP in a p53-dependent manner, an effect enhanced by Parc downregulation.[7] Taken together with the observation that Parc controls p53 subcellular trafficking and CDDP sensitivity by its cytoplasmic sequestration, these findings reveal tightly regulated control mechanisms for intracellular p53 localization.

13.3.4 Mitochondrial Action of p53: Interaction with Bcl-2 Family Members and MOMP

Mitochondrial outer membrane permeabilization (MOMP) is a crucial step in the apoptotic process, which is directly governed by pro-apoptotic Bcl-2 family members including Bax and Bak, and BH3-only proteins, including Bid, Bim, and PUMA.[84,85] p53 response elements are present in the promoter regions of these apoptotic factors, allowing for their upregulation during p53-induced cell death.[13] Under cellular stress, p53 also directly translocates to the mitochondria and participates in the induction of apoptosis both by interacting with pro-apoptotic Bcl-2 family members to induce MOMP and by forming an inhibitory complex with Bcl-2 and Bcl-XL to neutralize their anti-apoptotic effects.[86] Interestingly, the p53 DBD interacts directly with the interface of Bcl-2 protein. p53 mutants are incapable of Bcl-2 complex formation and are, therefore, defective in mitochondrial permeabilization.[87] In response to CDDP, p53 is targeted to the mitochondria to induce the release of cytochrome c (cyto c), second mitochondria-derived activator of caspase/Diablo homolog (smac/DIABLO), and apoptosis inducing factor (AIF), resulting in caspase-3 activation in chemosensitive OVCA cells, a response attenuated by Akt.[3,8,88]

13.4 INVOLVEMENT OF NO/sGC/cGMP/PKG SIGNALING PATHWAY IN THE REGULATION OF CDDP SENSITIVITY IN OVARIAN CANCER

13.4.1 NO/sGMP/PKG Pathway

The nitric oxide (NO)/cyclic GMP(cGMP)/cGMP-dependent protein kinase (protein kinase G [PKG]) pathway has recently become recognized as a central player in promoting cell proliferation and chemoresistance in human OVCA cells.[89–91] Endogenous NO can be produced by three different nitric oxide synthase (NOS) isoforms, NOS1 (also called neuronal NOS), NOS2 (also called inducible NOS), and NOS3 (also called endothelial NOS).[92] NOS1 and NOS3 produce NO at low physiological levels while NOS2 produces NO at high pathological levels.[92,93] At low physiological levels, NO tonically activates the heme-dependent soluble guanylyl cyclase,[94] elevating cGMP levels and causing continuous activation of the serine/threonine kinase PKG-I. The activated PKG-I then phosphorylates the downstream anti-apoptotic effectors, such as CREB and vasodilator-stimulated phosphoprotein (VASP), resulting in an increase in cell proliferation and decrease in apoptosis in many types of cells, including neural cells, vascular smooth muscle cells, and pancreatic islet cells.[95–98]

13.4.2 Activation of PKG-Iα and PKG-Iβ Isoforms Depends on the Levels of Endogenous NO

It has been previously reported that PKG-I plays both anti-apoptotic and pro-apoptotic roles in different types of cancer.[89–91,99] For examples, PKG-I was shown to be pro-apoptotic in colon cancer,[99] but exhibited an anti-apoptotic role in nonsmall cell lung cancer and OVCA cells.[89–91] Indeed, PKG exists in two isoforms, PKG-Iα and PKG-Iβ, which are ubiquitously expressed in most of mammalian cells.[96,99,100] PKG-Iα was shown to be expressed in OVCA, mesothelioma, nonsmall cell lung cancer, while PKG-Iβ was expressed in colon cancer.[89–91,99] Due to different enzymatic kinetics (K_{cat}) of the two PKG-I isoforms, NO can activate different isoforms when it exists in different cellular concentrations. Low levels of NO (0.01–1 nanomolar) can activate PKG-Iα while high levels of NO (1–50 nanomolar) can activate PKG-Iβ. We have found that the type of PKG-I isoform being activated may determine the role of PKG-I in tumorigenesis, and which isoform to be activated is dependent on the levels of cellular NO.[96,101]

13.4.3 Activation of PKG-Iα and Src in Ovarian Cancer

We have previously found that only the type Iα splice variant of PKG is expressed in two types of human OVCA cells.[90,91] Out of the two PKG isoforms, PKG-Iα is the more sensitive to stimulation by cGMP, and thus, is likely to be the only PKG isoform that is subsequently activated by the presence of low physiological levels of NO.[100,101] Activated PKG-Iα can then regulate the activities of its downstream anti-apoptotic effectors mentioned previously.[97,98] In addition, we have further discovered new crosstalk in OVCA between PKG-Iα and c-Src, the first proto-oncogene to be identified, resulting in enhanced PKG-Iα kinase activity. Activated PKG-Iα further enhances Src signaling, resulting in elevated levels of DNA synthesis and cell proliferation[91,102–104] and tumorigenesis in OVCA cells.

13.4.4 Involvement of NO/sGC/cGMP/PKG Signaling Pathway and p53 Regulation in CDDP Sensitivity

Both the NO/sGC/cGMP/PKG and p53 pathway are essential in the regulation of OVCA sensitivity.[89,90,105] However, the crosstalk between the two pathways in regulating CDDP-induced apoptosis in OVCA cells has only recently been demonstrated.[89,90] The mode of regulation is highly dependent on the presence of NOS isoforms and NO levels in the cell. We have previously demonstrated the differential regulation of three different NOS isoforms in two isogenic chemosensitive–chemoresistant OVCA cell line pairs.[90] The results showed that all three isoforms of

NOS are expressed in both cell lines, but their expression is differentially regulated at basal levels and by CDDP in both cell lines. Interestingly, our results suggested that NOS2 contributes to CDDP-induced apoptosis in chemosensitive cells, but NOS1 and NOS3 contribute to chemoresistance by suppressing CDDP-induced apoptosis in a p53-independent manner in chemoresistant cells. Treatment with an NO donor, S-nitroso-N-acetylpenicillamine (SNAP), elevated NO content and upregulated apoptosis in both cancer cell lines. Also, CDDP sensitization induced by high levels of NO in chemosensitive cells directly involves p53 upregulation.[90] In contrast, CDDP sensitization induced by inhibition of all three forms of NOS in chemoresistant cells did not change p53 levels. Thus, the role of p53 in CDDP sensitization appears to be different in OVCA cells with a different NO status.[90]

Overall, the NO/sGC/cGMP/PKG signaling pathway plays an essential role in regulating tumorigenesis and CDDP sensitivity in OVCA. It is likely that which NOS isoform is expressed, the levels of cellular NO produced, and which PKG-I isoform is expressed are the determinants of CDDP sensitivity in OVCA, whereas p53 is a direct mediator of high-level NO sensitization of CDDP-induced apoptosis.[89–91,95]

13.5 ROLE OF AKT AND mTOR IN CDDP CHEMORESISTANCE IN OVARIAN CANCER

13.5.1 PI3K/Akt Pathway in Chemoresistant Ovarian Cancer

Phosphoinositide-3 kinase (PI3K) is a phospholipid kinase, which is activated by several receptor tyrosine kinases in response to growth stimuli. Activated PI3K creates phosphatidylinositol 3,4,5-triphosphate (PIP_3) by phosphorylating the membrane lipid phosphatidylinositol 4,5-bisphosphate (PIP_2), thereby recruiting cytoplasmic PI3K targets to the plasma membrane for activation and further signaling.[106,107] The tumor suppressor phosphatase and tensin homolog (PTEN) regulate PI3K by dephosphorylating PIP_3 to PIP_2.[107]

The oncogenic serine/threonine kinase Akt, also known as protein kinase B (PKB), is an important downstream effector of the PI3K pathway. Akt is a family of proteins consisting of three members (Akt1, Akt2, and Akt3) that share similar structures and have high sequence homology. The structure of the three Akt isoforms is composed of the pleckstrin homology (PH) domain important for protein–protein interaction located in the amino terminal, followed by a catalytic domain necessary for Akt kinase activity, and a regulatory domain located in the carboxy terminal.[108] Akt is recruited to the plasma membrane by PIP_3[109] and activated through phosphorylation-dependent mechanism by the phosphoinositide-dependent kinase 1 (PDK1; Thr^{308})[110,111] and mammalian target of rapamycin complex 2 (mTORC2; Ser^{473}).[112,113]

Activated Akt has the ability to regulate numerous cellular pathways involved in apoptosis, survival, and proliferation. Akt regulates the protein stability of p53 and attenuates its function through dual phosphorylation and stabilization of MDM2 (Ser^{166} and Ser^{186}), which translocates into the nucleus and facilitates p53 ubiquitin-mediated degradation through the proteasomal pathway.[114,115] Conversely, p53 can regulate Akt activation by enhancing the transcription of the PI3K inhibitor PTEN, negatively regulating PI3K activity, and thereby, increasing p53 content and activation.[116,117]

Akt also modulates the activity of several other apoptosis-regulating proteins. Akt attenuates the expression of the pro-apoptotic proteins Bim and Fas ligand by phosphorylating and inhibiting the forkhead transcription factor 1 (FOXO-1; Thr^{32} and Ser^{253}), leading to its nuclear exclusion and inhibition of its transcriptional targets.[118] Akt phosphorylates and inhibits the pro-apoptotic protein BAD (Ser^{136}), thereby inhibiting the permeabilization of the outer mitochondrial membrane and release of mitochondrial death proteins by decreasing the binding of BAD with the anti-apoptotic protein Bcl-XL.[119] Akt also phosphorylates and inhibits caspase-9 (Ser^{196}).[120] We have demonstrated that Akt enhances the stability of the caspase-3 inhibitor X-linked inhibitor of apoptosis protein (XIAP; Ser^{87}), preventing XIAP auto-ubiquitination and subsequent proteasomal degradation.[121] We have also demonstrated that Akt activation in chemosensitive OVCA cells protected the anti-apoptotic protein FLIP from CDDP-induced, p53-mediated ubiquitination, and subsequent proteasomal degradation.[9] Furthermore, Akt regulates the mitochondrial pro-apoptotic protein AIF, which mediates caspase-independent CDDP-induced apoptosis through promoting DNA fragmentation and nuclear condensation. CDDP induces AIF mitochondrial release and nuclear accumulation in chemosensitive, but not chemoresistant, OVCA cells. Akt activation inhibited AIF mitochondrial release and nuclear accumulation in chemosensitive OVCA cells, while the downregulation of Akt activity in chemoresistant OVCA cells enhanced CDDP-induced AIF nuclear localization and apoptosis.[122] Akt indirectly activates the transcription factor NF-κB by facilitating inhibitor of κB (IκB) degradation.[123,124] Activated NF-κB is a known positive regulator of many anti-apoptotic and survival proteins, including PPM1D.[41]

Akt enhances cellular proliferation by relieving cell cycle arrest at both the G_1 and the G_2/M phases. Akt phosphorylates and inhibits the p53-responsive cyclin-dependent kinase inhibitor p21 (Thr^{145}), leading to p27 downregulation, ultimately resulting in the resumption of the cell cycle beyond the G_1 checkpoint.[125–127] Akt also phosphorylates and inhibits the G_2/M cell cycle regulator Chk1 (Ser^{280}), relieving cell cycle arrest at the G_2/M phase.[128]

Overexpression and/or activation of the PI3K/Akt survival pathway are associated with tumorigenesis in several human malignancies.[129–133] We have shown that Akt is a determinant of CDDP sensitivity and OVCA chemoresistance. We have also demonstrated that the activation of Akt attenuates p53 pro-apoptotic signaling, promoting chemoresistance and the survival of OVCA cells and that Akt downregulation sensitizes chemoresistant OVCA cells to CDDP-induced apoptosis in a p53-dependent manner. Furthermore, Akt activation in chemosensitive cells resulted in a significant decrease in p53-DNA binding in response to CDDP, inhibition of p53 Ser^{15} and Ser^{20} phosphorylation, and attenuation of CDDP-induced apoptosis.[4,9,134]

We have observed that Akt plays an important role in regulating the stability of PPM1D protein and increases its content in response to CDDP-induced DNA damage in OVCA cells. Akt inhibition in resistant OVCA cells did not change CDDP-induced PPM1D mRNA expression; however, it caused a significant downregulation of PPM1D content. Activated Akt overexpression attenuated PPM1D decrease in response to CDDP and significantly reduced CDDP-induced apoptosis in chemosensitive OVCA cells. In resistant OVCA cells with high Akt activity, PPM1D stability was enhanced in response to protein synthesis inhibition, while it significantly decreased in their sensitive counterparts following CDDP treatment. Furthermore, we have observed a significant decrease in PPM1D content following the inhibition of Akt activity in resistant cells (unpublished data). Our observations suggest a possible new mechanism by which Akt can attenuate the activity of several tumor suppressors and disrupt the DNA damage response to enhance chemoresistance through positive regulation of its newly discovered effector PPM1D.[10]

13.5.2 mTOR Pathway and Ovarian Cancer Chemoresistance

The mammalian target of rapamycin (mTOR) has emerged as a critical regulatory pathway of cellular metabolism, growth, proliferation, and survival. mTOR exists in two functionally distinct complexes, mTORC1 and mTORC2. mTORC1 is sensitive to rapamycin and controls protein synthesis and cellular metabolism, while mTORC2 is involved in cytoskeleton assembly and is also responsible for phosphorylation of Akt at Ser^{473} allowing full activation.[135] Conversely, Akt activates mTOR through direct phosphorylation at Ser^{2448}, through which Akt forms its own positive feedback loop to enhance its activation.[136] Signaling pathways for both mTOR complexes interconnect and influence each other via several key mediators, including Akt.

The interplay between Akt and mTOR complexes is essential for their cellular function. After phosphorylation by mTORC2, Akt activates mTORC1 by phosphorylating and inhibiting both tuberous sclerosis complex 2 (TSC2) and proline-rich protein (PRAS40), negative regulators of mTORC1.[137] Active mTORC1 elicits a negative feedback loop on Akt activity by influencing the responsiveness of its downstream effector, p70S6K1, to insulin receptor substrate 1 (IRS-1) and rictor, an mTORC2 component.[138] Since mTORC2 was found to be an activator of Akt by phosphorylating Ser^{473}, Akt activity is both positively and negatively controlled by mTOR. However, it is important to note that phosphorylation of Akt at Ser^{473} does not require Akt-dependent activation of mTORC1, and Akt cannot promote cell proliferation and oncogenic transformation in mTORC1-null cells.[138]

The mTOR signaling pathway is also regulated by other molecular events and stimuli including mitogens, hypoxia, amino acids, and intracellular energy levels.[139] One of the most clinical implications of Akt-independent mTOR activity is AMP-activated protein kinase (AMPK), a master metabolic regulator.[140] AMPK inhibits mTORC1 both directly and indirectly via TSC2 in response to low cellular energy levels. Therefore, reported AMPK activators such as metformin, AICAR, and A769662 may be promising therapeutic agents for cancers featuring dysregulation of mTOR signaling pathways.

mTOR signaling dysregulation exists in various cancers including OVCA and is frequently related to tumorigenesis, tumor growth, and metastasis. Aberration of the mTOR signaling pathway confers resistance to CDDP-based chemotherapy and adverse prognosis in OVCA patients.[141] The role of mTOR in chemoresistance is commonly relevant to other common mutational events in cancer such as those occurring in the epidermal growth factor receptor (EGFR), Ras, and Akt. p70S6K1 is the major downstream effector of mTORC1, promoting cancer cell proliferation, growth, and angiogenesis.[142] Therefore, mTORC1 is a logical molecular target for overcoming OVCA chemoresistance. Clinical studies in OVCA involving the rapamycin analog

RAD001 have shown its sensitization of ovarian tumors to CDDP treatment, prolonging mean survival time in a mouse model.[143,144] BEZ235, a dual PI3K/mTOR inhibitor, can also recapitulate the importance of mTORC1 in regulating cell proliferation in OVCA.[145] Other inhibitors have also been used to demonstrate this concept. Although mTORC1 and dual PI3K/mTOR inhibitors are effective in sensitizing cancer cells to chemotherapy, losing negative feedback from mTORC1 to Akt and a broad effect of dual PI3K/mTOR inhibitors remain major disadvantages. Therefore, development of a specific mTORC2 inhibitor could form an alternative approach for overcoming mTOR-mediated chemoresistance in OVCA since mTORC2 is known to promote cell survival through Akt, and associates with other kinases to promote metastasis and tumor formation in breast and colon cancers, respectively.[146,147]

The plausible molecular targets for the inhibition of mTORC2 function include mammalian stress-activated protein kinase-interacting protein (mSIN1), mTOR-associated protein LST8 (mLST8), and rictor. These proteins are required for the integrity of the complex, thereby enhancing tumor development and progression. Rictor also has other roles in cell migration and cancer cell metastasis.[146] Moreover, mTORC2 inhibitors may have an advantage over mTOR catalytic site inhibitors in that they do not perturb the negative feedback loop to IRS-1.[148] We have demonstrated that siRNA-mediated rictor knockdown can sensitize chemoresistant OVCA cells to CDDP-induced apoptosis (unpublished data). This result corroborates the possibility that development of an mTOR inhibitor, specifically targeting mTORC2, would provide a great impact on chemoresistant OVCA therapy.

13.6 FUNCTIONAL FOOD COMPOUNDS AS A NEW OPPORTUNITY FOR CANCER PATIENTS

13.6.1 Functional Food Compounds

The basic nutrients in our food supply can be broadly characterized as proteins, carbohydrates, fats, vitamins, and minerals, which are commonly viewed as the primary molecular input needed for the maintenance of cellular homeostasis. However, there exist other components present in foods that can modulate cellular status and human health. A variety of bioactive compounds have been identified in foods that provide beneficial health effects beyond basic nutrition. These substances can occur naturally in the organism of origin (e.g., plants, fungi, and animals) or arise during various food processing techniques such as heating, fermenting, drying, and enzymatic processing. Although these substances have in the past been regarded with little interest, numerous studies have enabled the growing recognition of these functional food compounds as having both health-promoting and disease-preventing functions.

In today's modern developed societies, health consciousness among the general public has increased rapidly. The extension of lifespan has been possible with a better understanding of chronic diseases such as cancer, diabetes, and heart disease, leading to an improving awareness of the relationship between health and diet. Functional foods are defined by the Institute of Medicine's Food and Nutrition Board as "any food or food ingredients that may provide a health benefit beyond the traditional nutrients it contains." There are multiple components in natural foods that are capable of producing a wide range of health-related phenomena which vary depending on the content, concentration, and bioavailability of the compound. Due to the extreme diversity of bioactive compounds found in nearly all food sources, there has been great interest in determining which of the compounds are most functional in the human body. Identifying proper functional compounds and their mechanisms of action could be highly beneficial in the prevention, reversal, and cure of many common diseases.

13.6.2 Functional Food Compounds as Chemopreventive and Therapeutic Agents

One of the recent major breakthroughs in the area of functional food science is the discovery of specific chemopreventive and chemotherapeutic effects of some compounds against cancer. Carcinogenesis is a dynamic process that involves many complex factors,[149] which may explain why no single molecular strategy has been widely effective. As a result, a focus on prevention rather than cure as an alternative approach to controlling cancer has received growing emphasis. Chemoprevention is defined as a range of pharmacological approaches used to arrest or reverse the process of cancer development before invasion and metastasis occur.[150] Since the process of carcinogenesis can require 20 years or more for certain cancers, the potential arises for suppression of tumors in their early, premalignant stages before they become lethal.

For many years, it was thought that functional food substances possess anticancer activity due mainly to their antioxidant properties; however, antioxidant effects alone do not account for all of the therapeutic effects observed, including the specific inhibition of signal transduction pathways and efficacy at low doses. Recent research suggests that compounds naturally occurring in foods can act with similar mechanistic properties to small molecule inhibitory drugs like Gleevec for leukemia and Iressa for lung cancer. The development and survival of cancer cells depends on signaling pathway dysregulation, which activates and maintains a malignant phenotype. Thus, any substances that can control abnormal cancerous signaling have the potential to influence and negate cancer growth.

Finding optimal functional foods with antitumor activity can aid in preventing the onset of cancer and save lives. Every food contains numerous organic compounds, although not all of them have identifiable bioactivity. In many cases, a functional food compound of therapeutic interest can be found in a number of food products. With the right functional food combinations there could be a better chance of controlling and eliminating the disease before it is diagnosed.

13.6.3 Functional Food Compounds as Signaling Inhibitors in Cancer Cells

Resveratrol is a stilbene found in grapes, red wine, peanuts, mulberry, and some other fruits and vegetables. It has been reported to inhibit cyclooxygenase-2 (COX-2), an inflammation-triggering enzyme known to play a major role in many cancers.[151] LTA_4H, Ref-1, and AP-1 are also well-reported targets of resveratrol that exhibit anticancer effects against various cancers including colon, pancreatic, and skin cancers.[152,153]

Quercetin is a flavonol present in red wine, onion, tomato, black/green tea, apples, and various berries, exhibiting strong preventive effects against cell transformation and tumor development through the suppression of Raf-1, MEK-1, and PI3K.[154,155] Quercetin possesses potent anti-inflammatory effects through the downregulation of COX-2 and NOS2, two critical factors in cancer development and sustenance.[156,157] Curcumin, the major curcuminoid in the spice turmeric, is an inhibitor of NF-κB, the p300/CREB-binding protein, and spleen tyrosine kinase. Curcumin exhibits preventive and therapeutic effects against leukemia, liver, breast, and colon cancers.[158]

Myricetin is found in various fruits and vegetables, including onions, berries, and grapes, as well as red wine. Myricetin suppresses UVB-induced COX-2 expression and skin tumors by inhibiting Fyn.[159] It was reported to inhibit angiogenesis by regulating PI3K and can also directly bind with Raf-1, MEK1, MKK4 and the JNK 1/signal transducer and activator of transcription 3 proteins, resulting in significant cancer preventive effects.[158,160]

Several isoflavones from soybean and its metabolites including genistein, 7,3′,4′-trihydroxyisoflavone (THIF), and equol have also been reported to possess strong chemopreventive effects. Genistein inhibits EGFR and DNA methyltransferase, while activating the retinoic acid receptor β, p16^{Ink4a} and the MGMT gene, causing suppression of esophageal, skin, and prostate cancers.[161,162] In addition, 7,3′,4′-THIF prevents neoplastic cell transformation and proliferation of epidermal cells by attenuating CDK2, CDK4, and PI3K. Equol directly inhibits MEK1, preventing cell transformation.[163,164]

Luteolin is a naturally occurring flavone in onion, broccoli, and celery that prevents cell transformation, inflammation, and skin cancer development. We have observed that luteolin exhibits strong inhibitory effects against Src and PKC-epsilon.[165] Furthermore, luteolin is an inhibitor of the tumor progression locus 2 serine/threonine kinase, suppressing tumor necrosis factor-alpha-induced COX-2 expression in JB6 mouse epidermal cells.[166]

13.6.4 Functional Food Compounds as Chemosensitizing Agents

While chemoprevention of OVCA may be the most ideal strategy for reducing the incidence of disease, in reality medical science is preoccupied with determining the most effective treatment strategies after it has been identified. One of the major enduring obstacles in OVCA treatment has been the failure to improve detection of the disease at initial stages when therapeutic intervention will have lasting effects. In contrast to breast cancer, which has benefited from successful public awareness campaigns and effective screening technology, diagnostic techniques for OVCA remain relatively obscure, largely due to a lack of symptoms.

Functional food compounds have potential application in chemoresistant OVCA therapy to tip the balance in favor of apoptosis by priming such pathways for more robust responses. For example, the platelet-derived growth factor (PDGF) and its receptor are commonly overexpressed in OVCA, leading to autocrine stimulation.[167] Imatinib is a monoclonal antibody that has been developed to target the PDGF receptor, but has so far been unsuccessful in clinical trials. This has been theorized to be due to the existence of a feedback loop regulated by the PI3K/Akt pathway. Akt is responsible for CDDP resistance in a number of OVCA cell lines, which has led to the development of a plethora of synthetic PI3K inhibitors, a prominent example being LY294002. The clinical development of LY294002 was indefinitely suspended due to its indirect targeting of unintended substrates. Our laboratory has observed that a number of functional food compounds purified from natural sources exhibit PI3K inhibitory ability with potency greater than LY294002 (unpublished data). Such compounds include the anthocyanin myricetin and the diarylheptanoid hirsutenone. X-ray crystallography data show that myricetin directly inhibits the ATP-binding pocket of PI3K's catalytic subunit, which is most likely its primary mechanism of attenuating Akt activation.[168] Such compounds may one day provide health care professionals with more flexible options for manipulation of the Akt pathway prior to or during CDDP treatment.

Tangeritin is a polymethoxylated citrus flavonoid that has been shown to sensitize multiple CDDP-resistant human OVCA cell lines via downregulation of the PI3K/Akt pathway.[169] While tangeritin alone had very little effect on OVCA cells, in combination with small doses of CDDP (3 μM), apoptosis was significantly induced, concurrent with caspase activation and poly (ADP-ribose) polymerase (PARP) cleavage. The tangeritin–CDDP combination also induced cell cycle arrest at the G_2/M phase in chemoresistant cells with a p53-mutant phenotype. The downregulation of the PI3K/Akt pathway was evident through downstream effects, with levels of NF-κB, GSK3-β, and phosphorylated BAD (Ser^{136}) all significantly reduced.

A major factor currently influencing prognosis in breast and ovarian cancers is the status of the breast cancer susceptibility gene (BRCA). Mutational damage in either BRCA1 or BRCA2 genes can lead to hereditary breast–ovarian cancer syndrome. PARP is an enzyme that repairs DNA single-strand breaks and is of particular importance for BRCA-deficient cancers.[170] PARP inhibition exacerbates BRCA deficiency, resulting in a higher frequency of DNA damage and chromosomal instability, which increases the likelihood of cell cycle arrest and apoptosis. There are numerous functional food compounds that target PARP activity and warrant further investigation. One such candidate that has received recent attention is epigallocatechin gallate (EGCG), the major polyphenolic compound found in green tea. EGCG treatment downregulates PARP levels and, interestingly, also targets other hallmarks of cancer, including angiogenesis, proliferation, and migration.[171]

Like all solid malignancies, ovarian tumors cannot survive without an adequate nutrient supply derived through angiogenesis. In the human ovary, angiogenesis is also important for follicular development and maturation during normal ovulation. This is accompanied by detectable changes in vascular endothelial growth factor (VEGF) levels throughout the menstrual cycle. Dysregulation of VEGFA has been detected in a number of human ovarian tumors, providing rationale for the development of bevacizumab, a monoclonal antibody that targets the VEGF receptor. Bevacizumab has had modest success in clinical trials, but complications have arisen during combination therapy, including gastrointestinal perforations. In such circumstances, the application of a functional food compound could be more appropriate. Dietary flavonoids including genistein and kaempferol have shown effective inhibition of VEGF activity in a range of OVCA cell lines.[172] In strategic combination with genotoxic agents, anti-angiogenic compounds may provide the extra burden necessary for cancer cells to activate apoptotic pathways. Another aspect of angiogenesis that could potentially be manipulated using food compounds is vascular remodeling to improve delivery of chemotherapeutic drugs to sites of action. This is especially applicable to strategies targeting the ovaries, due to their difficult surgical accessibility.

Resveratrol, the phytoalexin mentioned earlier, gained prominence after its potential therapeutic activity was demonstrated in a range of cancer cells. In addition to its primary inhibitory effects on signaling pathways, mouse models of angiogenesis have shown that resveratrol also inhibits neovascularization artificially induced by VEGF.[173] Acting through oral administration, it inhibits tumor growth, and in combination with CDDP or doxorubicin produces a shift to the left in dose–response curves when administered to OVCA cells.[174] Other studies have shown apoptosis-independent methods of resveratrol action, via the process of autophagocytosis (the process by which cells digest themselves in response to adverse conditions). Although resveratrol induces the formation of the apoptosome, the inhibition of its formation does not entirely abrogate cell death. Resveratrol-induced autophagosomes in OVCA cells have been detected by immunofluorescence and electron microscopy imaging.[175] This has important implications for the treatment of chemoresistant tumors, as autophagy can occur in the complete absence of a genotoxic agent.

Another functional food compound that brings a new perspective into the field is piceatannol, which is normally found in low concentrations in the skin of grapes.[176] We have found that very low concentration of piceatannol can improve the effects of CDDP is chemosensitive cells *in vitro*. Its action appears to be dependent on p53, whereby piceatannol enhances levels of p53 activation, detectable by increased levels in the nucleus, likely leading to the transcription of pro-apoptotic factors including NOXA. Treatment with piceatannol leads directly to XIAP degradation in both sensitive and resistant lines. The synergistic effects of piceatannol and CDDP were confirmed in a mouse OVCA xenograft model, whereby the dual treatment significantly reduced tumor size when compared to either agent alone (unpublished data). In physiological circumstances, piceatannol appears in the bloodstream after metabolic conversion of its primary form, resveratrol. Thus a new concept emerges, in that functional foods in their pure forms may elicit different effects when administered orally versus intravenously, due in part to pharmacodynamic effects occurring during absorption. Cytochrome p450 (CYP450) enzymes convert resveratrol into piceatannol, as well as many other polyphenols into their active metabolites. Dependent upon CYP450 genotype, patients may, therefore, have different capacities to effectively produce such active metabolites, resulting in varying bioavailability of the functional compound.

Recent studies of novel phytochemicals like piperlongumine (found in long pepper) have found that at least some of these compounds exhibit simultaneous effects on multiple oncogenic targets through reactive oxygen species generation.[177] This is especially important as inhibition of a single cascade can lead to cancer cell adaptation through upregulation of compensatory pathways.

13.7 CONCLUSION

Chronic human diseases like OVCA have proven to be highly complex and involve the dysregulation of multiple molecular pathways. While contemporary research often focuses on specific pathways, the "-omics" fields (including genomics, epigenomics, proteomics, metabolomics, etc.) tend to provide a more wholesome perspective of OVCA pathophysiology. These allow the examination of global differences at the molecular and cellular levels between OVCA patients, ultimately allowing a personalized approach to OVCA treatment. Personalized medicine is an important emerging concept in cancer therapy, whereby OVCA is not regarded as a single disease, but rather as a broad range of subtypes that vary from one patient to another and which could best be treated based on the molecular signatures of each patient.

For the improvement of detection techniques, further evolution in the characterization of OVCA is necessary. Most important is the development of appropriate biomarkers that can identify the presence of the disease and its subtypes. Cancer antigen 125 (CA125) has been proposed as one such marker detectable in the bloodstream, but its applicability is limited and not present in all patients. Another strategy could be the identification of circulating tumor cells, although not all tumor types may be appropriately detected. One of the more promising methods is tumor genotyping to detect common mutations. For example, BRCA-negative patients may benefit more from compounds targeting PARP activity. The routine collection of ascites fluid could also aid studies designed to determine how individual differences in the molecular signatures are used to develop a personalized medicinal approach.

Various functional food compounds have been identified to have chemopreventive and chemotherapeutic effects against diverse types of cancers. Further research to identify compounds with high efficacy and to elucidate their mechanisms of action will aid in the development of more personalized nutritional advice to protect individuals with cancer susceptibility. In addition, the development of supplementary products with safe and effective functional food extracts and genetically engineered foods may lead to improvements in chemotherapeutic strategies.

Natural food compounds have many benefits over standard artificial agents. Due to their long history of human consumption, they are more likely to be tolerated better than conventional chemotherapeutics, and thus could more readily be approved by regulatory bodies. Food compounds can be used in horizontal (against parallel signaling pathways) or vertical (multiple targets in the same pathway) inhibition to achieve maximal effects. The global effects of multiple food compounds could one day play critical roles in pushing the signaling balance toward pro-apoptotic decisions. However, the eventual application of functional food compounds for either OVCA chemoprevention or therapy awaits comprehensive *in vivo* studies. Conclusive data from clinical trials involving the use of functional food compounds remain elusive and warrant further investigation. There is also a need to develop an appropriate delivery method to enhance drug bioavailability at the tumor site. Further research into the effects of functional food compounds on oncogenic signaling will add knowledge to the collective understanding of OVCA chemoresistance, and lay the foundations for the development of novel strategies for this deadly disease.

ACKNOWLEDGMENTS

This work was supported by grants from the Canadian Institute of Health Research (MOP-15691) and the World Class University (WCU) program (R31-10056) through the National Research Foundation of Korea funded by the Ministry of Education, Science and Technology.

REFERENCES

1. www.cancer.ca/en/cancer-information/cancer-type/ovarain/statistics
2. Yap TA, Carden CP, and Kaye SB, Beyond chemotherapy: Targeted therapies in ovarian cancer. *Nat Rev Cancer*, 2009; 9(3): 167–181.
3. Fraser M, Leung B, Jahani-Asl A, Yan X, Thompson WE, and Tsang BK, Chemoresistance in human ovarian cancer: The role of apoptotic regulators. *Reprod Biol Endocrinol*, 2003; 1: 66.
4. Fraser M, Bai T, and Tsang BK, Akt promotes cisplatin resistance in human ovarian cancer cells through inhibition of p53 phosphorylation and nuclear function. *Int J Cancer*, 2008; 122(3): 534–546.
5. Honda R, Tanaka H, and Yasuda H, Oncoprotein MDM2 is a ubiquitin ligase E3 for tumor suppressor p53. *FEBS Lett*, 1997; 420(1): 25–27.
6. Jung YS, Qian Y, and Chen X, Examination of the expanding pathways for the regulation of p21 expression and activity. *Cell Signal*, 2010; 22(7): 1003–1012.
7. Woo MG, Xue K, Liu J, McBride H, and Tsang BK, Calpain-mediated processing of p53-associated parkin-like cytoplasmic protein (PARC) affects chemosensitivity of human ovarian cancer cells by promoting p53 subcellular trafficking. *J Biol Chem*, 2012; 287(6): 3963–3975.
8. Yang X, Fraser M, Moll UM, Basak A, and Tsang BK, Akt-mediated cisplatin resistance in ovarian cancer: Modulation of p53 action on caspase-dependent mitochondrial death pathway. *Cancer Res*, 2006; 66(6): 3126–3136.
9. Abedini MR, Muller EJ, Bergeron R, Gray DA, and Tsang BK, Akt promotes chemoresistance in human ovarian cancer cells by modulating cisplatin-induced, p53-dependent ubiquitination of FLICE-like inhibitory protein. *Oncogene*, 2010; 29(1): 11–25.
10. Ali AY, Abedini MR, and Tsang BK, The oncogenic phosphatase PPM1D confers cisplatin resistance in ovarian carcinoma cells by attenuating checkpoint kinase 1 and p53 activation. *Oncogene*, 2012; 31(17): 2175–2186.
11. Peng CY, Graves PR, Thoma RS, Wu Z, Shaw AS, and Piwnica-Worms H, Mitotic and G2 checkpoint control: Regulation of 14-3-3 protein binding by phosphorylation of Cdc25C on serine-216. *Science*, 1997; 277(5331): 1501–1505.
12. Chan TA, Hermeking H, Lengauer C, Kinzler KW, and Vogelstein B, 14-3-3Sigma is required to prevent mitotic catastrophe after DNA damage. *Nature*, 1999; 401(6753): 616–620.
13. Miyashita T and Reed JC, Tumor suppressor p53 is a direct transcriptional activator of the human bax gene. *Cell*, 1995; 80(2): 293–299.
14. Sax JK, Fei P, Murphy ME, Bernhard E, Korsmeyer SJ, and El-Deiry WS, BID regulation by p53 contributes to chemosensitivity. *Nat Cell Biol*, 2002; 4(11): 842–849.
15. Nakano K and Vousden KH, PUMA, a novel proapoptotic gene, is induced by p53. *Mol Cell*, 2001; 7(3): 683–694.
16. Park SY, Jeong MS, and Jang SB, In vitro binding properties of tumor suppressor p53 with PUMA and NOXA. *Biochem Biophys Res Commun*, 2012; 420(2): 350–356.

17. Moroni MC, Hickman ES, Lazzerini Denchi E, Caprara G, Colli E, Cecconi F, Müller H, and Helin K, Apaf-1 is a transcriptional target for E2F and p53. *Nat Cell Biol*, 2001; 3(6): 552–558.
18. Muller M, Wilder S, Bannasch D, Israeli D, Lehlbach K, Li-Weber M, Friedman SL, Galle PR, Stremmel W, Oren M, and Krammer PH, p53 activates the CD95 (APO-1/Fas) gene in response to DNA damage by anticancer drugs. *J Exp Med*, 1998; 188(11): 2033–2045.
19. Liu X, Yue P, Khuri FR, and Sun SY, p53 upregulates death receptor 4 expression through an intronic p53 binding site. *Cancer Res*, 2004; 64(15): 5078–5083.
20. Wu GS, Burns TF, McDonald ER 3rd, Jiang W, Meng R, Krantz ID, Kao G et al., KILLER/DR5 is a DNA damage-inducible p53-regulated death receptor gene. *Nat Genet*, 1997; 17(2): 141–143.
21. Abedini MR, Muller EJ, Brun J, Bergeron R, Gray DA, and Tsang BK, Cisplatin induces p53-dependent FLICE-like inhibitory protein ubiquitination in ovarian cancer cells. *Cancer Res*, 2008; 68(12): 4511–4517.
22. Pietsch EC, Sykes SM, McMahon SB, and Murphy ME, The p53 family and programmed cell death. *Oncogene*, 2008; 27(50): 6507–6521.
23. Concin N, Hofstetter G, Berger A, Gehmacher A, Reimer D, Watrowski R, Tong D, et al., Clinical relevance of dominant-negative p73 isoforms for responsiveness to chemotherapy and survival in ovarian cancer: Evidence for a crucial p53-p73 cross-talk in vivo. *Clin Cancer Res*, 2005; 11(23): 8372–8383.
24. Muller M, Schleithoff ES, Stremmel W, Melino G, Krammer PH, and Schilling T, One, two, three—p53, p63, p73 and chemosensitivity. *Drug Resist Updat*, 2006; 9(6): 288–306.
25. Concin N, Becker K, Slade N, Erster S, Mueller-Holzner E, Ulmer H, Daxenbichler G, et al., Transdominant DeltaTAp73 isoforms are frequently up-regulated in ovarian cancer. Evidence for their role as epigenetic p53 inhibitors in vivo. *Cancer Res*, 2004; 64(7): 2449–2460.
26. Al-Bahlani S, Fraser M, Wong AY, Sayan BS, Bergeron R, Melino G, and Tsang BK, P73 regulates cisplatin-induced apoptosis in ovarian cancer cells via a calcium/calpain-dependent mechanism. *Oncogene*, 2011; 30(41): 4219–4230.
27. Fiscella M, Zhang H, Fan S, Sakaguchi K, Shen S, Mercer WE, Vande Woude GF, O'Connor PM, and Appella E, Wip1, a novel human protein phosphatase that is induced in response to ionizing radiation in a p53-dependent manner. *Proc Natl Acad Sci USA*, 1997; 94(12): 6048–6053.
28. Lu X, Bocangel D, Nannenga B, Yamaguchi H, Appella E, and Donehower LA, The p53-induced oncogenic phosphatase PPM1D interacts with uracil DNA glycosylase and suppresses base excision repair. *Mol Cell*, 2004; 15(4): 621–634.
29. Yamaguchi H, Durell SR, Chatterjee DK, Anderson CW, and Appella E, The Wip1 phosphatase PPM1D dephosphorylates SQ/TQ motifs in checkpoint substrates phosphorylated by PI3K-like kinases. *Biochemistry*, 2007; 46(44): 12594–12603.
30. Lu X, Nguyen TA, Moon SH, Darlington Y, Sommer M, and Donehower LA, The type 2C phosphatase Wip1: An oncogenic regulator of tumor suppressor and DNA damage response pathways. *Cancer Metastasis Rev*, 2008; 27(2): 123–135.
31. Chuman Y, Yagi H, Fukuda T, Nomura T, Matsukizono M, Shimohigashi Y, and Sakaguchi K, Characterization of the active site and a unique uncompetitive inhibitor of the PPM1-type protein phosphatase PPM1D. *Protein Pept Lett*, 2008; 15(9): 938–948.
32. Yamaguchi H, Minopoli G, Demidov ON, Chatterjee DK, Anderson CW, Durell SR, and Appella E, Substrate specificity of the human protein phosphatase 2Cdelta, Wip1. *Biochemistry*, 2005; 44(14): 5285–5294.

33. Lu X, Ma O, Nguyen TA, Jones SN, Oren M, and Donehower LA, The Wip1 Phosphatase acts as a gatekeeper in the p53-Mdm2 autoregulatory loop. *Cancer Cell*, 2007; 12(4): 342–354.
34. Choi J, Appella E, and Donehower LA, The structure and expression of the murine wildtype p53-induced phosphatase 1 (Wip1) gene. *Genomics*, 2000; 64(3): 298–306.
35. Capasso H, Palermo C, Wan S, Rao H, John UP, O'Connell MJ, and Walworth NC, Phosphorylation activates Chk1 and is required for checkpoint-mediated cell cycle arrest. *J Cell Sci*, 2002; 115(Pt 23): 4555–4564.
36. Lu X, Nguyen TA, and Donehower LA, Reversal of the ATM/ATR-mediated DNA damage response by the oncogenic phosphatase PPM1D. *Cell Cycle*, 2005; 4(8): 1060–1064.
37. Bulavin DV, Demidov ON, Saito S, Kauraniemi P, Phillips C, Amundson SA, Ambrosino C et al., Amplification of PPM1D in human tumors abrogates p53 tumor-suppressor activity. *Nat Genet*, 2002; 31(2): 210–215.
38. Rauta J, Alarmo EL, Kauraniemi P, Karhu R, Kuukasjarvi T, and Kallioniemi A, The serine-threonine protein phosphatase PPM1D is frequently activated through amplification in aggressive primary breast tumours. *Breast Cancer Res Treat*, 2006; 95(3): 257–263.
39. Lu X, Nguyen TA, Zhang X, and Donehower LA, The Wip1 phosphatase and Mdm2: Cracking the "Wip" on p53 stability. *Cell Cycle*, 2008; 7(2): 164–168.
40. Zhang X, Lin L, Guo H, Yang J, Jones SN, Jochemsen A, and Lu X, Phosphorylation and degradation of MdmX is inhibited by Wip1 phosphatase in the DNA damage response. *Cancer Res*, 2009; 69(20): 7960–7968.
41. Lowe JM, Cha H, Yang Q, and Fornace AJ, Jr., Nuclear factor-kappaB (NF-kappaB) is a novel positive transcriptional regulator of the oncogenic Wip1 phosphatase. *J Biol Chem*, 2010; 285(8): 5249–5257.
42. Hershko T, Korotayev K, Polager S, and Ginsberg D, E2F1 modulates p38 MAPK phosphorylation via transcriptional regulation of ASK1 and Wip1. *J Biol Chem*, 2006; 281(42): 31309–31316.
43. Rossi M, Demidov ON, Anderson CW, Appella E, and Mazur SJ, Induction of PPM1D following DNA-damaging treatments through a conserved p53 response element coincides with a shift in the use of transcription initiation sites. *Nucleic Acids Res*, 2008; 36(22): 7168–7180.
44. Han HS, Yu E, Song JY, Park JY, Jang SJ, and Choi J, The estrogen receptor alpha pathway induces oncogenic Wip1 phosphatase gene expression. *Mol Cancer Res*, 2009; 7(5): 713–723.
45. Song JY, Han HS, Sabapathy K, Lee BM, Yu E, and Choi J, Expression of a homeostatic regulator, Wip1 (wild-type p53-induced phosphatase), is temporally induced by c-Jun and p53 in response to UV irradiation. *J Biol Chem*, 2010; 285(12): 9067–9076.
46. Chuman Y, Kurihashi W, Mizukami Y, Nashimoto T, Yagi H, and Sakaguchi K, PPM1D430, a novel alternative splicing variant of the human PPM1D, can dephosphorylate p53 and exhibits specific tissue expression. *J Biochem*, 2009; 145(1): 1–12.
47. Park HK, Panneerselvam J, Dudimah FD, Dong G, Sebastian S, Zhang J, and Fei P, Wip1 contributes to cell homeostasis maintained by the steady-state level of Wtp53. *Cell Cycle*, 2011; 10(15): 2574–2582.
48. Zhang J and Chen X, Novel role of Wip1 in p53-mediated cell homeostasis under non-stress conditions. *Cell Cycle*, 2011; 10(19): 3235.
49. Zhu YH and Bulavin DV, Wip1-dependent signaling pathways in health and diseases. *Prog Mol Biol Transl Sci*, 2012; 106: 307–325.
50. Zhu YH, Zhang CW, Lu L, Demidov ON, Sun L, Yang L, Bulavin DV, and Xiao ZC, Wip1 regulates the generation of new neural cells in the adult olfactory bulb through p53-dependent cell cycle control. *Stem Cells*, 2009; 27(6): 1433–1442.

51. Lambros MB, Natrajan R, Geyer FC, Lopez-Garcia MA, Dedes KJ, Savage K, Lacroix-Triki M et al., PPM1D gene amplification and overexpression in breast cancer: A qRT-PCR and chromogenic in situ hybridization study. *Mod Pathol*, 2010; 23(10): 1334–1345.
52. Satoh N, Maniwa Y, Bermudez VP, Nishimura K, Nishio W, Yoshimura M, Okita Y, Ohbayashi C, Hurwitz J, and Hayashi Y, Oncogenic phosphatase Wip1 is a novel prognostic marker for lung adenocarcinoma patient survival. *Cancer Sci*, 2011; 102(5): 1101–1106.
53. Wang P, Rao J, Yang H, Zhao H, and Yang L, Wip1 over-expression correlated with TP53/p14(ARF) pathway disruption in human astrocytomas. *J Surg Oncol*, 2011; 104(6): 679–684.
54. Li J, Yang Y, Peng Y, Austin RJ, van Eyndhoven WG, Nguyen KC, Gabriele T et al., Oncogenic properties of PPM1D located within a breast cancer amplification epicenter at 17q23. *Nat Genet*, 2002; 31(2): 133–134.
55. Hirasawa A, Saito-Ohara F, Inoue J, Aoki D, Susumu N, Yokoyama T, Nozawa S, Inazawa J, and Imoto I, Association of 17q21-q24 gain in ovarian clear cell adenocarcinomas with poor prognosis and identification of PPM1D and APPBP2 as likely amplification targets. *Clin Cancer Res*, 2003; 9(6): 1995–2004.
56. Saito-Ohara F, Imoto I, Inoue J, Hosoi H, Nakagawara A, Sugimoto T, and Inazawa J, PPM1D is a potential target for 17q gain in neuroblastoma. *Cancer Res*, 2003; 63(8): 1876–1883.
57. Fuku T, Semba S, Yutori H, and Yokozaki H, Increased wild-type p53-induced phosphatase 1 (Wip1 or PPM1D) expression correlated with downregulation of checkpoint kinase 2 in human gastric carcinoma. *Pathol Int*, 2007; 57(9): 566–571.
58. Castellino RC, De Bortoli M, Lu X, Moon SH, Nguyen TA, Shepard MA, Rao PH, Donehower LA, and Kim JY, Medulloblastomas overexpress the p53-inactivating oncogene WIP1/PPM1D. *J Neurooncol*, 2008; 86(3): 245–256.
59. Tan DS, Lambros MB, Rayter S, Natrajan R, Vatcheva R, Gao Q, Marchio C et al., PPM1D is a potential therapeutic target in ovarian clear cell carcinomas. *Clin Cancer Res*, 2009; 15(7): 2269–2280.
60. Shreeram S, Demidov ON, Hee WK, Yamaguchi H, Onishi N, Kek C, Timofeev ON et al., Wip1 phosphatase modulates ATM-dependent signaling pathways. *Mol Cell*, 2006; 23(5): 757–764.
61. Shreeram S, Hee WK, Demidov ON, Kek C, Yamaguchi H, Fornace AJ, Jr., Anderson CW, Appella E, and Bulavin DV, Regulation of ATM/p53-dependent suppression of myc-induced lymphomas by Wip1 phosphatase. *J Exp Med*, 2006; 203(13): 2793–2799.
62. Lu X, Nannenga B, and Donehower LA, PPM1D dephosphorylates Chk1 and p53 and abrogates cell cycle checkpoints. *Genes Dev*, 2005; 19(10): 1162–1174.
63. Fujimoto H et al., Regulation of the antioncogenic Chk2 kinase by the oncogenic Wip1 phosphatase. *Cell Death Differ*, 2006; 13(7): 1170–1180.
64. Yoda A, Xu XZ, Onishi N, Toyoshima K, Fujimoto H, Kato N, Oishi I, Kondo T, and Minami Y, Intrinsic kinase activity and SQ/TQ domain of Chk2 kinase as well as N-terminal domain of Wip1 phosphatase are required for regulation of Chk2 by Wip1. *J Biol Chem*, 2006; 281(34): 24847–24862.
65. Yoda A, Toyoshima K, Watanabe Y, Onishi N, Hazaka Y, Tsukuda Y, Tsukada J, Kondo T, Tanaka Y, and Minami Y, Arsenic trioxide augments Chk2/p53-mediated apoptosis by inhibiting oncogenic Wip1 phosphatase. *J Biol Chem*, 2008; 283(27): 18969–18979.
66. Carlessi L, Buscemi G, Fontanella E, and Delia D, A protein phosphatase feedback mechanism regulates the basal phosphorylation of Chk2 kinase in the absence of DNA damage. *Biochim Biophys Acta*, 2010; 1803(10): 1213–1223.
67. Pei D, Zhang Y, and Zheng J, Regulation of p53: A collaboration between Mdm2 and Mdmx. *Oncotarget*, 2012; 3(3): 228–235.

68. Bulavin DV, Phillips C, Nannenga B, Timofeev O, Donehower LA, Anderson CW, Appella E, and Fornace AJ, Jr., Inactivation of the Wip1 phosphatase inhibits mammary tumorigenesis through p38 MAPK-mediated activation of the p16(Ink4a)-p19(Arf) pathway. *Nat Genet*, 2004; 36(4): 343–350.
69. Takekawa M, Adachi M, Nakahata A, Nakayama I, Itoh F, Tsukuda H, Taya Y, and Imai K, p53-inducible wip1 phosphatase mediates a negative feedback regulation of p38 MAPK-p53 signaling in response to UV radiation. *EMBO J*, 2000; 19(23): 6517–6526.
70. Nguyen TA, Slattery SD, Moon SH, Darlington YF, Lu X, and Donehower LA, The oncogenic phosphatase WIP1 negatively regulates nucleotide excision repair. *DNA Repair*, 2010; 9(7): 813–823.
71. Oh KS, Bustin, M, Mazur, SJ, Appella, E, Kraemer, KH, UV-induced histone H2AX phosphorylation and DNA damage related proteins accumulate and persist in nucleotide excision repair-deficient XP-B cells. *DNA Repair*, 2011; 10(1): 5–15.
72. Abedini MR, Qiu Q, Yan X, and Tsang BK, Possible role of FLICE-like inhibitory protein (FLIP) in chemoresistant ovarian cancer cells in vitro. *Oncogene*, 2004; 23(42): 6997–7004.
73. Irmler M, Thome M, Hahne M, Schneider P, Hofmann K, Steiner V, Bodmer JL et al., Inhibition of death receptor signals by cellular FLIP. *Nature*, 1997; 388(6638): 190–195.
74. Micheau O, Thome M, Schneider P, Holler N, Tschopp J, Nicholson DW, Briand C, and Grutter MG, The long form of FLIP is an activator of caspase-8 at the Fas death-inducing signaling complex. *J Biol Chem*, 2002; 277(47): 45162–45171.
75. Mihara M, Erster S, Zaika A, Petrenko O, Chittenden T, Pancoska P, and Moll UM, p53 has a direct apoptogenic role at the mitochondria. *Mol Cell*, 2003; 11(3): 577–590.
76. Mihara M and Moll UM, Detection of mitochondrial localization of p53. *Methods Mol Biol*, 2003; 234: 203–209.
77. Dai C and Gu W, p53 post-translational modification: Deregulated in tumorigenesis. *Trends Mol Med*, 2010; 16(11): 528–536.
78. Li M, Chen D, Shiloh A, Luo J, Nikolaev AY, Qin J, and Gu W, Deubiquitination of p53 by HAUSP is an important pathway for p53 stabilization. *Nature*, 2002; 416(6881): 648–653.
79. Song MS, Song SJ, Kim SY, Oh HJ, and Lim DS, The tumour suppressor RASSF1A promotes MDM2 self-ubiquitination by disrupting the MDM2-DAXX-HAUSP complex. *EMBO J*, 2008; 27(13): 1863–1874.
80. Yuan J, Luo K, Zhang L, Cheville JC, and Lou Z, USP10 regulates p53 localization and stability by deubiquitinating p53. *Cell*, 2010; 140(3): 384–396.
81. Nikolaev AY, Li M, Puskas N, Qin J, and Gu W, Parc: A cytoplasmic anchor for p53. *Cell*, 2003; 112(1): 29–40.
82. Nikolaev AY and Gu W, PARC: A potential target for cancer therapy. *Cell Cycle*, 2003; 2(3): 169–171.
83. Mulhall JP, Barnas J, Kobylarz K, and Mueller A, p53-Associated Parkin-like cytoplasmic protein (Parc) short-interfering RNA (siRNA) alters p53 location and biology of Peyronie's disease fibroblasts. *BJU Int*, 2010; 106(11): 1706–1713.
84. Chipuk JE and Green DR, How do BCL-2 proteins induce mitochondrial outer membrane permeabilization? *Trends Cell Biol*, 2008; 18(4): 157–164.
85. Chipuk JE, Fisher JC, Dillon CP, Kriwacki RW, Kuwana T, and Green DR, Mechanism of apoptosis induction by inhibition of the anti-apoptotic BCL-2 proteins. *Proc Natl Acad Sci USA*, 2008; 105(51): 20327–20332.
86. Vaseva AV, Marchenko ND, Ji K, Tsirka SE, Holzmann S, and Moll UM, p53 opens the mitochondrial permeability transition pore to trigger necrosis. *Cell*, 2012; 149(7): 1536–1548.

87. Tomita Y, Marchenko N, Erster S, Nemajerova A, Dehner A, Klein C, Pan H, Kessler H, Pancoska P, and Moll UM, WT p53, but not tumor-derived mutants, bind to Bcl2 via the DNA binding domain and induce mitochondrial permeabilization. *J Biol Chem*, 2006; 281(13): 8600–8606.
88. Cregan SP, Fortin A, MacLaurin JG, Callaghan SM, Cecconi F, Yu SW, Dawson TM, Dawson VL, Park DS, Kroemer G, and Slack RS, Apoptosis-inducing factor is involved in the regulation of caspase-independent neuronal cell death. *J Cell Biol*, 2002; 158(3): 507–517.
89. Fraser M, Chan SL, Chan SS, Fiscus RR, and Tsang BK, Regulation of p53 and suppression of apoptosis by the soluble guanylyl cyclase/cGMP pathway in human ovarian cancer cells. *Oncogene*, 2006; 25(15): 2203–2212.
90. Leung EL, Fraser M, Fiscus RR, and Tsang BK, Cisplatin alters nitric oxide synthase levels in human ovarian cancer cells: Involvement in p53 regulation and cisplatin resistance. *Br J Cancer*, 2008; 98(11): 1803–1809.
91. Leung EL, Wong JC, Johlfs MG, Tsang BK, and Fiscus RR, Protein kinase G type Ialpha activity in human ovarian cancer cells significantly contributes to enhanced Src activation and DNA synthesis/cell proliferation. *Mol Cancer Res*, 2010; 8(4): 578–591.
92. Beckman JS and Koppenol WH, Nitric oxide, superoxide, and peroxynitrite: The good, the bad, and ugly. *Am J Physiol*, 1996; 271(5 Pt 1): C1424–1437.
93. Bellamy TC, Griffiths C, and Garthwaite J, Differential sensitivity of guanylyl cyclase and mitochondrial respiration to nitric oxide measured using clamped concentrations. *J Biol Chem*, 2002; 277(35): 31801–31807.
94. Ridnour LA, Thomas DD, Switzer C, Flores-Santana W, Isenberg JS, Ambs S, Roberts DD, and Wink DA, Molecular mechanisms for discrete nitric oxide levels in cancer. *Nitric Oxide*, 2008; 19(2): 73–76.
95. Cheng Chew SB, Leung PY, and Fiscus RR, Preincubation with atrial natriuretic peptide protects NG108–15 cells against the toxic/proapoptotic effects of the nitric oxide donor S-nitroso- N-acetylpenicillamine. *Histochem Cell Biol*, 2003; 120(3): 163–171.
96. Fiscus RR, Involvement of cyclic GMP and protein kinase G in the regulation of apoptosis and survival in neural cells. *Neurosignals*, 2002; 11(4): 175–190.
97. Fiscus RR, Lu L, Tu AW, Hao H, Yang L, and Wang X, Brain natriuretic peptide enhances the endothelium-independent cAMP and vasorelaxant responses of calcitonin gene-related peptide in rat aorta. *Neuropeptides*, 1998; 32(6): 499–509.
98. Johlfs MG and Fiscus RR, Protein kinase G type-Ialpha phosphorylates the apoptosis-regulating protein Bad at serine 155 and protects against apoptosis in N1E-115 cells. *Neurochem Int*, 2010; 56(4): 546–553.
99. Thompson WJ, Piazza GA, Li H, Liu L, Fetter J, Zhu B, Sperl G, Ahnen D, and Pamukcu R, Exisulind induction of apoptosis involves guanosine 3′,5′-cyclic monophosphate phosphodiesterase inhibition, protein kinase G activation, and attenuated beta-catenin. *Cancer Res*, 2000; 60(13): 3338–3342.
100. Fiscus RR, Rapoport RM, and Murad F, Endothelium-dependent and nitrovasodilator-induced activation of cyclic GMP-dependent protein kinase in rat aorta. *J Cyclic Nucleotide Protein Phosphor Res*, 1983; 9(6): 415–425.
101. Fiscus RR, Yuen JP, Chan SL, Kwong JH, and Chew SB, Nitric oxide and cyclic GMP as pro- and anti-apoptotic agents. *J Card Surg*, 2002; 17(4): 336–339.
102. LaFevre-Bernt M, Corbin JD, Francis SH, and Miller WT, Phosphorylation and activation of cGMP-dependent protein kinase by Src. *Biochim Biophys Acta*, 1998; 1386(1): 97–105.
103. Wong JC and Fiscus RR, Protein kinase G activity prevents pathological-level nitric oxide-induced apoptosis and promotes DNA synthesis/cell proliferation in vascular smooth muscle cells. *Cardiovasc Pathol*, 2010; 19(6): e221–231.

104. Wong JC and Fiscus RR, Essential roles of the nitric oxide (no)/cGMP/protein kinase G type-Ialpha (PKG-Ialpha) signaling pathway and the atrial natriuretic peptide (ANP)/cGMP/PKG-Ialpha autocrine loop in promoting proliferation and cell survival of OP9 bone marrow stromal cells. *J Cell Biochem*, 2011; 112(3): 829–839.
105. Fraser M, Leung B, Jahani-Asl A, Yan X, Thompson WE, and Tsang BK, Chemoresistance in human ovarian cancer: The role of apoptotic regulators. *Reprod Biol Endocrinol*, 2003; 1: 66.
106. Hu P, Mondino A, Skolnik EY, and Schlessinger J, Cloning of a novel, ubiquitously expressed human phosphatidylinositol 3-kinase and identification of its binding site on p85. *Mol Cell Biol*, 1993; 13(12): 7677–7688.
107. West KA, Castillo SS, and Dennis PA, Activation of the PI3K/Akt pathway and chemotherapeutic resistance. *Drug Resist Updat*, 2002; 5(6): 234–248.
108. Datta SR, Brunet A, and Greenberg ME, Cellular survival: A play in three Akts. *Genes Dev*, 1999; 13(22): 2905–2927.
109. Shirai T, Tanaka K, Terada Y, Sawada T, Shirai R, Hashimoto Y, Nagata S et al., Specific detection of phosphatidylinositol 3,4,5-trisphosphate binding proteins by the PIP3 analogue beads: An application for rapid purification of the PIP3 binding proteins. *Biochim Biophys Acta*, 1998; 1402(3): 292–302.
110. Alessi DR, James SR, Downes CP, Holmes AB, Gaffney PR, Reese CB, and Cohen P, Characterization of a 3-phosphoinositide-dependent protein kinase which phosphorylates and activates protein kinase Balpha. *Curr Biol*, 1997; 7(4): 261–269.
111. Alessi DR, Deak M, Casamayor A, Caudwell FB, Morrice N, Norman DG, Gaffney P et al., 3-Phosphoinositide-dependent protein kinase-1 (PDK1): Structural and functional homology with the Drosophila DSTPK61 kinase. *Curr Biol*, 1997; 7(10): 776–789.
112. Sarbassov DD, Ali SM, Sengupta S, Sheen JH, Hsu PP, Bagley AF, Markhard AL, and Sabatini DM, Prolonged rapamycin treatment inhibits mTORC2 assembly and Akt/PKB. *Mol Cell*, 2006; 22(2): 159–168.
113. Jacinto E, Facchinetti V, Liu D, Soto N, Wei S, Jung SY, Huang Q, Qin J, and Su B, SIN1/MIP1 maintains rictor-mTOR complex integrity and regulates Akt phosphorylation and substrate specificity. *Cell*, 2006; 127(1): 125–137.
114. Zhou BP, Liao Y, Xia W, Zou Y, Spohn B, and Hung MC, HER-2/neu induces p53 ubiquitination via Akt-mediated MDM2 phosphorylation. *Nat Cell Biol*, 2001; 3(11): 973–982.
115. Ogawara Y, Kishishita S, Obata T, Isazawa Y, Suzuki T, Tanaka K, Masuyama N, and Gotoh Y, Akt enhances Mdm2-mediated ubiquitination and degradation of p53. *J Biol Chem*, 2002; 277(24): 21843–21850.
116. Stambolic V, MacPherson D, Sas D, Lin Y, Snow B, Jang Y, Benchimol S, and Mak TW, Regulation of PTEN transcription by p53. *Mol Cell*, 2001; 8(2): 317–325.
117. Mayo LD, Dixon JE, Durden DL, Tonks NK, and Donner DB, PTEN protects p53 from Mdm2 and sensitizes cancer cells to chemotherapy. *J Biol Chem*, 2002; 277(7): 5484–5489.
118. Brunet A, Bonni A, Zigmond MJ, Lin MZ, Juo P, Hu LS, Anderson MJ, Arden KC, Blenis J, and Greenberg ME, Akt promotes cell survival by phosphorylating and inhibiting a Forkhead transcription factor. *Cell*, 1999; 96(6): 857–868.
119. Datta SR, Dudek H, Tao X, Masters S, Fu H, Gotoh Y, and Greenberg ME, Akt phosphorylation of BAD couples survival signals to the cell-intrinsic death machinery. *Cell*, 1997; 91(2): 231–241.
120. Cardone MH, Roy N, Stennicke HR, Salvesen GS, Franke TF, Stanbridge E, Frisch S, and Reed JC, Regulation of cell death protease caspase-9 by phosphorylation. *Science*, 1998; 282(5392): 1318–1321.
121. Dan HC, Sun M, Kaneko S, Feldman RI, Nicosia SV, Wang HG, Tsang BK, and Cheng JQ, Akt phosphorylation and stabilization of X-linked inhibitor of apoptosis protein (XIAP). *J Biol Chem*, 2004; 279(7): 5405–5412.

122. Yang X, Fraser M, Abedini MR, Bai T, and Tsang BK, Regulation of apoptosis-inducing factor-mediated, cisplatin-induced apoptosis by Akt. *Br J Cancer*, 2008; 98(4): 803–808.
123. Kane LP, Shapiro VS, Stokoe D, and Weiss A, Induction of NF-kappaB by the Akt/PKB kinase. *Curr Biol*, 1999; 9(11): 601–604.
124. Romashkova JA and Makarov SS, NF-kappaB is a target of AKT in anti-apoptotic PDGF signalling. *Nature*, 1999; 401(6748): 86–90.
125. Gesbert F, Sellers WR, Signoretti S, Loda M, and Griffin JD, BCR/ABL regulates expression of the cyclin-dependent kinase inhibitor p27Kip1 through the phosphatidylinositol 3-Kinase/AKT pathway. *J Biol Chem*, 2000; 275(50): 39223–39230.
126. Rossig L, Jadidi AS, Urbich C, Badorff C, Zeiher AM, and Dimmeler S, Akt-dependent phosphorylation of p21(Cip1) regulates PCNA binding and proliferation of endothelial cells. *Mol Cell Biol*, 2001; 21(16): 5644–5657.
127. Graff JR, Konicek BW, McNulty AM, Wang Z, Houck K, Allen S, Paul JD, Hbaiu A, Goode RG, Sandusky GE, Vessella RL, and Neubauer BL, Increased AKT activity contributes to prostate cancer progression by dramatically accelerating prostate tumor growth and diminishing p27Kip1 expression. *J Biol Chem*, 2000; 275(32): 24500–24505.
128. King FW, Skeen J, Hay N, and Shtivelman E, Inhibition of Chk1 by activated PKB/Akt. *Cell Cycle*, 2004; 3(5): 634–637.
129. Vivanco I and Sawyers CL, The phosphatidylinositol 3-Kinase AKT pathway in human cancer. *Nat Rev Cancer*, 2002; 2(7): 489–501.
130. Nicholson KM and Anderson NG, The protein kinase B/Akt signalling pathway in human malignancy. *Cell Signal*, 2002; 14(5): 381–395.
131. Testa JR and Bellacosa A, AKT plays a central role in tumorigenesis. *Proc Natl Acad Sci USA*, 2001; 98(20): 10983–10985.
132. Kandel ES and Hay N, The regulation and activities of the multifunctional serine/threonine kinase Akt/PKB. *Exp Cell Res*, 1999; 253(1): 210–229.
133. Cheng JQ, Godwin AK, Bellacosa A, Taguchi T, Franke TF, Hamilton TC, Tsichlis PN, and Testa JR, AKT2, a putative oncogene encoding a member of a subfamily of protein-serine/threonine kinases, is amplified in human ovarian carcinomas. *Proc Natl Acad Sci USA*, 1992; 89(19): 9267–9271.
134. Fraser M, Leung BM, Yan X, Dan HC, Cheng JQ, and Tsang BK, p53 is a determinant of X-linked inhibitor of apoptosis protein/Akt-mediated chemoresistance in human ovarian cancer cells. *Cancer Res*, 2003; 63(21): 7081–7088.
135. Efeyan A and Sabatini DM, mTOR and cancer: Many loops in one pathway. *Curr Opin Cell Biol*, 2010; 22(2): 169–176.
136. Nave BT, Ouwens M, Withers DJ, Alessi DR, and Shepherd PR, Mammalian target of rapamycin is a direct target for protein kinase B: Identification of a convergence point for opposing effects of insulin and amino-acid deficiency on protein translation. *Biochem J*, 1999; 344(Pt 2): 427–431.
137. Guertin DA and Sabatini DM, Defining the role of mTOR in cancer. *Cancer Cell*, 2007; 12(1): 9–22.
138. Bhaskar PT and Hay N, The two TORCs and Akt. *Dev Cell*, 2007; 12(4): 487–502.
139. Zoncu R, Efeyan A, and Sabatini DM, mTOR: From growth signal integration to cancer, diabetes and ageing. *Nat Rev Mol Cell Biol*, 2011; 12(1): 21–35.
140. Memmott RM and Dennis PA, Akt-dependent and -independent mechanisms of mTOR regulation in cancer. *Cell Signal*, 2009; 21(5): 656–664.
141. No JH, Jeon YT, Park IA, Kim YB, Kim JW, Park NH, Kang SB, Han JY, Lim JM, and Song YS, Activation of mTOR signaling pathway associated with adverse prognostic factors of epithelial ovarian cancer. *Gynecol Oncol*, 2011; 121(1): 8–12.
142. Jiang BH and Liu LZ, Role of mTOR in anticancer drug resistance: Perspectives for improved drug treatment. *Drug Resist Updat*, 2008; 11(3): 63–76.

143. Mabuchi S, Altomare DA, Cheung M, Zhang L, Poulikakos PI, Hensley HH, Schilder RJ, Ozols RF, and Testa JR, RAD001 inhibits human ovarian cancer cell proliferation, enhances cisplatin-induced apoptosis, and prolongs survival in an ovarian cancer model. *Clin Cancer Res*, 2007; 13(14): 4261–4270.
144. Mabuchi S, Kawase C, Altomare DA, Morishige K, Sawada K, Hayashi M, Tsujimoto M et al., mTOR is a promising therapeutic target both in cisplatin-sensitive and cisplatin-resistant clear cell carcinoma of the ovary. *Clin Cancer Res*, 2009; 15(17): 5404–5413.
145. Montero JC, Chen X, Ocana A, and Pandiella A, Predominance of mTORC1 over mTORC2 in the regulation of proliferation of ovarian cancer cells: Therapeutic implications. *Mol Cancer Ther*, 2012; 11(6): 1342–1352.
146. Ying X, Meng X, Wang S, Wang D, Li H, Wang B, Du Y, Liu X, Zhang W, and Kang T, Simultaneous determination of three polyphenols in rat plasma after orally administering hawthorn leaves extract by the HPLC method. *Nat Prod Res*, 2012; 26(6): 585–591.
147. Roulin D, Cerantola Y, Dormond-Meuwly A, Demartines N, and Dormond O, Targeting mTORC2 inhibits colon cancer cell proliferation in vitro and tumor formation in vivo. *Mol Cancer*, 2010; 9: 57.
148. Sparks CA and Guertin DA, Targeting mTOR: Prospects for mTOR complex 2 inhibitors in cancer therapy. *Oncogene*, 2010; 29(26): 3733–3744.
149. Nowell PC and Croce CM, Chromosomes, genes, and cancer. *Am J Pathol*, 1986; 125(1): 7–15.
150. Sporn MB, Carcinogenesis and cancer: Different perspectives on the same disease. *Cancer Res*, 1991; 51(23 Pt 1): 6215–6218.
151. Zykova TA, Zhu F, Zhai X, Ma WY, Ermakova SP, Lee KW, Bode AM, and Dong Z, Resveratrol directly targets COX-2 to inhibit carcinogenesis. *Mol Carcinog*, 2008; 47(10): 797–805.
152. Yang S, Irani K, Heffron SE, Jurnak F, and Meyskens FL, Jr., Alterations in the expression of the apurinic/apyrimidinic endonuclease-1/redox factor-1 (APE/Ref-1) in human melanoma and identification of the therapeutic potential of resveratrol as an APE/Ref-1 inhibitor. *Mol Cancer Ther*, 2005; 4(12): 1923–1935.
153. Oi N, Jeong CH, Nadas J, Cho YY, Pugliese A, Bode AM, and Dong Z, Resveratrol, a red wine polyphenol, suppresses pancreatic cancer by inhibiting leukotriene A(4)hydrolase. *Cancer Res*, 2010; 70(23): 9755–9764.
154. Lee KW, Kang NJ, Heo YS, Rogozin EA, Pugliese A, Hwang MK, Bowden GT, Bode AM, Lee HJ, and Dong Z, Raf and MEK protein kinases are direct molecular targets for the chemopreventive effect of quercetin, a major flavonol in red wine. *Cancer Res*, 2008; 68(3): 946–955.
155. Hwang MK, Song NR, Kang NJ, Lee KW, and Lee HJ, Activation of phosphatidylinositol 3-kinase is required for tumor necrosis factor-alpha-induced upregulation of matrix metalloproteinase-9: Its direct inhibition by quercetin. *Int J Biochem Cell Biol*, 2009; 41(7): 1592–1600.
156. Shen SC, Lee WR, Lin HY, Huang HC, Ko CH, Yang LL, and Chen YC, In vitro and in vivo inhibitory activities of rutin, wogonin, and quercetin on lipopolysaccharide-induced nitric oxide and prostaglandin E(2) production. *Eur J Pharmacol*, 2002; 446(1–3): 187–194.
157. Mutoh M, Takahashi M, Fukuda K, Matsushima-Hibiya Y, Mutoh H, Sugimura T, and Wakabayashi K, Suppression of cyclooxygenase-2 promoter-dependent transcriptional activity in colon cancer cells by chemopreventive agents with a resorcin-type structure. *Carcinogenesis*, 2000; 21(5): 959–963.
158. Kang NJ, Shin SH, Lee HJ, and Lee KW, Polyphenols as small molecular inhibitors of signaling cascades in carcinogenesis. *Pharmacol Ther*, 2011; 130(3): 310–324.

159. Jung SK, Lee KW, Byun S, Kang NJ, Lim SH, Heo YS, Bode AM, Bowden GT, Lee HJ, and Dong Z, Myricetin suppresses UVB-induced skin cancer by targeting Fyn. *Cancer Res*, 2008; 68(14): 6021–6029.
160. Jung SK, Lee KW, Byun S, Lee EJ, Kim JE, Bode AM, Dong Z, and Lee HJ, Myricetin inhibits UVB-induced angiogenesis by regulating PI-3 kinase in vivo. *Carcinogenesis*, 2010; 31(5): 911–917.
161. Akiyama T, Ishida J, Nakagawa S, Ogawara H, Watanabe S, Itoh N, Shibuya M, and Fukami Y, Genistein, a specific inhibitor of tyrosine-specific protein kinases. *J Biol Chem*, 1987; 262(12): 5592–5595.
162. Fang MZ, Chen D, Sun Y, Jin Z, Christman JK, and Yang CS, Reversal of hypermethylation and reactivation of p16INK4a, RARbeta, and MGMT genes by genistein and other isoflavones from soy. *Clin Cancer Res*, 2005; 11(19 Pt 1): 7033–7041.
163. Lee DE, Lee KW, Song NR, Seo SK, Heo YS, Kang NJ, Bode AM, Lee HJ, and Dong Z, 7,3′,4′-Trihydroxyisoflavone inhibits epidermal growth factor-induced proliferation and transformation of JB6 P+ mouse epidermal cells by suppressing cyclin-dependent kinases and phosphatidylinositol 3-kinase. *J Biol Chem*, 2010; 285(28): 21458–21466.
164. Kang NJ, Lee KW, Rogozin EA, Cho YY, Heo YS, Bode AM, Lee HJ, and Dong Z, Equol, a metabolite of the soybean isoflavone daidzein, inhibits neoplastic cell transformation by targeting the MEK/ERK/p90RSK/activator protein-1 pathway. *J Biol Chem*, 2007; 282(45): 32856–32866.
165. Byun S, Lee KW, Jung SK, Lee EJ, Hwang MK, Lim SH, Bode AM, Lee HJ, and Dong Z, Luteolin inhibits protein kinase C(epsilon) and c-Src activities and UVB-induced skin cancer. *Cancer Res*, 2010; 70(6): 2415–2423.
166. Kim JE, Son JE, Jang YJ, Lee DE, Kang NJ, Jung SK, Heo YS, Lee KW, and Lee HJ, Luteolin, a novel natural inhibitor of tumor progression locus 2 serine/threonine kinase, inhibits tumor necrosis factor-alpha-induced cyclooxygenase-2 expression in JB6 mouse epidermis cells. *J Pharmacol Exp Ther*, 2011; 338(3): 1013–1022.
167. Henriksen R, Funa K, Wilander E, Backstrom T, Ridderheim M, and Oberg K, Expression and prognostic significance of platelet-derived growth factor and its receptors in epithelial ovarian neoplasms. *Cancer Res*, 1993; 53(19): 4550–4554.
168. Walker EH, Pacold ME, Perisic O, Stephens L, Hawkins PT, Wymann MP, and Williams RL, Structural determinants of phosphoinositide 3-kinase inhibition by wortmannin, LY294002, quercetin, myricetin, and staurosporine. *Mol Cell*, 2000; 6(4): 909–919.
169. Arafa el SA, Zhu Q, Barakat BM, Wani G, Zhao Q, El-Mahdy MA, and Wani AA, Tangeretin sensitizes cisplatin-resistant human ovarian cancer cells through downregulation of phosphoinositide 3-kinase/Akt signaling pathway. *Cancer Res*, 2009; 69(23): 8910–8917.
170. Gudmundsdottir K and Ashworth A, The roles of BRCA1 and BRCA2 and associated proteins in the maintenance of genomic stability. *Oncogene*, 2006; 25(43): 5864–5874.
171. Siddiqui IA, Malik A, Adhami VM, Asim M, Hafeez BB, Sarfaraz S, and Mukhtar H, Green tea polyphenol EGCG sensitizes human prostate carcinoma LNCaP cells to TRAIL-mediated apoptosis and synergistically inhibits biomarkers associated with angiogenesis and metastasis. *Oncogene*, 2008; 27(14): 2055–2063.
172. Luo H, Jiang BH, King SM, and Chen YC, Inhibition of cell growth and VEGF expression in ovarian cancer cells by flavonoids. *Nutr Cancer*, 2008; 60(6): 800–809.
173. Brakenhielm E, Cao R, and Cao Y, Suppression of angiogenesis, tumor growth, and wound healing by resveratrol, a natural compound in red wine and grapes. *FASEB J*, 2001; 15(10): 1798–800.
174. Rezk YA, Balulad SS, Keller RS, and Bennett JA, Use of resveratrol to improve the effectiveness of cisplatin and doxorubicin: Study in human gynecologic cancer cell lines and in rodent heart. *Am J Obstet Gynecol*, 2006; 194(5): e23–26.

175. Opipari AW, Jr., Tan L, Boitano AE, Sorenson DR, Aurora A, and Liu JR, Resveratrol-induced autophagocytosis in ovarian cancer cells. *Cancer Res*, 2004; 64(2): 696–703.
176. Larrosa M, Tomas-Barberan FA, and Espin JC, The grape and wine polyphenol piceatannol is a potent inducer of apoptosis in human SK-Mel-28 melanoma cells. *Eur J Nutr*, 2004; 43(5): 275–284.
177. Raj L, Ide T, Gurkar AU, Foley M, Schenone M, Li X, Tolliday NJ et al., Selective killing of cancer cells by a small molecule targeting the stress response to ROS. *Nature*, 2011; 475(7355): 231–234.

14 Ovarian Cancer
A Bioepidemiological Approach

Kathryn Coe, Lisa M. Hess, and G. Marie Swanson

CONTENTS

14.1 INTRODUCTION

Ovarian cancer is the ninth most common cancer among women in the United States, but is the leading cause of gynecologic cancer-related death. Approximately 1 woman in every 72 women in the United States will be diagnosed with ovarian cancer during her lifetime, and a woman's risk of death from ovarian cancer is 1 in 95 (Howlader et al., 2012). In 2012, 22,280 U.S. women were diagnosed with ovarian cancer and 15,500 died from this disease (Siegel et al., 2012). The prognosis of advanced ovarian cancer is poor; however, 5-year survival rates from early-stage disease are greater than 90%. The majority of women diagnosed with ovarian cancer (more than 75%) have advanced stage disease (stage III–IV), which has less than 30% 5-year survival rate (Howlader et al., 2012).

Ovarian cancer was previously thought to be a silent killer; however, key symptoms have been identified that are associated with an undetected ovarian cancer. Unfortunately, these symptoms are nonspecific and despite an increased knowledge of the symptomology of early and advanced ovarian cancer, this has not translated to early diagnosis or to improved survival outcomes (Nagle et al., 2011). Survival is influenced by a number of prognostic factors, including disease stage and grade at diagnosis, residual disease following primary debulking surgery, and overall quality of life at diagnosis (Holschneider and Berek, 2000).

The factors associated with an increased risk of ovarian cancer diagnosis include nulliparity; age over 55 years; family history of ovarian cancer; genetic factors such as BRCA1/2 mutations; Lynch syndrome or hereditary nonpolyposis colorectal cancer (HNPCC syndrome); a personal history of breast, colorectal, or uterine cancer; and endometriosis. Protective factors include multiparity, tubal ligation, hysterectomy, and oral contraceptive use (Holschneider and Berek, 2000).

14.2 CARCINOGENESIS

Ovarian cancers comprise a very heterogeneous set of malignancies that affect the ovaries. These malignancies are categorized by cell type (e.g., epithelial, germ, or stromal cell cancers). More than 90% of all ovarian cancer diagnoses are epithelial cell cancers, which are the most likely cell type to become malignant and lead to premature mortality (Jelovac and Armstrong, 2011). Epithelial cancers are far from homogenous and encompass a variety of serous, endometrioid, mucinous, squamous, and clear cell types, as well as other mixed or undifferentiated forms, all of which have very different epidemiology, biology, cytogenetic features, outcomes, as well as distinct clinical patterns of growth and response to treatment (Karst and Drapkin, 2010). Serous carcinomas are the most common cell type of all ovarian cancer diagnoses, accounting for about 75% of all spontaneous epithelial ovarian cancers and practically all cancers associated with a germline BRCA mutation. Women with inherited BRCA mutations represent 10% of all serous epithelial ovarian cancer diagnoses, but few spontaneous ovarian cancers are associated with a somatic inactivation of BRCA (Merajver et al., 1995).

This complexity and heterogeneity are reflected in the vast array of abnormalities that have been identified to explain ovarian cancer carcinogenesis in various subsets of patients, including oncogene amplification, loss of heterozygosity, silencing of various tumor suppressor genes, hypermethylation, defects in mismatch repair, and microsatellite instability (Lalwani et al., 2011; Landen et al., 2008; Ricciardelli and Oehler, 2009). The cytogenetic complexity and multiple potential molecular abnormalities across the spectrum of ovarian cancers are not only daunting but also potentially represent a malignancy that one day may benefit from advances in personalized medicine and individualized therapy (Clouser et al., 2009). The development of molecularly targeted therapies has been challenged to date due to the lack of a common genetic or molecular pathway of carcinogenesis (Ricciardelli and Oehler, 2009).

This extreme heterogeneity among ovarian cancers has been a challenging barrier for researchers focusing on early detection and treatment of ovarian cancer. For many years, the ovarian surface epithelium was considered the cell of cancer initiation and development, yet no precancerous lesion has yet been identified. Since that time, it is now believed that most ovarian cancers originate from the fallopian tube (Salvador et al., 2009). Unlike many other cancers that follow a multistep progression to reach metastatic disease, ovarian cancers (particularly serous epithelial ovarian cancers) do not appear to follow this stepwise progression model and appear to be a class among themselves with regard to the various pathways to carcinogenesis.

More recently, scientists have found, similar to other zones of epithelial transition, that ovarian surface epithelium and the epithelial cells of the fimbriae may encompass a zone that is incompletely determined, that is, these epithelial cells represent an area of transition, where there is no clear or distinct line of differentiation from one epithelium to the other despite clear morphologic differences between the fallopian fimbriae and the ovary (Auersperg, 2010). These transitional zones are associated with a propensity for cancer development and progression in other regions of the body, such as the cervix. This is of important prognostic value, as well as having implications for prevention and early detection strategies. While these areas of epithelium may be considered a transitional zone, the fallopian tube is associated with serous tumors whereas the ovarian surface epithelium has the capacity to differentiate and follow many different pathways (Auersperg, 2010).

In the mid-2000s, two classes of ovarian cancer were proposed (type I and type II). Instead of categorizing tumors by histology or stage at diagnosis, they instead were organized into the more benign-behaving cancers (type I) and those tumors that are most likely to metastasize (type II). Type I tumors include those with low-grade features and slow growth (e.g., endometrioid, mucinous, low-grade serous tumors), whereas type II tumors are likely to rapidly progress, are high grade, and almost always serous. Increasing evidence supports the theory that type I ovarian cancers (e.g., low-grade serous, borderline, or mucinous tumors) originate in the ovarian surface epithelium, whereas type II ovarian cancers (e.g., most high-grade serous tumors) originate in the fimbrial epithelium of the fallopian tube.

Ovarian tumors are more likely to be diagnosed in advanced stages even if detected early, as it is not likely for any tumor to be confined to the ovary (i.e., stage I) when originating in the fallopian tube, which is already exterior to the ovary and where cells can easily include the peritoneum. The anatomical location of the cell of origin alone predisposes these cancers to be advanced due to the current staging systems, even if of relatively minimal volume (Karst and Drapkin, 2010). Therefore, early detection of the majority of type II ovarian cancers at a nonadvanced stage would likely be an impossibility, given that early and advanced disease are thought to be two separate and largely unique entities under these assumptions. Therefore, advanced cancer is hypothesized to be not simply due to progression of early disease but to be a separate type of ovarian cancer, biologically and otherwise.

14.3 DESCRIPTIVE EPIDEMIOLOGY OF CANCERS OF THE OVARY

Global incidence: Cancer incidence data from across the world are collected and reported by the World Health Organization and the International Association for Cancer Research. Incidence rates of cancers of the ovary vary considerably across the globe. The highest incidence rates occur in the United States and Europe (10.0–13.6 per 100,000 women). The lowest rates are seen among women in Africa and Asia (rates are particularly low in Algeria, Tunisia, Canada, and China) ranging from 2.1 to 4.8 per 100,000 women. Global variation, to some extent, is a result of true differences in incidence as well as variations in complete and accurate reporting of all newly diagnosed cases.

TABLE 14.1
Age-Adjusted Incidence and Mortality Rates of Ovarian Cancer by Race/Ethnicity in the United States, 2005–2009

Race	Incidence per 100,000	Mortality per 100,000
All races	12.7	8.2
White	13.4	8.6
Black/African American	9.8	6.8
Hispanic/Latina	11.3	5.9
Asian/Pacific Islander	9.8	5.0
American Indian/ Alaskan Native	11.2	6.8

Source: Howlader, N. et al. (eds), *SEER Cancer Statistics Review, 1975–2009*, Vintage 2009 Populations, Bethesda, MD, National Cancer Institute, http://seer.cancer.gov/csr/1975_2009_pops09/, based on November 2011 SEER data submission, posted to the SEER web site, 2012.

Incidence and mortality in the United States: As shown in Table 14.1, age-adjusted incidence of ovarian cancer varies by race/ethnicity in the United States. The highest rate occurs among White women and the lowest among Asian, Pacific Islander women.

Hispanic/Latina, American Indian, and African American women have a lower incidence of ovarian cancer than White women, which is also associated with a lower mortality rate (Howlader et al., 2012). The difference in incidence rates among racial/ethnic groups can be at least partially explained by reproductive histories, discussed in the next section, which in turn are influenced by culture.

In Table 14.2, time trends are shown for incidence and mortality in the United States. Incidence over time has declined about 6% for women younger than 65 and about 11% for those 65 and older. Overall, 5-year mortality has declined by about 20%. This is largely due to advancements in chemotherapeutic regimens that have prolonged the time that women live with their cancers and is not associated with any improvement in cure rates (Huang et al., 2008). Among women younger than 65, death due to ovarian cancer declined by about 45%, while among women 65 and older, there is an overall increase of about 6%.

As Table 14.2 shows, ovarian cancer incidence and mortality increase with age. The incidence rates are 3.2 per 100,000 for women aged 30–34; 9.0 per 100,000 for women aged 40–44; 21.1 per 100,000 for women aged 50–54; 34.0 per 100,000 for women aged 60–64; 45.7 per 100,000 for women aged 70–74; and 53.3 per 100,000 for women aged 80–84. Age-specific death rates for ovarian cancer have a similar pattern (SEER, 2011).

TABLE 14.2
Trends in Age-Adjusted Incidence and Mortality

Year of Diagnosis	All Ages	<65	65+
A. Incidence per 100,000			
1975	16.3	11.6	48.9
1988	15.3	9.6	54.7
1998	14.3	8.8	52.4
2009	12.7	7.9	46.0
B. Mortality per 100,000			
1975	9.9	5.8	37.6
1988	9.3	4.4	43.2
1998	8.7	3.7	43.6
2009	7.8	3.2	40.1

Source: SEER, http://seer.cancer.gov/csr/1975_2009_pops09/index.html, (accessed October 4, 2012), 2011.

TABLE 14.3
Five-Year Relative Survival Rate (%) by Age, Extent of Disease at Diagnosis, and Race Cancer of the Ovary, the United States, SEER Program 2002–2008

Extent of Disease at Diagnosis	All	Age <65		Age 65+	
		Black	White	Black	White
All	43.7	46.1	56.4	20.1	27.8
Localized	91.5	90.2	92.8	80.4	87.4
Regional	71.9	64.1	80.3	37.2	57.4
Distant	26.9	24.6	35.7	11.7	19.1

Survival in the United States: Ovarian cancer 5-year relative survival has improved over time, with the current (2002–2008) survival at 43.2% compared to 36.1% in 1975–1977. As shown in Table 14.3, 5-year relative survival declines as stage of disease at diagnosis is more advanced. At the same time, trends within age groups for White and Black women show that Black women have lower survival for each stage of disease at diagnosis within each age group. For Black women diagnosed with regional or distant ovarian cancer, survival is considerably lower than that observed among White women.

14.4 ANALYTIC EPIDEMIOLOGY OF CANCERS OF THE OVARY

14.4.1 Genetics and Family History

Approximately 10% of all ovarian cancers are associated with family history and inherited genetic factors, such as BRCA mutations (Claus et al., 1996). Family history of the disease is suspected if two or more first- or second-degree relatives have been diagnosed with ovarian cancer before age 50. As with other cancers, family history of cancer of the ovary also increases lifetime risk to about 5%–7% (Salehi et al., 2008). Women with a family history of ovarian cancer tend to be diagnosed with advanced serous epithelial cancers, the most common ovarian cancer.

Considerable research today is focused on the molecular epidemiology of cancers of the ovary, including hereditary mutations in BRCA1 and BRCA2, which are genes that normally work together to prevent breast and ovarian cancer. In some cases, however, a woman (or man) inherits a mutated or altered form of BRCA1 or BRCA2, and these mutations interfere with the normal activity of the gene, thus making these individuals more susceptible to both breast and ovarian cancer. There is a 50% chance that these mutations are passed on to offspring.

Studies focusing on genetics assess the general risk of women who carry a BRCA mutation, as well as the risk among selected subsets of women. Women of Ashkenazi Jewish ancestry, because they are more likely to have inherited and to carry a mutation in BRCA1 or BRCA2, are reported to be at greater risk of ovarian cancer (Daly and Obrams, 1998; Koifman and Koifman, 2001; Steinberg et al., 1998). Studies of two specific forms of the BRCA1 mutation found that among Ashkenazi Jewish women the prevalence of the BRCA1/2 mutation was approximately 1 in 40, while the overall prevalence of the mutation in the general population is estimated to be from 1 in 400 to 1 in 800 (Petrucelli et al., 2010). Antoniou et al. (2003), who pooled pedigree data from 22 population-based studies that were unselected for family history, found that the average risk of developing ovarian cancer among women with these mutations was 39% (95% CI: 18%–54%). Petrucelli et al. (2010), however, found that there is no exact risk estimate that can be applied to all individuals with these mutations.

14.4.2 Age and Fertility

Early menarche has been associated with an increased risk of ovarian cancer in a number of studies conducted in the United States and elsewhere (Wu et al., 1988). Late menopause also has been associated with a higher risk of ovarian cancer (Hildreth et al., 1981). The lifetime cumulative duration of ovulation may play a role in the risk of ovarian cancer, which is demonstrated by the protective effects of ovulation inhibition, such as by hysterectomy or oral contraceptive use. However, tubal ligation has also been associated with reduced risk of ovarian cancer, demonstrating that the relationship between fertility and ovulation in ovarian cancer remains unclear.

Research has consistently shown that risk of ovarian cancer declines with age at first pregnancy and total number of full-term pregnancies. Women who give birth to their first child at age 25 or younger have a decreased risk of ovarian cancer

(Daly and Obrams, 1998). Higher risk of ovarian cancer is associated with first childbirth after age 35 (Negri et al., 1991). Nulliparous women experience a higher risk of ovarian cancer (Negri et al., 1991). In a prospective cohort study of 31,377 Iowa women, age 55–69, nulliparous women with a family history of ovarian cancer were at much higher risk than were their parous counterparts (relative risk=2.7, 95% confidence interval: 1.1–6.6) (Vachon et al., 2002). There was an increased risk of ovarian cancer among nulliparous women when family history included first- and second-degree relatives with breast or ovarian cancer.

Multiparity appears to decrease the risk of ovarian cancer (Daly and Obrams, 1998). The Nurses Cohort Study of 121,700 women found that parity reduced ovarian cancer risk (odds ratio [OR]=0.84; 95% CI: 0.77–0.91 for each pregnancy) (Hankinson et al., 1995). A summary of seven case-control studies found that one full-term pregnancy had a significant reduction on ovarian cancer risk (OR=0.47) (John et al., 1993). Risk decreased as the number of births increased; after six full-term pregnancies, the odds ratio was 0.29, with a 95% confidence interval of 0.20–0.42. Risk declined by about 15% for each additional full-term pregnancy (Risch et al., 1994).

Women who have used oral contraceptives (OCs) have a reduced risk of ovarian cancer of about 30% and even women with pathogenic mutations in the BRCA1 and BRCA2 genes experience a reduced risk of ovarian cancer with OC use (Narod et al., 1998). OC use was protective among women with BRCA1 mutations (OR=0.5; 95% CI: 0.3–0.9) although not significant for BRCA2 mutation carriers (OR=0.4; 95% CI: 0.2–1.1) (Narod et al., 1998). Similarly, a population-based case-control study of 767 women also found that 4–8 years of OC use may reduce the risk of ovarian cancer by approximately 50% in women with a family history of the disease (Walker et al., 2002).

While women who have used oral contraceptives have a reduced risk, long-term use of hormone replacement therapy (HRT) or estrogen replacement therapy (ERT) may be associated with slightly elevated ovarian cancer risk. Women who have taken hormones to relieve symptoms of menopause may increase their risk of ovarian cancers by about 11% (Petrucelli et al., 2010; Salehi et al., 2008). Risk, however, appears to increase with increasing years of use (Riman et al., 2002), and short-term use has not been associated with an increased risk of ovarian cancer.

A prospective study of 211,581 healthy postmenopausal women in the United States evaluated women who had taken oral HRT or ERT after age 35 to compare ovarian cancer mortality with the effect of HRT (Rodriguez et al., 2001). Risk of ovarian cancer mortality was reported to be higher in HRT users at baseline and slightly higher for previous users than never users. Risk doubled with 10 years or more duration of use; however, only 66 of the 944 women who died of ovarian cancer had used HRT for at least 10 years.

Some research has found that the risk of ovarian cancer among women whose hormone replacement treatment included progestin was lower than for those whose HRT included estrogen only (Pearce et al., 2009). The risk among women with progestin included in their HRT remained elevated compared to women who did not have HRT; however, it is unknown if more frequent use of progestin would inhibit the effects of estrogen on cancer risk.

14.4.3 Medical Treatments

There are consistent data from studies of tubal ligation demonstrating reduced risk of ovarian cancer. A meta-analysis showed a reduction in risk of ovarian cancer of 34% among women who had tubal ligation and also observed that this protective effect remained for 10–14 years subsequent to having had this procedure (Cibula et al., 2011). Epidemiologic and other studies have shown that tubal ligation and prior hysterectomy are associated with a decreased risk of ovarian cancer. In a case-control study, Rosenblatt and Thomas (1996) found that the protective effect of tubal ligation was greatest in women of parity less than four; the protective effect was only for clear cell and endometrioid tumors. When Cramer et al. (1995) combined data from two case-control studies, they found that both tubal ligation and prior hysterectomy were protective.

An analysis of pooled interview data on infertility and the use of fertility drugs from eight case-control studies conducted in the United States, Denmark, Canada, and Australia found that nulligravid women who attempted to become pregnant for more than 5 years, compared with nulligravid women who attempted to become pregnant for less than 1 year, experienced a 2.7-fold increased risk of ovarian cancer (Ness et al., 2002). Some controversy remains surrounding the relationships among infertility, fertility drug use, and the risk of ovarian cancer (Sit et al., 2002). Pooled interview data of fertility drug use for more than 12 months found no association with ovarian cancer risk (Ness et al., 2002).

14.4.4 Diet, Physical Activity, and Obesity

These risk factors are highly intertwined in their potential to either increase or reduce the risk of any cancer, generally; but have yet to be understood in ovarian cancer, specifically. Recent studies have investigated the consumption of meat, fish, and tea and the relationship to ovarian cancer incidence. The Australian study of meat consumption found no overall risk associated with total meat consumption or the consumption of red meat, but did find elevated risk among women who consumed high levels of processed meat (Kolohdooz et al., 2010). They also found that high levels of consumption of fish and poultry were associated with a reduced risk of ovarian cancer. However, these studies were not able to determine any causal relationship.

Teas, along with many fruits and vegetables, contain flavonoids, which, according to experimental studies, have potential anticarcinogenic characteristics (Gates et al., 2007). The Swedish Mammography Cohort study (61,057 women between the ages of 46 and 76) found that consumption of tea was inversely associated with risk of ovarian cancer, after controlling for potential confounders (*P* for trend, .03) (Larsson and Wolk, 2005). Analysis of data from the Nurses' Health Study (121,701 women) found evidence that nonherbal tea consumption may be inversely associated with ovarian cancer (Gates et al., 2007). Chang et al. (2007), in an analysis of data from the *California Teacher's Study* (92,275 women), found that women who consumed over 3 mg of isoflavones per day experienced a 44% decrease in incidence of ovarian cancer, when compared with women who consumed less than 1 mg/day. Other researchers studying the effects of tea consumption and risk of ovarian cancer, however, have produced mixed results, with some showing reduced risk and some showing no association (Oppeneer and Robien, 2011). Chen et al. (2007) conducted a meta-analysis of two cohort and seven case-control studies to evaluate the relationship between tea consumption and ovarian cancer risk. This meta-analysis did not find any association between tea consumption and risk of ovarian cancer. None of these studies was designed to determine if there were any causal relationship between tea and ovarian cancer.

Physical activity has been hypothesized to be a protective factor against ovarian cancer. The results of a recent case-control study, a systematic review, and a meta-analysis, all carried out by a group of Australian cancer researchers, produced equivocal results. The case-control study showed small reductions in risk and no association, while the systematic review and meta-analysis found a small reduction in risk (Olsen et al., 2007).

Obesity and body weight have been studied as a risk factor for both the occurrence of ovarian cancer and the survival of women diagnosed with ovarian cancer. Obesity has been inconsistently shown to be associated with the risk of ovarian cancer (McLemore et al., 2009; Salehi et al., 2008). Some studies have found that obesity is associated with shorter survival time among women diagnosed with ovarian cancer (Yang et al., 2011), while other studies have found weight gain during treatment to be a prognostic indicator of improved survival (Hess et al., 2010). Current research is investigating the potential role of a healthy diet in combination with moderate physical activity in reducing the risk of recurrence following complete response to primary therapy (GOG-0225, Diet and Physical Activity Change or Usual Care in Improving Survival in Patients With Previously Treated Stage II, Stage III, or Stage IV Ovarian Epithelial Cancer, Fallopian Tube Cancer, or Primary Peritoneal Cancer). This study was designed based on preliminary evidence from the Women's Health Initiative (WHI), which found that women who adopted a low-fat diet had a significant 40% reduction in ovarian cancer risk (Prentice et al., 2007). In this study, lifestyle changes, but not necessarily the associated body weight changes, were related to the improved outcomes in ovarian cancer.

14.5 THEORY AND OVARIAN CANCER RISK

As ovarian cancers comprise a very heterogeneous set of malignancies, one would suspect that a single causal mechanism would not be sufficient to explain all types. It is, thus, not surprising that a number of hypotheses have been suggested to explain disease etiology, with incessant ovulation, gonadotropin, and inflammation hypotheses being the most frequently discussed. These theories are not mutually exclusive; they converge on ovulation and inflammation.

The incessant ovulation hypothesis, which was first formulated by Fathalla (1971) and then expanded by other researchers (e.g., Casagrande et al., 1979), proposes that the release of an oocyte during ovulation causes trauma to the ovarian surface epithelium that must be repaired; in the case of repeated ovulation, this repair must occur frequently, without adequate physiological rest. This repetitive cycle may result in cellular proliferation; the DNA damage and inflammatory cytokines associated with these processes contribute to the cells' susceptibility to neoplasia (Karst and Drapkin, 2010).

This theory is used to explain why multiparous women have a reduced risk of ovarian cancer compared to nonporous women. Other known protective factors, such as hysterectomy, lactation, and use of anovulant oral contraceptives, all pause the process of ovulation, giving the ovarian surface epithelium a period during which it does not experience this repeated physical damage. Factors known to increase risk, such as endometriosis, early menarche, late menopause, and nulliparity, as they are associated with more frequent ovulation and increased epithelial damage, also appear to support this theory. Under the incessant ovulation hypothesis, it was thought that the use of hormonal treatments for infertility would increase the risk of ovarian cancer. However, studies have observed no increased risk among women treated for infertility (Vlahos et al., 2010).

The gonadotropin hypothesis (see Biskind and Biskind, 1944, 1948; Cramer and Welch, 1983) was built upon Fathalla's incessant ovulation hypothesis. It was formulated to account for gaps that this theory was unable to explain—why infertile women receiving fertility medications and women with polycystic ovarian syndrome experience increased risk of ovarian cancer, and why progesterone-only oral contraceptives (which do not inhibit ovulation) are associated with a decreased risk. This theory proposed that stimulation of estrogen production via exposure to high levels of gonadotropic hormones, which occurs during menopause, ovulation, and infertility therapy that involves use of fertility-enhancing hormones (Salehi et al., 2008), leads to increased activation of the ovarian surface epithelium. This activation may lead to increased risk of epithelial ovarian cancers. Experiments with animals suggest that an excess of gonadotropin and stromal stimulation may result in increased risk for ovarian cancer by disturbing normal feedback inhibition between the ovary and the pituitary or by destroying ovarian follicles (Cramer and Welch, 1983). As this proposal alone was insufficient to explain the increased risk associated with circulating androgens, the hypothesis was expanded to include the increased risk associated with androgens and the decreased risk associated with progestin in the tumor microenvironment (Landen et al., 2008; Ricciardelli and Oehler, 2009).

The inflammation hypothesis was proposed based on data supporting an increased incidence of ovarian cancer among individuals with pelvic inflammatory disease, which cannot be explained by the incessant ovulation hypothesis. It is supported by epidemiologic evidence that suggests a decreased risk of ovarian cancer among chronic anti-inflammatory medication users, and it may explain the hypothesized protective role of tubal ligation (Ricciardelli and Oehler, 2009), perhaps by blocking the tubes and preventing cancer causing substances from entering the ovaries. Both endometriosis and ovulation (e.g., tissue reconstruction) are associated with a local inflammatory reaction, which involves rapid cell division, DNA excision and repair, oxidative stress, and high concentrations of cytokines and prostaglandins, all of which are established promoters of mutagenesis (Ness et al., 2000). This hypothesis also can help explain ovarian malignancies that are a consequence of inflammation in the ovarian epithelium, resulting from exposure to environmental toxicants.

However, while each of these hypotheses has supporting biologic and epidemiologic evidence, none of these hypotheses has been shown to be completely conclusive. None of the hypotheses have been shown to be fully proven as models of ovarian carcinogenesis. Each hypothesis appears to be relevant to a subset of these malignancies. Multiple factors seem to contribute to the initiation and progression of the disease. There is no unifying model that can encompass the breadth of ovarian cancers.

14.6 MODERN DARWINIAN THEORY, CULTURE, AND FEMALE REPRODUCTIVE HISTORIES

An understanding of Modern Darwinian Theory and human evolution can contribute to our understanding of ovarian cancer by forcing us to move our attention to ultimate, or evolutionary, factors rather than the proximate factors—internal mechanisms in the body—upon which rest the existing hypothesis for ovarian cancer etiology. An assumption underlying Modern Darwinian Theory is that we, like other species, were designed to reproduce. Traits that are adaptive—that is, traits produced by natural selection—have persisted because of the effects those traits (the phenotype) and the genes underlying those traits (the genotype) had, in the distant ancestral past, on survival and reproduction. We inherited, from our hunter-gatherer ancestors, genes that were selected over a great many generations and that reflect interactions between the gene and the environment in which those ancestors lived. As that environment has changed significantly, while it is assumed that natural selection has made few changes in the gene pool of humans during the past 10,000 years (Eaton et al., 1994), we will turn to anthropology and studies of the anatomy and physiology of early humans and studies of living hunter-gatherers, whose lifestyle best approximates that of our distant ancestors.

To understand an adaptation, it is important to pursue both ultimate and proximate explanations. Proximate explanations ask "how" questions; that is, they address the way that functionality is achieved often through external triggers (e.g., exposure to toxicant) and/or internal mechanisms—the genetic instructions provided by DNA, the release of a particular hormone, or the particular physiological reaction to a xenobiotic agent. Ultimate or evolutionary explanations, on the other hand, explain why certain inheritable traits were favored; that is, they address the "why" questions—What is the trait's evolutionary function (Alcock, 2009)? Proximate and ultimate explanations are not opposite ends of a continuum, they are complementary explanations.

To begin this discussion, we will look at ovarian malignancies across species; such comparative studies are commonly used in evolutionary biology to identify adaptations. When species that share a phylogenetic group (family, genus, species) differ, it is assumed that different selective pressures have produced divergence in traits. This is referred to as divergent evolution. Spontaneously developed ovarian malignancies, as Fathalla (1979) pointed out, are rare in mammals, including nonhuman primates (Siebold and Wolf, 1973). Some 90% of mammals are seasonal breeders, with the human being an exception (see Murdock et al., 2005). Ovarian tumors also are relatively rare in domesticated mammals, including cows, horses, and chickens (MacLachlan, 1987). Fathalla (1971: p. 163) attributed the human females' increased risk of ovarian cancer to the large number of ovulations they experience during a lifetime—human females, he wrote, have "extravagant and mostly purposeless ovulation." Although human females, like all mammals, do not ovulate frequently, they differ from many other mammalian females in that they have a much longer reproductive life. Thus, currently, a human female, over a lifetime, may experience more ovulary cycles.

Convergent evolution, on the other hand, can help explain why members of unrelated species (e.g., birds and mammals) might have acquired a similar biological trait. One species that is not closely related to humans and that does experience a high incidence of spontaneous ovarian cancer is the domestic fowl (*Gallus domesticus*) (Barua et al., 2009; Lee et al., 2012). Similarities between the reproductive physiology of hens and human females, which include the fact that the follicular development and ovulatory cycles are under the control of pituitary gonadotropins and ovarian steroids in both domestic fowl and humans (Robinson and Etches, 1986; Rodriguez-Burford et al., 2001), makes the hen an interesting model to be explored as a model for human ovarian cancer. Hens lay eggs frequently, and by the time a hen has completed 2 years of egg laying, she has ovulated about as many times as a woman approaching menopause. The incidence of ovarian cancer in hens rises dramatically with age, with a 4% incidence at age 2, which increases as high as 40% by age 6 (Zhuge et al., 2009). According to Hales et al. (2008), approximately half of all egg-laying hens, who ovulate nearly every day, develop ovarian cancer after 4 years.

The fact that hens, who frequently lay eggs, and human females, who experience many ovulatory cycles during their lifetime, both experience increased risk for ovarian malignancies, supports that that an increase in lifetime exposure to ovulation plays a role in ovarian cancer etiology. While it is not possible to identify with any precision the reproductive lifestyle of ancestral hens, the one thing that is certain is that the ancestors of hens lived in the wild. In birds we find a variety of reproductive strategies; some wild birds are seasonal breeders while others ovulate only when conditions are appropriate (Wallace, 1913). The domestication of hens could have led to a modification of their genotype through artificial selection so that they would produce more eggs than their ancestors did under wild conditions. This increase in ovulation and egg production, however, may be due simply to a change in the environment. When a hen's eggs are removed from the nest as fast as they are laid, a considerable increase in the number of eggs laid, an ovulations, will result (Pearl, 1912).

To describe the lifestyle of the human ancestress, we will draw on hundreds of ethnographies of hunter-gatherers, whose lifestyle best approximates that of our more distant ancestors. These ethnographies, published over the past 100 years, provide descriptions that indicate that the lifestyle of our ancestresses, including their reproductive patterns, differed significantly from our own. Their level of physical activity was high while diets, typically, were low in saturated fat and refined carbohydrates (Eaton et. al., 1988). Exposure to environmental factors that might promote inflammation, with the exception of smoke from fire or dust, did not occur. Humans, according to Gurven and Kaplan (2007), were designed to be hard-working and productive members of a social group until they began to approach seven decades, at which time senescence rapidly would begin to occur. The modal age at adult death for much of human evolution was, on average, 72 years, with a range of 68–72 years (Gurven and Kaplan, 2007).

The reproductive patterns of our ancestresses involved marrying early, soon after puberty and a reproductive developmental sequence that involved, with few interruptions, a series of pregnancies and lactation. Menopause, which is an adaptive trait found in few species outside of humans, would have given a woman a significant amount of time before senescence and death to rear her last offspring and to help her daughters rear theirs (Williams, 1957). Menstruation, rather than being a monthly event, was infrequent. While ancestral humans may have had more years during which ovulation was possible, ovulation still was a relatively rare event. Beginning soon after puberty, women were constantly pregnant or nursing a child (Coe and Steadman, 1995). Frequent nursing is known to suppress ovulation in hunter-gatherers (Konner and Worthman, 1980). While the ovarian cancer rates of women in hunter-gatherer societies are not known, we do know that women living a more traditional lifestyle (e.g., early pregnancy, multiparity, and breastfeeding) are less likely to get reproductive cancers (Coe and Steadman, 1995).

While this reproductive lifestyle probably did not change dramatically when humans moved to agriculture and a more sedentary lifestyle, it did change dramatically beginning around the time of the industrial revolution. When women entered the workplace, they began to marry and reproduce at older ages and to produce fewer offspring; they also were less likely to nurse their offspring. They also were likely to have been exposed to chemicals in the workplace, chemicals that had not been present in the ancestral environment. Increases in the chronic and deadly "diseases of civilization"—including ovarian cancer—may be associated with these behavioral and environmental changes (Eaton et al., 1988).

This evolutionary approach can account for data indicating that lower risk for ovarian cancer is experienced by women who follow the ancestral reproductive sequence (begin childbearing early, soon after the initiation of menses, are multiparous, and breastfeed their children for prolonged periods of time). It also can explain why women living a Westernized lifestyle, which involves changes in reproductive patterns, have higher rates of ovarian cancer, compared with women in non-Westernized societies. This hypothesis also can help explain why women who are infertile may be at high risk, and why women who delay reproduction, and/or are nulliparous, also experience a higher risk for ovarian cancer than do multiparous women.

This approach, however, also leads us to focus on the role that might be played by aging and senescence. We know that aging is associated with cellular malfunction and that cancer and a poorer prognoses after being diagnosed with cancer, are correlated with aging. Our understanding of the processes underlying the linkage between aging and cancer, however, is still minimal (Ahman et al., 2009). We know that aging is associated with inflammatory processes; however, it is not clear if aging leads to the inflammatory processes that result in chronic disease or if inflammation is the factor that induces both aging and chronic disease (Ahman et al., 2009).

Keeping in mind that the genes we have were selected in an environment in which there was little exposure to xenobiotic agents, a study of environmental toxicants is a very important arena for research, as such exposures can exacerbate hypersensitivity, autoimmunity, and pathological inflammation (Rooney et al., 2012). Xenobiotic agents serve as environmental initiators of inflammation, which can result in cell damage, elevations of cytokines and prostaglandins, and oxidative stress, all of which may be mutagenic. It is important to keep in mind that the initiation of the process leading to cancer depends not only on the receptivity of the cell but on exposure to a mutagenic substance.

14.7 SUMMARY

Ovarian cancer, which is the ninth most common cancer among women in the United States and the leading cause of gynecologic cancer-related death, is a very heterogeneous set of malignancies that affect the ovaries. The fact that the symptoms of ovarian cancer are often so vague, and seemingly unrelated to ovarian function, has made early diagnosis a challenge. The heterogeneity of the disease has made it more difficult to increase our understanding of this disease and identify effective methods for early detection. In this chapter, we have outlined the biology and epidemiology of ovarian cancer and reviewed the theoretical approaches taken to try to increase understanding of the disease. We have, thus, provided a summary of current thinking about ovarian cancer and its etiology and epidemiological profile.

REFERENCES

Ahman, A., Banerjee, S., Wang, Z., Kong, D., Majumdar, A., and Sakar, F. (2009) Aging and inflammation: Etiological culprits of cancer, *Current Aging Science*, 7: 174–186.

Alcock, J. (2009) *Animal Behavior*. Sunderland, MA: Sinauer Associates.

Antoniou, A. et al. (2003) Average risks of breast and ovarian cancer associated with BRCA1 or BRCA2 mutations detected in case series unselected for family history: A combined analysis of 22 studies, *American Journal of Human Genetics*, 72(5): 1117–1130.

Auersperg, N. (2010) The origin of ovarian carcinomas: A unifying hypothesis, *International Journal of Gynecologic Pathology*, 30: 12–21.

Barua, A., Bitterman, P., Abramowicz, J., Dirks, A., Bahr, J., Hales, D., Bradaric, M., Edassery, S., Rotmensch, J., and Luborsky, J. (2009) Histopathology of ovarian cancer in laying hens, a preclinical model of human ovarian cancer, *International Journal of Gynecological Cancer*, 19(4): 531–539.

Biskind, M. and Biskind, G. (1944) Development of tumors in the rat ovary after transplantation into the spleen, *Proceedings of the Society for Experimental Biology and Medicine*, 55: 176–179.

Biskind, M. and Biskind, G. (1948) Atrophy of the ovaries transplanted to the spleen in unilaterally castrated rates, *Science*, 108: 137–138.

Casagrande, J., Louie, E., Pike, M., Roy, S., Ross, R., and Henderson, B. (1979) "Incessant ovulation" and ovarian cancer, *Lancet*, 2: 170–173.

Chang, E.T. et al. (2007) Diet and risk of ovarian cancer in the California Teachers Study cohort, *American Journal of Epidemiology*, 165: 802–813.

Chen, Quansheng., Zhao, Jiewen., Fang, C. H., Wang, Dongmei (2007) Feasibility study on identification of green, black, and Oolong teas using near-infrared reflectance spectroscopy based on support vector machine (SV)M, *Spectrochimica Acta Part A: Molecular and Biomolecular Spectroscopy*, 66(3): 568–574.

Cibula, D., Widschwendter, M., Majek, O., and Dusek, L. (2011) Tubal ligation and the risk of ovarian cancer: Review and meta-analysis, *Human Reproduction Update*, 17(1): 55–67.

Claus, E.B., Schildkraut, J.M., Thompson, W.D., and Risch, N.J. (1996) The genetic attributable risk of breast and ovarian cancer. *Cancer*, 1(44): 2318–2324.

Clouser, M., Hess, L.M., and Chambers, S.K. (2009) Biomarker targets and novel therapeutics, *Cancer Treatment and Research*, 149: 85–105.

Coe, K. and Steadman, L. (1995) The human breast and the ancestral reproductive cycle: An inquiry into the etiology of breast cancer, *Human Nature*, 6(3): 197–220.

Cramer, D. and Welch, W. (1983) Determinants of ovarian cancer risk. II. Inferences regarding pathogenesis, *Journal of the National Cancer Institute*, 71: 717–721.

Cramer, D., Xu, H., and Harlow, B. (1995) Does "incessant" ovulation increase risk for early menopause, *American Journal of Obstetrics and Gynecology*, 2(1): 568–573.

Daly, M. and Obrams, G. (1998) Epidemiology and risk assessment for ovarian cancer, *Seminars in Oncology*, 25(3): 255–264.

Eaton, S. et al. (1994) Women's reproductive cancers in evolutionary context, *The Quarterly Review of Biology*, 69(3): 353–367.

Eaton, S. B., Konner, M., and Shostak, M. (1988) Stone agers in the fast lane: Chronic degenerative diseases in evolutionary perspective, *The American Journal of Medicine*, 84(4): 739–749.

Fathalla, M. (1971) Incessant ovulation—A factor in ovarian neoplasia? *Lancet*, 2(7716): 163.

Fathalla (1979) http://ac.els-cdn.com/S014067367192335X/1-s2.0-S014067367192335X-main.pdf?_tid=ff28a450-c228-11e2-af03-00000aacb35e&acdnat=1369149391_9cbac0823d9ac0fc1a1e8657990388bf (accessed May 21, 2013).

Gates, M., Tworoger, S., Hecht, J., De Vivo, I., Rosner, B., and Hankinson, S. (2007) A prospective study of dietary flavonoid intake and incidence of epithelian ovarian cancer, *International Journal of Cancer*, 121(1): 2225–2232.

Gurven, M. and Kaplan, H. (2007) Longevity among hunter-gatherers: A cross-cultural examination, *Population and Development Review*, 33(2): 321–335.

Hales, D., Zhuge, Y., Lagman, J., Ansenberger, K., Mahon, C., Barua, A., Luborshy, J., and Bahr, J. (2008) Cyclooxygenases expression and distribution in the normal ovary and their role in ovarian cancer in the domestic hen (Gallus domesticus), *Endocrine*, 33(3): 235–244.

Hankinson, S., Colditz, G., Hunter, D., Manson, J., Willett, W., Meir, L., Stampfer, M.J., and Speizer, F.L. (1995) Reproductive factors and family history of breast cancer in relation to plasma estrogen and prolactin levels in postmenopausal women in the Nurses' Health Study (United States), *Cancer Causes and Control*, 6(3): 217–224.

Hess, L.M., Barakat, R., Tian, C., Ozols, R.F., and Alberts, D.S. (2010) Weight change during chemotherapy as a potential prognostic factor for stage III epithelial ovarian carcinoma: A Gynecologic Oncology Group study, *Gynecologic Oncology*, 107(2): 260–265.

Hildreth, N., Kelsey, J., Livolsi, V., Fishcer, D., Holford, T., Mostow, E., Schwartz, P., and White, C. (1981) An epidemiologic study of epithelial carcinoma of the ovary, *American Journal of Epidemiology*, 114(3): 398–405.

Holschneider, C.H. and Berek, J.S. (2000) Ovarian cancer: Epidemiology, biology and prognostic factors, *Seminars in Surgical Oncology*, 19: 3–10.

Howlader, N. et al. (eds). (2012) *SEER Cancer Statistics Review, 1975–2009* (Vintage 2009 Populations). Bethesda, MD: National Cancer Institute. http://seer.cancer.gov/csr/1975_2009_pops09/, based on November 2011 SEER data submission, posted to the SEER web site (accessed May 21, 2013).

Huang, L. et al. (2008) Improved survival time: What can survival cure models tell us about population-based survival improvements in late-stage colorectal, ovarian, and testicular cancer? *Cancer*, 112(10): 2289–2230.

Jelovac, D. and Armstrong, D. (2011) Recent progress in the diagnosis and treatment of ovarian cancer, *CA: A Cancer Journal for Clinicians*, 61(3): 183–203.

John, E., Whittemore, A., Harris, R., Itnrye, J., and Collaborative Ovarian Cancer Group. (1993) Characteristics relating to ovarian cancer risk: Collaborative analysis of seven U.S. case-control studies. Epithelial ovarian cancer in black women, *Journal of National Cancer Institute*, 85(2):142–147.

Karst, A.M. and Drapkin, R. (2010) Ovarian cancer pathogenesis: A model in evolution, *Journal of Oncology*, Vol. 2010, Article ID 932371. Doi:10.1155/2010/2010/932371.

Koifman, S. and Koifman, R. (2001) Breast cancer mortality among Ashkenazi Jewish women in Sao Paulo and Porto Alegre, Brazil, *Breast Cancer Research*, 3: 270–275.

Kolohdooz, F., vanderPols, J., Bain, C., Marks, G., Hughes, M.C., Whiteman, D., and Webb, P. (2010) Diet and ovarian cancer: Results from two Australian case-control studies conducted 10 years apart, *American Journal of Clinical Nutrition*, 91: 1752–1763.

Konner, M. and Worthman, C. (1980) Nursing frequency, gonadal function and birth spacing among! Kung hunter-gatherers, *Science*, 207: 78–91.

Lalwani, N., Prasad, S.R., Vikram, R., Shanbhougue, A.K., Huettner, P.C., and Fasih, N. (2011) Histologic, molecular and cytogenetic features of ovarian cancers: Implications for diagnosis and treatment, *Radiographics*, 31(3): 625–646.

Landen, C.N., Birrer, M.J., and Sood, A.K. (2008) Early events in the pathogenesis of epithelial ovarian cancer, *Journal of Clinical Oncology*, 26(6): 995–1005. Available on line at http://jco.ascopubs.org/content/26/6/995.full.pdf+html (accessed May 21, 2013).

Larsson, S. and Wolk, A. (2005) Tea consumption and ovarian cancer risk in a population-based cohort, *Archives of Internal Medicine*, 165(22): 2683–2686.

Lee, J.Y., Jeong, W., Lim, W., Kim, J, Bazer, F.W., et al. (2012) Chicken pleiotrophin: Regulation of tissue specific expression by estrogen in the oviduct and distinct expression pattern in the ovarian Carcinomas. *PLoS ONE 7*(4): e34215. doi:10.1371/journal.pone.0034215 (accessed May 21, 2013).

MacLachlan, N.J. (1987) Ovarian disorders in domestic animals, *Environmental Health Perspectives*, 73: 27–33.

McLemore, M.R., Miaskowski, C., Aouizerat, B.E., Chen, L.-M., and Dodd, M.J. (2009) Epidemiological and genetic factors associated with ovarian cancer, *Cancer Nursing*, 32(4): 281–288.

Merajver, S. et al. (1995) Somatic mutations in the *BRCA1* gene in sporadic ovarian tumours, *Nature Genetics*, 9: 439–443.

Murdock, W., Van Kird, E., and Alexander, B. (2005) A brief communication; DNA damages in ovarian surface epithelial cells of ovulatory hens, *Experimental Biology and Medicine*, 230(6): 429–433.

Nagle, C.M. et al. (2011) Reducing time to diagnosis does not improve outcomes for women with symptomatic ovarian cancer, *Journal of Clinical Oncology*, 29(16): 2253–2258.

Narod, S. et al. (1998) Oral contraceptives and the risk of hereditary ovarian cancer, *New England Journal of Medicine*, 339: 424–428.

Negri, E., Franceschi, S., Tzonou, A., Booth, M., La Veccia, C., Parazzini, F., Beral, V., Boyle, P., and Trichopoulos, D. (1991) Pooled analysis of 3 European case-control studies: 1: Reproductive factors and the risk of epithelial ovarian cancer, *International Journal of Cancer*, 1(56): 50–56.

Ness, Roberta B. Cramer, Daniel W., Goodman, Marc T., Kjaer, Suzanne K., Mallin K., Mosgaard, Berit, Prudie, Davie, Risch, Harvey, Vergona, Ronald, and Wu, Anna (2002). Infertility, fertility drugs, and ovarian cancer: A pooled analysis of case-control studies. *American Journal of Epidemiology*, 155(3):217–224.

Nesse, R., Grisso, J., Cottreau, C., Klapper, J., Vergona, R., Wheeler, J., Morgan, M., and Schlesselman, J. (2000) Factors related to inflammation of the ovarian epithelium and risk of ovarian cancer, *Epidemiology*, 11(2): 111–117.

Olsen, C., Bain, C., Jordan, S., Nagle, C., Green, A., Whiteman, D., Webb, P., and Australian Ovarian Cancer Study Group. (2007) Recreational physical activity and epithelial ovarian cancer: A case-control study, systematic review, and meta-analysis, *Cancer Epidemiology Biomarkers & Prevention*, 16(11): 2321–2330.

Olsen, C., Green, A., Whiteman, D., Sadeqhi, S., Kohohdooz, F., and Webb, P. (2007) Obesity and the risk of epithelial ovarian cancer: A systematic review and meta-analysis, *European Journal of Cancer*, 43: 690–709.

Oppeneer, S. and Robien, K. (2011) Tea consumption and epithelial ovarian cancer risk: A systematic review of observational studies, *Nutrition and Cancer*, 63(6), 817–826.

Pearce, C.L., Chung, K., Pike, M., and Wu, A. H. (2009). Increases in ovarian cancer risk associated with menopausal estrogen therapy. *Cancer*, 115(3):531–539.

Pearl, R. (1912) The mode of inheritance of fecundity in the domestic fowl, *Journal of Experimental Zoology*, 13(2): 153–268.

Petrucelli, N., Daly, M., and Feldman, G.L. (2010) Hereditary breast and ovarian cancer due to mutations in BRCA1 and BRCA2, *Genetics in Medicine*, 12(5): 245–259.

Prentice, R.L. et al. (2007) Low-fat dietary pattern and cancer incidence in the Women's Health Initiative Dietary Modification Randomized Controlled Trial, *Journal of National Cancer Institute*, 99: 1534–1543.

Ricciardelli, C. and Oehler, M. (2009) Diverse molecular pathways in ovarian cancer and their clinical significance, *Maturitas*, 62: 270–275.

Riman, T., Dickman, P., Nilsson, S., Correia, N., Nordlinder, H., Magnusson, C., Weiderpass, E., and Persson, I. (2002) Hormone replacement therapy and the risk of invasive epithelial ovarian cancer in Swedish women, *Journal of the National Cancer Institute*, 94(78): 497–504.

Risch, M. et al. (1994) Parity, contraception, infertility and the risk of epithelial ovarian cancer, *American Journal of Epidemiology*, 140(7): 585–597.

Robinson, F. and Etches, R. (1986) Ovarian steroidogenesis during follicular maturation in the domestic fowl (*Gallus domesticus*), *Biology of Reproduction*, 35: 1096–1105.

Rodriguez-Burford, C. et al. (2001) Immunohistochemical expression of molecular markers in an avian model, *Gynecologic Oncology*, 81: 373–379.

Rodriguez, C., Patel, A.V., Calle, J., Jacob, E., and Thun, M. (2001) Estrogen replacement therapy and ovarian cancer mortality in a large prospective Study of US women, *Journal of the American Medical Association*, 285(11): 1460–1465.

Rooney, A.A., Luebke, R.W., Selgrade, M.K., and Germolec, D.R. (2012) Immunotoxicology and its application in risk assessment, *EXS*, 101: 251–287.

Rosenblatt, K. and Thomas, D. (1996) Reduced risk of ovarian cancer in women with a tubal ligation or hysterectomy. The World Health Organization Collaborative Study of Neoplasia and Steroid Contraceptives, *Cancer Epidemiology Biomarkers & Prevention*, 5: 933–935.

Salehi, F., Dunfield, L., Phillip, K.P., Krewski, D., and Banderhyden, B.C. (2008) Risk factors for ovarian. Cancer: An overview with emphasis on hormonal factors, *Journal of Toxicology and Environmental Health*, 11, 301–321.

Salvador, S., Gilks, B., Kobel, M., Huntsman, D., Rosen, B., Miller, D. (2009) The fallopian tube: Primary site of most pelvic high-grade serous carcinomas, *International Journal of Cancer*, 19(1): 58–64.

SEER (2011). Previous Version: Seer Cancer Statistics Review, 1975-2009 (Vintage 2009 Populations). Updated August 20, 2012. http://seer.cancer.gov/csr/1975_2009_pops09/index.html (accessed October, 4, 2012).

Siebold, H. and Wolf, R. (1973) Neoplasms and proliferative lesions in 1065 nonhuman primate necropsies, *Laboratory Animal Science*, 23: 533–539.

Siegel, R., Naishadham, D., and Jemal, A. (2012) Cancer statistics, 2012, *CA: A Cancer Journal for Clinicians*, 62(1): 10–29.

Sit, A., Modugno, F., Weissfield, J., Berga, S., and Ness, R. (2002) Hormone replacement therapy formulations and risk of epithelial ovarian carcinoma, *Gynecologic Oncology*, 86(2): 118–123.

Steinberg, K.K., Pernarelli, J.M., Marcus, M., Khoury, M.J., Schildraut, J., and Marchbanks, P.A. (1998) Increases risk for familial ovarian cancer among Jewish Women, *Genetic Epidemiology*, 15: 51–59.

Vachon, C.M., Mink, P., Janney, C.A., Sellers, T., Thomas, A., Cerhan, J., Hartmann, L., and Folsom, A. (2002) Association of parity and ovarian cancer risk by family history of breast or ovarian cancer in a population based study of postmenopausal women, *Epidemiology*, (1): 66–71.

Vlahos, N.F., Economopoulos, K.P., and Creatsas, G. (2010) Fertility drugs and ovarian cancer risk: A critical review of the literature, *Annals of the New York Academy of Sciences*, 1205: 214–219.

Wallace, C. (1913) The stimulation and inhibition of ovulation in birds and mammals, *Journal of Animal Behavior*, 3(3): 215–221.

Walker, G., Schlesselman, J., and Ness, R. (2002) Family history of cancer, Oral contraceptive use, and ovarian cancer risk, *Obstetrical and Gynecological Survey*, 57(5): 288–290.

Williams, G. C., (1957) Pleiotropy, natural selection, and the evolution of senescence, *Evolution*, 11: 398–411.

Wu, M. et al. (1988) Personal and environmental characteristics related to epithelial ovarian cancer.1. Reproductive and menstrual events and oral contraceptive use, *American Journal of Epidemiology*, 128(6): 1216–1227.

Yang, H., Yoon, C., Myung, S., and Park, S. (2011) Effect of obesity on survival of women with epithelial ovarian cancer: A systematic review and meta-analysis of observational studies, *International Journal of Gynecological Cancer*, 21: 1525–1532.

Zhuge, Y., Lagman, J., Ansenberger, K., Mahon, C., Daikoku, T., Dey, S., Bahr, J., and Hales, D. (2009) CYP1B1 expression in ovarian cancer in the laying hen *Gallus domesticus*, *Gynecological Oncology*, 112(1): 171–178.

Part IV

Risk Assessment

15 Assessing Ovarian Toxicity in Human Health Risk Assessment for Environmental Chemicals and Pharmaceuticals

Susan L. Makris and Wafa Harrouk

CONTENTS

ABBREVIATIONS

CDER	Center for Drug Evaluation and Research
EMEA	European Medicines Agency
EPA	U.S. Environmental Protection Agency
FDA	U.S. Food and Drug Administration
ICH	International Committee on Harmonization of Technical Requirements for Registration of Pharmaceuticals for Human Use
NTP	National Toxicology Program
OECD	Organisation for Economic Co-operation and Development
PDMA	Pharmaceuticals and Medical Devices Agency (Japan)

15.1 INTRODUCTION

For environmental agents and pharmaceuticals, reproductive toxicity has been defined as the occurrence of biologically adverse effects on the reproductive systems of females or males following exposure. The toxicity may be expressed as alterations to the female or male reproductive organs, the related endocrine system, or pregnancy outcomes. Manifestations can include adverse effects on puberty onset and attainment of full reproductive function, gamete production and transport, reproductive cycle normality, sexual behavior, fertility, implantation, gestation, parturition, lactation, pre- and postnatal development and growth, premature reproductive senescence, or modifications in other functions dependent on the integrity of the reproductive systems (EPA, 1996; ICH, 2000; OECD, 2008b). The main functions of the ovaries are (1) to produce ova (the eggs necessary for fertilization) and (2) to secrete steroid hormones, namely, estrogen during the follicular preovulatory phase of the female reproductive cycle and progesterone during the luteal or postovulatory phase of the cycle. Thus, any agent that targets the ovaries or the hormones they produce may be classified as an ovarian toxicant. Alterations can range from a reversible perturbation of the hormone levels (endocrine changes) to permanent damage such as follicular insufficiency or ovarian cancers. However, it should be noted that ovarian cancer is not a single disease. There are over 30 types/subtypes of malignancies, each with its unique histopathological appearance, biologic behavior, and possible etiology (Hildreth et al., 1981) (see Chapters 12 through 14).

In females, alteration of ovarian integrity may result in one or more adverse manifestations; thus, it is essential that ovarian morphology and function be assessed when screening environmental agents and pharmaceuticals for evidence of potential hazard to human health. Detection of ovarian toxicity in nonclinical testing paradigms is especially important because oocytes are generally considered to have no (or limited) (Johnson et al., 2004) regenerative ability and any abnormalities in the ovaries can be translated as an impairment of female reproductive capacity.

15.2 RISK ASSESSMENT

Risk assessment is the process by which scientific judgments are made concerning the potential for toxicity to occur in humans (EPA, 1996). The basic concepts

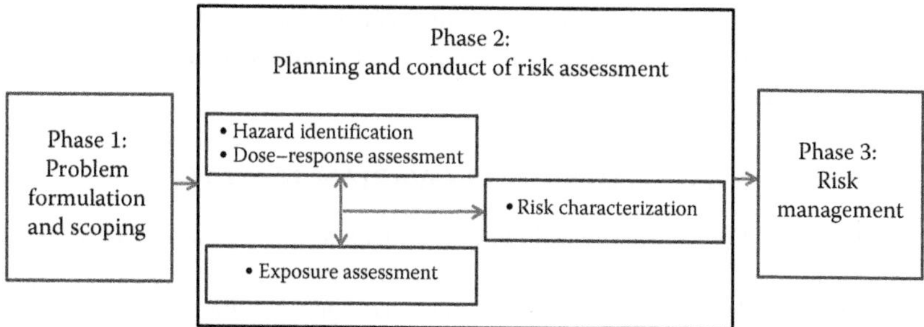

FIGURE 15.1 Basic components of the risk assessment framework. (From NRC, *Risk Assessment in the Federal Government: Managing the Process,* National Academy Press, Washington, DC, 1983; NRC, *Science and Decisions: Advancing Risk Assessment,* National Academies Press, Washington, DC, 2009.)

of the risk assessment paradigm were described by the National Research Council (NRC) as consisting of hazard identification, dose–response assessment, and exposure assessment (Figure 15.1) (NRC, 1983, 2009). These components contribute to the development of a risk characterization. This is an essential aspect of risk management, which falls within a broader social and regulatory context. The general framework of risk assessment as described by the NRC is applicable to both environmental agents and pharmaceuticals. Methods used to identify hazard, assess dose response, and characterize exposure have many commonalities for environmental agents and pharmaceuticals. However, approaches to risk management can be very dissimilar and will not be addressed here.

In the United States, the Environmental Protection Agency (EPA) and the Food and Drug Administration (FDA) have developed toxicity-specific risk assessment guidelines that are consistent with the principles described by the NRC. These guidelines include standard definitions and terminology, descriptions of the evaluation and interpretation of animal and human hazard data, dose–response evaluation, derivation of reference values, exposure assessment, and risk characterization and communication. For the EPA, two of these guidelines are particularly relevant to the assessment of noncancer reproductive risk. They are the *Guidelines for Developmental Toxicity Risk Assessment* (EPA, 1991) and the *Guidelines for Reproductive Toxicity Risk Assessment* (EPA, 1996). Additionally, the EPA has published guidelines for the assessment of carcinogenic risk: the *Guidelines for Carcinogen Risk Assessment* (EPA, 2005a) and the *Supplemental Guidance for Assessing Susceptibility from Early-Life Exposure to Carcinogens* (EPA, 2005b). In Europe, the Organisation for Economic Co-operation and Development (OECD) has also published guidance on testing and assessing chemicals for reproductive (and developmental) toxicity (OECD, 2008b). Likewise, for pharmaceuticals, standardized risk assessment guidance exists in the United States for noncancer reproductive risks (FDA, 2011) as well as for assessing carcinogenicity risks (ICH, 1995, 1997b). Similar approaches are followed in Europe (EMEA, 2008) for the evaluation and interpretation of developmental/reproductive toxicology and carcinogenicity data. Taken together, these peer-reviewed documents provide sound scientific principles and a conceptual framework that form the basis of harmonized reproductive (including developmental and cancer) risk assessment for environmental toxicants and pharmaceuticals.

15.3 HAZARD ASSESSMENT FOR OVARIAN TOXICITY

As illustrated in Figure 15.1, the identification of toxicological hazards and the characterization of the dose response for adverse outcomes are integral aspects of the human health risk assessment process. The general approach to this issue is similar for environmental chemicals and pharmaceuticals in that it relies upon the evaluation of all reliable data that demonstrate an association (or lack thereof) between exposures to a particular substance of interest and toxicological responses. Such responses can be specific to the level of the organism, system, organ, tissue, cell, or biochemical pathway. It is within that conceptual framework of evaluation that the subject of hazard identification and dose-response assessment for ovarian toxicity is discussed.

Much of the data that inform the hazard evaluation process are derived from animal toxicology studies. For environmental agents, a broad screening approach utilizing standardized protocols for controlled experiments in laboratory animals may be needed to identify toxicological targets. Alternatively, a more directed and iterative chemical-specific approach may be possible. This type of customized approach is typically used in the preclinical assessment of pharmaceuticals, and it is not precluded for environmental chemicals. Prior to conducting extensive mammalian *in vivo* studies, ancillary data are usually collected and considered for risk assessment. This can include background information on chemical class, physical–chemical properties, structure–activity relationships, and functional genomic and proteomic data, which can be useful in predicting potential for toxicities (Cabrera et al., 2011). *In vitro*, *ex vivo*, and nonmammalian (e.g., zebra fish, drosophila, Caenorhabditis elegans) assays may provide useful information on potential toxicological targets (Ellis-Hutchings et al., 2011) and/or mode of action (Abbott et al., 2011). A number of such assays are considered to be useful in identifying chemicals with the potential to disrupt the endocrine system, which plays a role in the integrity of the reproductive system (Laws et al., 2012). Considered holistically, all of this information can be useful in prioritizing further research and designing a thoughtful approach to hazard assessment that refines the testing strategy and reduces the number of experimental animals and other resources needed for this assessment. Depending on the outcome of the preliminary data, short-term mammalian studies are often used to identify high-dose toxicities to target organs or systems and are useful in selecting doses for the chronic toxicity testing. Toxicokinetic assays can be instrumental in refining study designs for further toxicological testing (Frantz et al., 1994; Wier, 2012).

The animal toxicology database typically includes a number of sensitive indicators of reproductive toxicity, including structural and functional biomarkers of effects on ovarian health and integrity. Outcomes of concern could be direct measures of ovarian toxicity (e.g., histopathological lesions in ovarian tissue or decreases

TABLE 15.1
Key Assumptions for Reproductive Toxicity Hazard and Dose-Response Assessment[a]

- An agent that produces an adverse reproductive effect in experimental animals is assumed to pose a potential threat to humans.
- Effects of xenobiotics on male and female reproductive processes are assumed generally to be similar unless demonstrated otherwise. For developmental outcomes, the specific effects in humans are not necessarily the same as those seen in the experimental species.
- In the absence of information to determine the most appropriate experimental species, data from the most sensitive species should be used.
- In the absence of information to the contrary, an agent that affects reproductive function in one sex is assumed to adversely affect reproductive function in the other sex.
- A nonlinear dose–response curve is assumed for reproductive toxicity.

Source: EPA, Guidelines for Reproductive Toxicity Risk Assessment, EPA/630/R-96/009, Risk Assessment Forum, Washington, DC, 1996, http://www.epa.gov/raf/pubhumanhealth.htm

[a] These assumptions are considered to be plausibly conservative and protective of public health (NRC, 1994).

in follicle counts), or they may be indirect (e.g., alterations in female reproductive hormones or disruptions in fertility). Adverse outcomes in animal studies are considered to be indicators of potential risk to humans. For environmental agents, key assumptions for hazard and dose–response assessment for reproductive toxicity are judiciously applied (see Table 15.1).

When available, epidemiology or clinical data can be particularly informative in human health assessments for environmental chemicals and pharmaceuticals. There are a number of human correlates for the female reproductive system end points assessed in animal toxicology studies. Some end points that are relevant to the evaluation of ovarian toxicity can be assessed noninvasively in humans; these can include measurement of hormone levels, menstrual cycle normality, and the timing of puberty (pubarche), first menses (menarche), and menopause. Evidence of reproductive failure in the human population, such as altered time to pregnancy, clinical infertility and subfertility, or spontaneous abortion (miscarriage) (Källén, 2012), may also be related to compromised ovarian health. In addition to these noncancer outcomes, evidence of an increase in the incidence of ovarian cancers in the human population may be associated with environmental or pharmaceutical exposures.

Specific considerations for dose–response evaluation and exposure assessment are not addressed here, since the focus of this chapter is on hazard identification for ovarian toxicity. The following text addresses issues specific to environmental chemicals and pharmaceuticals and provides examples of substances that have been shown to target the ovary.

15.4 SCREENING ENVIRONMENTAL AGENTS FOR OVARIAN TOXICITY

15.4.1 Approaches to Testing Environmental Agents

In general, human exposure to environmental agents (e.g., industrial chemicals, pollutants, pesticides) is unintended. Nevertheless, there is a general recognition that some human exposure to these substances is likely to occur. In order to assess risk resulting from such exposures, toxicological information is generated. The studies that are considered essential to adequate screening for adverse reproductive toxicity are often specified by regulation, or the principles that guide such decisions are embodied within regulations. For example, for registering food-use and nonfood-use conventional, antimicrobial, and biologic pesticides, the U.S. Environmental Protection Agency, Office of Pesticide Programs, requires the submission of specific toxicology studies, as listed in the Federal Insecticide, Fungicide, and Rodenticide Act (FIFRA) (EPA, 2007). For industrial chemicals, legally binding test rules are negotiated between the EPA and chemical registrants in accordance with the Toxic Substances Control Act (TSCA). Overall, in regard to ovarian toxicity, the toxicology bioassays typically used in screening environmental chemicals for potential adverse health effects will include an evaluation of morphological and functional consequences of short-, intermediate-, and/or long-term exposures at various life stages.

15.4.2 Testing Guidelines for Environmental Chemicals

Toxicology testing guidelines (i.e., recommended study protocols) are available for environmental chemical assessment. EPA and OECD study guidelines are harmonized through a formal process of protocol development and publication. The use of harmonized test methods is addressed in an OECD Council Decision on Mutual Acceptance of Data. Mutual data acceptance means that "data generated in the testing of chemicals in an OECD Member country (or some nonmember economies) in accordance with OECD Test Guidelines and OECD principles of Good Laboratory Practice shall be accepted in other Member countries (or nonmember economies) for purposes of assessment and other uses relating to the protection of man and the environment" (OECD, 2008a). Since the United States is an OECD member country, studies conducted using EPA and OECD guidelines are reciprocally accepted. This principle of harmonization between OECD and EPA testing guidelines facilitates consistency in test methods used across multiple laboratories, countries, and scientific and regulatory organizations. The NTP, which is a U.S. interagency nonregulatory research program, evaluates the toxicology of agents of public health concern, conducts studies, and publishes the resulting study reports (general toxicology/carcinogenicity, developmental toxicology, and reproductive toxicology) on their website (http://ntp-server.niehs.nih.gov/).

15.4.3 Ovarian End Points Evaluated in Guideline Screening Studies for Environmental Chemicals

Table 15.2 summarizes ovarian end points that are assessed in EPA, OECD, and NTP toxicological testing guidelines that are typically used in screening environmental chemicals. Most of these studies are conducted in laboratory rodents. In the table, the protocols are grouped by type (i.e., general toxicological screening, reproductive toxicity testing, and *in vivo* endocrine assays). Guideline protocols that do not focus on female reproductive system outcomes and end points are not included in this table. Examples of such guideline protocols are the developmental neurotoxicity study (EPA, 1998k; OECD, 2007a), the dominant lethal assay (OECD, 1984; EPA, 1998j), the Hershberger assay (EPA, 2009a; OECD, 2009e), and metabolism and toxicokinetics studies (EPA, 1998l; OECD, 2010). Some in-life data collected in toxicology studies can provide information about normal functioning of the ovary. For example, hormone measurements, the age of vaginal opening (a pubertal indicator of sexual maturation in the rodent), and the timing and regularity of estrous cycles, mating, and fertility can be linked to ovarian (dys)function. In some cases, these functional and developmental outcomes may be influenced by other systemic toxicological responses and may be difficult to interpret. Postmortem assessment of the ovaries can include organ weights, macroscopic observations at necropsy, histopathological evaluation of fixed and stained tissue sections, quantitative assessment of ovarian follicles by type, and corpora lutea counts (in pregnant females). In general, short- and long-term toxicology testing protocols focus primarily on the postmortem evaluation of organs and tissues, while reproductive and endocrine toxicity testing protocols provide a broader assessment that includes a number of sensitive life stage-related developmental and functional end points.

Methodologies for female reproductive system assessment in laboratory animal models have a long history of use and validation in research and regulatory testing. Numerous publications address in-life measurements such as mating/sexual behavior (Cooper et al., 1993a), assessment of implantation (Cummings, 1993), serum hormone levels (Davis, 1993; Goldman and Cooper, 1993), estrous cycle evaluation (Cooper et al., 1993b; Goldman et al., 2007), and the evaluation of vaginal patency (Beckman and Feuston, 2003; OECD, 2008b). Likewise, standards for postmortem evaluation of female reproductive system tissues and the interpretation of lesions, including neoplasms, have been extensively addressed in the literature (Manson and Mattson, 1992; Peluso, 1992; Peluso and Gordon, 1992; Davis, 1993; Davis et al., 1999; Chen et al., 2003; Vanderhyden et al., 2003), including for the histopathological evaluation of reproductive organs following exposures to endocrine disrupting chemicals (OECD, 2009a).

Follicular toxicity is an important aspect of the histopathological evaluation of female reproductive tissues. Since the primordial follicles present at birth are the source from which all growing follicles and ovulated oocytes will be derived, a depletion of primordial follicles can have important consequences for reproductive success. As shown in Table 15.2, a quantitative assessment of ovarian follicles is recommended in the reproduction and fertility effects study (i.e., two-generation reproduction study) (EPA, 1998f; OECD, 2001b) and the extended one-generation reproductive toxicity study (OECD, 2011). Inclusion of this end

TABLE 15.2
Ovary Evaluation Specified by Toxicological Testing Guidelines for Environmental Chemicals

		In-Life				Postmortem					
Guideline Name	**Guideline No.**	**Hor**	**VO**	**Cyc**	**Mat/Fert**	**Wt**	**Mac**	**Mic**	**CL**	**PFC**	**References**
Subacute studies											
Repeated-dose 28-day oral toxicity study in rodents	OPPTS 870.3050	NS	NA	NS	NA	NS	NS	X	NA	NS	EPA (2000a)
	OECD 407	NS	NA	(X)	NA	X	X	X	NA	NS	OECD (2009b)
21-/28-day dermal toxicity	OPPTS 870.3200	NS	NA	NS	NA	X	X	X	NA	NS	EPA (1998c)
	OECD 410	NS	NA	NS	NA	NS	X	NS	NA	NS	OECD (1981a)
28-day inhalation toxicity	OECD 412	NS	NA	NS	NA	NS	X	X	NA	NS	OECD (2009c)
14-day toxicity[a]	NA[b]	NS	NA	NS	NA	NS	X	NS	NA	NS	(www.ntp.org)
Subchronic studies											
90-day oral toxicity in rodents	OPPTS 870.3100 OECD 408	NS	NA	NS	NA	X	X	X	NA	NS	EPA (1998a) and OECD (1998a)
90-day oral toxicity in nonrodents	OPPTS 870.3150 OECD 409	NS	NA	NS	NA	X	X	X	NA	NS	EPA (1998b) and OECD (1998b)
90-day dermal toxicity	OPPTS 870.3250	NS	NA	NS	NA	X	X	X	NA	NS	EPA (1998d)
	OECD 411	NS	NA	NS	NA	NS	X	X	NA	NS	OECD (1981b)
90-day inhalation toxicity	OECD 413	NS	NA	NS	NA	X	X	X	NA	NS	OECD (2009d)
13-week toxicity[a,c]	NA[b]	NS	NA	X	NA	NS	X	NS	NA	NS	(www.ntp.org)
Chronic studies											
Chronic toxicity	OPPTS 870.4100 OECD 452	NS	NA	NS	NA	X	X	X	NA	NS	EPA (1998g) and OECD (2009g)
Carcinogenicity	OPPTS 870.4200	NS	NA	NS	NA	X	X	X	NA	NS	EPA (1998h)
	OECD 451	NS	NA	NS	NA	(X)	X	X	NA	NS	OECD (2009f)
Combined chronic toxicity/carcinogenicity	OPPTS 870.4300 OECD 453	NS	NA	NS	NA	X	X	X	NA	NS	EPA (1998i) and OECD (2009h)
Combined chronic toxicity/carcinogenicity testing of respirable fibrous particles	OPPTS 870.8355	NS	NA	NS	NA	X	X	NS	NA	NS	EPA (2001)

2-year study[a,c]	NA[b]	NS	NA	NS	NA	NS	X	X	NA	NS	(www.ntp.org)
Reproductive toxicity studies											
Reproduction/developmental toxicity screening test	OPPTS 870.3550 OECD 421	NS	NS	NS	X	NS	X	X	X	X [d]	EPA (2000a) and OECD (1995)
Combined repeated-dose toxicity study with the reproduction/developmental toxicity screening test	OPPTS 870.3650 OECD 422	NS	NS	NS	X	NS	X	X	X	X [d]	EPA (2000b) and OECD (1996)
One-generation reproduction study	OECD 415	NS	NS	NS	X	NS	X	(X)	NS	NS	OECD (1983)
Prenatal developmental toxicity study	OPPTS 870.3700[e] OECD 414	NS	NS	NS	NA	NS	X	NS	X	NS	EPA (1998e), OECD (2001a), and NTP (2011)
Reproduction and fertility effects	OPPTS 870.3800 OECD 416	NS	X	X	X	X	X	X	NS	X	EPA (1998f) and OECD (2001b)
Extended one-generation reproductive toxicity study	OECD 443	X	X	X	X	X	X	X	X	X	OECD (2011)
Reproductive assessment by continuous breeding (RACB)	NA[b]	X	X	X	X	X	X	X	X	(X)	Chapin and Sloane (1997) and NTP (2011)
In vivo endocrine assays											
Uterotrophic assay[f]	OPPTS 890.1600 OECD 440	NS	NA	NS	NA	NS	NS	NS	NA	NS	OECD (2007b) and EPA (2009c)
Pubertal development and thyroid function in intact juvenile/peripubertal female rats	OPPTS 890.1450	NS	X	X	NA	X	NS	X	X [d]	X [d]	EPA (2009b)

Note: X, recommended for evaluation; (X), optional evaluation; NS, not specified; NA, not applicable.

Note: Hor, hormone measures; VO, vaginal opening; Cyc, estrous cyclicity (vaginal smears); Mat/Fert, mating or fertility; Wt, ovary weight (wet); Mac, macroscopic pathological evaluation at necropsy; Mic, microscopic histopathological evaluation of fixed and stained tissue sections; CL, corpora lutea counts, PFC, primordial follicle counts.

[a] Applies to oral, inhalation, or dermal route of administration.

[b] NTP study designs are not assigned guideline numbers.

[c] Animals assigned to study are derived from a perinatal study (www.ntp.org).

[d] Qualitative (not quantitative) assessment of ovarian follicles.

[e] NTP specifies the use of OPPTS 870.3700 for developmental toxicity testing.

[f] Optional testing in either sexually immature or ovariectomized adult female rodents.

point in the guidelines was based upon published studies demonstrating that follicular counts were a sensitive means of evaluating ovarian toxicity (Mattison et al., 1983; Takizawa et al., 1984; Weitzman et al., 1992; Flaws et al., 1994) and a number of NTP studies that showed the feasibility of assessing follicle counts in reproductive toxicity bioassays using continuous breeding (Bolon et al., 1997). Detailed strategies for sectioning and counting the follicles have been proposed (Smith et al., 1991; Bolon et al., 1997; Bucci et al., 1997; Heindel, 1998;); however, the testing guidelines do not specify the exact procedures to use. A collaborative review of ovarian toxicity evaluation in repeated-dose and fertility studies (Sanbuissho et al., 2009) included ovarian follicle evaluations using immunohistochemical staining for proliferating cell nuclear antigens (PCNAs) and found that this technique was useful to detect small follicles (Yoshida et al., 2009). Some experts believe that careful qualitative histopathological evaluation of the ovary, in conjunction with hormonal, estrous cyclicity, and reproductive outcome data, will be sufficiently sensitive to detect ovarian toxicants (Regan et al., 2005) and that follicular quantification is not necessary. Nevertheless, unpublished studies submitted to the U.S. EPA for pesticide registration have identified several chemicals for which ovarian counts were significantly decreased in the two-generation reproduction studies, although no qualitative histopathology follicular findings were reported in the same studies.

15.4.4 Examples of Environmental Chemicals That Have Been Shown to Target the Ovary

Both in-life and postmortem end points assessed in guideline toxicity screening studies (Table 15.2) are likely to detect a variety of adverse outcomes to the female reproductive system, including morphological and functional alterations to the developing and adult ovary. Histopathological evaluation of reproductive organs in rodent chronic/carcinogenicity studies can detect evidence of ovarian cancer. Noncancer effects can include altered sexual differentiation of the brain or other developmental abnormalities that affect attainment of puberty or adult reproductive function, disruption of the neuroendocrine control of hormones in adults, or depletion of primordial or small follicles through advanced follicular atresia. The following are some examples of environmental chemicals that elicit ovarian toxicity in rodent studies. This is not intended to be an exhaustive list of ovarian toxicants nor a systematic review of all studies identifying ovarian toxicity. Instead, it is presented to illustrate a variety of chemical classes, adverse end points, susceptible life stages, and modes of action that have been reported in the published literature:

- *Thiram*, a dithiocarbamate pesticide, inhibits the luteinizing hormone (LH) surge in rats, thereby inhibiting ovulation, when administered by a single injection of ≥25 mg/kg during a sensitive period prior to initiation of the surge (Stoker et al., 1993). It has been proposed that the mode of action for this outcome involves the inhibition of dopamine-β-hydroxylase, which affects norepinephrine synthesis (a neurotransmitter that plays an important role in the hypothalamic regulation of pituitary function).

- Treatment of adult rats with 2 g/kg of the plasticizer *di-(2-ethylhexyl) phthalate (DEHP)* causes decreased serum estradiol levels. Evidence suggests that the DEHP active metabolite, mono-(2-ethylhexyl) phthalate (MEHP), acts through a receptor-mediated signaling pathway to suppress estradiol production in the ovary, leading to anovulation (Lovekamp-Swan and Davis, 2003). It has been suggested that the mode of action may involve DEHP treatment-related decreased circulating thyroxine levels and a subsequent disruption of the hypothalamic–pituitary–ovarian axis (Sekiguchi et al., 2006). In a 2-week repeated-dose study with DEHP, histopathological lesions (vacuolation of stromal cells) were observed at 300 mg/kg/day, with increased large atretic follicles noted at ≥1000 mg/kg/day. In 4-week repeated-dose and fertility studies, decreased corpora lutea, prolonged and irregular estrous cycles, and decreased fertility were observed at 3000 mg/kg/day (the highest dose tested) (Takai et al., 2009).
- *Atrazine*, a chlorotriazine herbicide, was found to disrupt the ovulatory LH and prolactin surges in rats by altering hypothalamic regulation of the pituitary gland (Cooper et al., 2007). At doses of ≥50 mg/kg/day, altered estrous cycles, including persistent estrus, were observed in young adult rats. Administration of atrazine and its metabolic by-products to pubertal rats (i.e., on postnatal days 22–41) resulted in delayed vaginal opening and irregular estrous cycles at ≥50 mg/kg/day, decreased ovarian weights at ≥100 mg/kg/day, and decreased corpora luteum development with a 1.6-fold increase in the average number of atretic follicles at 200 mg/kg/day (Laws et al., 2000, 2003). The disrupted estrous cyclicity and histopathological findings were confirmed in a 2-week gavage study in adult rats; atrazine treatment at 300 mg/kg/day resulted in prolonged diestrus, loss of currently formed corpora lutea, decreased numbers of previously formed corpora lutea, increased large-sized atretic follicles, and swelling of previously formed luteal cells (Shibayama et al., 2009).
- Following exposures of rats to *diuron*, a urea-derived pesticide, from gestation day 12 until postnatal day 51, reductions in ovarian weight and corpora lutea were observed at a dose of 1250 ppm on postnatal day 75 (Grassi et al., 2011), suggesting ovarian toxicity. In this study, there were no observed treatment-related effects on the timing of vaginal opening or in estrous cyclicity.
- The estrogenic pesticide *methoxychlor* was found to target ovarian antral follicles in adult mice administered intraperitoneal injections of ≥64 mg/kg/day for 20 or 30 days (Paulose et al., 2012). An observed 50% increase in follicular atresia did not affect overall fertility of the mice in this study.
- Treatment with the plasticizer *di(2-ethylhexyl)adipate (DEHA)* for 2 or 4 weeks resulted in increased atresia of large follicles, decreased currently formed corpora lutea, and follicular cysts at ≥1000 mg/kg/day (Wato et al., 2009). In a fertility study with DEHA, conducted by the same research group, increased mean estrous cycle length and postimplantation loss were also observed at ≥1000 mg/kg/day.

- *1,3-Butadiene* is a highly volatile gas used in the manufacture of synthetic rubber and thermoplastic resins (reviewed in EPA [2002]). Targeted ovarian toxicity was observed after chronic inhalation exposures to 1,3-butadiene. In a chronic inhalation study in mice (NTP, 1993), ovarian atrophy was observed at ≥6.25 ppm, and significant incidences of benign or malignant granulosa cell tumors were observed at ≥62.5 ppm after 103 weeks of exposure (EPA, 2002).
- *4-Vinylcyclohexene* (a dimer of 1,3-butadiene) and its mono- and diepoxide metabolites, which are released into the environment during the manufacture of rubber products, insecticides, and flame retardants, have been shown to cause destruction of small preantral (i.e., primordial and primary) follicles in ovaries of mice and rats by accelerating the process of atresia via apoptotic signaling (Hoyer et al., 2001; Hoyer and Sipes, 2007). Mice are more sensitive than rats to this outcome, due to species-related differences in the metabolism of 4-vinylcyclohexene to its active metabolites, although the age of treatment (immature/peripubertal vs. adult/aged rodents) with the diepoxide did not affect the ability of the chemical to destroy oocytes in primordial and primary follicles (Flaws et al., 1994; Muhammad et al., 2009). Repeated-dose (2- and 4-week) studies with intraperitoneal administration of 4-vinylcyclohexene diepoxide (VCD) in rats found decreases in small follicles at 80 mg/kg/day after 2 weeks of treatment and at ≥20 mg/kg/day after 4 weeks of treatment (Ito et al., 2009). Estrous cyclicity was not affected by intraperitoneal injection of VCD in the fertility study (Kodama et al., 2009). Chronic (105-week) gavage administration of mice with 4-vinylcyclohexene identified granulosa cell hyperplasia and neoplasms at ≥200 mg/kg/day (the lowest dose tested) (NTP, 1986).
- *7,12-Dimethylbenz(a)anthracene (DMBA)*, a polycyclic aromatic hydrocarbon and component of cigarette smoke, is a reproductive toxicant in mice. Weitzman and colleagues administered single intraperitoneal injections of 0.1, 1, or 10 mg/kg DMBA to mice, producing a dose-dependent decrease in ovarian volume and number of corpora lutea, consistent with toxicity to growing and resting follicles (Weitzman et al., 1992).
- In NTP reproductive toxicity assessments, ovarian follicle counts were significantly decreased for *2,2-bis(bromoethyl)-1,3 propanediol, methoxyacetic acid,* and *ethylene glycol monomethyl ether (EGME)* (Heindel, 1998). EGME was also evaluated in 2- and 4-week repeated-dose studies and a fertility study that administered the test substance for 2 weeks prior to mating, during mating, and until gestation day 6 (Dodo et al., 2009). Continuous diestrus, hypertrophy of the corpora lutea with decreased cellular debris indication apoptosis, and increased PCNA-negative large atretic follicles were observed in the repeated-dose studies at ≥100 mg/kg/day. These findings were considered suggestive of suppressed ovulation due to hypertrophic corpora lutea and were supported by the results of the fertility study, which demonstrated irregular estrous cycles, prolonged mating periods, lower pregnancy rates, and decreased corpora lutea of pregnancy at the same treatment level.

In spite of the likelihood that guideline studies will be able to detect a variety of toxicological effects on the ovary, information gaps may still exist for the female reproductive hazard characterization for environmental agents. One particularly notable example is the lack of adequate assessment of reproductive senescence. Those studies that assess reproductive function do not retain the adult females into old age as do chronic/carcinogenicity studies, yet the chronic/carcinogenicity studies do not assess estrous cyclicity. Therefore, treatment-related acceleration of primordial follicle depletion in the ovary could lead to reproductive failure at an earlier age than occurs in control females and is generally considered predictive of that potential outcome. However, early reproductive senescence might not be observed using the current testing paradigm.

15.5 SCREENING PHARMACEUTICALS FOR OVARIAN TOXICITY

15.5.1 Approaches to Testing Pharmaceuticals

In contrast to the human exposure to environmental agents, human exposure to pharmaceuticals usually occurs by design in order to treat a specific human condition or ailment. Each drug product is tested for a specific human indication, which stipulates the dose and duration of the exposure as well as the human population that will be using the drug product. Consequently, testing for each pharmaceutical is uniquely designed to address specific concerns about that drug. Prior to exposing humans to specific drug formulations, a stepwise process involving an evaluation of both animal and human efficacy and safety information is followed before proceeding to the next phase of drug development (phases 1, 2, 3, and 4; Figure 15.2). The goals of the nonclinical safety evaluation generally include a characterization of toxic effects with respect to end points such as target organs, dose dependence, and relationship to exposure. This information is used to estimate an initial safe starting dose and the maximal tolerated dose range for the human trials. Nonclinical studies also help identify potential adverse effects that can be monitored in clinical trials. The nonclinical safety assessment for marketing approval of a pharmaceutical usually includes (among others) pharmacology studies, general toxicity studies, toxicokinetic and nonclinical pharmacokinetic studies, reproduction toxicity studies, genotoxicity studies, and, for drugs that are intended for a chronic duration of use, an assessment of carcinogenic potential.

Phase 1: Screening for safety and tolerability, pharmacokinetics, pharmacodynamics, and early measurement of drug activity

Phase 2: Explore therapeutic efficacy in patients

Phase 3: Demonstrate or confirm therapeutic benefit

Phase 4: Post-approval therapeutic use studies

FIGURE 15.2 Phases of clinical development. (From ICH, E8: General consideration for clinical trials, ICH Harmonized Tripartite Guideline. http://www.ich.org/fileadmin/Public_Web_Site/ICH_Products/Guidelines/Efficacy/E8/Step4/E8_Guideline.pdf, 1997a.)

15.5.2 Testing Guidelines for Pharmaceuticals

Similar to the understanding between EPA and OECD, a formal process of guidance development and publication exists between the FDA and the International Conference on Harmonization of Technical Requirements for Registration of Pharmaceuticals for Human Use (ICH). The nonclinical program follows recommended standards, which are generally harmonized with other regions (Europe, Japan, and Canada). The nonclinical aspects followed by FDA per the understanding with the ICH are similar to those indicated in the guidelines recommended by EPA and OECD for environmental agents, in terms of study design, study conduct, and in the risk assessments that are obtained from the study analysis.

15.5.3 Ovarian End Points Assessed for Pharmaceutical Products

As a part of the development of drugs for human use, the FDA's Center for Drug Evaluation and Research (CDER) recommends a standard battery of toxicity testing using study designs intended to identify potential toxicity that can occur with the administration of a test drug to reproductive organs such as the ovary. If a signal is detected during the nonclinical testing paradigm, a risk assessment is usually performed, taking into consideration factors such as the indication, target population, route of exposure, duration, and exposure multiples for the expected clinical population. Ovarian toxicity is captured in the developmental and reproductive toxicity studies (DART) conducted according to ICH guideline S5A (ICH, 2000). In the United States, the data are interpreted according to the FDA CDER reproductive and developmental toxicity integration guidance (FDA, 2011). Ovarian toxicity end points are also obtained from the repeated-dose toxicity testing in rodents/nonrodents per ICH M3(R2) (ICH, 2009) and from carcinogenicity bioassays in rodents as per ICH S1A (ICH, 1995) and ICH S1B (ICH, 1997b). The ovarian end points assessed in these study types are summarized in Table 15.3 and discussed in more detail in the succeeding text.

15.5.4 Ovarian End Points Assessed in Developmental and Reproductive Toxicity (DART) Studies for Pharmaceuticals

A battery of tests designed to determine if a drug potentially impairs fertility or affects fetal and neonatal development is generally required for market approval. The goal of the pre- and postnatal developmental toxicity studies is to evaluate embryo/fetal viability, teratogenicity, and sexual maturation and fertility in male and female offspring, along with general growth and organ development and other functional (primarily neurobehavioral) end points. Some developmental stages (e.g., gestational, neonatal, peripubertal) are particularly sensitive to agents that impact the ovaries and their function.

15.5.5 Ovarian End Points Assessed in Repeated-Dose Toxicity Studies for Pharmaceuticals

Nonclinical safety assessment for new drugs intended to be used chronically typically includes repeated-dose toxicology studies in two species, where animals

TABLE 15.3
Ovarian End Points Captured for Pharmaceutical Ingredients in Nonclinical Testing

Study Name	Guidance	In-Life	Postmortem			References
			Wt	Mac	Mic	
Subacute studies: 28-day rodent general toxicity	ICH M3(R2)	NS	X	X	X	ICH (2009)
Chronic studies: 6-month rodent general toxicity	ICH M3(R2)	NS	X	X	X	ICH (2009)
Chronic studies: 9-month nonrodent general toxicity	ICH M3(R2)	NS	X	X	X	ICH (2009)
Carcinogenicity rodent studies: 2-year rat/mouse lifetime bioassay	ICH S1A	NS	X	X	X	ICH (1995)
Fertility and reproduction studies: rodent	ICH S5(R2)	NS	X	X	X	ICH (2000)
Embryo fetal development: rodent/ nonrodent	ICH S5(R2)	NS	X	X	X	ICH (2000)
Pre-/postnatal development: rodent	ICH S5(R2)	NS	X	X	X	ICH (2000)

Note: X, recommended for evaluation; NS, not specified.
Note: Wt, ovary weight (wet); Mac, macroscopic pathological evaluation at necropsy; Mic, microscopic histopathological evaluation of fixed and stained tissue sections.

are exposed to a range of drug concentrations spanning clinically equivalent doses to high level doses. Toxicity data obtained from repeated-dose, short-term (14 days, 1 month studies), subchronic toxicity testing (3 months in rodents, 6 months in nonrodents) and chronic studies (6 months in rodents, 9 months in nonrodents) contain information regarding the effect of the treatment on the ovaries of treated animals. Traditional end points include ovarian weights, macroscopic observations at necropsy, and histopathological evaluation of fixed and stained tissue sections. Depending on the outcomes of the previously mentioned standard toxicity tests, additional mechanistic nonclinical studies may be necessary to more fully characterize the impact of a given drug on the health of the ovaries. In addition to the end points of mating and fertility parameters, which are closely monitored in the reproductive and developmental studies, additional mechanistic studies may be conducted to help elucidate the biologic basis for ovarian toxicity. These studies could involve measurement of hormone levels (e.g., estrogen, follicle stimulating hormone, LH, or progesterone), ovarian follicular counting, and estrous cyclicity evaluation during the in-life portion of the study, as well as counting corpora lutea postmortem. Special attention is usually paid to toxic findings obtained as a result of suprapharmacological effects of the drug in question. For example, estrogenic drugs can produce effects such as increased ovarian weight and stimulation, increased uterine weight and endometrial stimulation, mammary gland stimulation, decreased thymus weight and involution, and increased bone mineral density.

Estrogenic hormone receptor antagonists and androgenic drugs tend to have the opposite effect on reproductive organs.

15.5.6 Ovarian End Points Assessed in Carcinogenicity Studies for Pharmaceuticals

The 2-year bioassay studies that are usually conducted in rodents (mice, rats) represent an important source of information about the chronic effects of exposure of the ovaries to new drugs. While the goal of these studies is to assess the effects of drugs for carcinogenic potential, organ changes including weights and histopathology are assessed that provide information about the noncancer effects of the drug on the ovaries. For example, the effect of persistent disruption of the hypothalamic–pituitary adrenal/gonadal/thyroidal axis(es) can result in various tumors that are seen in these assays (ICH, 1997b).

15.5.7 Pharmaceuticals Demonstrating Ovarian Toxicity

In the following, we provide examples of drugs that have been shown to affect the structure or function of the ovaries in animal models. A number of these drugs are classified as oncology drug products (e.g., cyclophosphamide, doxorubicin, busulfan, and cisplatin), all of which have shown ovarian toxicity findings.

Another group of drugs that affects the steroid hormones that are directly or indirectly produced by the ovaries are also provided in the following and include tamoxifen, diethylstilbestrol (DES), medroxyprogesterone acetate (MPA), mifepristone, and anastrozole.

Besides the suprapharmacological effects seen for the antineoplastic agents and the steroid hormone agents, there are a number of drugs whose primary pharmacology does not lend support to a role in contributing to ovarian toxicity; these include peroxisome proliferator-activated receptor (PPAR), alpha and gamma dual agonists, indomethacin, bromocriptine, chlorpromazine hydrochloride, and sulpiride. Further studies into these agents' mechanism of action to explain the toxic effect on the ovaries will not be explored in this chapter:

- A repeated-dose toxicity study conducted in the rat with *cyclophosphamide*, a chemotherapeutic and immunotherapeutic alkylating agent, identified a number of ovarian toxicity findings (Sato et al., 2009a). Increases in large-sized atretic follicles and atrophy of corpora lutea were observed in the 20 mg/kg/day group after 4 weeks of treatment. In a female fertility study, the numbers of implantations were slightly decreased, and corpora lutea of pregnancy were not observed in the 20 mg/kg/day group. A dose-dependent increase in the incidence of postimplantation loss was observed, and no abnormalities were noted in the estrous cycle and mating in all treated groups.
- *Doxorubicin*, an anthracycline agent, which is used as a chemotherapy agent, has been shown to be toxic to the ovaries both in animal models and in treated women (Meirow, 1999). Recent studies point to a role of apoptosis

in doxorubicin-induced ovarian toxicity, as has been shown by positive staining of terminal deoxynucleotidyl transferase dUTP nick end labeling (TUNEL) and active caspase-3 in histological examination of treated ovaries in mice. A single injection of doxorubicin resulted in a major reduction in both ovarian size and weight that lasted up to 1 month posttreatment. A dramatic reduction in ovulation rate was observed 1 week after treatment, followed by a partial recovery at 1 month. In addition, a significant reduction in the population of secondary and primordial follicles was noted 1 month following treatment (Ben-Aharon et al., 2010).

- *Busulfan* is an antineoplastic agent that targets small follicles (primordial and primary follicles) (Sakurada et al., 2009). In a 2-week study, all rats treated with busulfan showed normal estrous cyclicity and no toxicological changes in weight or histopathology of the ovaries. In a 4-week study, a decrease in small follicles was found histopathologically in 1/10 rats, even at 0.5 mg/kg/day, and in 4/10 rats at 1.5 mg/kg/day. PCNA immunohistochemistry of the follicles confirmed the decrease in number of small follicles at 1.5 mg/kg/day. In a female fertility study, increases in dead embryos and postimplantation loss were found in rats at 1.5 mg/kg/day.
- *Cisplatin*, a cancer chemotherapeutic agent that forms cross-links with DNA, caused a decrease in large follicles, an increase in atresia of medium and large follicles, and/or a decrease in currently formed corpora lutea in rats administered 1.0 or 2.0 mg/kg/day for 2 weeks. Decreases in small and/or large follicles and an increase in atresia of large follicles were observed in animals receiving 0.25 or 0.5 mg/kg/day for 4 weeks (Nozaki et al., 2009).
- Short-term studies with *tamoxifen*, an antiestrogenic oncology drug, identified a number of histological findings in the ovaries of rats (Tsujioka et al., 2009). These included increases in large atretic follicles, increases in interstitium cells, and absence of newly formed corpus lutea at 0.2 mg/kg/day in a 2-week study and at 0.03 and 0.2 mg/kg/day in a 4-week study. The treatment with tamoxifen induced estrogenic and antiestrogenic reactions in the uterus, while mucinous degeneration was detected in the vagina.
- *DES*, a classical endocrine-active agent and reproductive toxicant, causes various abnormalities in the female reproductive organs of mice when exposure takes place prenatally. Ovarian toxicity includes morphological changes such as the absence of corpora lutea, hypertrophy of interstitial tissue, and hemorrhagic cysts (Tenenbaum and Forsberg, 1985) and polyovular follicles (where a single follicle contains two or more oocytes). Studies conducted in 5-day old C57BL/6J mice indicated that DES may suppress follicle development and decrease the number of follicles in the ovaries of neonatal mice through its action on estrogen receptors (Kim et al., 2009).
- *MPA*, a synthetic progesterone, resulted in ovarian toxicity in both pregnant and nonpregnant rats following either a 2- or 4-week-treatment period. The number of MPA-treated nonpregnant female rats with irregular estrous cycles increased in number, and a decrease in ovarian weight was observed at 2 and 10 mg/kg/day in both duration groups (2 and 4 weeks). Histopathological examination revealed an increased number of large atretic

follicles and decreases in currently formed corpora lutea. In the female fertility study where pregnant rats were dosed from 2 weeks prior to mating until gestation day 7, the number of animals with an irregular estrous cycle and elongation of mean estrous cycle increased at 0.4 mg/kg/day, with no changes in fertility. A decreased number of copulating animals and a decreased gestation rate with low preimplantation loss were observed in the 2.0 mg/kg/day treatment group, and no copulation was observed in the group treated with 10 mg/kg/day (Ohtake et al., 2009).

- *Mifepristone*, a progesterone receptor antagonist, resulted in persistent estrus in the vaginal smears and the presence of multiple cysts in the ovaries at necropsy, increases in luteinized cysts and hypertrophy of previously formed corpora lutea in ovaries of rats receiving 20 mg/kg/day or more for 2 or 4 weeks. In a female fertility study, reproductive findings were not seen in the ovaries but were noted in the vagina (persistent vaginal cornification seen at 20 mg/kg/day) and the fertility outcome (all of the animals were completely infertile when dosed with 20 mg/kg/day during the postcoital period) and in implantation loss. An increase in preimplantation losses was observed in the animals treated with 20 mg/kg/day during the precoital phase, while treatment with 4 mg/kg/day mifepristone during the postcoital phase induced an increase in postimplantation losses at dose levels of 0, 0.8, 4, and 20 mg/kg/day from >2 weeks before copulation to postcoital day 7 (Tamura et al., 2009).
- An association of ovarian cancers with hormone replacement therapy (HRT) has been reported in several studies. (1) In a British study, the use of HRT among postmenopausal women was found to be associated with an increased risk of developing ovarian cancer. The incidence of ovarian cancer increased with increasing duration of use and the type of HRT used. The study reported that HRT with estrogen only had a higher association with ovarian cancer than HRTs using estrogen–progesterone combinations (Beral et al., 2007). (2) A Swedish study reported that estrogen use alone and estrogen–progestin used sequentially (progestin used on average 10 days/month) may be associated with an increased risk for ovarian cancer. In contrast, estrogen–progestin used continuously (progestin used on average 28 days/month) seemed to confer no increased ovarian cancer risk (Riman et al., 2002). (3) A National Cancer Institute study found that women who used estrogen replacement therapy after menopause were at increased risk for ovarian cancer compared to women who never used hormone therapy (Lacey et al., 2002).
- *Anastrozole*, a potent inhibitor of aromatase, is a rate-limiting enzyme in transforming androgens to estrogens. In the ovary, aromatase expression is detected in the granulosa cell and is essential for the maturation of follicles. In a repeated-dose toxicity study in rats, large abnormal atretic follicles, follicular cysts, a decrease in corpus luteum and depletion of developing corpus luteum were observed in the 1 and/or 50 mg/kg/day groups of both the 2- and 4-week studies in a histopathological examination of the ovaries (Shirai et al., 2009).

- Another example of a pharmaceutical that results in ovarian toxicity is an unidentified *PPAR alpha/gamma dual agonist* where ovarian toxicity was described following repeated-dose general toxicity study (2- and 4-week toxicity studies) and in a female fertility study. The ovarian toxicity findings from the repeated-dose testing included an increase in atresia of large follicles, a decrease in corpora lutea, and an increase in stromal cells. The fertility study revealed a decrease in the pregnancy rate among rats treated at the high dose (100 mg/kg/day) and a decrease in the number of corpora lutea, implantations, and live pups at the mid and high doses (40 and 100 mg/kg/day) (Sato et al., 2009b).
- *Indomethacin* is a nonselective inhibitor of cyclooxygenase (COX)-1 and COX-2, which are involved in prostaglandin synthesis from arachidonic acid. It is used as a nonsteroidal anti-inflammatory drug (NSAID) and an arylalkanoic acid class analgesic. Indomethacin has been thought to inhibit ovulation by acting directly and specifically on the preovulatory follicles of rat ovaries, where prostaglandin synthesis is markedly increased. In a general toxicity study, unruptured follicles or luteinized cysts were observed histopathologically in the 4 mg/kg/day group in both 2- and 4-week studies. In addition, follicular cysts were found in the 4 mg/kg/day group in the 4-week study (Tsubota et al., 2009).
- *Bromocriptine* has been in clinical use primarily for treatment of hyperprolactinemia and Parkinson's disease. Bromocriptine-induced hypoprolactinemia alters corpus luteum formation and ovary function in female rats. In a 2-week repeated-dose toxicity study, increase of ovarian weights was observed at 2 mg/kg/day. In the 4-week repeated-dose toxicity study, ovarian weights were increased at 0.4 and 2 mg/kg/day. The number of corpora luteum was increased in the 0.4 and 2 mg/kg/day groups of the 2- and 4-week repeated-dose toxicity studies. Bromocriptine did not affect estrous cyclicity in 2- and 4-week repeated dosing (Kumazawa et al., 2009).
- *Chlorpromazine HCl*, an antipsychotic drug, has been shown to cause ovarian toxicity in repeated-dose toxicity studies. In 2- and 4-week toxicity studies in the rat, ovarian weights were decreased at >10 mg/kg/day, and an increase in large atretic follicles was observed histopathologically at >3 mg/kg/day and >10 mg/kg/day in the 2- and 4-week studies, respectively. In addition, decreased uterine weights and/or atrophic findings in the uterus and vagina at 30 mg/kg/day and >10 mg/kg/day, mucification in the vaginal epithelium, and alveolar hyperplasia in the mammary gland at >3 mg/kg/day and >10 mg/kg/day were seen in the 2- and 4-week studies, respectively. Irregular estrous cycles were seen at >3 mg/kg/day and >10 mg/kg/day in the 2- and 4-week studies (Izumi et al., 2009).
- *Sulpiride*, a D2 antagonist, is used as an antipsychotic drug for the treatment of psychosis and depression. Antipsychotic drugs such as sulpiride or haloperidol may induce hyperprolactinemia. In ovarian histology of the 2-week rat toxicity study, increases in atretic follicles were seen at ≥1 mg/kg/day and increases in follicular cysts at ≥10 mg/kg/day. In the 4-week study, these findings were seen at ≥1 mg/kg day, and a decrease in large follicles

was seen at ≥10 mg/kg/day. Increased body weight gain was observed at ≥10 mg/kg/day in the 2- and 4-week studies. Treated females exhibited development of mammary alveolus by sulpiride-induced hyperprolactinemia. In the fertility study, sulpiride-treated females showing persistent diestrus resulted in successful mating, and almost all females were assessed to be pregnant. However, increased implantation loss was observed at ≥10 mg/kg/day, a finding which was attributed to the adverse effect of sulpiride on oocyte development, which can be one of the causes of ovulatory dysfunction including anovulation in humans and animals (Ishii et al., 2009).

15.6 SUMMARY

This chapter has discussed the assessment of ovarian toxicity for use in human health risk assessment. Issues specific to the evaluation of environmental agents and of pharmaceuticals in preclinical developmental have been described, with special emphasis on the types of studies that are typically utilized in a regulatory context. A limited review of some environmental chemicals and pharmaceuticals that have been shown to cause ovarian toxicity demonstrates the importance of identifying potential ovarian toxicity when assessing human risk to xenobiotic exposures.

DISCLAIMER

The views expressed in this chapter are those of the authors and do not necessarily represent the views or policies of the U.S. EPA or the U.S. FDA.

REFERENCES

Abbott, B. D., Rosen, M. B., Watkins, A. M. and Wood, C. R. 2011. Approaches for evaluation of mode of action. In: Hood, R. D. (ed.) *Developmental and Reproductive Toxicology: A Practical Approach.* 3rd ed. New York: Informa Healthcare.

Beckman, D. A. and Feuston, M. 2003. Landmarks in the development of the female reproductive system. *Birth Defects Res B Dev Reprod Toxicol,* 68: 137–143.

Ben-Aharon, I., Bar-Joseph, H., Tzarfaty, G., Kuchinsky, L., Rizel, S., Stemmer, S. M. and Shalgi, R. 2010. Doxorubicin-induced ovarian toxicity. *Reprod Biol Endocrinol,* 8: 20.

Beral, V., Bull, D., Green, J. and Reeves, G. 2007. Ovarian cancer and hormone replacement therapy in the Million Women Study. *Lancet,* 369: 1703–1710.

Bolon, B., Bucci, T. J., Warbritton, A. R., Chen, J. J., Mattison, D. R. and Heindel, J. J. 1997. Differential follicle counts as a screen for chemically induced ovarian toxicity in mice: Results from continuous breeding bioassays. *Fundam Appl Toxicol,* 39: 1–10.

Bucci, T. J., Bolon, B., Warbritton, A. R., Chen, J. J. and Heindel, J. J. 1997. Influence of sampling on the reproducibility of ovarian follicle counts in mouse toxicity studies. *Reprod Toxicol,* 11: 689–696.

Cabrera, R. M., Wlodarczyk, B. J. and Finnell, R. H. 2011. Functional genomics and proteomics in developmental and reproductive toxicology. In: Hood, R. D. (ed.), *Developmental and Reproductive Toxicology: A Practical Approach.* 3rd ed. New York: Informa Healthcare.

Chapin, R. E. and Sloane, R. A. 1997. Reproductive assessment by continuous breeding: Evolving study design and summaries of ninety studies. *Environ Health Perspect,* 105 Suppl 1: 199–205.

Chen, V. W., Ruiz, B., Killeen, J. L., Cote, T. R., Wu, X. C. and Correa, C. N. 2003. Pathology and classification of ovarian tumors. *Cancer,* 97: 2631–2642.

Cooper, R. L., Goldman, J. M. and Stoker, T. E. 1993a. Measuring sexual behavior in the female rat. In: Heindel, J. J. and Chapin, R. E. (eds.) *Methods in Toxicology, Part B, Female Reproductive Toxicology*. New York: Academic Press, Inc.

Cooper, R. L., Goldman, J. M. and Vandenbergh, J. G. 1993b. Monitoring of the estrous cycle in the laboratory rodent by vaginal lavage. In: Heindel, J. J. and Chapin, R. E. (eds.) *Methods in Toxicology, Part B, Female Reproductive Toxicology*. New York: Academic Press, Inc.

Cooper, R. L., Laws, S. C., Das, P. C., Narotsky, M. G., Goldman, J. M., Lee Tyrey, E. and Stoker, T. E. 2007. Atrazine and reproductive function: Mode and mechanism of action studies. *Birth Defects Res B Dev Reprod Toxicol,* 80: 98–112.

Cummings, A. M. 1993. Assessment of Implantation in the Rat. In: Heindel, J. J. and Chapin, R. E. (eds.) *Methods in Toxicology, Part B, Female Reproductive Toxicology*. New York: Academic Press, Inc.

Davis, B. J. 1993. Ovarian target cell toxicity. In: Heindel, J. J. and Chapin, R. E. (eds.) *Methods in Toxicology, Part B, Female Reproductive Toxicology*. New York: Academic Press, Inc.

Davis, B. J., Dixon, D. and Herbert, R. A. 1999. Ovary, oviduct, uterus, cervix, and vagina. In: Maronpot, R. R. (ed.), *Pathology of the Mouse*. Vienna, IL: Cache River Press.

Dodo, T., Taketa, Y., Sugiyama, M., Inomata, A., Sonoda, J., Okuda, Y., Mineshima, H., Hosokawa, S. and Aoki, T. 2009. Collaborative work on evaluation of ovarian toxicity. 11) Two- or four-week repeated-dose studies and fertility study of ethylene glycol monomethyl ether in female rats. *J Toxicol Sci,* 34 Suppl 1: SP121–128.

Ellis-Hutchings, R. G., de Jong, E., Piersma, A. H. and Carney, E. W. 2011. In vitro screening methods for developmental toxicity. In: Hood, R. D. (ed.), *Developmental and Reproductive Toxicology: A Practical Approach*. 3rd ed. New York: Informa Healthcare.

EMEA. 2008. Guideline on Risk Assessment of Medicinal Products on Human Reproduction and Lactation: From Data to Labelling. London, U.K.: Committee for Medicinal Products for Human Use (CHMP). http://www.ema.europa.eu/docs/en_GB/document_library/Scientific_guideline/2009/09/WC500003307.pdf

EPA. 1991. *Guidelines for Developmental Toxicity Risk Assessment, EPA/600/FR-91/001*. Washington, DC: Risk Assessment Forum, http://www.epa.gov/raf/pubhumanhealth.htm

EPA. 1996. *Guidelines for Reproductive Toxicity Risk Assessment, EPA/630/R-96/009*. Washington, DC: Risk Assessment Forum, http://www.epa.gov/raf/pubhumanhealth.htm

EPA. 1998a. *OPPTS 870.3100: 90-Day Oral Toxicity in Rodents, Health Effects Test Guidelines*. Washington, DC: EPA 712-C-98-199.

EPA. 1998b. *OPPTS 870.3150: 90-Day Oral Toxicity in Nonrodents, Health Effects Test Guidelines*. Washington, DC: EPA 712-C-98-200.

EPA. 1998c. *OPPTS 870.3200: 21/28-Day Dermal Toxicity, Health Effects Test Guidelines*. Washington, DC: EPA 712-C-98-201.

EPA. 1998d. *OPPTS 870.3250: 90-Day Dermal Toxicity, Health Effects Test Guidelines*. Washington, DC: EPA 712-98-202.

EPA. 1998e. OPPTS 870.3700: Prenatal Developmental Toxicity Study, Health Effects Test Guidelines. Washington, DC: EPA 712-C-98-207.

EPA. 1998f. OPPTS 870.3800: Reproduction and Fertility Effects, Health Effects Test Guidelines. Washington, DC: EPA 712-C-98-208.

EPA. 1998g. OPPTS 870.4100: Chronic Toxicity, *Health Effects Test Guidelines*. Washington, DC: EPA 712-C-98-210.

EPA. 1998h. OPPTS 870.4200: Carcinogenicity, Health Effects Test Guidelines. Washington, DC: EPA 712-C-98-211.

EPA. 1998i. *OPPTS 870.4300: Combined Chronic Toxicity/Carcinogenicity, Health Effects Test Guidelines*. Washington, DC: EPA 712-C-98-212.

EPA. 1998j. *OPPTS 870.5450: Rodent Dominant Lethal Assay, Health Effects Test Guidelines*. Washington, DC: EPA 712-C-98-227.

EPA. 1998k. *OPPTS 870.6300: Developmental Neurotoxicity Study, Health Effects Test Guidelines*. Washington, DC: EPA 712-C-98-239.

EPA. 1998l. *OPPTS 870.7485: Metabolism and Pharmacokinetics, Health Effects Test Guidelines*. Washington, DC: EPA 712-C-98-244.

EPA. 2000a. *OPPTS 870.3050: Repeated Dose 28-Day Oral Toxicity Study in Rodents, Health Effects Test Guidelines*. Washington, DC: EPA 712-C-00-366.

EPA. 2000b. *OPPTS 870.3650: Combined Repeated Dose Toxicity Study with the Reproduction/Developmental Toxicity Screening Test, Health Effects Test Guidelines*. Washington, DC: EPA 712-C-00-368.

EPA. 2001. *OPPTS 870.8355: Combined Chronic Toxicity/Carcinogenicity Testing of Respirable Fibrous Particles, Health Effects Test Guidelines*. Washington, DC: EPA 712-C-01-358.

EPA. 2002. *Health Assessment of 1,3-Butadiene, EPA/600/P-98/001F, Office of Research and Development*. Washington, DC: National Center for Environmental Assessment. http://www.epa.gov/iris/supdocs/butasup.pdf.

EPA. 2005a. *Guidelines for Carcinogen Risk Assessment, EPA/630/P-03/001F*. Washington, DC: Risk Assessment Forum, http://www.epa.gov/raf/publications/pdfs/CANCER_GUIDELINES_FINAL_3-25-05.PDF

EPA. 2005b. *Supplemental Guidance for Assessing Susceptibility from Early-Life Exposure to Carcinogens, EPA/630/R-03/003F*. Washington, DC: Risk Assessment Forum, http://www.epa.gov/raf/publications/pdfs/childrens_supplement_final.pdf

EPA. 2007. 40 CFR parts 9 and 158. Pesticides; data requirements for conventional chemicals; final rule. October 26, 2007. *Federal Register*, 72: 60934–60988.

EPA. 2009a. *OPPTS 890.1400: Hershberger Bioassay, Endocrine Disruptor Screening Program Test Guidelines*. Washington, DC: EPA 740-C-09-008.

EPA. 2009b. *OPPTS 890.1450: Pubertal Development and Thyroid Function in Intact Juvenile/Peripubertal Female Rats, Endocrine Disruptor Screening Program Test Guidelines*. Washington, DC: EPA 740-C-09-009.

EPA. 2009c. *OPPTS 890.1600: Uterotrophic Assay, Endocrine Disruptor Screening Program Test Guidelines*. Washington, DC: EPA 740-C-09-0010.

FDA. 2011. *Guidance for Industry, Reproductive and Developmental Toxicities—Integrating Study Results to Assess Concerns*. http://www.fda.gov/downloads/Drugs/GuidanceComplianceRegulatoryInformation/Guidances/UCM079240.pdf (accessed May, 2013).

Flaws, J. A., Doerr, J. K., Sipes, I. G. and Hoyer, P. B. 1994. Destruction of preantral follicles in adult rats by 4-vinyl-1-cyclohexene diepoxide. *Reprod Toxicol*, 8: 509–514.

Frantz, S. W., Beatty, P. W., English, J. C., Hundley, S. G. and Wilson, A. G. 1994. The use of pharmacokinetics as an interpretive and predictive tool in chemical toxicology testing and risk assessment: A position paper on the appropriate use of pharmacokinetics in chemical toxicology. *Regul Toxicol Pharmacol*, 19: 317–337.

Goldman, J. M. and Cooper, R. L. 1993. *Assessment of Toxicant-Induced Alterations in the Luteinizing Hormone Control of Ovulation in the Rat. Methods in Toxicology, Part B, Female Reproductive Toxicology*. New York: Academic Press, Inc.

Goldman, J. M., Murr, A. S. and Cooper, R. L. 2007. The rodent estrous cycle: Characterization of vaginal cytology and its utility in toxicological studies. *Birth Defects Res B Dev Reprod Toxicol*, 80: 84–97.

Grassi, T. F., Guerra, M. T., Perobelli, J. E., de Toledo, F. C., da Silva, D. S., De Grava Kempinas, W. and Barbisan, L. F. 2011. Assessment of female reproductive endpoints in Sprague-Dawley rats developmentally exposed to Diuron: potential ovary toxicity. *Birth Defects Res B Dev Reprod Toxicol*, 92: 478–486.

Heindel, J. J. 1998. Oocyte quantification and ovarian histology. In: Daston, G. and Kimmel, C. (eds.) *An Evaluation and Interpretation of Reproductive Endpoints for Human Health Risk Assessment*. Washington, DC: ILSI Press.

Hildreth, N. G., Kelsey, J. L., LiVolsi, V. A., Fischer, D. B., Holford, T. R., Mostow, E. D., Schwartz, P. E. and White, C. 1981. An epidemiologic study of epithelial carcinoma of the ovary. *Am J Epidemiol,* 114: 398–405.

Hoyer, P. B., Devine, P. J., Hu, X., Thompson, K. E. and Sipes, I. G. 2001. Ovarian toxicity of 4-vinylcyclohexene diepoxide: A mechanistic model. *Toxicol Pathol,* 29: 91–99.

Hoyer, P. B. and Sipes, I. G. 2007. Development of an animal model for ovotoxicity using 4-vinylcyclohexene: A case study. *Birth Defects Res B Dev Reprod Toxicol,* 80: 113–125.

ICH. 1995. *S1A: The Need for Carcinogenicity Studies of Pharmaceuticals, ICH Harmonized Tripartite Guideline*. http://www.ich.org/fileadmin/Public_Web_Site/ICH_Products/Guidelines/Safety/S1A/Step4/S1A_Guideline.pdf (accessed May, 2013).

ICH. 1997a. *E8: General Consideration for Clinical Trials, ICH Harmonized Tripartite Guideline*. http://www.ich.org/fileadmin/Public_Web_Site/ICH_Products/Guidelines/Efficacy/E8/Step4/E8_Guideline.pdf (accessed May, 2013).

ICH. 1997b. *S1B: Testing for Carcinogenicity of Pharmaceuticals, ICH Harmonized Tripartite Guideline*. http://www.ich.org/fileadmin/Public_Web_Site/ICH_Products/Guidelines/Safety/S1B/Step4/S1B_Guideline.pdf (accessed May, 2013).

ICH. 2000. *S5(R2): Detection of Toxicity to Reproduction for Medicinal Products & Toxicity to Male Fertility, ICH Harmonized Tripartite Guideline*. http://www.ich.org/fileadmin/Public_Web_Site/ICH_Products/Guidelines/Safety/S5_R2/Step4/S5_R2__Guideline.pdf (accessed May, 2013).

ICH. 2009. *M3(R2): Guidance on Nonclinical Safety Studies for the Conduct of Human Clinical Trials and Marketing Authorization for Pharmaceuticals, ICH Harmonized Tripartite Guideline*. http://www.ich.org/fileadmin/Public_Web_Site/ICH_Products/Guidelines/Multidisciplinary/M3_R2/Step4/M3_R2__Guideline.pdf (accessed May, 2013).

Ishii, S., Ube, M., Okada, M., Adachi, T., Sugimoto, J., Inoue, Y., Uno, Y. and Mutai, M. 2009. Collaborative work on evaluation of ovarian toxicity. 17) Two- or four-week repeated-dose studies and fertility study of sulpiride in female rats. *J Toxicol Sci,* 34 Suppl 1: SP175–188.

Ito, A., Mafune, N. and Kimura, T. 2009. Collaborative work on evaluation of ovarian toxicity. 4) Two- or four-week repeated dose study of 4-vinylcyclohexene diepoxide in female rats. *J Toxicol Sci,* 34 Suppl 1: SP53–58.

Izumi, Y., Watanabe, T., Awasaki, N., Hikawa, K., Minagi, T. and Chatani, F. 2009. Collaborative work on evaluation of ovarian toxicity. 16) Effects of 2 or 4 weeks repeated dose studies and fertility study of Chlorpromazine hydrochloride in rats. *J Toxicol Sci,* 34 Suppl 1: SP167–174.

Johnson, J., Canning, J., Kaneko, T., Pru, J. K. and Tilly, J. L. 2004. Germline stem cells and follicular renewal in the postnatal mammalian ovary. *Nature,* 428: 145–150.

Källén, B. 2012. Human Studies—Epidemiologic techniques in developmental and reproductive toxicology. In: Hood, R. D. (ed.), *Developmental and Reproductive Toxicology: A Practical Approach*. 3rd ed. New York: Informa Healthcare.

Kim, H., Hayashi, S., Chambon, P., Watanabe, H., Iguchi, T. and Sato, T. 2009. Effects of diethylstilbestrol on ovarian follicle development in neonatal mice. *Reprod Toxicol,* 27: 55–62.

Kodama, T., Yoshida, J., Miwa, T., Hasegawa, D. and Masuyama, T. 2009. Collaborative work on evaluation of ovarian toxicity. 4) Effects of fertility study of 4-vinylcyclohexene diepoxide in female rats. *J Toxicol Sci,* 34 Suppl 1: SP59–63.

Kumazawa, T., Nakajima, A., Ishiguro, T., Jiuxin, Z., Tanaharu, T., Nishitani, H., Inoue, Y., Harada, S., Hayasaka, I. and Tagawa, Y. 2009. Collaborative work on evaluation of ovarian toxicity. 15) Two- or four-week repeated-dose studies and fertility study of bromocriptine in female rats. *J Toxicol Sci,* 34 Suppl 1: SP157–165.

Lacey, J. V., Jr., Mink, P. J., Lubin, J. H., Sherman, M. E., Troisi, R., Hartge, P., Schatzkin, A. and Schairer, C. 2002. Menopausal hormone replacement therapy and risk of ovarian cancer. *JAMA,* 288: 334–341.

Laws, S. C., Ferrell, J. M., Stoker, T. E. and Cooper, R. L. 2003. Pubertal development in female Wistar rats following exposure to propazine and atrazine biotransformation by-products, diamino-S-chlorotriazine and hydroxyatrazine. *Toxicol Sci,* 76: 190–200.

Laws, S. C., Ferrell, J. M., Stoker, T. E., Schmid, J. and Cooper, R. L. 2000. The effects of atrazine on female wistar rats: An evaluation of the protocol for assessing pubertal development and thyroid function. *Toxicol Sci,* 58: 366–376.

Laws, S. C., Riffle, B. W., Stoker, T. E., Goldman, J. M., Wilson, V., Gray, L. E., Jr. and Cooper, R. L. 2012. The U.S. EPA Endocrine Disruptor Screening Program: The Tier 1 screening battery. In: Hood, R. D. (ed.), *Developmental and Reproductive Toxicology: A Practical Approach.* 3rd ed. New York: Informa Healthcare.

Lovekamp-Swan, T. and Davis, B. J. 2003. Mechanisms of phthalate ester toxicity in the female reproductive system. *Environ Health Perspect,* 111: 139–145.

Manson, J. M. and Mattson, B. A. 1992. Susceptibility of the ovary to toxic substances. In: Mohr, U., Dungworth, D. L. and Capen, C. C. (eds.) *Pathobiology of the Aging Rat.* Washington, DC: ILSI Press.

Mattison, D. R., Shiromizu, K. and Nightingale, M. S. 1983. Oocyte destruction by polycyclic aromatic hydrocarbons. *Am J Ind Med,* 4: 191–202.

Meirow, D. 1999. Ovarian injury and modern options to preserve fertility in female cancer patients treated with high dose radio-chemotherapy for hemato-oncological neoplasias and other cancers. *Leuk Lymphoma,* 33: 65–76.

Muhammad, F. S., Goode, A. K., Kock, N. D., Arifin, E. A., Cline, J. M., Adams, M. R., Hoyer, P. B., Christian, P. J., Isom, S., Kaplan, J. R. and Appt, S. E. 2009. Effects of 4-vinylcyclohexene diepoxide on peripubertal and adult Sprague-Dawley rats: Ovarian, clinical, and pathologic outcomes. *Comp Med,* 59: 46–59.

Nozaki, Y., Furubo, E., Matsuno, T., Fukui, R., Kizawa, K., Kozaki, T. and Sanzen, T. 2009. Collaborative work on evaluation of ovarian toxicity. 6) Two- or four-week repeated-dose studies and fertility study of cisplatin in female rats. *J Toxicol Sci,* 34 Suppl 1: SP73–81.

NRC. 1983. *Risk Assessment in the Federal Government: Managing the Process.,* Washington, DC: National Academy Press.

NRC. 1994. *Science and Judgement in Risk Assessment.* Washington, DC: Taylor & Francis.

NRC. 2009. *Science and Decisions: Advancing Risk Assessment.* Washington, DC: National Academies Press.

NTP. 1986. *Toxicology and Carcinogenesis Studies of 4-Vinylcyclohexene (CAS No. 100-40-3) in F344/N Rats and B6C3F1 Mice (Gavage Studies).* Research Triangle Park, NC: *NTP TR 303.* http://ntp.niehs.nih.gov/ntp/htdocs/LT_rpts/tr303.pdf#search=4-vinylcyclohexene

NTP. 1993. *Toxicology and Carcinogenesis Studies of 1,3-Butadiene (CAS No. 106-99-0) in B6C3F1 Mice (Inhalation Studies).* Research Triangle Park, NC: NTP TR 434. http://ntp.niehs.nih.gov/ntp/htdocs/LT_rpts/tr434.pdf#search=1,3-butadiene%20TR-434.

NTP. 2011. *Specifications for the Conduct of Studies to Evaluate the Reproductive and Developmental Toxicity of Chemical, Biological and Physical Agents in Laboratory Animals for the National Toxicology Program (NTP).* http://ntp.niehs.nih.gov/ntp/Test_Info/FinalNTP_ReproSpecsMay2011_508.pdf (accessed May, 2013).

OECD. 1981a. *Test No. 410: Repeated Dose Dermal Toxicity: 21/28-Day Study.* Paris, France: OECD Guidelines for the Testing of Chemicals.

OECD. 1981b. *Test No: 411: Subchronic Dermal Toxicity: 90-Day Study.* Paris, France: OECD Guidelines for the Testing of Chemicals.

OECD. 1983. *Test No. 415: One-Generation Reproduction Toxicity Study.* Paris, France: OECD Guidelines for the Testing of Chemicals.

OECD. 1984. *Test No. 478: Genetic Toxicology: Rodent Dominant Lethal Test.* Paris, France: OECD Guidelines for the Testing of Chemicals.

OECD. 1995. *Test No. 421: Reproduction/Developmental Toxicity Screening Test.* Paris, France: OECD Guidelines for the Testing of Chemicals.

OECD. 1996. *Test No. 422: Combined Repeated Dose Toxicity Study with the Reproduction/Developmental Toxicity Screening Test.* Paris, France: OECD Guidelines for the Testing of Chemicals.

OECD. 1998a. *Test No. 408: Repeated Dose 90-Day Oral Toxicity Study in Rodents.* Paris, France: OECD Guidelines for the Testing of Chemicals.

OECD. 1998b. *Test No. 409: Repeated Dose 90-Day Oral Toxicity Study in Non-Rodents.* Paris, France: OECD Guidelines for the Testing of Chemicals.

OECD. 2001a. *Test No. 414: Prenatal Developmental Toxicity Study.* Paris, France: OECD Guidelines for the Testing of Chemicals.

OECD. 2001b. *Test No. 416: Two-Generation Reproduction Toxicity.* Paris, France: OECD Guidelines for the Testing of Chemicals.

OECD. 2007a. *Test No. 426: Developmental Neurotoxicity Study.* Paris, France: OECD Guidelines for the Testing of Chemicals.

OECD. 2007b. *Test No. 440: Uterotrophic bioassay in rats: A Short-Term Screening Assay for Oestrogenic Properties.* Paris, France: OECD Guidelines for the Testing of Chemicals.

OECD. 2008a. *Questions & Answers Regarding the OECD Test Guidelines Programme* (TGP). OECD Test Guidelines Programme. http://www.oecd.org/dataoecd/52/33/40728679.doc (accessed May, 2013).

OECD. 2008b. *Series on Testing and Assessment, Number 43, Guidance Document on Mammalian Reproductive Toxicity Testing and Assessment.* Paris, France: *ENV/JM/MONO(2008)16*, http://www.oecd.org/document/30/0,3343,en_2649_34377_1916638_1_1_1_1,00.html

OECD. 2009a. *Series on Testing and Assessment, Number 106, Guidance Document for Histologic Evaluation of Endocrine and Reproductive Tests in Rodents, ENV/JM/MONO(2009)11.* Paris, France: http://www.oecd.org/env/chemicalsafetyandbiosafety/testingofchemicals/seriesontestingandassessmentpublicationsbynumber.htm

OECD. 2009b. *Test No. 407: Repeated Dose 28-Day Oral Toxicity Study in Rodents.* Paris, France: OECD Guidelines for the Testing of Chemicals.

OECD. 2009c. *Test No. 412: Subacute Inhalation Toxicity: 28-Day Study.* Paris, France: OECD Guidelines for the Testing of Chemicals.

OECD. 2009d. *Test No. 413: Subchronic Inhalation Toxicity: 90-Day Study.* Paris, France: OECD Guidelines for the Testing of Chemicals.

OECD. 2009e. *Test No. 441: Hershberger Bioassay in Rats: A Short-Term Screening Assay for (Anti)Androgenic Properties.* Washington, DC: OECD Guideline for the Testing of Chemicals.

OECD. 2009f. *Test No. 451: Carcinogenicity Studies.* Paris, France: OECD Guidelines for the Testing of Chemicals.

OECD. 2009g. *Test No. 452: Chronic Studies.* Paris, France: OECD Studies for the Testing of Chemicals.

OECD. 2009h. *Test No. 453: Combined Chronic Toxicity/Carcinogenicity Studies.* Paris, France: ECD Guidelines for the Testing of Chemicals

OECD. 2010. *Test No. 417: Toxicokinetics.* Paris, France: OECD Guidelines for the Testing of Chemicals.

OECD. 2011. *Test No. 443: Extended One-Generation Reproduction Toxicity Study.* Paris, France: OECD Guidelines for the Testing of Chemicals. Paris.

Ohtake, S., Fukui, M. and Hisada, S. 2009. Collaborative work on evaluation of ovarian toxicity. 1) Effects of 2- or 4-week repeated-dose administration and fertility studies with medroxyprogesterone acetate in female rats. *J Toxicol Sci,* 34 Suppl 1: SP23–29.

Paulose, T., Tannenbaum, L. V., Borgeest, C. and Flaws, J. A. 2012. Methoxychlor-induced ovarian follicle toxicity in mice: Dose and exposure duration-dependent effects. *Birth Defects Res B Dev Reprod Toxicol,* 95: 219–224.

Peluso, J. J. 1992. Morphologic and physiologic features of the ovary. In: Mohr, U., Dungworth, D. L. and Capen, C. C. (eds.) *Pathobiology of the Aging Rat.* Washington, DC: ILSI Press.

Peluso, J. J. and Gordon, L. R. 1992. Nonneoplastic and Neoplastic changes in the ovary. In: Mohr, U., Dungworth, D. L. and Capen, C. C. (eds.) *Pathobiology of the Aging Rat.* Washington, DC: ILSI Press.

Regan, K. S., Cline, J. M., Creasy, D., Davis, B., Foley, G. L., Lanning, L., Latendresse, J. R., Makris, S., Morton, D., Rehm, S. and Stebbins, K. 2005. STP position paper: Ovarian follicular counting in the assessment of rodent reproductive toxicity. *Toxicol Pathol,* 33: 409–412.

Riman, T., Dickman, P. W., Nilsson, S., Correia, N., Nordlinder, H., Magnusson, C. M., Weiderpass, E. and Persson, I. R. 2002. Hormone replacement therapy and the risk of invasive epithelial ovarian cancer in Swedish women. *J Natl Cancer Inst,* 94: 497–504.

Sakurada, Y., Kudo, S., Iwasaki, S., Miyata, Y., Nishi, M. and Masumoto, Y. 2009. Collaborative work on evaluation of ovarian toxicity. 5) Two- or four-week repeated-dose studies and fertility study of busulfan in female rats. *J Toxicol Sci,* 34 Suppl 1: SP65–72.

Sanbuissho, A., Yoshida, M., Hisada, S., Sagami, F., Kudo, S., Kumazawa, T., Ube, M., Komatsu, S. and Ohno, Y. 2009. Collaborative work on evaluation of ovarian toxicity by repeated-dose and fertility studies in female rats. *J Toxicol Sci,* 34 Suppl 1: SP1–22.

Sato, M., Shiozawa, K., Uesugi, T., Hiromatsu, R., Fukuda, M., Kitaura, K., Minami, T. and Matsumoto, S. 2009a. Collaborative work on evaluation of ovarian toxicity. 7) Effects of 2- or 4-week repeated dose studies and fertility study of cyclophosphamide in female rats. *J Toxicol Sci,* 34 Suppl 1: SP83–89.

Sato, N., Uchida, K., Nakajima, M., Watanabe, A. and Kohira, T. 2009b. Collaborative work on evaluation of ovarian toxicity. 13) Two- or four-week repeated dose studies and fertility study of PPAR alpha/gamma dual agonist in female rats. *J Toxicol Sci,* 34 Suppl 1: SP137–146.

Sekiguchi, S., Ito, S., Suda, M. and Honma, T. 2006. Involvement of thyroxine in ovarian toxicity of di-(2-ethylhexyl) phthalate. *Ind Health,* 44: 274–279.

Shibayama, H., Kotera, T., Shinoda, Y., Hanada, T., Kajihara, T., Ueda, M., Tamura, H., Ishibashi, S., Yamashita, Y. and Ochi, S. 2009. Collaborative work on evaluation of ovarian toxicity. 14) Two- or four-week repeated-dose studies and fertility study of atrazine in female rats. *J Toxicol Sci,* 34 Suppl 1: SP147–155.

Shirai, M., Sakurai, K., Saitoh, W., Matsuyama, T., Teranishi, M., Furukawa, T., Sanbuissho, A. and Manabe, S. 2009. Collaborative work on evaluation of ovarian toxicity. 8) Two- or four-week repeated-dose studies and fertility study of Anastrozole in female rats. *J Toxicol Sci,* 34 Suppl 1: SP91–99.

Smith, B. J., Plowchalk, D. R., Sipes, I. G. and Mattison, D. R. 1991. Comparison of random and serial sections in assessment of ovarian toxicity. *Reprod Toxicol,* 5: 379–383.

Stoker, T. E., Goldman, J. M. and Cooper, R. L. 1993. The dithiocarbamate fungicide thiram disrupts the hormonal control of ovulation in the female rat. *Reprod Toxicol,* 7: 211–218.

Takai, R., Hayashi, S., Kiyokawa, J., Iwata, Y., Matsuo, S., Suzuki, M., Mizoguchi, K., Chiba, S. and Deki, T. 2009. Collaborative work on evaluation of ovarian toxicity. 10) Two- or four-week repeated dose studies and fertility study of di-(2-ethylhexyl) phthalate (DEHP) in female rats. *J Toxicol Sci,* 34 Suppl 1: SP111–119.

Takizawa, K., Yagi, H., Jerina, D. M. and Mattison, D. R. 1984. Murine strain differences in ovotoxicity following intraovarian injection with benzo(a)pyrene, (+)-(7R,8S)-oxide, (-)-(7R,8R)-dihydrodiol, or (+)-(7R,8S)-diol-(9S,10R)-epoxide-2. *Cancer Res,* 44: 2571–2576.

Tamura, T., Yokoi, R., Okuhara, Y., Harada, C., Terashima, Y., Hayashi, M., Nagasawa, T., Onozato, T., Kobayashi, K., Kuroda, J., and Kusama, H. 2009. Collaborative work on evaluation of ovarian toxicity. 2) Two- or four-week repeated dose studies and fertility study of mifepristone in female rats. *J Toxicol Sci,* 34 Suppl 1: SP31–42.

Tenenbaum, A. and Forsberg, J. G. 1985. Structural and functional changes in ovaries from adult mice treated with diethylstilboestrol in the neonatal period. *J Reprod Fertil,* 73: 465–477.

Tsubota, K., Kushima, K., Yamauchi, K., Matsuo, S., Saegusa, T., Ito, S., Fujiwara, M., Matsumoto, M., Nakatsuji, S., Seki, J. and Oishi, Y. 2009. Collaborative work on evaluation of ovarian toxicity. 12) Effects of 2- or 4-week repeated dose studies and fertility study of indomethacin in female rats. *J Toxicol Sci,* 34 Suppl 1: SP129–136.

Tsujioka, S., Ban, Y., Wise, L. D., Tsuchiya, T., Sato, T., Matsue, K., Ikeda, T., Sasaki, M. and Nishikibe, M. 2009. Collaborative work on evaluation of ovarian toxicity. 3) Effects of 2- or 4-week repeated-dose toxicity and fertility studies with tamoxifen in female rats. *J Toxicol Sci,* 34 Suppl 1: SP43–51.

Vanderhyden, B. C., Shaw, T. J. and Ethier, J. F. 2003. Animal models of ovarian cancer. *Reprod Biol Endocrinol,* 1: 67.

Wato, E., Asahiyama, M., Suzuki, A., Funyu, S. and Amano, Y. 2009. Collaborative work on evaluation of ovarian toxicity. 9) Effects of 2- or 4-week repeated dose studies and fertility study of di(2-ethylhexyl)adipate (DEHA) in female rats. *J Toxicol Sci,* 34 Suppl 1: SP101–109.

Weitzman, G. A., Miller, M. M., London, S. N. and Mattison, D. R. 1992. Morphometric assessment of the murine ovarian toxicity of 7,12-dimethylbenz(a)anthracene. *Reprod Toxicol,* 6: 137–141.

Wier, P. J. 2012. Use of toxicokinetics in developmental and reproductive toxicology. In: Hood, R. D. (ed.), *Developmental and Reproductive Toxicology: A Practical Approach.* 3rd ed. New York: Informa Healthcare.

Yoshida, M., Sanbuissyo, A., Hisada, S., Takahashi, M., Ohno, Y. and Nishikawa, A. 2009. Morphological characterization of the ovary under normal cycling in rats and its viewpoints of ovarian toxicity detection. *J Toxicol Sci,* 34 Suppl 1: SP189–197.

Testing guidelines or study descriptions are available at the following website addresses:

USEPA Health Effects Test Guidelines: http://www.epa.gov/occspp/pubs/frs/publications/Test_Guildelines/series870.htm

USEPA Endocrine Disruptor Screening Program Test Guidelines: http://www.epa.gov/ocspp/pubs/frs/publications/Test_Guidelines/series890.htm

OECD Guidelines for the Testing of Chemicals: http://miranda.sourceoecd.org/vl=670229/cl=13/nw=1/rpsv/cw/vhosts/oecdjournals/1607310x/v1n4/contp1-1.htm

NTP Descriptions of Study Types: http://ntp.niehs.nih.gov/?objectid=72015D9F-BDB7-CEBA-F4EB4F9BF507820

CICH Guidelines: http://www.ich.org/products/guidelines.html (with links to FDA, EMEA, and PMDA guidelines)

Index

D

E

R

S

Printed and bound by CPI Group (UK) Ltd, Croydon, CR0 4YY
21/10/2024
01777044-0011